CHLAMYDIA

Edited by **Mihai Mares**

Chlamydia
Edited by Mihai Mares

Published by InTech

Janeza Trdine 9, 51000 Rijeka, Croatia

Publishing Process Manager Romina Skomersic

Technical Editor Teodora Smiljanic

Cover Designer InTech Design Team

Additional hard copies can be obtained from orders@intechopen.com

Chlamydia, Edited by Mihai Mares
p. cm.
ISBN 978-953-51-0470-4

For EU product safety concerns:
IN TECH d.o.o., Prolaz Marije Krucifikse Kozulić 3, 51000 Rijeka, Croatia,
info@intechopen.com or visit our website at intechopen.com.

Meet the editor

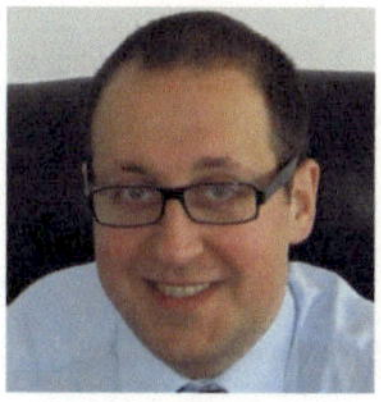

Dr Mihai Mareș received his PhD degree in Microbiology at "Gr. T. Popa" University of Medicine and Pharmacy from Iași-Romania (2005) and had the postgraduate training at University VII Denis-Diderot, Pasteur Institute, and Pitié-Salpêtrière Hospital – Paris (France), Complutense University – Madrid (Spain) and Karolinska Institute – Stockholm (Sweden). His areas of interest are represented by medical mycology and human reproduction, with researches emphasis on new antimicrobial molecules and microbial induced infertility, respectively. He has recently entered in the dynamic field of antimicrobial resistance, his group being the first in the country that deals with the surveillance of quinolones resistance in food borne pathogens and genital mycoplasmas. He has served as consultant for several pharmaceutical companies in the past few years. Currently, Dr. Mareș is Associate Professor of Medical Mycology and Head of Antimicrobial Chemotherapy Laboratory at Ion Ionescu de la Brad University – Iași (Romania). He is also Head of Andrology Laboratory at Origyn Fertility Center and President of the Romanian Society of Medical Mycology and Mycotoxicology.

Contents

Preface

Despite its sixty-years age, *Chlamydia* is not an obsolete pathogen. Moreover, it became a multifaceted pathogen capable of easy spreading in human populations. Last decades have not brought a significant decrease of *Chlamydia* infection prevalence in general population, even after the implementation of various prevention or educational programs.

Among the *Chlamydiaceae* taxa, *Chlamydia trachomatis* is the most important species from epidemiological point of view and it causes pelvic inflammatory disease, ectopic pregnancy, infertility due to the fallopian tube obstruction, infections in neonates, epididymis and joint illness in men. Worldwide, it is estimated that six million of people suffer from post-trachoma blindness and almost 90 million become sexually infected each year by this species. The consequences of chlamydial infection on conceiving ability are often very seriously and the chronic evolution of disease is an unfavorable prognosis factor. Alongside *Mycoplasma genitalium* - considered " a new *Chlamydia*", *Chlamydia trachomatis* is responsible for the most cases of pelvic inflammatory diseases – a chronic condition that affects an important segment of sexually active women population.

Another public health important topic is the involvement of *Chlamydia pneumoniae* in atherosclerosis development. It is also an insidious and chronic condition, difficult to deal with.

Taking into account the epidemiological characteristics and the physical consequences of infection, *Chlamydia* can be regarded as a silent "plague" of modern times and more efforts must be done worldwide to manage it.

This book contains an updated review of all-important issues concerning the chlamydial infection. It comprises 18 chapters grouped in four major parts dealing with etiology and pathogenicity, clinical aspects, diagnosis and prevention. New molecular findings about the pathogen ability to assure its intracellular persistence and the host immune response during infection are also extensively treated.

More than fifty medical specialists have contributed as co-authors to this complex editorial approach, each of them adding his/her experience and knowledge to improve our capacity to control an important infection. I would like to express my gratitude and appreciation to all of them, and last but not least, to all those who assisted me in the project.

Dr. Mihai Mares, PhD
Head of Andrology Laboratory, Origyn Fertility Center,
Associate Professor, Department of Public Health,
"Ion Ionescu de la Brad" University, Iasi,
Romania

Part 1

Epidemiology and Pathogenesis of Chlamydia Infections

1

Molecular Epidemiology of *Chlamydia trachomatis* Urogenital Infection

Virginia Sánchez Monroy and José D´Artagnan Villalba-Magdaleno
Military School of Graduate, University of the Mexican Army and Air Force
Military Medical School, University of the Mexican Army and Air Force
Universidad del Valle de México, Campus Chapultepec
México

1. Introduction

Each year an estimated 340 million new cases of curable sexually transmitted infections occur worldwide, with the largest proportion in the region of South and South East Asia, followed by subSaharan Africa and Latin America and the Caribbean (WHO, 2006). *Chlamydia trachomatis* infections are the most prevalent sexually transmitted bacteria infections recognized throughout the world. World Health Organization (WHO, 2001) estimated that there were 92 million new cases worldwide in 1999 and the incidence of infection has continued to increase each year in both industrialized and developing countries. *C. trachomatis* is now recognized as one the most common sexually transmissible bacterial infections among persons under than 25 years of age living in industrialized nations such as the United States, where the rate of prevalence runs at 4.2% (Miller et al., 2004).

The vast majority of published clearly, show that E, D, F and G, genotypes are isolated from urogenital tract infections with most frequency, however genotypes have yet to be consistently associated with disease severity or even disease phenotype and there is little knowledge of possible *Chlamydia* virulence factors, their expression and how they affect disease severity.

2. Characteristics of bacteria cell

According to the reclassification of the order *Chlamydiales* in 1999, the family *Chlamydiaceae* is now divided in two genera, *Chlamydia* and *Chlamydophila* (Everett., et al 1999).The genus *Chlamydia* comprises the species *C. trachomatis, C. suis* and *C. muridarum.*

C. trachomatis are obligate intracellular parasites, possess an inner and outer membrane similar to gram-negative bacteria and a lipopolysaccharide (LPS) but do not have a peptidoglycan layer. Have many characteristics of free-living bacteria, and their metabolism follows the same general pattern; the main difference is their little capacity for generating energy. It has been shown that *Chlamydiaceae* are auxotrophic for ATP, GTP and UTP but not for CTP. (Tipples & McClarty, 1993).

C. tracomatis, is an exclusively human pathogen, with a tropism conjuntival and urogenital, was originally identified by their accumulation of glycogen in inclusions and their sensitivity to sulfadiazine. Based on the type of disease produced, *C. trachomatis* has been divided into biovars, including the lymphogranuloma venereum (LGV) biovar and the trachoma biovar, associated with human conjunctival or urogenital columnar epithelium infections. The original Wang and Grayston classification (Wang & Grayston, 1970) defined 15 *C. trachomatis* serovars, based on antigenic differences, designated A-K and L1-L3, which differ by the antigenicity of their major outer membrane protein (MOMP), codified by gene *omp1*. In addition to these serovars, numerous variants have been characterized. Serovars A, B, Ba and C, infect mainly the conjunctiva and are associated with endemic trachoma; serovars D, Da, E, F, G, Ga, H, I, J and K are predominantly isolated from the urogenital tract and are associated with sexually transmitted diseases (STD), inclusion conjunctivitis or neonatal pneumonitis in infants born to infected mothers. Serovars L1, L2, L2a and L3 can be found in the inguinal lymph nodes and are associated with LGV (Table 1).

Biovar	Serovar	Diseases
Trachoma	A, B, Ba, C	trachoma
	D, E, F, G, H, I, J, K, Da, Ia	STD, conjuntivitis and pneumonitis
GV	L1-L2, L2a, L3	LGV

Table 1. Biovar and diseased caused by *C. trachomatis*

The genome sequencing projects have shown that *Chlamydia* has a relatively small chromosome at between 1.04 and 1.23 Mbp and contains between 894 and 1130 predicted protein-coding genes. The fully sequence *C. trachomatis* genome consist of a chromosome of approximately 1.0 Mbp plus an extrachromosomal plasmid of approximately 7.5 kbp, with a total of approximately 900 likely protein-coding genes (Read et al., 2000; Carlson et al., 2005) Table 2.

Characteristics	Dates
Genome size (pb)	1042519
Genes	894
Plasmid/phage size (bp)	7493
GC%	41.3
No. ORFs	894
No. tRNAs	37
No. rRNA operons	2
% non-coding	9.9

Table 2. Sequences and annotated of *C. trachomatis* D genome

The transcriptional profile of the *C. trachomatis* genome has been analysed by microarrays and RT-PCR (Douglas & Hatch, 2000; Shen et al., 2000). The microarrays and RT-PCR analysis has showed that 71% or 612 of the 894 genes of C. *trachomatis* continue to be expressed throughout the development cycle, while the others are temporally expressed (Nicholson et al., 2003). Analysis of the profiles of the temporally expressed genes has difficulties in classifying, because of the contrasting results of microarrays analysis on C. *trachomatis* by different groups (Belland et al., 2004; Nicholson et al., 2003).

3. The developmental cycle

C. *trachomatis* is a small obligate intracellular bacterium, has two developmental stages: -the extracellular elementary body (EB) and -the intracellular reticulate body (RB). EB is the infectious form metabolically inactive (EB), in this stage; the bacteria are in a state similar to that of an endospore, where the outer membrane is resistant to the environment and allows it to exist without a host cell. EB measured from 200 to 400 nm in diameter, is antigenic, non-proliferative, contains few ribosomes, is toxic in cell cultures, and is susceptible to penicillin, resistant to trypsin, osmotic shock and mechanical shock. While RB is intracellular, measured from 500 to 1500 nm in diameter, is not infective or antigenic, is proliferative, contains many ribosomes, is not toxic and is not inhibited by penicillin, is susceptible to trypsin, osmotic shock and mechanical shock.

The eukaryotic cell becomes infected when an EB adheres to the cytoplasmic membrane. The adhesion of EBs to cells is due to multiple weak specific ligand interactions, perhaps involving several molecules. There is evidence that MOMP binds to a heptaran-sulphate receptor on the host cell. The EB penetrates into the cell by endocytosis, remaining within a parasitophorous vacuole also termed inclusion or phagosome. By 2 h after infection within the phagosome EB begin differentiating into RB. Over the next several hours, RB increase in number and in size. RB can be observed dividing by binary fission by 12 h postinfection (hpi). After 18 to 24 h, the numbers of RB are maximized, and increasing numbers of RB begin differentiating back to EB, which accumulate within the lumen of the inclusion as the remainder of the RB continue to multiply. Depending on the species or strain, lysis or release from the infected cell occurs approximately 48 to 72 hpi.

4. The Infection with *C. trachomatis*

The C. *trachomatis* infects columnar epithelial cells of the ocular and urogenital mucosae. These infections have a significant impact on human health worldwide, causing trachoma, the leading cause of preventable blindness, and sexually transmitted diseases (STD) that include pelvic inflammatory disease and tubal factor infertility (Schachter, 1978; Brunham et al., 1988). Chlamydial STDs are also risk factors in cervical squamous cell carcinoma and HIV infection (Chesson & Pinkerton, 2000; Mbizvo et al., 2001).

Trachoma is one of the commonest infectious causes of blindness. The disease starts as an inflammatory infection of the eyelid and evolves to blindness due to corneal opacity. Despite long-standing control efforts, it is estimated that more than 500 million people are at high risk of infection, over 140 million persons are infected and about 6 million are blind in Africa, the Middle East, Central and South East Asia, and countries in Latin America. Trachoma is a communicable disease of families, with repeated reinfection occurring among family members. Transmission is driven by sharing of ocular secretions among young children in family or community groups, facilitated by the ubiquitous presence of flies. The disease is particularly prevalent and severe in rural populations living in poor and arid areas of the world where people have limited access to water and facial hygiene is poor. Visual loss from trachoma is 2-3-times more common in women than men and is a major cause of disability in affected communities, attacking the economically important middle-aged female population. Global elimination of trachoma as a disease of public health importance has been targeted by WHO for 2020.

The most common site of *C. trachomatis* infection is the urogenital tract. In men, it is the commonest cause of non-gonococcal urethritis and epididymitis however are asymptomatic in approximately 50% of men (Karam et al., 1986; Zimmerman et al., 1990). Urethritis is secondary to *C. trachomatis* infection in approximately 15 to 55 percent of men. Symptoms, if present, include a mild to moderate, clear to white urethral discharge. This is best observed in the morning, before the patient voids. Untreated chlamydial infection can spread to the epididymis. Patients usually have unilateral testicular pain with scrotal erythema, tenderness, or swelling over the epididymis. Men with asymptomatic infection serve as carriers of the disease, spreading the infection while only rarely suffering long-term health problems.

In women, chlamydial infection can lead to a serious reproductive morbidity. Infection of the lower genital tract occurs in the endocervix. It can cause an odorless, mucoid vaginal discharge, typically with no external pruritus. Some women develop urethritis; symptoms may consist of dysuria without frequency or urgency. Ascending infection that causes acute salpingitis with or without endometritis, also known as pelvic inflammatory disease (PID), whose long-term consequences are chronic pain, ectopic pregnancy and tubal factor infertility (Stamm, 1999). The 80% of the genital infections are asymptomatic and without clinical evidence of complications and appear to spontaneously resolve, although there only is limited knowledge about the clinical factors that influence the duration of untreated, uncomplicated genital infections (Zimmerman et al., 1990). These infections tend to be chronic and recurring and associated with scarring complications possibly related to hypersensitivity mechanisms.

A *C. tracomatis* infection can infect different mucosal linings, with the majority of cases in the urogenital tract but also the rectum, oropharynx and conjunctiva. Rectal chlamydial infection is often observed in men who have sex with men (Kent et al., 2005; Annan et al., 2009). Contamination of the hands with genital discharge may also lead to conjunctival infection following contact with the eyes. Babies born to mothers with infection of their genital tract frequently present with chlamydial eye infection within a week of birth (chlamydial "*ophthalmia neonatorum*"), and may subsequently develop pneumonia. Furthermore, an existing chlamydial infection increases the risk of contracting HIV (Joyee et al., 2005) and/or Herpes simplex infections (Freeman et al., 2006). This is especially true with the *Lymphogranuloma venereum* (LGV) disease, an invasive and frequently ulcerative chlamydial infection involving lymphatic tissue. LGV occurs only sporadically in North America, but it is endemic in many parts of the developing countries and represent a major risk factor for HIV acquisition (Blank et al., 2005; Schachter & Moncada, 2005; Cai et al., 2010). In addition, it was found that Chlamydial infection can be associated with human papillomavirus (Oh et al., 2009) and gonorrhea in a 20% of men and 42 % of women (Lyss et al., 2003; Srifeungfung et al., 2009).

5. Detection methods for *C. trachomatis*

Diagnosis of chlamydial infection is even more difficult in asymptomatic and in chronic or persistent infections where the pathogen load would be low. The large pools of asymptomatic infected people are not only at the risk of developing serious long-term sequelae but would also transmit the infection. The development of methods of detection in the laboratory highly sensitive and specific of nucleic acid amplification tests (NAATs) has been an important advance in the ability to conduct population-base screening programmes to prevent complications.

The assays that are used for diagnosis of *C. trachomatis* include conventional diagnostic methods and NAATs. Conventional diagnostic methods involve the isolation by cell culture and application of biochemical and immunological tests to identify. The cell culture is time consuming and laborious, and it has been in many laboratories replaced by antigen detection methods such as enzyme immunoassays (EIA), direct immunofluorescence assays (DFA) and DNA/RNA detection. EIA tests detect chlamydial LPS with a monoclonal or polyclonal antibody while DFA depending on the commercial product used detected LPS or MOMP component. DFA with a *C. trachomatis*-specific anti-MOMP monoclonal antibody is considered highly specific (Cles et al., 1988). DNA/RNA detection is based on the hybridization and its use is suitable for simple and fast diagnosis.

The NAATs includes polymerase chain reaction (PCR), ligase chain reaction (LCR), retrotranscription-PCR (RT-PCR) and real time-PCR. In these probes different DNA or RNA regions are used as target sequences for amplification. The major target sequences are located in cryptic plasmid, *omp1* gene and rRNAs. The cryptic plasmid is present in approximately 10 copies in each *C. trachomatis* organism (Hatt et al., 1988), reason for which some authors suggested that amplification of *C. trachomatis* plasmid DNA is more sensitive (Mahony et al., 1992). However, some studies suggest that plasmid-free variants of *C. trachomatis* may on rare occasions be present in clinical samples (An et al., 1992). Comparative studies of the NAATs suggest that the sensitivity and specificity are quite similar, but of screening tests for *C. trachomatis* NAATs are more sensitive than non-NAATs (Poulakkainen et al., 1998; Ostergaard, 1999; Van Dyck et al., 2001, Black, 1997).

6. Prevalence

The prevalence of urogenital *C. trachomatis* determinate with NAATs from different parts of the world published in the present year and the 2010 is summarized in the table 3. These reports show that the prevalence is high and independent of the country, urban or rural ubication.

Studies amongst clinically healthy population have shown a prevalence rate equal or major to 4%. Two reports show lower prevalence rate of 0.9 % in United States of America (Jordan et al., 2011) and Germany (Desai et al., 2011) for population of military and adolescent students respectively, and the higher prevalence rates are for students in China with 8.8% (Hsieh et al., 2010) and young people in England with 8.3% (Skidmore et al., 2011).

Country	Population studied	% Prevalence	Reference
		Clinically healthy population	
Switzerland	Young male offenders	2%	Haller et al., 2011
England	Young people	8.3%	Skidmore et al., 2011
Croatia	Young adults	6.3%	Božičević et al., 2011
Australia	Young international backpackers	3.5%	Davies et al., 2011
United States of America	Military	0.9 %	Jordan et al., 2011
Germany	Adolescents	0.9%	Desai et al., 2011
United States of America	Adults	5.8%	Jenkins et al., 2011
England	Students	3.41%	Aldeen et al., 2010
Spain	Adolescents and young adult women	4%	Corbeto et al., 2010
Perú	Adults	4.95%	Canchihuaman et al., 2010
United States of America	Athletes	2.7%	Hennrikus et al., 2010
France	General population	2.2%	Goulet et al., 2010
United States of America	General population	1.0%	Chai et al., 2010
Japan.	Students	8.1%	Imai et al., 2010
Switzerland	Undocumented immigrants	5.8%	Jackson et al., 2010
China	Students	8.8%	Hsieh et al., 2010
		Population visiting health services	
United States of America	Pregnant women	4.3%	Roberts et al., 2011
United States of America	Symptomatic adolescent women	19.7%	Goyal et al., 2011
Holland	Pregnant women	3.9%	Rours et al., 2011
Brazil	Women	4.0%	Rodrigues et al., 2011
Brazil	Pregnant women	25.7%	Ramos et al., 2011
Guinea	Women	12.6%	Månsson et al., 2010
United States of America	Women in family planning clinics	10.3%	Gaydos et al., 2011
India	Women	23.0%	Patel et al., 2010
Brazil	Men	13.1%	Barbosa et al., 2010
United States of America	Women with rectal infections	17.5 %	Hunte et al., 2010
Turkey	Pregnant women	7.3%	Aydin et al., 2010
Uganda	Women	7.8%	Darj et al., 2010
Korea	Women with overactive bladder symptoms	7.1%	Lee et al., 2010
Italy	Infertile couples	8.2%	Salmeri et al., 2010
South Africa	Men with urethritis	12.3%	Le Roux et al., 2010

Country	Population studied	% Prevalence	Reference
		high-risk population	
England	Female sex workers	6.8%	Platt et al., 2011
Pakistan	Female sex workers	7.7 %	Khan et al., 2011
China	Men who have sex with men	24%	Li et al., 2011
China	Female sex workers	17.4%	Jin et al., 2011
Indonesia	Female sex workers	37%	Silitonga et al., 2011
Indonesia	Female sex workers	27%	Mawu et al., 2011
Korea	Female rape victims.	28.85%	Jo et al., 2011
Spain	Injecting Drug Users	2.3%	Folch et al., 2011
Switzerland	Adults in a prison	8.3%	Steiner et al., 2010
United States of America	HIV patients	23.93%	Chkhartishvili et al., 2010
France	High-risk population	28%	Fresse et al., 2010
Korea	Female sex workers	12.8%	Lee et al., 2010
Kenia	Fishermen with STI	3.2%	Kwena et al., 2010
Tunisia	Female sex workers	72.9%	Znazen et al., 2010
Indonesia	Female sex workers	43.5%	Tanudyaya et al., 2010
Bangladesh	Female sex workers	2.5%	Huq et al., 2010

Table 3. Prevalence of *C. trachomatis* from different parts of the world published 2010–2011

The reports for the population that visiting health services shown average prevalence rate 11.7%, that ranges from of 4% to 25.7% in Brazil (Rodrigues et al., 2011; Ramos et al., 2011).

The higher prevalence rate reported are for the high-risk population with average of 21.6%; that ranges from of 2.5% in Bangladesh (Huq et al., 2010) up to 72.9% in Tunesia (Znazen et al., 2010) amongst female sex workers.

7. *C. trachomatis* genotypes

C. trachomatis comprises distinct serogroups and serovars. Different genotyping methods are used for determination of circulating *C. trachomatis* serovars within a population can provide information on the epidemiology and pathogenesis of infection, including mapping sexual networks, can allow for monitoring treatment success, and may play a role in developing strategies for improved disease control, such as vaccine design.

Different genotyping methods are available to differentiate between the serovars, and are mainly based on the diversity of the *omp1* gene, which encodes for the MOMP, an antigenically complex that displays serovar, serogroup, and species specificities (Baehr et al., 1988; Stephens et al., 1982). The MOMP is present in all human pathogenic *Chlamydia* species, contains four variable domains designated VS1, VS2, VS3, and VS4 that vary considerably between the species (Stephens et al., 1987; Yuan et al., 1989).

The genotyping methods are basically of two types: Immunological and molecular methods.

The Immunological methods are based in the use of polyvalent and specific monoclonal antibodies that recognized epitopes located on the MOMP of *C. trachomatis*. These methods have been replaced by molecular methods, which are better in specificity and sensitivity.

The molecular methods are based in nucleic acid amplification techniques and are of two types, i) methods that analyzed the *omp1* gene and ii) methods that analyzed several genes.

In methods that analyzed *omp1* gene the amplication products of the *omp1*-PCR are analyzed by restriction fragment length polymorphism (RFLP), nucleotide sequencing, array assay and Real-Time PCR.

In RFLP technical the amplication products of the *omp1*-PCR are cleaved with restriction endonuclease, this test is simple, rapid and its results show a high level of agreement with the results serotyping (Morré et al., 1998)

In array assay the amplication products of the *omp1*-PCR are analyzed by Southern blot hybridization using different DNA probes. These tests are rapid and accurately and also discriminate among multiple genotypes in one clinical specimen (Ruettger et al., 2011; Huang et al., 2008).

The nucleotide sequences of *omp1* show clearly mutations, variants of *omp1* and therefore providing evidence for existence of numerous subspecies. This method has a higher resolution than serotyping and RFLP (Morre et al., 1998), and has been considerate as gold standard for *C. trachomatis* genotyping (Sturm-Ramirez et al., 2000; Watson et al., 2002). However is still very laborious and not suitable for typing the isolates from a large number of clinical samples. A drawback is the difficulties in resolving mixed infections because peaks from different PCR products will be superposed in the chromatograms from sequencing reactions (Pedersen et al., 2009).

In genotyping by real time is evaluated with Taq Man probes in multiplex the *omp-1* gene, the test is specific and convenient for the rapid routine-diagnostic with capacity to detect mixed infections.

The methods that analyzed several genes are system based on hypervariable regions identified as housekeeping genes and polymorphic membrane protein genes. These methods have showed that are capable of identifying high intraserotype variation and greater genetic diversity in comparison to use *omp1* alone. Two types of methods have been described multilocus sequence typing (MLST), which analyzed candidate target regions by PCR and Sequencing (Klint et al., 2007) and the multi-locus variable number tandem repeat (VNTR) analysis and *omp1* or "MLVA-*omp1*"analized VNTR and *omp1* sequencing together (Pedersen 2008).

8. Genotyping for *C. trachomatis*

The vast majority of published data analyzed mainly with DNA sequencing of *omp1* clearly, show that E, D, F and G, genotypes are isolated from urogenital tract infections with most frequency, but prevalence of individual genotypes has been reported to differ by age, sex, geographic region and racial groups as is summary in the table 4, as studies in China, Holland and Australia from men who have sex with men, which G genotype was more frequent (Li et al., 2011; Quint et al., 2011; Twin et al., 2010). Studies also have shown that nearly of 60% of all typing of clinical isolates in different parts of the world report almost five different genotypes.

Country	Population studied	Genotype found, in descending order of prevalence	Reference
Greece	Men with urethritis	F, E, D, G, B, K, H	Psarrakos et al., 2011
China	Men who have sex with men	G, D, J	Li et al., 2011
Holland	Men who have sex with men	G/Ga, D/Da, J, LGV, L2	Quint et al., 2011
Mexico	Infertile women	F , E, G, K, D, H, LGV L2	De Haro-Cruz et al., 2011
Brasil	Youths and adults	E, F, D, I, J, G, K, H, B	Machado et al., 2011
England	Adults women	D, E, F	Wang et al., 2011
China	Adults	D, F, G, H, J, K	Tang et al., 2011
Australia	Men who have sex with men	D, G, J	Twin et al., 2010
Iran	Women symptomatic	E, F, D/Da, K, I, G, H, J	Taheri et al., 2010
China	Patients attending the STD clinic	E, F, G, D	Yang et al., 2010
Greece	Men with urethritis	E, G, F, Ja, D	Papadogeorgakis et al., 2010
Hungary	Female sex workers	D, E, F, G, H, I	Petrovay et al., 2009
Spain	Adults infected	E, D, G, F, B, H, I, J, K, LGV L2	Piñeiro et al., 2009
Costa Rica	Young women	E, F, D/Da, I/Ia	Porras et al., 2008
Australia	Heterosexual communities	E, F, J/Ja, D/Da, G, K	Bandea et al., 2008
England	Patients attending a genitourinary medicine clinic	E, F, D	Jalal et al., 2007
Brazil	Women attending the STD clinic	D, E, F, K	Lima et al., 2007
China	Women attending the STD clinic and female sex workers	E, F, G, D	Gao et al., 2007
China	Male attending the STD clinic	D, Da, F, K, J, G, H	Yu et al., 2007
Korea	Female sex workers	E, F, G, D, H, J	Lee et al., 2006
China	Clinical specimens	E, D, Da, F, J, K, G, H, Ba	Hsu et al., 2006
Africa	Volunteer students	E, F	Ngandjio et al., 2003
Iceland	Population attending the STD clinic	E, D, J, F, K, G, H, I	Jónsdóttir et al., 2003
India	females with urogenital infections	D, E, F	Singh et al., 2003
Stockholm	Youth health center	E, F, K, D	Sylvan et al., 2002

Country	Population studied	Genotype found, in descending order of prevalence	Reference
Sweden	patients attending the STD clinic	E, F, G, H	Jurstran et al., 2001
Thailand	Pregnant women	F, D, H, K, E, Ia, B, Ja, G	Bandea et al., 2001
Senegal	Female sex workers	E, D/Da, G, F, Ia, K	Sturm-Ramirez et al., 2000
Holland	Adults symptomatic or asyntomatic	D, E, F, Ga, K	Morré et al., 2000

Table 4. Distribution of *C. trachomatis* genotypes from different parts of the world

However MOMP differences and genotypes have yet to be consistently associated with disease severity or even disease phenotype and there is little knowledge of possible *Chlamydia* virulence factors, their expression and how they affect disease severity (Byrne, 2010).

9. Conclusion

Sexually transmitted infections (STI) are responsible for human suffering and carry significant economic costs. Many STI are entirely attributable to unsafe sex. Disease burden linked to unsafe sex amounted in 2004 to 70 millions disability-adjusted life years (DALYs) worldwide, of which 52 million were accounted for by developing countries. Unsafe sex ranked second among the 10 leading risk factor causes of DALYs worldwide, and third among the leading causes of DALYs in developing countries.

Lack of education and communication are contributing factors for the increase in new cases of *Chlamydia*. Also, the stigma surrounding sexually transmitted disease has hindered us in limiting the spread of this disease. Since *Chlamydia* is such a widespread disease, more government funded educational resources should be available to assist individuals in getting information and proper medical attention. Parents also need to be responsible for communicating with their children before a problem exists. If people are properly educated, the spread of *Chlamydia* should decline.

10. References

Aldeen, T.; Jacobs, J.; Powell, R. (2010). Screening university students for genital chlamydial infection: another lesson to learn. *Sexual Health,* Vol.7, No.4, (December 2010), pp. 491-494, ISSN 1449-8987.

An, Q.; Radcliffe, G.; Vassallo, R.; Buxton, D.; O'Brien, W.; Pelletier, D.; Weisburg, W.; Klinger, J.; Olive, D. (1992). Infection with a plasmid-free variant *Chlamydia* related to *Chlamydia trachomatis* identified by using multiple assays for nucleic acid detection. *Journal of Clinical Microbiology,* Vol.30, No.11, (November 1992) pp. 2814-2821, ISSN 1098-660X

Annan, N.; Sullivan, A.; Nori, A.; Naydenova, P.; Alexander, S.; McKenna, A.; Azadian, B.; Mandalia, S.; Rossi, M.; Ward, H.; Nwokolo, N. (2009). Rectal chlamydia--a reservoir of undiagnosed infection in men who have sex with men. *Sexually Transmitted Infections,*Vol.85, No.3, (June 2009) pp. 176-179, ISSN 1472-3263

Aydin, Y.; Atis, A.; Ocer, F.; Isenkul, R. (2010). Association of cervical infection of *Chlamydia trachomatis, Ureaplasma urealyticum* and *Mycoplasma hominis* with peritoneum colonisation in pregnancy. *Journal of Obstetrics and Ginecology,* Vol.30, No.8, (November 2010) pp. 809-812, ISSN 1364-6893

Baehr, W.; Zhang, Y.; Joseph, T.; Su, H.; Nano, F.; Everett, K.; Caldwell, H. (1988). Mapping antigenic domains expressed by *Chlamydia trachomatis* major outer membrane protein genes. *Proccedings of the National Academy of Sciences of the United States of America,* Vol.85, No.11, (June 1988) pp. 4000-4004, ISSN 1091-6490

Bandea, C.; Debattista, J.; Joseph, K.; Igietseme, J.; Timms, P.; Black, C. (2008). *Chlamydia trachomatis* serovars among strains isolated from members of rural indigenous communities and urban populations in Australia. *Journal of Clinical Microbiology,* Vol.46, No.1, (January 2001) pp. 355-356, ISSN 1098-660X

Bandea, C.; Kubota, K.; Brown, T.; Kilmarx, P.; Bhullar, V.; Yanpaisarn, S.; Chaisilwattana, P.; Siriwasin, W.; Black, C. (2001). Typing of *Chlamydia trachomatis* strains from urine samples by amplification and sequencing the major outer membrane protein gene (*omp1*). *Sexually Transmitted Infections,* Vol.77, No.6, (December 2001) pp. 419-422, ISSN 1472-3263

Barbosa, M.; Moherdaui, F.; Pinto, V.; Ribeiro, D.; Cleuton,M.; Miranda, A. (2010). Prevalence of *Neisseria gonorrhoeae* and *Chlamydia trachomatis* infection in men attending STD clinics in Brazil. *Revista da Sociedade Brasileira de Medicina Tropical,* Vol.43, No.5, (September-October 2010), pp. 500-503, ISSN 1678-9849

Belland, R.; Ojcius, D.; Byrne, G. (2004). *Chlamydia. Nature Reviews Microbiology,* Vol.2, No.7, (July 2004) pp. 530-531, ISSN 1740-1534

Black, C. (1997). Current methods of laboratory diagnosis of *Chlamydia trachomatis* infections. *Clinical Microbiology,* Vol.10, No.1, (January 1997) pp. 160-184, ISSN 1098-6618

Blank, S.; Schillinger, J.; Harbatkin, D. (2005). Lymphogranuloma venereum in the industrialised world. *Lancet,* Vol.365, No.9471, (May 2005) pp. 1607-1608, ISSN 1474-547X

Božičević, I.; Grgić, I.; Židovec-Lepej, S.; Čakalo, J.; Belak-Kovačević, S.; Štulhofer, A.; Begovac, J. (2011). Urine-based testing for *Chlamydia trachomatis* among young adults in a population-based survey in Croatia: feasibility and prevalence. *BMC Public Health,* Vol.14, No.11, (April) pp.230, ISSN 1471-2458

Brunham, R.; Binns, B.; Guijon, F.; Danforth, D.; Kosseim, M.; Rand, F.; McDowell, J.; Rayner, E. (1988). Etiology and outcome of acute pelvic inflammatory disease. *The Journal of Infectious Diseases,* Vol.158, No.3, (September 1988) pp. 510-517, ISSN 1537-6613

Byrne G. (2010). *Chlamydia trachomatis* strains and virulence: rethinking links to infection prevalence and disease severity. *The Journal of Infectious Diseases,* Vol.201, Suppl No.2:, (January 2010) pp. S126-S133, ISSN 1537-6613

Cai, L.; Kong, F.; Toi, C.; van Hal, S.; Gilber, G. (2010). Differentiation of *Chlamydia trachomatis* lymphogranuloma venereum-related serovars from other serovars using multiplex allele-specific polymerase chain reaction and high-resolution melting analysis. *International Journal of STD &AIDS,* Vol.21, No.11, (February 2010) pp. 101-104, ISSN 1758-1052

Canchihuaman, F.; Carcamo, C.; Garcia, P.; Aral S.; Whittington, W.; Hawes, S.; Hughes, J.; Holmes, K. (2010). Non-monogamy and risk of infection with *Chlamydia trachomatis* and *Trichomonas vaginalis* among young adults and their cohabiting partners in Peru. *Sexually transmitted Infections,* Vol.86, Suppl No.3, (December 2010), pp. 3:iii37-3:iii44, ISSN 1472-3263

Carlson, J.; Porcella, S.; McClarty, G.; Caldwell, H. (2005). Comparative genomic analysis of Chlamydia trachomatis oculotropic and genitotropic strains. *Infection and Immunity,* Vol.73, No.10, (October 2005) pp. 6407-6418, ISSN 1098-5522

Chai, S.; Aumakhan, B.; Barnes, M.; Jett-Goheen, M.; Quinn, N.; Agreda, P.; Whittle, P.; Hogan, T.; Jenkins, W.; Rietmeijer, C.; Gaydos C. (2010). Internet-based screening for sexually transmitted infections to reach nonclinic populations in the community: risk factors for infection in men. *Sexually Transmitted Diseases,* Vol.37, No.12, (December 2010) pp. 756-763, ISSN 1537-4521

Chesson, H. & Pinkerton, S. (2000). Sexually transmitted diseases and the increased risk for HIV transmission: implications for cost-effectiveness analyses of sexually transmitted disease prevention interventions. *Journal of Acquired Immune Deficiency Syndromes,* Vol.24, No.1, (May 2000) pp. 48-56, ISSN 1944-7884

Chkhartishvili, N.; Dvali, N.; Khechiashvili, G.; Sharvadze, L.; Tsertsvadze, T. (2010). High seroprevalence of *Chlamydia trachomatis* in newly diagnosed human immunodeficiency virus patients in georgia. *Georgian Medical News,* Vol.189, (December 2010), pp. 12-16, ISSN 1512-0112

Cles, L.; Bruch, K.; Stamm, W. (1988). Staining characteristics of six commercially available monoclonal immunofluorescence reagents for direct diagnosis of Chlamydia trachomatis infections. *Journal of Clinical Microbiology,* Vol.26, No.9, (September 1988) pp. 1735-1737, ISSN 1098-660X

Corbeto, E.; Lugo, R.; Martró, E.; Falguera, G.; Ros, R.; Avecilla, A.; Coll, C.; Saludes, V.; Casabona, J. (2010). Epidemiological features and determinants for *Chlamydia trachomatis* infection among women in Catalonia, Spain. *International Journal of STD &AIDS,* Vol.21, No.10, (October 2010) pp. 718-722, ISSN 1758-1052

Darj, E.; Mirembe, F.; Råssjö, E. (2010). STI-prevalence and differences in social background and sexual behavior among urban and rural young women in Uganda. *Sexual & Reproductive Healthcare,* Vol.1, No.3, (August 2010), pp. 111-115, ISSN 1877-5764

Davies, S.; Karagiannis, T.; Headon, V.; Wiig, R.; Duffy, J. (2011). Prevalence of genital chlamydial infection among a community sample of young international backpackers in Sydney, Australia. *International Journal of STD &AIDS,* Vol.22, No.3, (March 2011) pp. 160-164, ISSN 1758-1052

Dean, D.; Bruno, W.; Wan, R.; Gomes, J.; Devignot, S.; Mehari, T.; de Vries, H.; Morré, S.; Myers, G.; Read, T.; Spratt, B. (2009). Predicting phenotype and emerging strains among *Chlamydia trachomatis* infections. *Emerging Infectious Diseases,* Vol.15, No.9, (September 2009) pp. 1385-1394, ISSN 1080-6059

De Haro-Cruz, M.; Deleón-Rodríguez, I.; Escobedo-Guerra, M.; López-Hurtado, M.; Arteaga -Troncoso, G.; Ortiz-Ibarra. F.; Guerra-Infante, F. (2011). Genotyping of *Chlamydia trachomatis* from endocervical specimens of infertile Mexican women. *Enfermedades Infecciosas y Microbiologia Clinica,* Vol.29, No.2, (February 2011), pp. 102-108, ISSN 1578-1852

Desai, S.; Meyer, T.; Thamm, M.; Hamouda, O.; Bremer, V. (2011). Prevalence of *Chlamydia trachomatis* among young German adolescents, 2005-06. *Sexual Health,* Vol.8, No.1, pp. 120-122, ISSN 1449-8987

Douglas, A. & Hatch, T. (2000). Expression of the transcripts of the sigma factors and putative sigma factor regulators of *Chlamydia trachomatis* L2. *Gene,* Vol.247, No.1-2, (April 2000) pp. 209-214, ISSN 1879-0038

Everett, K.; Bush, R.; Andersen, A. (1999). Emended description of the order *Chlamydiales,* proposal of Parachlamydiaceae fam. nov. and Simkaniaceae fam. nov., each containing one monotypic genus, revised taxonomy of the family *Chlamydiaceae,* including a new genus and five new species, and standards for the identification of organisms. *International Journal of Systematic Bacteriology,* Vol.49, Pt No.2, (April 1999) pp. 415-440, ISSN 0020-7713

Folch, C.; Casabona, J.; Brugal, M.; Majó, X.; Esteve, A.; Meroño, M.; Gonzalez, V. (2011). Sexually Transmitted Infections and Sexual Practices among Injecting Drug Users in Harm Reduction Centers in Catalonia. *European Addiction Research,* Vol.17, No.5, (July 2011) pp. 271-278, ISSN 1421-9891

Freeman, E.; Weiss, H.; Glynn, J.; Cross, P.; Whitworth, J.; Hayes, R. (2006). Herpes simplex virus 2 infection increases HIV acquisition in men and women: systematic review and meta-analysis of longitudinal studies. *Acquired immune deficiency syndrome,* Vol.20, No.1, (January 2006) pp. 73-83, ISSN 1473-5571

Fresse, A.; Sueur, J.; Hamdad, F. (2010). Diagnosis and follow-up of genital chlamydial infection by direct methods and by detection of serum IgG, IgA and secretory IgA. *Indial Journal of Medical Microbiology,* Vol.28, No.4, (October-December 2010), pp. 326-33144, ISSN 1998-3646

Gao, X.; Chen, X.; Yin, Y.; Zhong, M.; Shi, M.; Wei, W.; Chen, Q.; Peeling, R.; Mabey, D. (2007). Distribution study of *Chlamydia trachomatis* serovars among high-risk women in China performed using PCR-restriction fragment length polymorphism genotyping. *Journal of Clinica Microbiology,* Vol.45, No.4, (February 2007) pp. 1185-1189, ISSN 1098-660X

Gaydos, C.; Barnes, M.; Aumakhan, B.; Quinn, N.; Wright, C.; Agreda, P.; Whittle, P.; Hogan T. (2011). *Chlamydia trachomatis* age-specific prevalence in women who used an internet-based self-screening program compared to women who were screened in family planning clinics. *Sexually Transmitted Diseases,* Vol.38, No.2, (February 2011), pp. 74-78, ISSN 1537-4521

Goulet, V.; de Barbeyrac, B.; Raherison, S.; Prudhomme, M.; Semaille, C.; Warszawski, J.; CSF group. (2010). Prevalence of *Chlamydia trachomatis*: results from the first national population-based survey in France. *Sexual Transmitted Infections,* Vol.86, No.4, (August 2010) pp. 263-270, ISSN 1472-3263

Goyal, M.; Hayes, K.; McGowan, K.; Fein, J.; Mollen C. (2011). Prevalence of *Trichomonas vaginalis* Infection in Symptomatic Adolescent Females Presenting to a Pediatric

Emergency Department. *Academic Emergency Medicine* , Vol.18, No.7, (July 1990) pp. 763-766, ISSN 1553-2712

Haller, D.; Steiner, A.; Sebo, P.; Gaspoz, J.; Wolff, H. (2011). *Chlamydia trachomatis* infection in males in a juvenile detention facility in Switzerland. *Swiss Medical Weekly,* Vol.141, (July 2011), ISSN 1424-3997

Hatt, C.; Ward, M.; Clarke, I. (1988). Analysis of the entire nucleotide sequence of the cryptic plasmid of *Chlamydia trachomatis* serovar L1. Evidence for involvement in DNA replication. *Nucleic Acids Research,* Vol.16, No.9, (May 1988) pp. 4053-4067, ISSN 1362-4962

Hennrikus, E.; Oberto, D.; Linder, J.; Rempel, J.; Hennrikus, N. (2010). Sports preparticipation examination to screen college athletes for *Chlamydia trachomatis. Medicine and Sciece in Sports and Exercise,* Vol.42, No.4, (April 2010), pp. 683-688, ISSN 1530-0315

Hsieh, Y.; Shih, T.; Lin, H.; Hsieh, T.; Kuo, M.; Lin, C.; Gaydos, C. (2010). High-risk sexual behaviours and genital chlamydial infections in high school students in Southern Taiwan. *International Journal of STD &AIDS,* Vol.21, No.4, (April 2010) pp. 253-259, ISSN 1758-1052

Hsu, M.; Tsai, P.; Chen, K.; Li, L.; Chiang, C.; Tsai, J.; Ke, L.; Chen, H.; Li, S. (2006). Genotyping of *Chlamydia trachomatis* from clinical specimens in Taiwan. *Journal of Medical Microbiology,* Vol.55, Pt No.3, (March 2006) pp. 301-308, ISSN 1473-5644

Huang, C.; Wong, W.; Li, L.; Chang, C.; Chen, B.; Li, S. (2008). Genotyping of Chlamydia trachomatis by microsphere suspension array. *Journal of Clinical Microbiology,* Vol.46, No.3, (Mar 2008), pp. 1126-1128, ISSN 1098-660X

Hunte, T.; Alcaide, M.; Castro, J. (2010). Rectal infections with chlamydia and gonorrhoea in women attending a multiethnic sexually transmitted diseases urban clinic. *International Journal of STD &AIDS,* Vol.21, No.12, (December 2010) pp. 819-822, ISSN 1758-1052

Huq, M.; Chawdhury, F.; Mitra, D.; Islam, M.; Salahuddin, G.; Das, J.; Rahman, M. (2010). A pilot study on the prevalence of sexually transmitted infections among clients of brothel-based female sex workers in Jessore, Bangladesh. *International Journal of STD &AIDS,* Vol.21, No.4, (April 2010) pp. 300-301, ISSN 1758-1052

Imai, H.; Nakao, H.; Shinohara, H.; Fujii, Y.; Tsukino, H.; Hamasuna, R.; Osada, Y.; Fukushima, K.; Inamori, M.; Ikenoue, T.; Katoh T. (2010). Population-based study of asymptomatic infection with *Chlamydia trachomatis* among *International Journal of STD &AIDS,* Vol.21, No.5, (May 2010) pp. 362-366, ISSN 1758-1052

Jackson, Y.; Sebo, P.; Aeby, G.; Bovier, P.; Ninet, B.; Schrenzel, J.; Sudre, P.; Haller, D.; Gaspoz, J.; Wolff, H. (2010). Prevalence and associated factors for *Chlamydia trachomatis* infection among undocumented immigrants in a primary care facility in Geneva, Switzerland: a cross-sectional study. *Journal of Immigrant and Minority Health,* Vol.12, No.6, (December 2010) pp. 909-9144, ISSN 1557-1920

Jalal, H.; Stephen, H.; Bibby, D.; Sonnex, C.; Carne, C. (2007). Molecular epidemiology of genital human papillomavirus and *Chlamydia trachomatis* among patients attending a genitourinary medicine clinic - will vaccines protect? *International Journal of STD &AIDS,* Vol.18, No.9, (September 2010) pp. 617-621, ISSN 1758-1052

Jenkins, W.; Rabins, C.; Barnes, M.; Agreda, P.; Gaydos, C. (2011). Use of the internet and self-collected samples as a sexually transmissible infection intervention in rural Illinois communities. *Sexual Health*, Vol.8, No.1, (March 2011), pp. 79-85, ISSN 1449-8987

Jin, X.; Chan, S.; Ding, G.; Wang, H.; Xu, J.; Wang, G.; Chang, D.; Reilly, K.; Wang, N. (2011). Prevalence and risk behaviours for *Chlamydia trachomatis* and *Neisseria gonorrhoeae* infection among female sex workers in an HIV/AIDS high-risk area. *International Journal of STD &AIDS*, Vol.22, No.2, (February 2011) pp. 80-84, ISSN 1758-1052

Jo, S.; Shin, J.; Song, K.; Kim, J.; Hwang, K.; Bhally H. (2011). Prevalence and Correlated Factors of Sexually Transmitted Diseases-*Chlamydia*, *Neisseria*, *Cytomegalovirus*-in Female Rape Victims. *The Journal of Sexual Medicine*, Vol.8, No.8, (August 2011) pp. 2317-2326, ISSN 1743-6109

Jónsdóttir, K.; Kristjánsson, M.; Hjaltalín, O.; Steingrímsson, O. (2003). The molecular epidemiology of genital *Chlamydia trachomatis* in the greater Reykjavik area, Iceland. *Sexually transmitted diseases*, Vol.30, No.3, (March 2003), pp. 249-256, ISSN 1537-4521

Jordan, N.; Lee, S.; Nowak, G.; Johns, N.; Gaydos, J. (2011). *Chlamydia trachomatis* reported among U.S. active duty service members, 2000-2008. *Military Medicine*, Vol.176, No.3, (March 2011), pp. 312-319, ISSN 1930-613X

Joyee, A.; Thyagarajan, S.; Reddy, E.; Venkatesan, C.; Ganapathy, M. (2005). Genital chlamydial infection in STD patients: its relation to HIV infection. *Indian Journal of Medical Microbiology*, Vol.23, No.1, (January 2005) pp. 37-40, ISSN 1998-3646

Jurstrand, M.; Falk,L.; Fredlund, H.; Lindberg, M.; Olcén, P.; Andersson, S.; Persson, K.; Albert, J.; Bäckman, A. (2001). Characterization of *Chlamydia trachomatis omp1* genotypes among sexually transmitted disease patients in Sweden. *Journal of Clinical Microbiology*, Vol.39, No.11, (November 2001), pp. 3915-3919, ISSN 1098-660X

Karam, G.; Martin, D.; Flotte, T.; Bonnarens, F.; Joseph, J.; Mroczkowski, T.; Johnson, W. (1986). Asymptomatic *Chlamydia trachomatis* infections among sexually active men. (1986). *The Journal of Infectious Diseases*, Vol.154, No.5, (November 1986) pp.900-903, ISSN 1537-6613

Kent, C.; Chaw, J.; Wong, W.; Liska, S.; Gibson, S.; Hubbard, G.; Klausner, J. (2005). Prevalence of rectal, urethral, and pharyngeal chlamydia and gonorrhea detected in 2 clinical settings among men who have sex with men: San Francisco, California, 2003. *Clinical Infectious Diseases*, Vol.41, No.1, (July 2005) pp. 67-74, ISSN 1537-6591

Khan, M.; Unemo, M.; Zaman, S.; Lundborg, C. (2011). HIV, STI prevalence and risk behaviours among women selling sex in Lahore, Pakistan. *BMC Infectious Diseases*, Vol.11, No.1, (May 2011), pp. 119, ISSN 1471-2334

Klint, M.; Fuxelius, H.; Goldkuhl, R.; Skarin, H.; Rutemark, C.; Andersson, S.; Persson, K.; Herrmann, B. (2007). High-resolution genotyping of *Chlamydia trachomatis* strains by multilocus sequence analysis. *Journal of Clinical Microbiology*, Vol.45, No.5, (May 2007), pp. 1410-1414, ISSN 1098-660X

Kwena, Z.; Bukusi, E.; Ng'ayo, M.; Buffardi, A.; Nguti, R.; Richardson, B.; Sang, N.; Holmes K. (2010). Prevalence and risk factors for sexually transmitted infections in a high-risk occupational group: the case of fishermen along Lake Victoria in Kisumu, Kenya. *International Journal of STD &AIDS,* Vol.21, No.10, (October 2010) pp. 708-713, ISSN 1758-1052

Lee, G.; Park,J.; Kim, S.; Yoo, C.; Seong, W. (2006). *OmpA* genotyping of *Chlamydia trachomatis* from Korean female sex workers. *The Journal of Infection,* Vol.52, No.6, (June 2006), pp. 451-454, ISSN 1532-2742

Lee, J.; Jung, S.; Kwon, D.; Jung, M.; Park, B. (2010). Condom Use and Prevalence of Genital Chlamydia trachomatis Among the Korean Female Sex Workers. *Epidemiology and Health,* Vol.32, (August 2010) pp. e2010008, ISSN 2092-7193

Lee, Y.; Kim, J.; Kim, J.; Park, W.; Choo, M.; Lee, K. (2010). Prevalence and treatment efficacy of genitourinary mycoplasmas in women with overactive bladder symptoms. *Korean Journal of Urology,* Vol.51, No.9, (September 2010) pp. 625-630, ISSN 2005-6745

Le Roux, M.; Ramoncha, M.; Adam, A.; Hoosen A. (2010). A etiological agents of urethritis in symptomatic South African men attending a family practice. *International Journal of STD &AIDS,* Vol.21, No.7, (July 2010) pp. 477-481, ISSN 1758-1052

Li, J.; Cai, Y.; Yin, Y.; Hong, F.; Shi, M.; Feng, T.; Peng, R.; Wang, B.; Chen, X. (2011). Prevalence of anorectal *Chlamydia trachomatis* infection and its genotype distribution among men who have sex with men in Shenzhen, China. *Japanese Journal of Infectious Diseases,* Vol.64, No.2, pp. 143-146, ISSN 1344-6304

Lima, H.; Oliveira, M.; Valente, B.; Afonso, D.; Darocha, W.; Souza, M.; Alvim, T.; Barbosa-Stancioli, E.; Noronha, F. (2007). Genotyping of *Chlamydia trachomatis* from endocervical specimens in Brazil. *Sexually transmitted diseases,* Vol.34, No.9, (September 2007), pp. 709-717, ISSN 1537-4521

Lyss, S.; Kamb, M.; Peterman, T.; Moran, J.; Newman, D.; Bolan, G.; Douglas, J.; Iatesta, M.; Malotte, C.; Zenilman, J.; Ehret, J.; Gaydos, C.; Newhall, W. Project RESPECT Study Group. (2003). *Chlamydia trachomatis* among patients infected with and treated for *Neisseria gonorrhoeae* in sexually transmitted disease clinics in the United States. *Annals of Internal Medicine,* Vol.139, No.3, (August 2003) pp. 178-185, ISSN 1539-3704

Machado, A.; Bandea, C.; Alves, M.; Joseph, K.; Igietseme, J.; Miranda, A.; Guimarães, E.; Turchi, M.; Black, C. (2011). Distribution of *Chlamydia trachomatis* genovars among youths and adults in Brazil. *Journal of Medical Microbiology,* Vol.60, Pt No.4, (April 2011), pp. 472-476, ISSN 1473-5644

Mahony, J.; Luinstra, K.; Sellors, J; Jang, D.; Chernesky MA. (1992). Confirmatory polymerase chain reaction testing for *Chlamydia trachomatis* in first-void urine from asymptomatic and symptomatic men. *Journal of Clinical Microbiology,* Vol.30, No.9, (September 1992) pp. 2241-2245, ISSN 1098-660X

Månsson, F.; Camara, C.; Biai, A.; Monteiro, M.; da Silva Z.; Dias, F.; Alves, A.; Andersson, S.; Fenyö, E.; Norrgren, H.; Unemo, M. (2010). High prevalence of HIV-1, HIV-2 and other sexually transmitted infections among women attending two sexual health clinics in Bissau, Guinea-Bissau, West Africa. *International Journal of STD &AIDS,* Vol.21, No.9, (September 2010) pp. 631, ISSN 1758-1052

Mawu, F.; Davies, S.; McKechnie, M.; Sedyaningsih, E.; Widihastuti, A.; Hillman, R. (2011). Sexually transmissible infections among female sex workers in Manado, Indonesia, using a multiplex polymerase chain reaction-based reverse line blot assay. *Sexual Health,* Vol.8, No.1, (March 2011) pp. 52-60, ISSN 1449-8987

Mbizvo, E.; Msuya, S.; Stray-Pedersen, B.; Sundby, J.; Chirenje, M.; Hussain, A. (2001). HIV seroprevalence and its associations with the other reproductive tract infections in asymptomatic women in Harare, Zimbabwe. *International Journal of STD &AIDS,* Vol.12, No.8, (August 2001) pp.524-531, ISSN 1758-1052

Miller, W.; Ford, C.; Morris, M.; Handcock, M.; Schmitz, J.; Hobbs, M.; Cohen, M.; Harris, K.; Udry, J. (2004). Prevalence of chlamydial and gonococcal infections among young adults in the United States. *The Journal of the American Medical Association,* Vol.291, No.18, (May 2004) pp. 2229-2236, ISSN 1538-3598

Morré, S.; Meijer, C.; Munk, C.; Krüger-Kjaer, S.; Winther, J.; Jørgensens, H.; van Den Brule, A. (2000). Pooling of urine specimens for detection of asymptomatic *Chlamydia trachomatis* infections by PCR in a low-prevalence population: cost-saving strategy for epidemiological studies and screening programs. *Journal of Clinical Microbiology,* Vol.38, No.4, (April 2000) pp. 1679-1680, ISSN 1098-660X

Morré, S.; Ossewaarde, J.; Lan, J.; van Doornum, G.; Walboomers, J.; MacLaren, D.; Meijer, C.; van den Brule, A. (1998). Serotyping and genotyping of genital *Chlamydia trachomatis* isolates reveal variants of serovars Ba, G, and J as confirmed by *omp1* nucleotide sequence analysis. *Journal of Clinical Microbiology,* Vol.36, No.2, (February 1998) pp. 345-351, ISSN 1098-660X

Ngandjio, A.; Clerc, M.; Fonkoua, M.; Thonnon, J.; Njock, F.; Pouillot, R.; Lunel, F.; Bebear, C.; De Barbeyrac, B.; Bianchi, A. (2003). Screening of volunteer students in Yaounde (Cameroon, Central Africa) for *Chlamydia trachomatis* infection and genotyping of isolated C. trachomatis strains. *Journal of Clinical Microbiology,* Vol.41, No.9, (September 2003), pp. 4404-4407, ISSN 1098-660X

Nicholson, T.; Olinger, L.; Chong, K.; Schoolnik, G.; Stephens R. (2003). Global stage-specific gene regulation during the developmental cycle of *Chlamydia trachomatis. Journal of Bacteriology,* Vol.185, No.10, (May 2010) pp. 3179-3189, ISSN 1098-5530

Oh, J.; Franceschi, S.; Kim, B.; Kim, J.; Ju, Y.; Hong, E.; Chang, Y.; Rha, S.; Kim, H.; Kim, J.; Kim, C.; Shin, H. (2009). Prevalence of human papillomavirus and *Chlamydia trachomatis* infection among women attending cervical cancer screening in the Republic of Korea. *European Journal Cancer Prevention,* Vol.18, No.1, (February 2009), pp. 56-61, ISSN 1473-5709

Ostergaard L. (1999). Diagnosis of urogenital *Chlamydia trachomatis* infection by use of DNA amplification. *Acta pathologica, microbiologica, et immunologica Scandinavica,* Vol.89, No.5, pp. 36, ISSN 1362-4962

Papadogeorgakis, H.; Pittaras, T.; Papaparaskevas, J.; Pitiriga, V.; Katsambas, A.; Tsakris A. (2010). *Chlamydia trachomatis* serovar distribution and *Neisseria gonorrhoeae* coinfection in male patients with urethritis in Greece. *Journal of Clinical Microbiology,* Vol.48, No.6, (June 2001) pp. 2231-2234, ISSN 1098-660X

Patel, A.; Sachdev, D.; Nagpal, P.; Chaudhry, U.; Sonkar, S.; Mendiratta, S.; Saluja D. (2011). Prevalence of *Chlamydia* infection among women visiting a gynaecology outpatient department: evaluation of an in-house PCR assay for detection of *Chlamydia trachomatis. Annals of Clinical Microbiology and Antimicrobials,* Vol.9, No.24, (September 2011), ISSN 1476-0711

Pedersen, L.; Herrmann, B.; Moller, J.; (2009). Typing Chlamydia trachomatis: from egg yolk to nanotechnology. FEMS immunology and medical microbiology, Vol.55, No.2, (March 2009), pp. 120-130, ISSN 1574-695X

Pedersen, L.; Podenphant, L.; Moller, J. (2008). Highly discriminative genotyping of Chlamydia trachomatis using omp1 and a set of variable number tandem repeats. Clinical Microbiology and Infection, Vol.14, No.7, (July 2008), pp. 644-652, ISSN 1469-0691

Petrovay, F.; Balla, E.; Németh, I.; Gönczöl, E. (2009). Genotyping of *Chlamydia trachomatis* from the endocervical specimens of high-risk women in Hungary. *Journal of Medical Microbiology,* Vol.58, Pt No.6, (June 2010), pp. 760-764, ISSN 1473-5644

Piñeiro, L.; Montes, M.; Gil-SetasA.; Camino X.; Echeverria.; Cilla G. (2009). Genotyping of *Chlamydia trachomatis* in an area of northern Spain. *Enfermedades Infecciosas y Microbiologia Clinica,* Vol.27, No.8, (October 2009), pp. 462-464, ISSN 1578-1852

Platt, L.; Grenfell, P.; Bonell, C.; Creighton, S.; Wellings, K.; Parry, J.; Rhodes T. (2011). Risk of sexually transmitted infections and violence among indoor-working female sex workers in London: the effect of migration from Eastern Europe. *Sexually transmitted Infections,* Vol.86, No.5, (August 2011), pp. 377-384, ISSN 1472-3263

Porras, C.; Safaeian, M.; González, P.; Hildesheim, A.; Silva, S.; Schiffman, M.; Rodríguez, A.; Wacholder, S.; Freer, E.; Quint, K.; Bratti, C.; Espinoza, A.; Cortes, B.; Herrero, R.; Costa Rica HPV Vaccine Trial (CVT) Group. (2008). Epidemiology of genital *Chlamydia trachomatis* infection among young women in Costa Rica. *Sexually transmitted diseases,* Vol.35, No.5, (May 2008), pp. 461-468, ISSN 1537-4521

Psarrakos, P.; Papadogeorgakis, E.; Sachse, K.; Vretou, E. (2011). *Chlamydia trachomatis ompA* genotypes in male patients with urethritis in Greece - Conservation of the serovar distribution and evidence for mixed infections with *Chlamydophila abortus. Molecular and Cellular Probes,* Vol.25, No.1, (August 2011), pp. 168-173, ISSN 1096-1194

Puolakkainen, M.; Hiltunen-Back, E.; Reunala, T.; Suhonen, S.; Lähteenmäki, P.; Lehtinen, M.; Paavonen, J. (1998). Comparison of performances of two commercially available tests, a PCR assay and a ligase chain reaction test, in detection of urogenital *Chlamydia trachomatis* infection. *Journal of Clinical Microbiology,* Vol.36, No.6, (June 1998) pp. 1489-1493, ISSN 1098-660X

Quint, K.; Bom, R.; Quint, W.; Bruisten, S.; van der Loeff, M.; Morré S.; de Vries, H. (2011). Anal infections with concomitant *Chlamydia trachomatis* genotypes among men who have sex with men in Amsterdam, the Netherlands. *Sexual Transmitted BMC Infectious Diseases,* Vol.11, No.63, (March 2011), ISSN 1471-2334

Ramos, B.; Polettini, J.; Marcolino, L.; Vieira, E.; Marques, M.; Tristão, A.; Nunes, H.; Rudge, M.; Silva, M. (2011). Prevalence and risk factors of *Chlamydia trachomatis* cervicitis in pregnant women at the genital tract infection in obstetrics unit care at Botucatu Medical School, São Paulo State University-UNESP, Brazil. *Journal Low Genital Trac Disease,* Vol.15, No.1, (January 2011) pp. 20-24, ISSN 1526-0976

Read, T.; Brunham, R.; Shen, C.; Gill, S.; Heidelberg, J.; White, O.; Hickey, E.; Peterson, J.; Utterback, T.; Berry,K.; Bass, S.; Linher, K.; Weidman, J.; Khouri, H.; Craven, B.; Bowman, C.; Dodson, R.; Gwinn, M.; Nelson, W.; DeBoy, R.; Kolonay, J.; McClarty, G.; Salzberg, S.; Eisen, J.; Fraser, C. (2000). Genome sequences of *Chlamydia trachomatis* MoPn and *Chlamydia pneumoniae* AR39. *Nucleic Acids Research,* Vol.28, No.6, (March 2000) pp. 1397-1406, ISSN 1362-4962

Roberts, S.; Sheffield, J.; McIntire, D.; Alexander, J. (2011). Urine screening for *Chlamydia trachomatis* during pregnancy. *Obstetrics Gynecology. Military Medicine,* Vol.117, No.4, (April 2011), pp. 883-885, ISSN 1873-233X

Rodrigues, M.; Fernandes, P.; Haddad, J.; Paiva, M.; Souza, Mdo.; Andrade, T.; Fernandes A. (2011). Frequency of *Chlamydia trachomatis, Neisseria gonorrhoeae, Mycoplasma genitalium, Mycoplasma hominis* and *Ureaplasma* species in cervical samples. *Journal of Obstetrics and Ginecology,* Vol.31, No.3, pp. 237-241, ISSN 1364-6893

Rours, G.; Duijts, L.; Moll, H.; Arends, L.; de Groot, R,; Jaddoe, V.; Hofman, A.; Steegers, E.; Mackenbach, J.; Ott, A.; Willemse, H.; van der Zwaan, E.; Verkooijen, R.; Verbrugh, H. (2011). *Chlamydia trachomatis* infection during pregnancy associated with preterm delivery: a population-based prospective cohort study. *European Journal of Epidemiology,* Vol.26, No.6, (May 2011) pp. 493-502, ISSN 1573-7284

Ruettger, A.; Feige, J.; Slickers, P.; Schubert, E.; Morré, S.; Pannekoek, Y.; Herrmann, B.; de Vries, H.; Ehricht, R.; Sachse, K. (2011). Genotyping of *Chlamydia trachomatis* strains from culture and clinical samples using an ompA-based DNA microarray assay. *Molecular and Cellular,* Vol.25, No.1, (February 2011), pp. 19-27, ISSN 1096-1194

Salmeri, M.; Santanocita, A.; Toscano, M.; Morello, A.; Valenti, D.; La Vignera, S.; Bellanca, S.; Vicari, E.; Calogero A. (2010). *Chlamydia trachomatis* prevalence in unselected infertile couples. *Systems Biology in Reproductive Medicine,* Vol.56, No.6, (December 2010) pp. 450-456, ISSN 1939-6376

Schachter, J. (1978). Chlamydial infections (first of three parts). *The New England Journal Medicine.,* Vol.298, No.8, (February 1978) pp. 428-435, ISSN 1533-4406

Schachter, J. & Moncada J. (2005). Lymphogranuloma venereum: how to turn an endemic disease into an outbreak of a new disease? Start looking. *Sexually Transmitted Diseases,* Vol.32, No.6, (June 2005) pp. 331-332, ISSN 1537-4521

Shen, L.; Shi, Y.; Douglas, A.; Hatch, T.; O'Connell, C.; Chen, J.; Zhang, Y. (2000). Identification and characterization of promoters regulating tuf expression in *Chlamydia trachomatis* serovar F. *Archives of Biochemimistry and Biophysics,* Vol.379, No.1, (July 2000) pp. 46-56, ISSN 1096-0384

Silitonga, N.; Davies, S.; Kaldor, J.; Wignall, S.; Okoseray, M. (2011). Prevalence over time and risk factors for sexually transmissible infections among newly-arrived female sex workers in Timika, Indonesia. *Sexual Health,* Vol.8, No.1, (March 2011) pp. 61-64, ISSN 1449-8987

Singh, V.; Salhan, S.; Das, B.; Mittal, A. (2003). Predominance of *Chlamydia trachomatis* serovars associated with urogenital infections in females in New Delhi, India. *Journal of Clinical Microbiology,* Vol.41, No.6, (June 2003), pp. 2700-2702, ISSN 1098-660X

Skidmore, S.; Copley, S.; Cordwell, D.; Donaldson, D.; Ritchie, D.; Spraggon, M. (2011). Positive nucleic acid amplification tests for *Neisseria gonorrhoeae* in young people tested as part of the National Chlamydia Screening Programme. *International Journal of STD &AIDS,* Vol.22, No.7, (July 2010) pp. 398-399, ISSN 1758-1052

Srifeungfung, S.; Roongpisuthipong, A.; Asavapiriyanont, S.; Lolekha, R.; Tribuddharat,C.; Lokpichart, S.; Sungthong, P.; Tongtep, P. (2009). Prevalence of *Chlamydia trachomatis* and *Neisseria gonorrhoeae* in HIV-seropositive patients and gonococcal antimicrobial susceptibility: an update in Thailand. *Japanese Journal of Infectious Diseases,* Vol.62, No.6, (November 2009), pp. 467-470, ISSN 1344-6304

Sylvan, S.; Von Krogh, G.; Tiveljung, A.; Siwerth, B.; Henriksson, L.; Norén, L.; Asp, A.; Grillner, L. (2002). Screening and genotyping of genital *Chlamydia trachomatis* in urine specimens from male and female clients of youth-health centers in Stockholm County. *Sexually Transmitted Diseases,* Vol.29, No.7, (July 2002), pp. 379-386, ISSN 1537-4521

Stamm, W. (1999). *Chlamydia trachomatis* is infections of the adult. In sexually transmitted disease 3rd edition. Edited by: Holmes KK, Sparling PF, Mardh PA. McGraw-Hill , 407-422, ISBN 978-0070296886 New York, United States of America.

Steiner, A.; Haller, D.; Elger, B.; Sebo, P.; Gaspoz, J.; Wolff, H. (2010). *Chlamydia trachomatis* infection in a Swiss prison: a cross sectional study. *Swiss Medical Weekly,* Vol.140, (November 2010) pp. w13126, ISSN 1424-3997

Stephens, R.; Sanchez-Pescador, R.; Wagar E.; Inouye, C.; Urdea M. (1987). Diversity of *Chlamydia trachomatis* major outer membrane protein genes. *Journal of Bacteriology,* Vol.169, No.9, (September 1987) pp. 3879-3885, ISSN 1098-5530

Stephens R.; Tam, M.; Kuo, C.; Nowinski, R. (1982). Monoclonal antibodies to *Chlamydia trachomatis*: antibody specificities and antigen characterization. *Journal of Immunity,* Vol.128, No.3, (March 1982) pp. 1083-1089, ISSN 1550-6606

Sturm-Ramirez, K.; Brumblay, H.; Diop, K.; Guèye-Ndiaye, A.; Sankalé, J.; Thior, I.; N'Doye, I.; Hsieh, C.; Mboup, S.; Kanki, P. (2000). Molecular epidemiology of genital *Chlamydia trachomatis* infection in high-risk women in Senegal, West Africa. *Journal of Clinical Microbiology,* Vol.38, No.1, (January 2000) pp. 138-145, ISSN 1098-660X

Taheri, B.; Motamedi, H.; Ardakani, M. (2010). Genotyping of the prevalent *Chlamydia trachomatis* strains involved in cervical infections in women in Ahvaz, Iran. *Journal of Medical Microbiology,* Vol.59, Pt No.9, (September 2010), pp. 1023-1028, ISSN 1473-5644

Tang, J.; Zhou, L.; Liu, X.; Zhang, Ch.; Zhao, Y.; Wang Y. (2011). Novel multiplex real-time PCR system using the SNP technology for the simultaneous diagnosis of *Chlamydia trachomatis, Ureaplasma parvum* and *Ureaplasma urealyticum* and genetic typing of serovars of *C. trachomatis* and *U. parvum* in NGU. *Molecular and Cellular Probes,* Vol.25, No.1, (February 2011), pp. 55-59, ISSN 1096-1194

Tanudyaya, F.; Rahardjo, E.; Bollen, L.; Madjid, N.; Daili, S.; Priohutomo, S.; Morineau, G.; Nurjannah, Roselinda, Anartati A.; Purnamawati, K.; Mamahit, E. (2010).

Prevalence of sexually transmitted infections and sexual risk behavior among female sex workers in nine provinces in Indonesia, 2005. *The Southeast Asian Journal of Tropical Medicine and Public Health,* Vol.41, No.2, (Marchr 2010) pp. 463-473, ISSN 0125-1562

Tipples, G. & McClarty, G. (1993). The obligate intracellular bacterium *Chlamydia trachomatis* is auxotrophic for three of the four ribonucleoside triphosphates. *Molecular Microbiology,* Vol.25, No.1, (June 1993), pp. 1096-1194, ISSN 1365-2958

Twin, J.; Moore, E.; Garland, S.; Stevens, M.; Fairley C.K; Donovan, B.; Rawlinson, W.; Tabrizi, S. (2010). *Chlamydia trachomatis* Genotypes Among Men Who Have Sex With Men in Australia. *Sexually Transmitted Diseases,* (November 2010), ISSN 1537-4521

Van Dyck, E.; Ieven, M.; Pattyn, S.; Van Damme, L.; Laga, M. (2001). Detection of *Chlamydia trachomatis* and *Neisseria gonorrhoeae* by enzyme immunoassay, culture, and three nucleic acid amplification tests. *Journal of Clinical Microbiology,* Vol.39, No.5, (May 2001) pp. 1751-1756, ISSN 1098-660X

Wang, S. & Grayston J. (1970). Immunologic relationship between genital TRIC, lymphogranuloma venereum, and related organisms in a new microtiter indirect immunofluorescence test. *American Journal of Ophthalmology,* Vol.70, No.3, (September 1970) pp. 367-374, ISSN 1879-1891

Wang, Y.; Skilton, R.; Cutcliffe, L.; Andrews, E.; Clarke, I.; Marsh, P. (2011). Evaluation of a high resolution genotyping method for *Chlamydia trachomatis* using routine clinical samples. *Public Library of Science one,* Vol.6, No.2, (February 2011) pp. e16971, ISSN 1932-6203

Watson E.; Templeton, A.; Russell, I.; Paavonen, J.; Mardh, P.; Stary, A.; Pederson, B. (2002). The accuracy and efficacy of screening tests for *Chlamydia trachomatis*: a systematic review. *Journal of Medical Microbiology,* Vol.51, No.12, (December 2002) pp. 1021-1031, ISSN 1473-5644

World Health Organization. Prevention and control of sexually transmitted infections: draft global strategy. [http://www.who.int]. WHO, 2006.

World Health Organization. Global prevalence and incidence of selected curable sexually transmissible disease: overview and estimates. Genoveva. WHO, 2001.

Yang, B.; Zheng, H.; Feng, Z.; Xue, Y.; Wu, X.; Huang, J.; Xue X.; Jiang H. (2010). The prevalence and distribution of *Chlamydia trachomatis* genotypes among sexually transmitted disease clinic patients in Guangzhou, China, 2005-2008. *Japanese Journal of Infectious Diseases,* Vol.63, No.5, (September 2010) pp. 342-345, ISSN 1344-6304

Yu, M.; Li, L.; Li, S.; Tang, L.; Tai, Y.; Chen, K. (2007). Molecular epidemiology of genital chlamydial infection among male patients attending an STD clinic in Taipei, Taiwan. *Sexually transmitted diseases,* Vol.34, No.8, (August 2007), pp. 570-573, ISSN 1537-4521

Yuan, Y.; Zhang, Y.; Watkins, N.; Caldwell, H. (1989). Nucleotide and deduced amino acid sequences for the four variable domains of the major outer membrane proteins of the 15 *Chlamydia trachomatis* serovars. *Infection and Immunity,* Vol.57, No.4, (April 1989) pp. 1040-1049, ISSN 1098-5522

Zimmerman, H.; Potterat, J.; Dukes, R.; Muth, J.; Zimmerman, H.; Fogle, J.; Pratts, C. (1990). Epidemiologic differences between chlamydia and gonorrhea. *American Journal of Public Health,* Vol.80, No.11, (November 1990) pp. 1338-1342, ISSN 1541-0048

Znazen, A.; Frikha-Gargouri, O.; Berrajah, L.; Bellalouna, S.; Hakim, H.; Gueddana, N.; Hammami, A. (2010). Sexually transmitted infections among female sex workers in Tunisia: high prevalence of *Chlamydia trachomatis. Sexual Transmitted Infections,* Vol.86, No.7, (December 2010) pp. 500-5005, ISSN 1472-3263

2

Host-Pathogen Co-Evolution: *Chlamydia trachomatis* Modulates Surface Ligand Expression in Genital Epithelial Cells to Evade Immune Recognition

Gerialisa Caesar[1], Joyce A. Ibana[2], Alison J. Quayle[2] and Danny J. Schust[1]
[1]*Department of Obstetrics, Gynecology and Women's Health, University of Missouri School of Medicine, Columbia, MO*
[2]*Department of Microbiology, Immunology and Parasitology, Louisiana State University Health Sciences Center, New Orleans, LA*
USA

1. Introduction

Chlamydia trachomatis (*C. trachomatis*) is an obligate intracellular bacterium that causes significant human disease (Everett, Bush et al. 1999). This pathogen is usually categorized by its major outer membrane protein (MOMP) antigen, and serovars D though K infect the mucosal columnar epithelial cells of the urogenital tract (Linhares and Witkin 2010). Though *C. trachomatis* infection can be treated using several antibiotic regimens, the World Health Organization considers it to be the world's most common bacterial sexually transmitted disease, infecting approximately 90 million people worldwide (Gerbase, Rowley et al. 1998). In 2010, the Center for Disease Control reported the rate of chlamydial infection in women as 592.2 cases per 100,000 in the US. In contrast, only 219.3 cases per 100,000 men were reported(CDC 2010). Clearly there remains an urgent need for improved risk assessment tools, disease prevention strategies, reliable screening regimens and efficacious treatments if we are to control this highly prevalent disease.

Clinical presentation and disease sequelae after sexual transmission of *C. trachomatis* (serovars D-K) differ between men and women. In men, *C. trachomatis* infection is most typically symptomatic, is a common cause for urethritis and the much rarer syndrome of epididymitis(Peipert 2003), and is occasionally associated with impaired fertility(Idahl, Abramsson et al. 2007; Joki-Korpela, Sahrakorpi et al. 2009). *C. trachomatis* most commonly infects the endocervix in women, but the great majority (70-90%) of cases are asymptomatic(Peipert 2003). Natural history studies indicate individuals can spontaneously clear *C. trachomatis* infection, but this can take several months to several years(Dean, Suchland et al. 2000). Importantly, infection in women may be complicated by ascending infection and endometritis and/or salpingitis {reviewed in (Brunham and Rey-Ladino 2005)}. Pelvic inflammatory disease (PID) is a too frequent end result of chlamydial infection of the female lower genital tract. While the final syndrome is most certainly multibacterial, *Neisseria gonorrheae* and *C. trachomatis* are frequent inciting factors (Paavonen and Lehtinen 1996). PID is an ascending genital infection from the cervix to the upper genital tract with infectious spill into the female peritoneal cavity. The disease can result in scarring and pelvic organ disfigurement that lead to increases in ectopic pregnancy rates, tubal factor infertility (Hellstrom, Schachter et al. 1987) and possibly early pregnancy wastage (Witkin 1999). If left untreated during pregnancy, chlamydial genital infections in women have been associated with preterm delivery (Rours, Duijts et al. 2011).

2. Developmental cycle of *Chlamydia trachomatis*

Chlamydia exhibits a predominantly biphasic developmental cycle, differentiating between a metabolically inactive but infectious elementary body (EB) and a replicating and metabolically active, but non-infectious, reticulate body (RB) (Nelson, Virok et al. 2005; Linhares and Witkin 2010). Attachment and entry of EBs into permissive cells are critical steps in chlamydial development, but the molecules and mechanisms utilized in these processes are not well understood. Several bacterial ligands have been implicated as adhesins, and include heparin sulfate-like proteins, MOMP, OmcB, glycoproteins and Hsp70 (reviewed by Hackstadt 1999). The host factor/s involved in attachment is/are likely proteinacious, and the host cytoplasmic chaperone protein disulfide isomerase (PDI) has been strongly implicated as a structural requirement for attachment of multiple serovars, as well as necessary for entry (Davis, Raulston et al. 2002; Conant and Stephens 2007; Abromaitis and Stephens 2009). After EB internalization, *Chlamydia*-derived vesicles mature into a specialized parasitophorous vacuole termed an inclusion, which is nonfusogenic with lysosomal and endosomal membranes (Fields, Fischer et al. 2002; Carabeo, Mead et al. 2003; Hybiske and Stephens 2007a; Hybiske and Stephens 2007b). The exact mechanisms involved in the differentiation of the chlamydial EB into a RB remain incompletely described, but morphological investigations have demonstrated decondensation of chromatin occurs early in the process and supports the transition from a metabolically inert EB to a metabolically active RB (Beatty, Byrne, et al. 1993; Beatty, Morrison, et al. 1995; Belland, Zhong et al. 2003) Elegant investigations using transcriptional profiling have listed chaperonin, metabolite translocation, metabolite interconversion, endosomal trafficking, and inclusion membrane modification genes to be among the first to be activated (immediate early genes) during this transition (Belland, Zhong, et al. 2003; AbdelRahman and Belland 2005). As might have been predicted, these genes fall into categories required for pathogen acquisition of nutrients and for inhibiting fusion of the chlamydial inclusion with the host cell lysosomal pathway. Inside the inclusion, the elementary bodies differentiate into reticulate bodies that, in turn, divide rapidly via binary fission. RB condense back into EB and completion of the chlamydial cell cycle results in EB release by host cell lysis or extrusion (Todd and Caldwell 1985; ; Hybiske and Stephens 2007b). Secondary differentiation of RB back into EB involves late gene expression and includes genes that direct recondensation of chromosomes, production of the outer membrane complex and even a number of genes previously described as immediate early genes (Nicholson, Olinger et al. 2003; AbdelRahman and Belland 2005). This latter finding appears to suggest that the EB is readying itself for its next cycle of attack. Newly-released, re-differentiated EB are thence able to infect nearby epithelial cells.

3. Chlamydial persistence

The term "persistence" has been used to describe an alternative *in vitro* pattern of chlamydial growth during which the bacteria cannot be cultivated, but remain viable for extended periods of time (Beatty, Belanger et al. 1994; Belland, Nelson et al. 2003). Persistence is characterized by the presence of large, morphologically aberrant RB within the inclusion (Beatty, Morrison et al. 1995). While the chlamydial chromosomes can continue to divide in these aberrant RB *in vitro*, replication by binary fission does not occur nor does re-differentiation into EB (Beatty, Morrison et al. 1995). To date, there is no direct evidence that persistence occurs *in vivo*. That said, *in vivo* persistence is suggested by several clinical findings. Firstly investigators have shown that chlamydial antigens and nucleic acids can be detected in tissues that do not support cultivable growth (Holland, Hudson et al. 1992; Patton, Askienazy-Elbhar et al. 1994). Second, multiple, same-serovar recurrent *C. trachomatis* infections have been observed in a cohort of women over a 2-5 year period despite antibiotic treatment (Dean, Suchland et al. 2000) . Thirdly, gynecologic and primary care clinicians frequently encounter recurrent chlamydial disease when re-infection is highly unlikely (e.g., no longer sexually active; prior tubal ligation surgery) again suggesting long-term dormancy of chlamydial forms. The induction of persistence has been implicated in chlamydial immune evasion and pathogenesis (Beatty, Byrne et al. 1993; Beatty, Byrne et al. 1994; Beatty, Morrison et al. 1994). We hypothesize that the ability of *C. trachomatis* to enter into a persistent growth form *in vivo* might represent a balance between host and pathogen struck through many years of co-evolution. The fact that persistent chlamydial forms are non-infectious could limit their immune detection for extended periods of time, and thereby limit immune-mediated damage. The fact that persistent chlamydial forms can be rapidly induced to return to the typical developmental cycle with removal of growth stressors *in vitro* (Beatty, Morrison et al. 1995; Belland, Nelson et al. 2003) would also suggest bacteria could successfully survive what might otherwise be lethal exogenous or host-induced stressors.

A variety of stressors can cause *C. trachomatis* to enter into persistent growth *in vitro*. These include exposure to antibiotics such as penicillin and ampicillin, interferon gamma (IFNγ) and nutrient depletion (Clark, Schatzki et al. 1982; Beatty, Byrne et al. 1993; Belland, Nelson et al. 2003; Wyrick 2010). While most *in vitro* persistence models are in transformed cell lines, persistent chlamydial forms have recently been induced in primary human endocervical epithelial cell cultures using ampicillin (Wang, Frohlich et al. 2011). While ampicillin and penicillin are not used in treatment of chlamydial infections, it has been noted that the widespread use of these antibiotics for control of other infections could inadvertently encourage the development of persistent forms in infected, undiagnosed individuals (Wyrick 2010). It is also a possibility that improper dosage and exposure duration of appropriate antibiotics for treatment of *C. trachomatis* may divert chlamydial organisms into the persistence pathway; indeed the presence of morphologic variants of *C. trachomatis* has been documented in the genital tissues of a small proportion of men and women treated with azithromycin (Bragina, Gomberg et al. 2001).

Cytokines secreted by local phagocytes, NK cells and T cells are important in immune defense against infection. These same cytokines, however, may also be implicated in disease pathogenesis. For many pathogens, including *C. trachomatis,* IFNγ plays an important role in resolution of infection (Marks, Tam et al. 2010; Agrawal, Bhengraj et al. 2011; Matthews, Wilkinson et al. 2011; Ohman, Tiitinen et al. 2011; Patel, Stefanidou et al. 2011). The role of IFNγ in chlamydial clearance is complicated by the fact that inflammation can damage host cells and IFNγ itself can also drive persistence (Beatty, Belanger et al. 1994). IFNγ exposure induces the expression of indoleamine 2,3-dioxygenase (IDO) in various types of epithelial cells (Feng and Taylor 1989). The IFNγ-mediated induction of IDO facilitates the catabolism of tryptophan to kynurenine (Beatty, Belanger et al. 1994). *C. trachomatis* is a tryptophan auxotroph, and continuous exposure to IFNγ at inhibitory concentrations results in the eradication of the bacteria (Byrne and Krueger, 1983). However, exposure to sub-inhibitory IFNγ concentrations, which may be a likely scenario *in vivo,* induces chlamydial organisms to enter a persistent phase, with characteristic aberrant inclusions and the presence of small, non-replicating RB (Byrne and Krueger 1983). A potential therapeutic problem associated with IFNγ-induced persistence is the reduced bactericidal activity of doxycycline against these aberrant growth forms as demonstrated by Reveneau et al., *in vitro* (Reveneau, Crane et al. 2005). We (Ibana, Nagamatsu et al. 2011) have recently demonstrated that levo-methyl-tryptophan (L-1MT), an IDO inhibitor, prevents IFNγ-induced *C. trachomatis* persistence without resulting in productive multiplication of the bacterium. L-1MT also improved the efficacy of doxycycline against the IFNγ-induced *C. trachomatis* persistent forms, and may thus provide a novel approach to clear doxycycline-resistant forms of the bacterium.

Although persistence has not been definitively demonstrated *in vivo, in vitro* modeling has suggested a role for persistent chlamydial forms in disease pathogenesis. While synthesis of many of the antigenic outer membrane antigens is decreased in *in vitro* persistence models (Beatty, Morrison et al. 1995), persistent organisms do replicate their chromosomal material and they remain metabolically active (Belland, Nelson et al. 2003). In fact, persistent organisms induced by IFNγ and penicillin exposure continue to produce and secrete the 60 kDa chlamydial heat shock protein, CHSP60 (Beatty, Byrne et al. 1993; Beatty, Morrison et al. 1995; Linhares and Witkin 2010). Although circulating antibodies against *C. trachomatis* membrane associated proteins (MOMPs) have been linked to infertility, the presence of anti-CHSP60 antibodies appears to be more sensitive and specific for the disease (Linhares and Witkin 2010; Stephens, Aubuchon et al. 2011). The presence of anti-CHSP60 IgA antibodies in the cervical secretions of women undergoing IVF has been associated with decreased live birth rates (Witkin 1999) and the presence of circulating IgG to CHSP60 in women with prior ectopic pregnancy has been linked repeat ectopic pregnancy and other adverse pregnancy outcomes (Sziller, Fedorcsak, et al 2008). To explain these findings, it has been hypothesized that prolonged exposure to CHSP60 may break tolerance to the human HSP60 that is normally expressed by normal human embryos (Linhares and Witkin 2010, Stephens, Aubuchon et al. 2011).

4. Pathogen immune evasion

Millions of years of co-evolution have benefitted many pathogens and their hosts. Constantly changing pathogenic challenges allowed hosts to develop efficient, effective, redundant and advanced immune systems. The evolving host has driven the successful pathogen to develop strategies to evade detection by the host immune systems. At times, immune detection is evaded just long enough to enable a complete pathogen replication cycle with spread of progeny to surrounding cells. For other pathogens, immune evasion allows for prolonged and even lifelong pathogen persistence.

Exogenous pathogens, whether they are viral or bacterial, typically encounter several barriers to infection and successful pathogens have adapted to breech these barriers. For most pathogens, the first of these obstacles involves surviving in a local mucosal

Immune Effector Cell Type	Host Cell Ligand	Immune Cell Ligand	Function of Mucosal Immune Cell	Mechanism of Pathogen Recognition	*C. Trachomatis* Evasion Strategy
CD8+ T cell recognition (adaptive immunity)	MHC class I	T cell receptor	Response to altered self or to cytosolic, pathogen - derived antigens	IDO induces IFNγ-mediated increases in host MHC class I expression at the cell surface	CPAF-mediated degradation of RFX-5, which is essential for IFNγ-induced MHC class I expression Amino-terminal CPAF fragment (CPAFn) directly involved
CD4+ T cell recognition (adaptive immunity)	MHC class II	T cell receptor	Response to extracellular/ endosomal pathogens	IFNγ increases MHC class II (HLA-DR) expression on infected host cells	CPAF-mediated degradation of USF1, a transcription factor important for MHC class II expression. Carboxy-terminal fragment (CPAFc) directly involved
Natural Killer Cell recognition (innate immunity)	MHC class I (non-antigen dependent)	Killer inhibitory receptors (KIRs; inhibitory) NKG2D (activating) others	Self/non-self recognition; Absence of self signals abnormality Innate immunity	Altered expression of self MHC class I recognized by NK expressed inhibitory KIRs Altered expression of MICA recognized by NK cell expressed activating NKG2D	MICA expression altered only in directly-infected cells
Natural Killer T cells (innate immunity)	CD1d	Vα24-JαQ/Vβ11 Invariant T cell receptor	Response to lipid-derived antigens.	CD1d molecule recognizes NKT cell receptor and produces IFNγ. IFNγ catabolizes tryptophan and aids in clearing *C. trachomatis* infection	CPAF and cellular proteasome - mediated degradation of host MHC class I and CD1d surface expression CPAF binds directly to the CD1d cytoplasmic tail

Table 1. MHC and MHC-like ligands modulated by C. trachomatis to evade immune detection

microenvironment and crossing the mucosal epithelial barrier. The common gastrointestinal bacterium, *Heliobacter pylori,* is particularly adept at this. *H. pylori* express a variety of colonization factors, including outer membrane adhesins, which allow the bacteria to survive in the acidic and mucus-filled gastrointestinal lumen and attach to epithelial cell surfaces (Fischer, Prassl et al. 2009). Once the epithelial barrier has been breached, pathogens must next surmount innate immune detection. Such detection includes recognition by the host complement system and by host macrophages, dendritic cells, monocytes, neutrophils and eosinophils (Ploegh 1998). The latter includes recognition through, among others, Toll-like receptors (TLRs), nucleotide-binding and oligomerization domain (NOD)-like receptors and helicases (Xiao 2010). Several bacteria, including *Salmonella enterica, Escherichia coli* and several *Brucella* species use molecular mimicry to evade host immune signaling and the innate immune recognition and clearance mediated by these cell surface receptors (Xiao 2010). Successful pathogens must next subvert, at least temporarily, those immune cells that straddle innate and adaptive immune functionality, including natural killer (NK) and natural killer T (NKT) cells (**Table 1, Figure 1**). Finally pathogens that have survived the previous obstacles will encounter the host adaptive immune response involving B and T cells and both immediate and memory responses. Intracellular pathogens, including most viruses, have developed a wide variety of immune evasion strategies. For example the human herpesviruses are characterized by their ability to establish latency in immunocompetent human hosts, often with infrequent or absent symptomatology. These DNA viruses comprise a large group of related pathogens with well-described but variable mechanisms for abrogating presentation of virus-derived antigens to host immune cells via major histocompatibility (MHC) class I molecules (Tortorella, Gewurz et al. 2000; Horst, Ressing et al. 2011). Extracellular pathogens are more likely to target antigen presentation by MHC class II molecules.

Historically, it was thought that chlamydial antigens were retained within the inclusion. More recent studies, however, have reported that both CD4+ and CD8+ T cells respond to chlamydial-derived antigens (Grotenbreg, Roan et al. 2008; Roan and Starnbach 2008; Finco, Frigimelica et al. 2011) suggesting that MHC class I and MHC class II antigen presentation are both involved in chlamydial recognition and that antigen cross-presentation or autophagy could be important in chlamydial clearance and possibly in chlamydial pathogenesis (Finco, Frigimelica et al 2011). We now know that chlamydial antigens access the host cell cytosol through a variety of mechanisms (Cocchiaro and Valdivia 2009). Wyrick et al. have shown in an elegant series of experiments that chlamydial antigens are present in the cytosol attached to vesicles that have everted from the *C. trachomatis* inclusion (Giles, Whittimore et al. 2006) and that *C. trachomatis* antigens can traffic to the endoplasmic reticulum (ER) of infected epithelial cells (Giles and Wyrick 2008). Interestingly, some of the chlamydial antigens that trafficked to the ER were seen to co-localize with the MHC-like molecule CD1d (see below) (Wyrick 2010). Others have shown that proteins such as the chlamydial outer membrane complex protein B (OmcB) (Qi, Gong et al. 2011) and the chlamydia protease, CPAF (see below), are present in the host cell cytosol (Sharma, Bosnic et al. 2004; Kawana, Quayle et al. 2007), the latter being secreted through a Sec-dependent pathway (Chen, Lei et al. 2010). *C. trachomatis* also uses the type III secretory system (T3SS) to move bacterial virulence proteins from EB into the host cytosol (Clifton, Fields et al. 2004; Hower, Wolf et al. 2009). Not surprisingly, *C. trachomatis* has devised immune evasion strategies to subvert host recognition of infection via MHC class I and MHC class II. While several additional mechanisms for pathogen evasion of host clearance have been reported

(Betts, Wolf et al. 2009), we will concentrate here on *C. trachomatis* immune evasion via modulation of those surface-expressed ligands important in antigen presentation.

5. Downregulation of MHC class I and II

Chlamydial avoidance of adaptive immune responses involving $CD8^+$ T cells and $CD4^+$ T cell recognition (Van Voorhis, Barrett et al. 1996; Kelly, Walker et al. 2000; Rank, Bowlin et al. 2000) can involve pathogen-driven suppression of host cell surface expression of IFNγ-inducible MHC class I and II molecules at the site of infection (Fruh, Ahn et al. 1997). The major histocompatibility complex (MHC) is a polymorphic and polygenic host DNA region used by cells to produce and present 8-10 amino acid, self- and pathogen-derived peptides at the host cell surface. Altered self peptides (e.g., from neoplastic change) and pathogen-derived peptides are antigenic and induce host immune response. The two most prominent products encoded by the MHC in humans are referred to as MHC class I and class II molecules (**Figure 1**). Each provides information to the host immune system on antigenic insults, although these insults conventionally differ in location. MHC class I molecules bind and present peptides at the host cell surface that are derived from altered self or from intracellular pathogens (typically within the host cytosol). In contrast, MHC class II molecules bind and present peptides from extracellular pathogens, whose destruction and processing typically occurs within the host cell endosome (Germain 1986). This relative dichotomy is challenged by the classical description of inclusion-sequestered chlamydia-derived antigens. As discussed above, there are many descriptions of cytosolic and extracellular (Campbell, Larsen et al. 1998) chlamydial antigens that now explain the detection of CD4+ and CD8+ T cell responses to chlamydial antigens (**Figure 1**).

The expression of MHC class I molecules on epithelial cells is up-regulated by IFNγ during most infections (Maudsley and Morris 1989). RFX, a transcription complex that binds to the promoter region of MHC class I and class II molecules is important for both constitutive and IFNγ-inducible MHC class I expression in chlamydia infected cells (van den Elsen and Gobin 1999). Zhong, et al (Zhong, Liu et al. 2000) were the first to show that degradation of RFX5 occurred in cells infected with *C. trachomatis* L serovars and that such degradation inhibited both constitutive and IFNγ-inducible MHC class I expression in infected cells. As predicted, cells from patients deficient in RFX 5, a sub-unit of RFX, exhibit reduced IFNγ-mediated induction of MHC class I expression (Gobin, Peijnenburg et al. 1998).

Chlamydia has also evolved a strategy for inhibiting IFNγ-inducible MHC class II expression. Here the pathogen degrades a ubiquitously expressed transcription factor required for IFNγ-mediated induction of the MHC Class II trans-activator (CIITA), called upstream stimulatory factor 1 (USF1) (Zhong, Fan et al. 1999). USF1 is a non-DNA-binding co-activator required for MHC class II expression (Chang, Fontes et al. 1994). A more detailed mechanism for this degradation was put forth with the discovery of its more generalized role in MHC degradation and is now known to involve a chlamydia-encoded proteasome-like activity factor (CPAF). CPAF is present in the cytosol of chlamydia-infected cells and is primarily responsible for the degradation of RFX5 and USF1 and subsequent down regulation of surface MHC class I and II expression, respectively. The active components of CPAF are a dimer consisting of a 29kDa amino-terminal fragment (CPAFn) and a 35KDa carboxy-terminal fragment (CPAFc). Activity of the CPAFn fragment has been shown to be responsible for degradation of RFX5 (Zhong, Fan et al. 2001). With the very recent description of a specific inhibitor of CPAF (Bednar, Jorgensen et al. 2011) it is

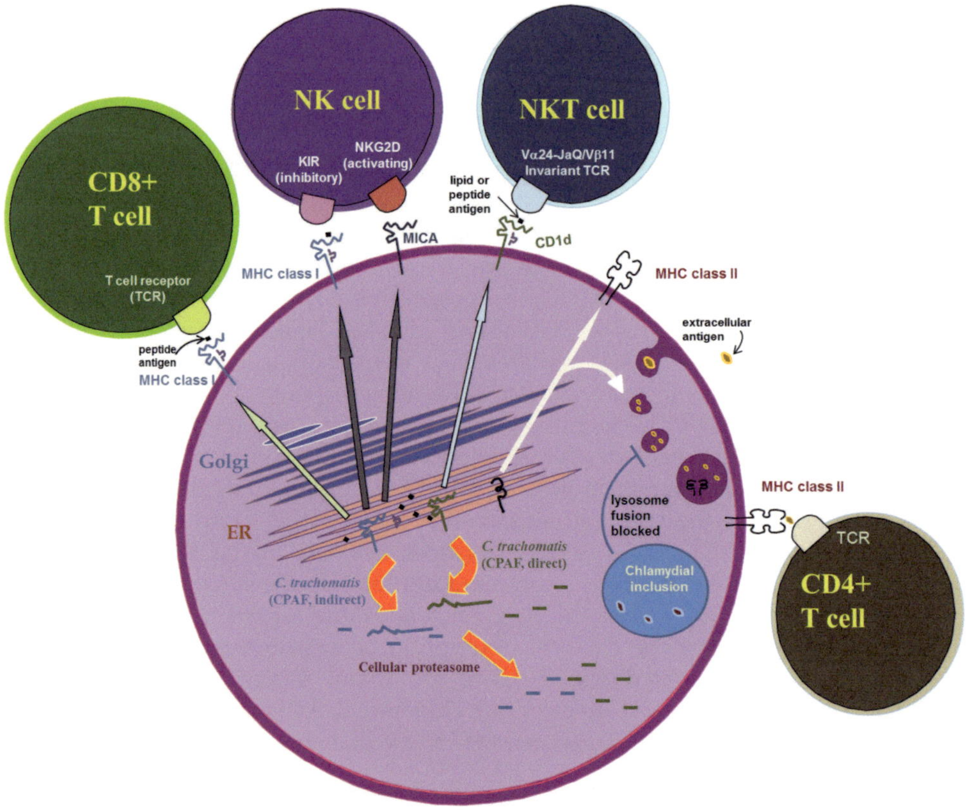

Fig. 1. Presentation of chlamydial antigens. Cytosolic antigens are degraded by the cellular proteasome into 8-10 amino acid peptide fragments that are actively transported into the lumen of the endoplasmic reticulum (ER). These antigenic peptides (depicted as short black lines) are loaded into the peptide binding groove of the MHC class I heavy chain. Heavy chains containing peptide associate with an invariant chain, β_2-microglobulin, and are processed thru the Golgi apparatus for stable expression at the host cell surface. Here, MHC class I molecules interact with T cell receptors (TCRs) on CD8+ T cells or with immunoglobulin-like killer inhibitory receptors (antigen independent) on natural killer (NK) cells (antigen dependent). The MHC class I-related protein A (MICA) is also processed through the secretory pathway for type-2 proteins, but is expressed at the cell surface in the absence of β_2-microglobulin or antigenic peptide. Here MICA can bind to activating receptors on the NK cell (antigen independent). Lipid-derived antigens are presented on the cell surface by the MHC-like molecule, CD1d which is also stably expressed as a trimer of heavy chain, β_2-microglobulin and antigen. CD1d presents antigen to natural killer T (NKT) cells bearing an invariant Vα24-JαQ/Vβ11 TCR. Extracellular antigens bind to MHC class II molecules for presentation at the cell surface. The MHC class II molecule is processed thru the secretory pathway for direct expression at the cells surface or for transfer into the endocytic pathway. Extracellular peptides can enter the MHC class II antigen-binding groove on cell-surface-expressed MHC class II directly or after displacement from other cell surface antigen-presenting molecules. More commonly, antigen loading of MHC class II occurs within the endocytic pathway. Although chlamydiae actively prevent fusion of their intracellular inclusions with the endocytic pathway, CD4+ T cells do respond to chlamydial antigens.

expected that much more will be learned about CPAF and about chlamydial pathogenesis and prevention in the coming years.

6. Production of CPAF and effects on CD1d

CPAF also interacts with the antigen presenting molecule, CD1d (Skold and Behar 2003). CD1d is similar in structure to MHC class I molecules. Like MHC class I and class II molecules, CD1 can present peptide antigens, although these peptides are typically quite hydrophobic (Boes, Stoppelenburg et al. 2009). Unlike MHC products, CD1d is monogenic and has fairly limited polymorphism. CD1d most commonly presents lipid-derived antigens from self- and pathogen-derived sources to natural killer T (NKT) cells (Porcelli 1995). CD1d molecules recognize an invariant Vα24-JαQ/Vβ11 T cell receptor expressed by human NKT cells (Porcelli, Gerdes et al. 1996; Zhou 2007). CD1d recognition by invariant NKT cells results in the production of large amounts of both IL-4 and IFNγ by the NKT cell that is suggested to play a role in TH1/TH2 differentiation of CD4+ T helper cells. (Taniguchi and Nakayama 2000). Using an immortalized penile urethra-derived epithelial cell line developed in our laboratory, we have demonstrated that *C. trachomatis* infection decreases cell surface expression of CD1d (**Figure 2**) (Kawana, Quayle et al. 2007). This effect was

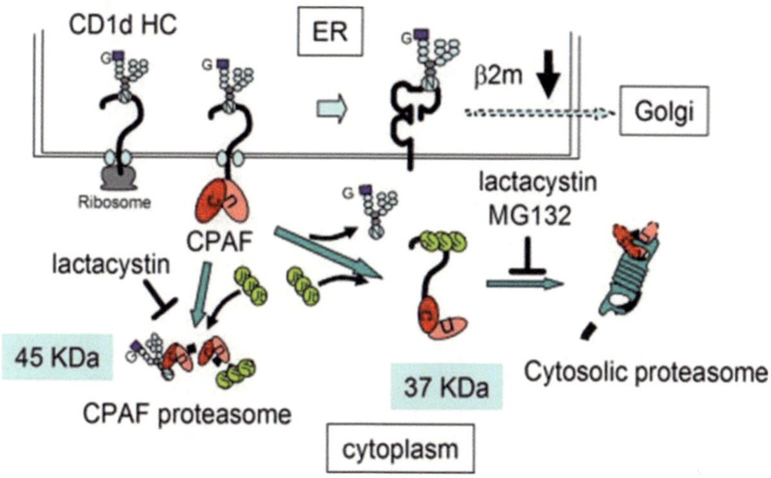

Fig. 2. Putative proteolytic degradation pathways for CD1d HCs upon *C. trachomatis infection*. In *C. trachomatis*-infected cells, β2m-unassembled CD1d HC forms accumulate in the ER due to degradation of RFX5 by CPAF. CPAF secreted from the chlamydial inclusion into the cytosol interacts with the CD1d HC via the cytoplasmic tail of CD1d and CPAF is ubiquitinated. The binding of CPAF triggers dislocation of the 45-kDa immature glycosylated form of CD1d into the cytosol. One proteolytic pathway involves the conventional cellular proteasome. Glycosylated CD1d HC is ubiquitinated in the cytosol (ubiquitin ligase), and deglycosylated (peptide N-glycosidase) to create the 37-kDa , non-glycosylated CD1d molecule. CPAF and the ubiquitinated, deglycosylated CD1d HC are degraded by the cytosolic proteasome. The alternative proteolytic pathway involves CPAF-mediated degradation. The 45-kDa immature glycosylated CD1d HC interacts with CPAF. CPAF targets the CD1d HC for degradation by a proteolytic activity distinct from that of the cytosolic proteasome. Green symbols indicate multiubiquitins. Kawana, et. al., *J Biol Chem* 2001; 282(10): 7368-7375. Reproduced with permission.

again linked to the proteasomal activity of CPAF. CPAF binds to the cytoplasmic tail of the nascent CD1d heavy chain and targets it for degradation by a CPAF-mediated pathway and via a pathway that includes the ubiquitination and deglycosylation steps integral to the conventional unfolded protein response (Kawana, Quayle et al. 2007). The immunoevasive targeting of CD1d is not unique to *C. trachomatis*. We have also shown that cell surface expression of CD1d is reduced *in vitro* and *in vivo* in human papillomavirus (HPV)-positive cells (Miura, Kawana et al. 2010). This effect can be isolated to the presence of the E5 proteins of HPV subtype 6 and HPV subtype 16, it occurs at a post-transcriptional level and it is mediated by proteasomal degradation.

In addition to known expression on standard antigen-presenting cells, CD1d is found on alternative APCs, including intestinal epithelial cells (Blumberg, Terhorst et al. 1991), epidermal keratinocytes (Bonish, Jullien et al. 2000) and basal and suprabasal cells of the vaginal, ectocervical, and penile urethral epithelia (Kawana, Matsumoto et al. 2008). In contrast, limited expression of CD1d was seen in human endocervical and endometrial tissues, the former representing the major cellular target for *C. trachomatis* in the female genital tract. *In vitro* exposure of genital tract cells to IFNγ increased cell surface expression of CD1d in all cells studied, although the strongest induction was seen in those cells that expressed CD1d at the highest levels *in vivo*. Through these studies, Kawana, et. al. (Kawana, Matsumoto et al. 2008) were the first to place a functional significance on *C. trachomatis*-mediated reductions in cell surface expression of CD1d. Antibody-induced cross-linking of CD1d on penile urethral epithelial cells induces the secretion of IL-12 and IL-15. Cross-linking induced Th1 cytokine production was abrogated in penile urethral cells infected with *C. trachomatis* (Kawana, Matsumoto et al. 2008). A relative deficiency in CD1d baseline expression in the human endocervix and poor IFNγ-induced CD1d expression in penile urethral cells may make these sites particularly susceptible to pathogen transmission.

7. Effects of *C. trachomatis* on surface ligand expression in directly-infected and bystander cells

Although we and others had previously reported on *C. trachomatis*-mediated inhibition of IFNγ-inducible MHC class I and II expression and Cd1d expression (Zhong, Fan et al. 1999; Zhong, Liu et al. 2000; Zhong, Fan et al. 2001; Kawana, Quayle et al. 2007; Kawana, Matsumoto et al. 2008), all published experiments had been conducted via bulk analysis of mixed populations of infected cells and non-infected bystander cells. Transmission of *C. trachomatis* to the epithelial cells in the genital tract after *in vivo* exposure likely results in only a small population of infected cells. Some *in vitro* protocols exist that can result in infection of a very high proportion of *C. trachomatis*-infected epithelial cells, but this does not reflect *in vivo* infection characteristics. Other infection protocols used for *in vitro* study of host immune response to *C. trachomatis* infection result in a mixed population of *C. trachomatis*-exposed cells and uninfected, bystander cells. Bulk analysis of these mixed populations, however, dilutes changes that may occur in only one of these subpopulations. We hypothesized that separation of these cellular subpopulations, when combined with side-by-side analyses, would allow a more inclusive and accurate assessment of the overall impact of *C. trachomatis* on host epithelial cell immune response.

We have recently completed and published our first investigation on *C. trachomatis* immune evasion strategies that stratified cells by infection status to allow independent assessment of immune cell ligands on infected and uninfected host epithelial cells in a single culture (Ibana, Schust et al. 2011). Using flow cytometry to separate *C. trachomatis*-infected cells from those non-infected bystander cells, we were able to investigate the possible indirect effects of soluble factors released during *C. trachomatis* infection on uninfected cells. We hypothesized that investigating the effects of *C. trachomatis* in both infected and uninfected bystander cells would promote a better understanding of the immunological milieu induced by *C. trachomatis* at the local site of infection and concentrated our initial efforts on the MHC class I molecule.

Natural killer (NK) cells and CD8+ T cells are important components of the host cellular immune defense against intracellular microorganisms (**Figure 1**). Each of these immune cell subpopulations can mediate their protective immune activities via two mechanisms: (1) direct cytolysis and (2) secretion of IFNγ and other cytokines [reviewed in (Trinchieri 1989). Direct cytolytic activities are induced by the interaction of cell surface receptors on NK cells and CD8+ T cells with the ligands expressed on the surface of target cells. CD8+ T cells can lyse target cells that express cognate antigens presented by the target cell MHC class I molecule. The immunologic activity of NK cells results from a summation of signals mediated through NK cell-expressed activating and inhibitory receptors (Moretta et al. 2001). Unlike those of CD8+ T cells, NK cell ligand-mediated interactions are typically antigen-independent. While MHC class I products bind to an inhibitory class of NK cell killer immunoglobulin-like receptors (KIRs) to aid in self/non-self recognition, other ligands on host cells can bind to activating NK cell receptors. One such molecule, the target cell-expressed MHC class I-related protein A (MICA), primarily functions as a ligand for the NK cell activating receptor, NKG2D (Bauer, Groh et al. 1999). It is well-documented that modulation of the expression of these ligands on host cells is one of the primary strategies that intracellular microorganisms use to evade immune cell recognition. Intracellular microorganisms that can diminish surface expression of MHC class I by their host cells are more impervious to CD8+ T cell activity. However, the loss of MHC class I at the cell surface may make the infected host cells more susceptible to cytolytic NK cell activity when the interacting NK cell expresses a predominance of activating NK cell receptors (Ljunggren and Karre 1990) In short, co-evolution alongside human pathogens may have driven the development of host NK cells to counter the ability of some intracellular pathogens to evade immune detection via downregulation of host MHC class I expression.

By examining directly-infected and uninfected bystander cells separately, we have shown that MHC class I downregulation in the presence of *C. trachomatis* is mediated by direct and indirect (soluble) factors (Ibana, Schust et al. 2011) In contrast, we now have preliminary data suggesting that MICA expression is altered in *C. trachomatis*-infected cells but not in bystander, uninfected cells (Ibana, Aiyar et al. 2012). *C. trachomatis* infection of epithelial cells alters two well-documented characteristics of infected cultures: (a) their immune cells ligand expression (Soderlund and Kihlstrom 1982; Zhong, Fan et al. 1999; Zhong, Liu et al. 2000; Kawana, Quayle et al. 2007; Ibana, Nagamatsu et al. 2011) and (b) the extent and nature of epithelial cell chemokine and cytokine secretion (Rasmussen, Eckmann et al. 1997). Changes in the cell surface expression of immune cell ligands on epithelial cells at the local site of *C. trachomatis* infection may reflect the susceptibility of these cells to host immune cell mediated activities, while the secretion of soluble factors can facilitate the migration of host immune cells to the infected site. We hypothesize that these soluble factors may play an important role in the cross-talk between *C. trachomatis*-infected cells and neighboring uninfected cells. We are presently in the process of further defining the host soluble factor or factors that may be responsible for the decrease in MHC class I surface expression on uninfected-bystander cells in *C. trachomatis* serovar D-infected endocervical epithelial cell (A2EN) cultures, and suspect there may be several factors involved.

8. MHC class I expression after infection with genital and disseminating *C. trachomatis* serovars

As a corollary to these observations, we find it intriguing to comment on reports showing that a lymphogranuloma venereum (LGV) serovar of *C. trachomatis*, which causes a disseminated form of infection, utilizes CPAF to downregulate both constitutive and IFNγ-induced MHC class I expression in cervical epithelial (HeLa) cells (Zhong, Liu et al. 2000; Zhong, Fan et al. 2001). This finding was interpreted by the investigators to represent an important mechanism for immune evasion of CD8+ T cell recognition by *C. trachomatis*. We have confirmed the LGV modulation of MHC class I in our own experiments (**Figure 3**) However, using *C. trachomatis* serovar D, which causes local infection within the female genital tract, we have seen that the level of MHC class I down regulation is less than after serovar LGV infection and that IFNγ attenuates the down-modulation of MHC class I expression in *C. trachomatis*-infected cells and in bystander, uninfected cells (Ibana, Schust et al. 2011). Rather, MHC class I expression in IFNγ-exposed cells remains similar to that in mock-infected controls (**Figure 3**).

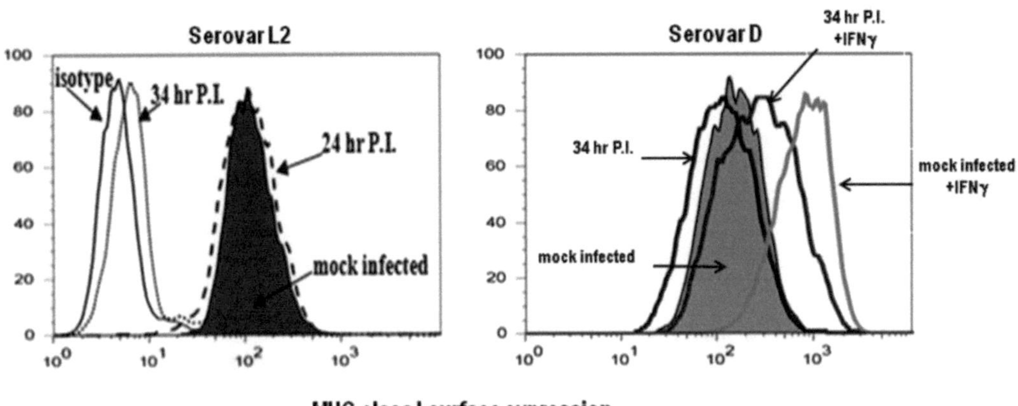

Fig. 3. MHC class I modulation after exposure to non-disseminating (serovar D) and disseminating (serovar L2) genital *C. trachomatis*. Primary-like endocervical epithelial cells (A2EN) were infected with *C. trachomatis* serovar L2 or serovar D. Surface MHC class I expression was quantitated in chlamydial-LPS-positive cells gated by flow cytometry. A dramatic decrease in the surface expression of MHC class I was observed in A2EN cells infected with serovar L2 at 34 hours post infection (hpi); those infected with serovar D exhibited much smaller decreases in MHC class I expression. Although the IFNγ-induced increase in MHC class I was noted in both infected and uninfected cells, it was attenuated with *C. trachomatis* serovar D infection.

These results may suggest that genital *C. trachomatis* serovars do not utilize evasion of CD8+ T cell recognition via MHC class I modulation to the extent that disseminating serovars do. Supporting our observations are reports that chlamydia-specific CD8+ T cells are fully capable of lysing epithelial cells infected with genital serovars of *C. trachomatis* (Roan and Starnbach 2006; Grotenbreg, Roan et al. 2008). Others have noted differences *in vitro* in the innate immune responses to genital *C. trachomatis* serovar E and disseminating *C. trachomatis* serovar L2 infection of HeLa cells (Dessus-Babus, Knight et al. 2000). *In vivo*, the former results in local or ascending infection with canalicular spread along genital mucosal surfaces. In contrast, disseminating chlamydial disease is a sub-mucosal infection with rapid spread to regional lymph nodes (Schachter and Osoba 1983). *In vitro*, the release of the anti-inflammatory cytokine IL-11 was increased in HeLa cells infected with *C. trachomatis* serovar L2 when compared to cells infected with the non-disseminating genital serovar E (Dessus-Babus, Knight et al. 2000). Although the mechanism for differences in MHC class I modulation between the Serovar D- and LGV-infected cells remains unknown, this observation may also help to explain the localization of infection with genital *C. trachomatis* serovars but disseminated disease after infection by LGV serovars and certainly warrants further investigations. Since MHC class I down-regulation is linked to CPAF activity (Zhong, Liu et al. 2000; Zhong, Fan et al. 2001), this could be a protein of interest, as would other secreted chlamydial proteins.

9. Conclusions

Host-pathogen co-evolution drives adaptations in each partner that ensure survival of the host and propagation of the pathogen. This often involves sophisticated methods of injury evasion but neither the host nor the pathogen typically acquires complete protection. Rather, compromises are met that partially benefit both partners. For *C. trachomatis* and its human host, this balance could be typified by the concept of chlamydial persistence. Persistent growth *in vitro* is promoted by exogenous growth conditions that are stressful to the pathogen, but re-initiation of the productive growth cycle occurs when these stressors are removed. Although there is currently no direct human *in vivo* evidence for chlamydial persistence due to the very challenging nature of these types of investigations, we have postulated that this phenomenon may protect the host from relatively prolonged and/or intense immune-induced pathologies. On the other hand, chlamydial persistence may also provide a mechanism that enables the pathogen to establish prolonged infection and re-infection even though this may be disadvantageous to some hosts over time. From this perspective, persistence may be perceived as an adaptation that may facilitate long-term association of pathogen and host.

While a precarious balance must be struck between *C. trachomatis* and its host, we have here concentrated on several ways in which *C. trachomatis* evades host immune detection through modulation of surface ligands involved in antigen presentation. Since host response to chlamydial infections involves innate and adaptive immune cells, we have addressed mechanisms by which chlamydia can evade destruction by CD4+ and CD8+ T cells, as well as NK and NKT cells. We have reviewed data generated by ourselves and others on modulation of surface expression of MHC class I, MHC class II, CD1d and MICA. While the majority of these modulations appear to be advantageous only for the infecting pathogen, we have recently begun to look at direct and soluble mediators of these effects and their temporal initiation post-infection in an effort to better understand the host response to immune evasion. Finally, we have begun to dissect serovar-specific differences in host cell surface ligand modulation as a means of gaining a more complete understanding of the pathogenesis of localized, ascending and disseminating infections with genital *C. trachomatis*. Continued study of host-pathogen interactions should help us to better address the epidemiology of *C. trachomatis* infection and to develop more effective disease treatment and prevention paradigms.

10. References

Abromaitis, S. and R. S. Stephens (2009). "Attachment and entry of Chlamydia have distinct requirements for host protein disulfide isomerase." *PLoS Pathog* 5(4): e1000357.

AbdelRahman, Y. M. and R. J. Belland (2005). "The chlamydial developmental cycle". *FEMS Microbiol Rev* 29:949-959.

Agrawal, T., A. R. Bhengraj, et al. (2011). "Expression of TLR 2, TLR 4 and iNOS in Cervical Monocytes of Chlamydia trachomatis-infected Women and Their Role in Host Immune Response." *Am J Reprod Immunol.* 66(6):534-543.

Bauer, S., V. Groh, et al. (1999). "Activation of NK cells and T cells by NKG2D, a receptor for stress-inducible MICA." *Science* 285(5428): 727-729.

Beatty, W. L., T. A. Belanger, et al. (1994). "Role of tryptophan in gamma interferon-mediated chlamydial persistence." *Ann N Y Acad Sci* 730: 304-306.

Beatty, W. L., G. I. Byrne, et al. (1993). "Morphologic and antigenic characterization of interferon gamma-mediated persistent Chlamydia trachomatis infection in vitro." *Proc Natl Acad Sci U S A* 90(9): 3998-4002.

Beatty, W. L., G. I. Byrne, et al. (1994). "Repeated and persistent infection with Chlamydia and the development of chronic inflammation and disease." *Trends Microbiol* 2(3): 94-98.

Beatty, W. L., R. P. Morrison, et al. (1994). "Persistent chlamydiae: from cell culture to a paradigm for chlamydial pathogenesis." *Microbiol Rev* 58(4): 686-699.

Beatty, W. L., R. P. Morrison, et al. (1995). "Reactivation of persistent Chlamydia trachomatis infection in cell culture." *Infect Immun* 63(1): 199-205.

Bednar, M. M., I. Jorgensen, et al. (2011). "Chlamydia Protease-like Activity Factor (CPAF): Characterization of Proteolysis Activity in vitro and Development of a Nanomolar Affinity CPAF Zymogen-Derived Inhibitor." *Biochemistry.* 50(35):7441-7443.

Belland, R. J., D. E. Nelson, et al. (2003). "Transcriptome analysis of chlamydial growth during IFN-gamma-mediated persistence and reactivation." *Proc Natl Acad Sci U S A* 100(26): 15971-15976.

Belland, R.J., G. Zhong, et al. (2003). "Genomic transcriptional profiling of the developmental cycle of Chlamydia trachomatis." *Proc Natl Acad Sci USA* 100(14):8478-8483.

Betts, H. J., K. Wolf, et al. (2009). "Effector protein modulation of host cells: examples in the Chlamydia spp. arsenal." *Curr Opin Microbiol* 12(1): 81-87.

Blumberg, R. S., C. Terhorst, et al. (1991). "Expression of a nonpolymorphic MHC class I-like molecule, CD1D, by human intestinal epithelial cells." *J Immunol* 147(8): 2518-2524.

Boes, M., A. J. Stoppelenburg, et al. (2009). "Endosomal processing for antigen presentation mediated by CD1 and Class I major histocompatibility complex: roads to display or destruction." *Immunology* 127(2): 163-170.

Bonish, B., D. Jullien, et al. (2000). "Overexpression of CD1d by keratinocytes in psoriasis and CD1d-dependent IFN-gamma production by NK-T cells." *J Immunol* 165(7): 4076-4085.

Bragina, E. Y., M. A. Gomberg, et al. (2001). "Electron microscopic evidence of persistent chlamydial infection following treatment." *J Eur Acad Dermatol Venereol* 15(5): 405-409.

Brunham, R. C. and J. Rey-Ladino (2005). "Immunology of Chlamydia infection: implications for a Chlamydia trachomatis vaccine." *Nat Rev Immunol* 5(2): 149-161.

Byrne, G. I. and D. A. Krueger (1983). "Lymphokine-mediated inhibition of Chlamydia replication in mouse fibroblasts is neutralized by anti-gamma interferon immunoglobulin." *Infect Immun* 42(3): 1152-1158.

Campbell, S., J. Larsen, et al. (1998). "Chlamydial elementary bodies are translocated on the surface of epithelial cells." *Am J Pathol* 152(5): 1167-1170.

Carabeo, R. A., D. J. Mead, et al. (2003). "Golgi-dependent transport of cholesterol to the Chlamydia trachomatis inclusion." *Proc Natl Acad Sci U S A* 100(11): 6771-6776.

CDC. (2010). "2009 Sexually transmitted disease surveillance." from http://www.cdc.gov/std/stats09/chlamydia.htm.

Chang, C. H., J. D. Fontes, et al. (1994). "Class II transactivator (CIITA) is sufficient for the inducible expression of major histocompatibility complex class II genes." *J Exp Med* 180(4): 1367-1374.

Chen, D., L. Lei, et al. (2010). "Characterization of Pgp3, a Chlamydia trachomatis plasmid-encoded immunodominant antigen." *J Bacteriol* 192(22): 6017-6024.

Clark, R. B., P. F. Schatzki, et al. (1982). "Ultrastructural effect of penicillin and cycloheximide on Chlamydia trachomatis strain HAR-13." *Med Microbiol Immunol* 171(3): 151-159.

Clifton, D. R., K. A. Fields, et al. (2004). "A chlamydial type III translocated protein is tyrosine-phosphorylated at the site of entry and associated with recruitment of actin." *Proc Natl Acad Sci U S A* 101(27): 10166-10171.

Cocchiaro, J. L. and R. H. Valdivia (2009). "New insights into Chlamydia intracellular survival mechanisms." *Cell Microbiol* 11(11): 1571-1578.

Conant, C. G. and R. S. Stephens (2007). "Chlamydia attachment to mammalian cells requires protein disulfide isomerase." *Cell Microbiol* 9(1): 222-232.

Davis, C. H., J. E. Raulston, et al. (2002). "Protein disulfide isomerase, a component of the estrogen receptor complex, is associated with Chlamydia trachomatis serovar E attached to human endometrial epithelial cells." *Infect Immun* 70(7): 3413-3418.

Dean, D., R. J. Suchland, et al. (2000). "Evidence for long-term cervical persistence of Chlamydia trachomatis by omp1 genotyping." *J Infect Dis* 182(3): 909-916.

Dessus-Babus, S., S. T. Knight, et al. (2000). "Chlamydial infection of polarized HeLa cells induces PMN chemotaxis but the cytokine profile varies between disseminating and non-disseminating strains." *Cell Microbiol* 2(4): 317-327.

Everett, K. D., R. M. Bush, et al. (1999). "Emended description of the order Chlamydiales, proposal of Parachlamydiaceae fam. nov. and Simkaniaceae fam. nov., each containing one monotypic genus, revised taxonomy of the family Chlamydiaceae, including a new genus and five new species, and standards for the identification of organisms." *Int J Syst Bacteriol* 49 Pt 2: 415-440.

Feng, G. S. and M. W. Taylor (1989). "Interferon gamma-resistant mutants are defective in the induction of indoleamine 2,3-dioxygenase." *Proc Natl Acad Sci U S A* 86(18): 7144-7148.

Fields, K. A., E. Fischer, et al. (2002). "Inhibition of fusion of Chlamydia trachomatis inclusions at 32 degrees C correlates with restricted export of IncA." *Infect Immun* 70(7): 3816-3823.

Finco, O., E. Frigimelica, et al. (2011). "Approach to discover T- and B-cell antigens of intracellular pathogens applied to the design of Chlamydia trachomatis vaccines." *Proc Natl Acad Sci U S A* 108(24): 9969-9974.

Fischer, W., S. Prassl, et al. (2009). "Virulence mechanisms and persistence strategies of the human gastric pathogen Helicobacter pylori." *Curr Top Microbiol Immunol* 337: 129-171.

Fruh, K., K. Ahn, et al. (1997). "Inhibition of MHC class I antigen presentation by viral proteins." *J Mol Med (Berl)* 75(1): 18-27.

Gerbase, A. C., J. T. Rowley, et al. (1998). "Global epidemiology of sexually transmitted diseases." *Lancet* 351 Suppl 3: 2-4.

Germain, R. N. (1986). "Immunology. The ins and outs of antigen processing and presentation." *Nature* 322(6081): 687-689.

Giles, D. K., J. D. Whittimore, et al. (2006). "Ultrastructural analysis of chlamydial antigen-containing vesicles everting from the Chlamydia trachomatis inclusion." *Microbes Infect* 8(6): 1579-1591.

Giles, D. K. and P. B. Wyrick (2008). "Trafficking of chlamydial antigens to the endoplasmic reticulum of infected epithelial cells." *Microbes Infect* 10(14-15): 1494-1503.

Gobin, S. J., A. Peijnenburg, et al. (1998). "The RFX complex is crucial for the constitutive and CIITA-mediated transactivation of MHC class I and beta2-microglobulin genes." *Immunity* 9(4): 531-541.

Grotenbreg, G. M., N. R. Roan, et al. (2008). "Discovery of CD8+ T cell epitopes in Chlamydia trachomatis infection through use of caged class I MHC tetramers." *Proc Natl Acad Sci U S A* 105(10): 3831-3836.

Hellstrom, W. J., J. Schachter, et al. (1987). "Is there a role for Chlamydia trachomatis and genital mycoplasma in male infertility?" *Fertil Steril* 48(2): 337-339.

Holland, S. M., A. P. Hudson, et al. (1992). "Demonstration of chlamydial RNA and DNA during a culture-negative state." *Infect Immun* 60(5): 2040-2047.

Horst, D., M. E. Ressing, et al. (2011). "Exploiting human herpesvirus immune evasion for therapeutic gain: potential and pitfalls." *Immunol Cell Biol* 89(3): 359-366.

Hower, S., K. Wolf, et al. (2009). "Evidence that CT694 is a novel Chlamydia trachomatis T3S substrate capable of functioning during invasion or early cycle development." *Mol Microbiol* 72(6): 1423-1437.

Hybiske, K. and R. S. Stephens (2007a). "Mechanisms of Chlamydia trachomatis entry into nonphagocytic cells." *Infect Immun* 75(8): 3925-3934.

Hybiske, K. and R. S. Stephens (2007b). "Mechanisms of host cell exit by the intracellular bacterium Chlamydia." *Proc Natl Acad Sci U S A* 104(27): 11430-11435.

Ibana J. A., A. Aiyar, et al. (2012). "Modulation of MICA on the surface of *Chlamydia trachomatis*-infected endocervical epithelial cells promotes NK cell-mediated killing." *FEMS Immunol Med Microbiol* (in press).

Ibana, J. A., T. Nagamatsu, et al. (2011). "Attenuation of IDO1 activity by 1-methyl tryptophan blocks IFNγ-induced *Chlamydia trachomatis* persistence in human epithelial cells." *Infect Immun* 79(11):4425-4437.

Ibana, J. A., D. J. Schust, et al. (2011). "Chlamydia trachomatis immune evasion via downregulation of MHC class I surface expression involves direct and indirect mechanisms." *Infect Dis Obstet Gynecol* 2011: 420905.

Idahl, A., L. Abramsson, et al. (2007). "Male serum Chlamydia trachomatis IgA and IgG, but not heat shock protein 60 IgG, correlates with negatively affected semen characteristics and lower pregnancy rates in the infertile couple." *Int J Androl* 30(2): 99-107.

Joki-Korpela, P., N. Sahrakorpi, et al. (2009). "The role of Chlamydia trachomatis infection in male infertility." *Fertil Steril* 91(4 Suppl): 1448-1450.

Kawana, K., J. Matsumoto, et al. (2008). "Expression of CD1d and ligand-induced cytokine production are tissue specific in mucosal epithelia of the human lower reproductive tract." *Infect Immun* 76(7): 3011-3018.

Kawana, K., A. J. Quayle, et al. (2007). "CD1d degradation in Chlamydia trachomatis-infected epithelial cells is the result of both cellular and chlamydial proteasomal activity." *J Biol Chem* 282(10): 7368-7375.

Kelly, K. A., J. C. Walker, et al. (2000). "Differential regulation of CD4 lymphocyte recruitment between the upper and lower regions of the genital tract during Chlamydia trachomatis infection." *Infect Immun* 68(3): 1519-1528.

Linhares, I. M. and S. S. Witkin (2010). "Immunopathogenic consequences of Chlamydia trachomatis 60 kDa heat shock protein expression in the female reproductive tract." *Cell Stress Chaperones* 15(5): 467-473.

Ljunggren, H. G. and K. Karre (1990). "In search of the 'missing self': MHC molecules and NK cell recognition." *Immunol Today* 11(7): 237-244.

Marks, E., M. A. Tam, et al. (2010). "The female lower genital tract is a privileged compartment with IL-10 producing dendritic cells and poor Th1 immunity following Chlamydia trachomatis infection." *PLoS Pathog* 6(11): e1001179.

Matthews, K., K. A. Wilkinson, et al. (2011). "Predominance of interleukin-22 over interleukin-17 at the site of disease in human tuberculosis." *Tuberculosis (Edinb).*

Maudsley, D. J. and A. G. Morris (1989). "Regulation of IFN-gamma-induced host cell MHC antigen expression by Kirsten MSV and MLV. I. Effects on class I antigen expression." *Immunology* 67(1): 21-25.

Miura, S., K. Kawana, et al. (2010). "CD1d, a sentinel molecule bridging innate and adaptive immunity, is downregulated by the human papillomavirus (HPV) E5 protein: a possible mechanism for immune evasion by HPV." *J Virol* 84(22): 11614-11623.

Nelson, D. E., D. P. Virok, et al. (2005). "Chlamydial IFN-gamma immune evasion is linked to host infection tropism." *Proc Natl Acad Sci U S A* 102(30): 10658-10663.

Nicholson, T. L., L. Olinger, et al. (2003). "Global stage-specific gene regulation during the developmental cycle of Chlamydia trachomatis." *J Bacteriol* 185(10):3179-3189.

Ohman, H., A. Tiitinen, et al. (2011). "Cytokine gene polymorphism and Chlamydia trachomatis-specific immune responses." *Hum Immunol* 72(3): 278-282.

Paavonen, J. and M. Lehtinen (1996). "Chlamydial pelvic inflammatory disease." *Hum Reprod Update* 2(6): 519-529.

Patel, M., M. Stefanidou, et al. (2011). "Dynamics of cell-mediated immune responses to cytomegalovirus in pediatric transplantation recipients." *Pediatr Transplant* (epub July 18). 10(1):18-28.

Patton, D. L., M. Askienazy-Elbhar, et al. (1994). "Detection of Chlamydia trachomatis in fallopian tube tissue in women with postinfectious tubal infertility." *Am J Obstet Gynecol* 171(1): 95-101.

Peipert, J. F. (2003). "Clinical practice. Genital chlamydial infections." *N Engl J Med* 349(25): 2424-2430.

Ploegh, H. L. (1998). "Viral strategies of immune evasion." *Science* 280(5361): 248-253.

Porcelli, S., D. Gerdes, et al. (1996). "Human T cells expressing an invariant V alpha 24-J alpha Q TCR alpha are CD4- and heterogeneous with respect to TCR beta expression." *Hum Immunol* 48(1-2): 63-67.

Porcelli, S. A. (1995). "The CD1 family: a third lineage of antigen-presenting molecules." *Adv Immunol* 59: 1-98.

Qi, M., S. Gong, et al. (2011). "A Chlamydia trachomatis OmcB C-terminal fragment is released into the host cell cytoplasm and is immunogenic in humans." *Infect Immun* 79(6): 2193-2203.

Rank, R. G., A. K. Bowlin, et al. (2000). "Characterization of lymphocyte response in the female genital tract during ascending Chlamydial genital infection in the guinea pig model." *Infect Immun* 68(9): 5293-5298.

Rasmussen, S. J., L. Eckmann, et al. (1997). "Secretion of proinflammatory cytokines by epithelial cells in response to Chlamydia infection suggests a central role for epithelial cells in chlamydial pathogenesis." *J Clin Invest* 99(1): 77-87.

Reveneau, N., D. D. Crane, et al. (2005). "Bactericidal activity of first-choice antibiotics against gamma interferon-induced persistent infection of human epithelial cells by Chlamydia trachomatis." *Antimicrob Agents Chemother* 49(5): 1787-1793.

Roan, N. R. and M. N. Starnbach (2006). "Antigen-specific CD8+ T cells respond to Chlamydia trachomatis in the genital mucosa." *J Immunol* 177(11): 7974-7979.

Roan, N. R. and M. N. Starnbach (2008). "Immune-mediated control of Chlamydia infection." *Cell Microbiol* 10(1): 9-19.

Rours, G. I., L. Duijts, et al. (2011). "Chlamydia trachomatis infection during pregnancy associated with preterm delivery: a population-based prospective cohort study." *Eur J Epidemiol* 26(6): 493-502.

Schachter, J. and A. O. Osoba (1983). "Lymphogranuloma venereum." *Br Med Bull* 39(2): 151-154.

Sharma, J., A. M. Bosnic, et al. (2004). "Human antibody responses to a Chlamydia-secreted protease factor." *Infect Immun* 72(12): 7164-7171.

Skold, M. and S. M. Behar (2003). "Role of CD1d-restricted NKT cells in microbial immunity." *Infect Immun* 71(10): 5447-5455.

Soderlund, G. and E. Kihlstrom (1982). "Physicochemical surface properties of elementary bodies from different serotypes of chlamydia trachomatis and their interaction with mouse fibroblasts." *Infect Immun* 36(3): 893-899.

Stephens, A.J., M. Aubuchon, et al. (2011) "Antichlamydial antibodies, human fertility and pregnancy wastage." *Inf Dis Obstet Gynecol* (e-pub ahead of print).

Sziller, I., P. Fedorcsak, et al. (2008). "Circulating antibodies to a conserved epitope of the Chlamydia trachomatis 60-kDa heat shock protein is associated with decreased spontaneous fertility rate in ectopic pregnant women treated by salpingectomy." *Am J Reprod Immunol* 59:99-104.

Taniguchi, M. and T. Nakayama (2000). "Recognition and function of Valpha14 NKT cells." *Semin Immunol* 12(6): 543-550.

Todd, W. J. and H. D. Caldwell (1985). "The interaction of Chlamydia trachomatis with host cells: ultrastructural studies of the mechanism of release of a biovar II strain from HeLa 229 cells." *J Infect Dis* 151(6): 1037-1044.

Tortorella, D., B. E. Gewurz, et al. (2000). "Viral subversion of the immune system." *Annu Rev Immunol* 18: 861-926.

Trinchieri, G. (1989). "Biology of natural killer cells." *Adv Immunol* 47: 187-376.

van den Elsen, P. J. and S. J. Gobin (1999). "The common regulatory pathway of MHC class I and class II transactivation." *Microbes Infect* 1(11): 887-892.

Van Voorhis, W. C., L. K. Barrett, et al. (1996). "Analysis of lymphocyte phenotype and cytokine activity in the inflammatory infiltrates of the upper genital tract of female macaques infected with Chlamydia trachomatis." *J Infect Dis* 174(3): 647-650.

Wang, J., K. J. Frohlich, et al. (2011). "Altered protein secretion of Chlamydia trachomatis in persistently infected human endocervical epithelial cells." *Microbiology*. 157(Pt 10):2759-2771.

Witkin, S. S. (1999). "Immunity to heat shock proteins and pregnancy outcome." *Infect Dis Obstet Gynecol* 7(1-2): 35-38.

Wyrick, P. B. (2010). "Chlamydia trachomatis persistence in vitro: an overview." *J Infect Dis* 201 Suppl 2: S88-95.

Xiao, T. S. (2010). "Subversion of innate immune signaling through molecular mimicry." *J Clin Immunol* 30(5): 638-642.

Zhong, G., P. Fan, et al. (2001). "Identification of a chlamydial protease-like activity factor responsible for the degradation of host transcription factors." *J Exp Med* 193(8): 935-942.

Zhong, G., T. Fan, et al. (1999). "Chlamydia inhibits interferon gamma-inducible major histocompatibility complex class II expression by degradation of upstream stimulatory factor 1." *J Exp Med* 189(12): 1931-1938.

Zhong, G., L. Liu, et al. (2000). "Degradation of transcription factor RFX5 during the inhibition of both constitutive and interferon gamma-inducible major histocompatibility complex class I expression in chlamydia-infected cells." *J Exp Med* 191(9): 1525-1534.

Zhou, D. (2007). "OX40 signaling directly triggers the antitumor effects of NKT cells." *J Clin Invest* 117(11): 3169-3172.

3

Manipulation of Host Vesicular Trafficking and Membrane Fusion During *Chlamydia* Infection

Erik Ronzone, Jordan Wesolowski and Fabienne Paumet
Department of Microbiology and Immunology, Thomas Jefferson University
USA

1. Introduction

Chlamydia infections are associated with a wide range of diseases. *C. trachomatis* (serovars A, B, Ba and C) causes trachoma, the world's leading cause of infectious blindness. Serovars D through K are most commonly associated with sexually transmitted diseases and can cause infertility in women if left untreated [Paavonen and Eggert-Kruse, 1999]. Sexually transmitted diseases (STDs) are prevalent in every society in the world, including in developed countries (United States Centers for Disease Control [CDC]). Therefore, they represent a serious public health concern. Public programs aimed at increasing people's awareness of the risks these pathogens pose have helped in controlling the spread of disease. Nevertheless, *Chlamydia* is still the most frequently reported STD in the United States. In 2009, 1.2 million new cases of *Chlamydia* infections were reported in the United States alone, but the actual number of infections is estimated to be higher due to a large number of unreported cases (CDC). Vaccination is the gold standard for disease prevention, but despite years of research, no vaccines exist for bacterial STDs. The typical course of treatment for *Chlamydia* infections involves the use of antibiotics, but there is emerging evidence that non-specific antibacterial agents can cause lasting damage to an individual by adversely affecting the homeostasis of the microbiota, which is the collection of bacteria that positively affect normal human functioning [Stewardson et al., 2011].

The *Chlamydia* life cycle consists of two distinct stages: the elementary body (EB) and the reticulate body (RB) stages. They are characterized by differences in morphology, metabolism, and infectivity [Tamura et al., 1971]. Elementary bodies are metabolically inactive but infectious (**Figure 1-right**). Extensive disulphide cross-linking of cysteine-rich outer membrane proteins allows the EBs to survive outside the host cell [Hackstadt et al., 1985]. Upon coming in contact with a host cell, the EB is endocytosed into a plasma membrane-derived phagosome in which it eventually differentiates into a larger, metabolically active (but non-infectious) organism called a reticulate body. The RB remodels the phagosome in a multi-step process that is still incompletely understood (see **Figure 1-right**). This remodeled phagosome is called an *inclusion* and is distinguished by the presence of bacterial virulence-associated proteins (also known as *effectors*) on its surface in addition to host proteins that are not normally found on typical phagosomes. The remodeling process involves the action of a Type 3 Secretion System (T3SS) [Stephens et al., 1998]. Pharmacological inhibition of T3SS proteins halts the translocation of certain bacterial proteins into the inclusion membrane [Muschiol et al., 2006].

Chlamydia express bacterial effectors on the inclusion, including proteins of largely uncharacterized function called inclusion proteins, or Incs [Li et al., 2008; Rockey et al., 1995; Scidmore and Hackstadt, 2001]. Inc family members are found across species of Chlamydiae but do not share a high level of sequence homology. They do, however, share several structural features including a characteristic bi-lobed N-terminal transmembrane domain [Bannantine et al., 2000] and a cytosolic C-terminal domain capable of interacting with host proteins [Rockey et al., 1997]. These interactions are discussed in further detail below. Inc proteins likely play a major role in bacterial pathogenesis. However, their exact roles in infection remain unclear, largely due to the lack of genetic techniques to easily and rapidly generate targeted knockouts of these genes.

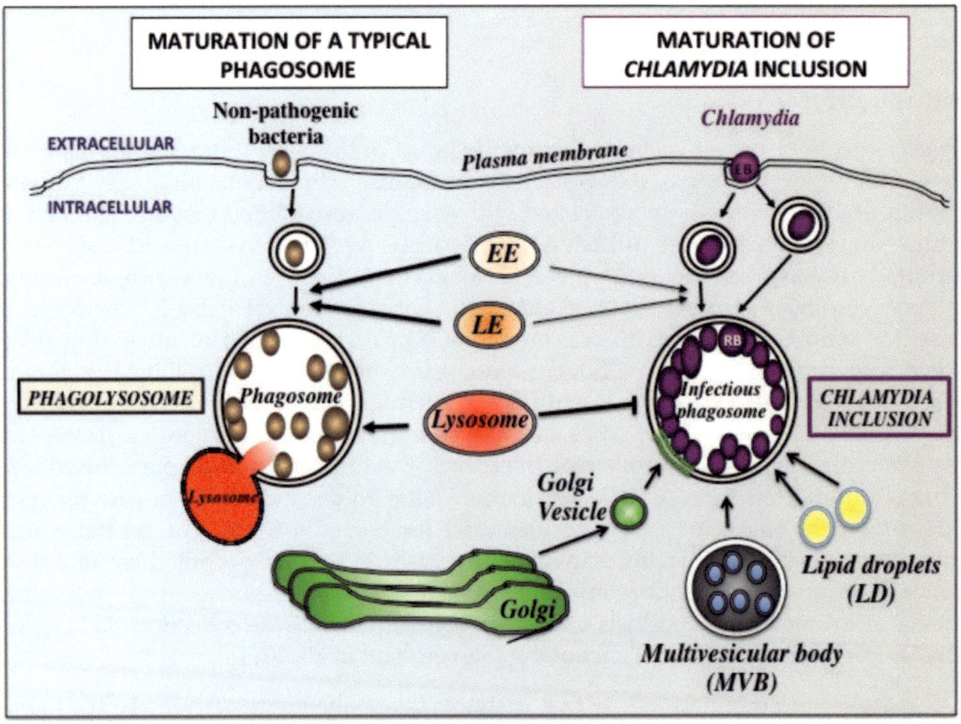

Fig. 1. Comparison of Typical Phagosomal Maturation and Maturation of *Chlamydia* Phagosomes (Inclusions). (Left) A typical phagosome fuses with early and late endocytic compartments and gradually acidifies. Upon fusion with the lysosome, it becomes a phagolysosome and the bacteria inside are destroyed. (Right) *Chlamydia* elementary bodies are internalized into separate phagosomes. In the case of *C. trachomatis*, these phagosomes eventually fuse with each other into a large inclusion. Inside the cell, the *Chlamydia* inclusion interacts with early and late endocytic compartments, but avoids fusing with lysosomes. In addition, it promotes fusion with Golgi-derived vesicles, lipid droplets (LD), and multi-vesicular bodies (MVB) to acquire host nutrients. The *Chlamydia* inclusions do not greatly acidify as in typical phagosomes.

Chlamydiae possess a highly condensed genome consisting of just over 1 million bases. This genome lacks many genes and gene networks essential for metabolism [Stephens et al., 1998]. As a result, Chlamydiae are obligate intracellular bacteria and must adapt to thrive under extremely challenging conditions inside host cells. In particular, the pathogen has to co-opt host resources such as nutrients, proteins, or lipids for its own use without triggering immune defenses or killing the host. To this end, Chlamydiae have evolved sophisticated mechanisms to support their intracellular lifestyle. For example, *Chlamydia* inclusions appear to fuse with a select set of host vesicles while avoiding fusion with other organelles—namely lysosomes (**Figure 1- Right**) [Fields and Hackstadt, 2002]. Fusion with the host vesicles likely results in the delivery of vital bioactive compounds that the bacteria then use to support its growth and survival inside the cell. However, the metabolic pathways involved in the utilization of host compounds are incompletely understood. Inclusions do not maturate to phagolysosomes (**Figure 1-Right**), that is to say they do not display markers specific to lysosomes [reviewed in [Fields and Hackstadt, 2002]], in contrast to many non-pathogenic bacteria (**Figure 1-Left**). By inhibiting interactions with the endocytic pathway, Chlamydiae are able to evade destruction by innate immune defenses. How the bacteria accomplish this task is the subject of intense research.

Chlamydia infection is a complex process involving many factors. In this chapter, we will review data that suggest that *Chlamydia* inclusions selectively promote fusion with Golgi-derived vesicles, lipid droplets, and multivesicular bodies while avoiding fusion with the lysosomal compartments. We will look at how *Chlamydia spp.* remodel their inclusion using a Type 3 Secretion System and discuss new research that aims at understanding host vesicle re-trafficking at the molecular level.

2. The *Chlamydia* inclusion is a remodeled version of the phagosome

In healthy individuals, innate immune cells can recognize and destroy invading bacteria using phagocytosis [Metchnikoff, 1891]. Bacteria are rapidly internalized into a special organelle called a *phagosome* that successively fuses with early and late endosomes resulting in acidification of the phagosome. During the final step of maturation, the acidified phagosome fuses with lysosomes to become a phagolysosome (**Figure 1-Left**) [Botelho and Grinstein, 2011]. Inside the phagolysosome, bacteria are destroyed through the action of proteases, hydrolytic enzymes and toxic compounds such as reactive oxygen species [Botelho and Grinstein, 2011]. Chlamydiae however, avoid this degradative pathway altogether (**Figure 1-Right**). At no point during infection are lysosomal markers found on the inclusion membrane [Fields and Hackstadt, 2002]. This observation suggests that *Chlamydia* modify the inclusion membrane to render it undetectable to lysosomes thus allowing it to avoid fusion with those compartments and eventual acidification.

2.1 *Chlamydia* modify the phosphatidylserine content of the inclusion they inhabit

One way to remodel the phagosomal membrane is by manipulating its lipid composition. A recent report looked at the localization of phosphatidylserine (PS) on phagosomes of inert and biologically active materials [Yeung et al., 2009]. Using a novel protein probe (referred to as Lact-C2) for membrane charge and lipid composition, the authors determined that PS contributes significantly to the lipid content of phagosomes. During *Chlamydia* infection however, Lact-C2 was found on the inclusion of *C. trachomatis* at only 6 hours post infection (hpi). At 18hpi, there was little or no Lact-C2 detected on the inclusion suggesting that *C. trachomatis* reorganized the lipid content of its inclusion. At this point, it is impossible to conclude with certainty what mechanisms are employed by the bacteria to alter the cellular distribution of PS.

In addition to remodeling the lipid composition of phagosomes, intracellular bacteria such as *Chlamydia* also modify the proteins on the membrane surface. It has been established that *Chlamydia* employs a Type 3 Secretion System to deliver bacterial proteins into the inclusion membrane and the host cytosol [Hueck, 1998; Subtil et al., 2001].

2.2 Secretion of *Chlamydia* proteins by a type 3 secretion system is necessary to protect the inclusion

Type 3 Secretion Systems (T3SS) are multimeric bacterial needle-like superstructures found in many Gram-negative pathogenic bacteria. T3SS allow for the transport of effectors through the bacterial membranes and across a eukaryotic membrane [Worrall et al., 2011]. The genome sequence of *C. trachomatis* reveals three distinct gene clusters containing open reading frames (ORFs) encoding putative gene products that show significant homology to known T3SS proteins from *Yersinia spp*. These genes include the pore-forming complex YscC, the structural components of the inner membrane complex YscJ, YscR, YscS, YscT, and YscU, and the ATPase YscN and its binding partner YscL [Stephens et al., 1998] (**Figure 2A**). The *Chlamydia* protein CopB is found on the inclusion membrane and is believed to be a translocator operating as the gateway for effectors to enter the host [Peters et al., 2007].

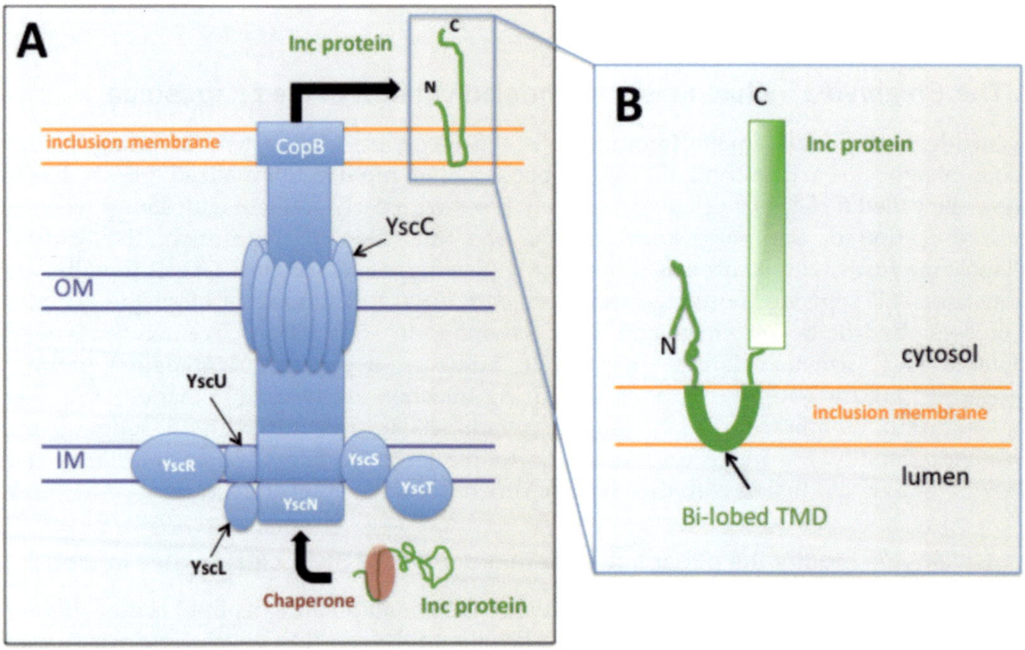

Fig. 2. *Chlamydia* Type 3 Secretion System. (A) The Type 3 Secretion System (T3SS) shuttles proteins from the bacterial cytoplasm into the host cytosol or inclusion membrane. Shown here is a schematic depicting the transport of an inclusion protein from the bacterial cytoplasm where it is bound to a chaperone protein, to the inclusion membrane through the T3SS. OM = outer membrane (bacteria); IM = inner membrane (bacteria). (B) Schematic representation of a typical inclusion protein (Inc). The N-terminal peptide faces the cytosol. The bi-lobed transmembrane domain inserts twice into the bilayer, allowing the C-terminal peptide to face the cytosol as well.

Secretion systems are mostly known for their ability to inject soluble effectors into the host cytosol, however they are also capable of shuttling proteins containing hydrophobic transmembrane domains (**Figure 2**). The inability to genetically insert recombinant fusion proteins into *Chlamydia* has necessitated the use of heterologous systems to study proteins secreted by a *Chlamydia* T3SS. Dautry-Varsat and co-workers demonstrated that the inclusion membrane proteins IncA, IncB, IncC, along with Cpn0026, Cpn0146, Cpn0308, Cpn0367, and Cpn0585 from *C. pneumoniae* are transported through a T3SS in *Shigella flexneri* [Subtil et al., 2001]. The N-terminal domains of these proteins were fused to a *cya* (adenylate cyclase) reporter gene and secretion was measured by western blotting supernatant and pellet fractions. These experiments demonstrated that the secretion signal was encoded in the N-terminal region of the *Chlamydia* protein. Interestingly, all of the proteins mentioned above with the exception of IncB and IncC contain N-terminal bi-lobed transmembrane domains. This led to the speculation that the secretion signal may be located in that region (**Figure 2B**). Follow-up studies using the same heterologous system identified fifteen *C. trachomatis* proteins shown to localize to the inclusion membrane (as measured by immunofluoresence microscopy) and to be secreted by the *S. flexneri* T3SS [Dehoux et al., 2011].

The sequencing of the *C. trachomatis* genome [Stephens et al., 1998] allowed *Chlamydia* research to enter the bioinformatics age. One of the first efforts to predict inclusion membrane proteins (Inc) used the bi-lobed transmembrane domain architecture as a criterion for localization to the inclusion [Bannantine et al., 2000]. This was based on the observation that IncA, IncB, and IncC each contained this unusual motif and were identified as being on the inclusion membrane. The authors of this study found forty-six ORFs in the *C. trachomatis* genome encoding for proteins predicted to possess a bi-lobed transmembrane domain, seventy ORFs were found in the genome of *C. pneumonia*, and twenty-three ORFs were found in both organisms. To confirm localization to the inclusion membrane, immunofluorescence was employed using antibodies directed against six of the identified putative proteins including CT484, CT223, CT229, CT233, CT442, and CT288 (**Table 1**). Only CT484 was undetectable by this method.

Inc Protein	Reference	**Inc Protein**	Reference
IncA	[Subtil et al., 2005]	**CT288**	[Subtil et al., 2005]
IncC	[Subtil et al., 2005]	**CT358**	[Dehoux et al., 2011]
IncD	[Subtil et al., 2005]	**CT440**	[Dehoux et al., 2011]
IncE	[Subtil et al., 2005]	**CT442**	[Subtil et al., 2005]
IncG	[Subtil et al., 2005]	**CT850**	[Dehoux et al., 2011]
CT223	[Subtil et al., 2005]	**Cpn0146**	[Dehoux et al., 2011]
CT226	[Dehoux et al., 2011]	**Cpn0186**	[Subtil et al., 2001]
CT228	[Dehoux et al., 2011]	**Cpn0308**	[Subtil et al., 2001]
CT229	[Subtil et al., 2005]	**Cpn0585**	[Subtil et al., 2001]
CT249	[Dehoux et al., 2011]	**Cpn1027**	[Dehoux et al., 2011]

Table 1. *Chlamydia* Inc Proteins Secreted by a Type 3 Secretion System. List of putative inclusion-bound bacterial proteins that are translocated through a Type 3 Secretion System. Proteins beginning with "CT" are from *C. trachomatis* and proteins beginning with "Cpn" are from *C. pneumoniae*. IncA,C,D,E, and G are from *C. trachomatis*.

This concept was extended when Zhong and colleagues investigated the intracellular location of fifty putative *C. trachomatis* inclusion membrane proteins [Li et al., 2008]. Antibodies were raised to putative Incs fused to either red fluorescent protein (RFP) or glutathione-S-transferase (GST). These antibodies were later used to confirm localization to the inclusion membrane. In total, twenty-two proteins were visible on the inclusion, seven were located within the inclusion, and twenty-one were undetectable by immunofluorescence.

Further evidence for a T3SS in *Chlamydia* has come in the form of pharmacologic inhibition of putative secretion-associated proteins. The compound INP0400, an inhibitor of the T3SS in *Y. pseudotuberculosis*, was shown to inhibit *Chlamydia* growth in cell lines when administered early during infection. For example, there was a decrease of the accumulation of 14-3-3β, a host phosphoserine-binding protein, around the inclusion, indicative of little or no IncG reaching the inclusion membrane [Muschiol et al., 2006]. The 14-3-3 family of proteins includes numerous members implicated in a myriad of pathways including apoptosis and tumor suppression [Morrison, 2009]. When INP0400 was added to cell culture media during the mid-cycle phase of infection, IncA function was apparently abrogated as multiple small inclusions were observed. The occurrence of multiple small inclusions (as opposed to one large inclusion) is indicative of a defective IncA protein [Fields et al., 2002; Hackstadt et al., 1999; Suchland et al., 2000]. The loss of functional IncA was attributed to a loss of translocation to the inclusion membrane as a result of the compound [Muschiol et al., 2006]. These findings are significant because they demonstrate the existence of an INP0400-sensitive protein or protein complex in *Chlamydia* likely to be a T3SS component.

2.3 Inclusion proteins can be post-translationally modified by the Host

The study of *Chlamydia* infection has largely focused on gross morphological changes during bacterial challenge. Re-organization of certain host markers and/or organelles implicates secreted bacterial effectors as being responsible for the observed phenotype. More recently, the role played by the inclusion in these phenomena has become more apparent. A complete identification of the inclusion proteome has still not been achieved. This could be due to the fact that (1) the proteome is likely to be dependent on the species of *Chlamydia*, the host cell or both; (2) it is dynamic and changes with length or phase of infection; (3) it is subject to the sensitivity and limitations of the techniques used to study it. Nevertheless, we can learn some basic facts about *Chlamydia*-host interactions through the study of known inclusion proteins. IncA and IncG for example, are two relatively well-studied proteins, each with identified binding partners. Importantly, discoveries regarding these two proteins have provided a starting point for the study of other inclusion proteins.

IncA was the first *Chlamydia* protein found on the inclusion membrane [Rockey et al., 1995]. Since then, IncA has been studied in relative depth. Microinjection experiments demonstrated that the soluble domain of IncA from *C. psittaci* is exposed to the host cytoplasm and that a host kinase is responsible for phosphorylating IncA [Rockey et al., 1997]. The function of IncA phosphorylation is unclear. *C. trachomatis* IncA is not known to be phosphorylated and no kinase for *C. psittaci* IncA has been identified [Fields and Hackstadt, 2002]. Furthermore, *C. trachomatis* IncA-mediated inhibition of endosomal fusion (discussed in detail below) was not reported to depend on phosphorylation [Paumet et al., 2009]. In contrast, *C. caviae* IncA was shown to be phosphorylated at serine 17, and this post translational modification was required for the inhibition of *C. caviae* inclusion development in cell lines [Alzhanov et al., 2004]. These differences, though not mutually exclusive, highlight the biological diversity among Chlamydiae.

IncG is another Inc protein phosphorylated by the host [Scidmore and Hackstadt, 2001]. A yeast two-hybrid screen using *C. trachomatis* IncG as a bait revealed that the phosphoserine-binding protein 14-3-3β binds the C-terminal region of IncG. Green fluorescent protein (GFP)-tagged 14-3-3β localized to the inclusion membrane in infected HeLa cells thus confirming the physiological relevance of this interaction. Serine 166 was determined to be a phosphorylation site as a mutation of this residue to alanine changed the electrophoretic mobility of IncG, consistent with a change in phosphorylation state. The S166A mutation abolishes interaction between IncG and 14-3-3β in a yeast two-hybrid assay. As for IncA, the kinase responsible for phosphorylating IncG is unknown. That both yeast and human cells apparently phosphorylate the same residue on IncG strongly suggests that the kinase is conserved from yeast to humans. Of course, the data do not rule out the possibility of multiple kinases being able to modify IncG.

Why *Chlamydia* would need to traffic 14-3-3β to the inclusion membrane is unknown. One possibility is that it helps form a multi-protein complex at the inclusion-cytoplasm interface. Another possibility is that IncG sequesters 14-3-3β to the inclusion and prevents it from functioning in its normal location in the cell. In any case, the finding that a *Chlamydia* protein is able to interact with 14-3-3β is significant because it implicates a connection between the inclusion and host cell cycle regulation. It should be pointed out that the interaction between 14-3-3β and IncG appears specific to *C. trachomatis* as the antibodies used to probe IncG on the inclusion of *C. trachomatis* strains A, B, Ba, C, D, E, F, G, H, I, J, K, L1, L2, and L3 did not cross-react with that of other species (namely *C. psittaci* and *C. pneumoniae*) [Scidmore and Hackstadt, 2001].

To date, phosphorylation is the only post-translational modification detected on Inc proteins. Additional modifications, such as glycosylation, would certainly be interesting, as it would extend the variability and functions of the bacterial effectors and possibly highlight new pathways manipulated by Chlamydiae. As molecular biology techniques become more sophisticated and comprehensive, we will be able to better probe these types of questions in the future.

In addition to modifying the phagosome they inhabit with the insertion of bacterial proteins through the T3SS, *Chlamydia* also manipulate the host proteins and lipids in order to change the nature of this compartment. They accomplish these modifications by (1) hijacking vesicles from the Golgi apparatus, (2) fusing with the multivesicular bodies and (3) corrupting host lipid droplets (see **Figure 1-Right,** and the following sections for more details).

3. Evidence for the fusion of Golgi vesicles with the inclusion membrane

The Golgi apparatus is the site of intracellular sorting of cargo. A variety of proteins—including members of the Rab and SNARE families—regulate trafficking between the Golgi and the different intracellular compartments or the plasma membrane [Conibear and Stevens, 1998]. The specific distribution of these proteins ensures a high degree of processivity and organization in cargo sorting [McNew et al., 2000; Paumet et al., 2005;

Paumet et al., 2004]. Perturbations of this network result in aberrant localization of cargo to incorrect compartments. One hallmark of *Chlamydia* infection is the disruption of vesicular trafficking and the redirection of exocytic vesicles to the inclusion [Hackstadt et al., 1995; Heinzen et al., 1996]. The delivery of lipidic cargo to the inclusion likely gives *Chlamydia* access to nutrients required for its intra-inclusion survival. In addition, this may give the inclusion a Golgi-like identity, helping it to escape the degradative pathway. However, there is experimental evidence showing that withholding lipids does not starve and/or kill the pathogen, but rather destabilizes the inclusion thus weakening the infection [Robertson et al., 2009].

3.1 Host-derived sphingomyelin is a key component of *Chlamydia* development

Direct evidence for an interaction between the inclusion and Golgi vesicles first came in 1995 when a derivative of the fluorescent Golgi marker {N-[7-(4-nitrobenzo-2-oxa-1,3-diazole)]}aminocaproylsphingosine (C6-NBD-ceramide) was shown to localize to the inclusion in a brefeldin A-sensitive manner [Hackstadt et al., 1995]. Brefeldin A inhibits cis-to-trans Golgi trafficking. Interestingly, Brefeldin A abrogated the association of the C6-NBD-ceramide with the inclusion leading to the conclusion that Chlamydiae intercept exocytic vesicles coming from the trans-Golgi network as opposed to the cis-Golgi face. The lipid species in question was determined to be sphingomyelin based on thin layer chromatographic analysis of purified inclusions. Later, Beatty and colleagues discovered that chemical inhibition of sphingomyelin acquisition in infected cells led to a corresponding loss of inclusion membrane integrity characterized by the absence of homotypic (inclusion-inclusion) fusion. In addition, they observed the premature differentiation from RBs to EBs, their early release, and a decrease in the ability of the bacteria to reactivate after reaching a persistent infection [Robertson et al., 2009]. Next, the authors inhibited host sphingomyelin synthesis at different steps during the metabolic pathway and analyzed the effects these compounds had on *Chlamydia* development. They found that pharmacologic inhibition by myriocin, which inhibits serine palmitoyltransferase (SPT) [Johnson et al., 2004], or fumonisin B1, which inhibits sphingosine N-acyltransferase downstreatm of SPT [Schroeder et al., 1994], correlated with the presence of multiple small inclusions in the cells tested [Robertson et al., 2009]. Addition of either dihydroceramide or sphingosine (two metabolites whose levels are negatively affected by myriocin) to the culture media restored normal inclusion morphology, validating that host sphingolipid synthesis is required for normal inclusion development. *Chlamydia* grown in cell lines with a nonfunctional SPT display defects similar to myriocin-treated cells. Complementation of the SPT proteins restores normal bacterial growth and development. Interestingly, subversion of Golgi-derived vesicles may actually occur through the hijacking of multivesicular bodies (MVBs) as treatment of infected cells with the MVB inhibitor U18666A disrupted the progression of the inclusion and produced phenotypes similar to that seen with myriocin treatment and SPT depletion [Robertson et al., 2009]. We discuss the manipulation of the MVBs by *Chlamydia* in section 4. In summary, these data strongly support that host-derived lipids, particularly sphingomyelin, are essential for *Chlamydia*. Interferring with this process results in apparently dysfunctional inclusion membranes.

3.2 Acquisition of Golgi-associated Rab proteins by the inclusion

Rab proteins are members of a large family of proteins (Ras-like proteins) conserved across eukaryotes. They regulate many aspects of membrane trafficking from specificity and tethering to fusion [Hutagalung and Novick, 2011]. Rabs are found in either a soluble or membrane bound form (**Figure 3**). They are attached to membranes via lipid anchors. In addition, they can be found in an "inactive" (GDP[1]-bound) or "active" (GTP[2]-bound) state. The activation state of Rabs is controlled by GEPs (guanine nucleotide exchange proteins) and GAPs (GTPase activating proteins). GEPs exchange GDP for GTP thus setting Rabs to an "active" state, whereas GAPs cause Rabs to hydrolyze the bound GTP to GDP causing them to enter an "inactive" state [Pfeffer, 2001; Segev, 2001].

During *Chlamydia* infection, Rabs involved in Golgi membrane fusion are found on the inclusion. Scidmore and colleagues analyzed the subcellular localization of eight Rabs (Rab1, 4, 5, 6, 7, 9, 10, 11) in cells infected with *Chlamydia* and found that the recruitment of specific Rabs to the inclusion was dependent on the species of *Chlamydia* [Rzomp et al., 2003]. During *C. trachomatis* infection, overexpressed Rabs1, 4, 6 and 11 relocate to the inclusion membrane as visualized by fluorescent microscopy [Rzomp et al. 2003]. The association between Rab6 and the inclusion appears specific to *C. trachomatis* since Rab6 was not found on the inclusion when cells were infected with either *C. muridarum* or *C. pneumoniae*. Rab10 however, seemed to localize only to the inclusions of *C. muridarum* and *C. pneumoniae* but not to that of *C. trachomatis*. Interestingly, the presence of Rabs on the inclusion was not dependent on intact microtubules, as inhibition of microtubules by nocodazole did not affect Rab acquisition.

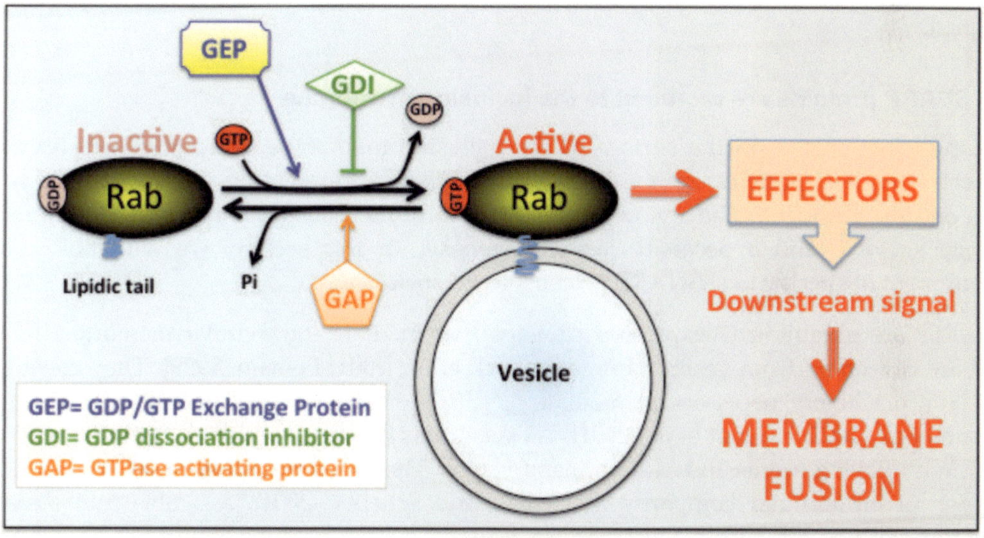

Fig. 3. Rab Proteins Regulate Membrane Fusion Through GTP Hydrolysis. (Left) Rabs are inactive when bound to GDP. A network of regulatory proteins coordinates activation or inhibition of Rab activity. GTP Exchange Proteins (GEPs) replace bound GDP with GTP and activate the Rab protein (Right). GDP Dissociation Inhibitors (GDIs) keep the Rab bound to GDP and locked in the inactive state. Once activated, Rab GTPases recruit effector proteins that act on downstream targets to promote membrane tethering and fusion. Afterwards, a GTPase Activating Protein (GAP) stimulates the GTPase activity of the Rab GTPase, which in turn hydrolyzes bound GTP to GDP and enters an inactive state.

[1] GDP: Guanosine diphosphate
[2] GTP: Guanosine triphosphate

Of the proteins found to associate with the inclusion, Rabs1, 6, and 10 are intimately involved in Golgi trafficking. Another Golgi Rab protein, Rab14, was later shown to localize to the *C. trachomatis* inclusion [Capmany and Damiani, 2010]. This localization was dependent on prenylation of Rab14 and occurred approximately 10-18 hours post-infection. Blocking bacterial protein synthesis with chloramphenicol treatment ablated the association between the inclusion and Rab14 suggesting that inclusion proteins are involved in Rab14 acquisition. IncA is detectable approximately 10-12 hours post infection and does not seem to be the main effector for Rab14 acquisition because incubation of infected cells at 32°C, which is known to block IncA expression on the inclusion surface [Fields et al., 2002], did not adversely affect the detection of Rab14 on the inclusion [Capmany and Damiani, 2010]. Notably, expression of the dominant negative (soluble) form of Rab14 inhibited *Chlamydia* growth most likely by blocking transport of sphingolipids to the inclusion.

The recruitment of Rab proteins likely acts to facilitate selective fusion between the inclusion and other intracellular compartments. One possible mechanism is the formation of tethering complexes that tie the inclusion to another vesicle or organelle. Rabs have been shown to be present in tethering complexes mediated by the formation of scaffolding complexes or by the action of coiled-coils [Hutagalung & Novick 2011]. It is interesting to note that several inclusion proteins are predicted to form coiled-coils. However, their structures are yet to be defined.

3.3 SNARE proteins are recruited to the inclusion membrane

The proteins located on the surface of the inclusion membrane, including both bacterial effectors and host proteins, are unique because of their position at the interface between the host and the pathogen. The abnormal composition of the *Chlamydia* inclusion membrane is key to survival and a necessity for pathogenesis. In this section, we will look at the recruitment of specific host SNARE proteins to the inclusion.

SNAREs are ubiquitously expressed proteins that mediate intracellular membrane fusion and are conserved from yeast to humans [Bock et al., 2001; Pelham, 1999]. They constitute the core machinery necessary to mediate specific membrane fusion [McNew et al., 2000; Parlati et al., 2002; Paumet et al., 2001]. As such, they are key regulators of all intracellular vesicle trafficking events and cargo transport steps. These proteins, present on the surface of almost all intracellular compartments [Chen and Scheller, 2001], assemble into a stable complex. As a result, both membranes are brought in a close apposition until fusion occurs (**Figure 4**). SNAREs are divided into two broad categories depending on their relative locations: *target-* (t-SNAREs) and *vesicle-* (v-SNAREs) SNAREs. Whereas the v-SNARE is always a single protein, the t-SNARE is composed of three subunits, one heavy chain and two light chains [Fukuda et al., 2000]. Notice that both light chains can be encoded in one or two separate proteins. A typical SNARE protein encodes a coiled-coil SNARE domain containing a heptad repeat motif spanning approximately 70 amino acids, and a C-terminal site that anchors it to a membrane. The SNARE domain contains a polar or charged residue located in the middle of the domain (also known as "zero-layer" [Fasshauer et al., 1998]) (see **Figure 5A**). The C-terminal anchoring site can be a simple hydrophobic transmembrane domain or a palmitoylation site.

Fusion specificity is largely encoded in the partnering of cognate SNARE proteins [McNew et al., 2000; Parlati et al., 2002; Paumet et al., 2001; Paumet et al., 2004]. Altogether, their characteristics designate SNAREs as excellent markers to determine the identity and activity of individual compartments in intracellular transport. Therefore, manipulation of individual SNARE proteins or of the complex itself may help intracellular pathogens to subvert normal trafficking patterns. As such, the recruitment of host SNAREs would afford the pathogen the ability to manipulate vesicular trafficking during infection.

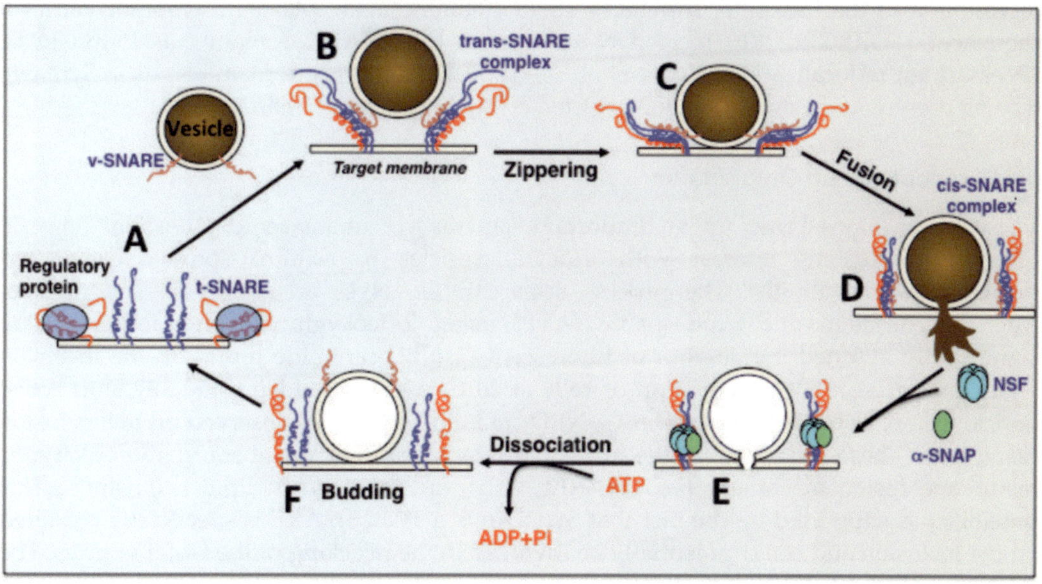

Fig. 4. Diagram of SNARE-Mediated Fusion. (A) In resting cells, SNARE proteins interact with effector proteins that control their availability. (B) Following a stimulatory signal, the t-SNARE proteins interact to form a complex that in turn binds the v-SNARE. As a result, a *trans*-SNARE complex forms (four-helix bundle) between t-SNAREs on the target membrane and a v-SNARE on the vesicle. (C) As the SNARE complex zippers from N- to C-terminal, the space between the opposing membranes decreases. (D) Fusion occurs when both bilayers merge and form a fusion pore. Following fusion, the *trans*-SNARE complex becomes a *cis*-SNARE complex (so called because all the SNAREs are now located on the same membrane). (E) The cis-SNARE complex is disassembled by NSF, an ATPase bound to its co-factor α-SNAP at the level of the SNARE motifs. (F) ATP hydrolysis dissociates the four-helix bundle, and the SNARE proteins are trafficked back to their original cellular compartments.

Syntaxin 6 is a SNARE protein that localizes to the trans-Golgi network (TGN) and likely plays a role in mediating the fusion of Golgi-derived vesicles with endosomes and/or lysosomes [Bock et al., 1997]. Recently, Hackstadt and co-workers showed that Syntaxin 6 relocates to the inclusion in a 18 hours post-infection [Moore et al., 2011]. Neither Syntaxin 4 nor Syntaxin 16 were found to localize to the inclusion suggesting that the recruitment of Syntaxin 6 was specific. Furthermore, the re-location of Syntaxin 6 to the inclusion is conserved among several species including *C. trachomatis*, *C. muridarum*, *C. caviae*, and *C. pneumoniae*. Treatment of the infected host cells with chloramphenicol to inhibit bacterial protein synthesis abrogated trafficking of Syntaxin 6 to the inclusion suggesting that bacterial effectors are necessary to induce this recruitment. The depletion of Syntaxin 6 by siRNA did not significantly affect the development of the inclusion nor change the recruitment of sphingomyelin to the inclusion [Moore et al., 2011]. Therefore, the role f Syntaxin6 during *Chlamydia* infection remains unclear.

SNARE domains mediate protein-protein interactions between SNAREs and are required for fusion. Interestingly, the SNARE domain of Syntaxin 6 was not required for the recruitment to the inclusion. Instead, a small 10-amino acid "plasma membrane retrieval sequence" (TDRYGRLDRE) located N-terminal to the SNARE domain was found to be necessary for re-localization [Moore et al., 2011]. Deletion of this domain results in Syntaxin 6 being present in the cytosol in non-infected cells [Watson and Pessin, 2000].

3.4 Perspectives on Golgi fusion

These observations bring up an important, and as yet unanswered, question: how do *Chlamydia* inclusions interact with exocytic vesicles to acquire sphingomyelin and presumably other lipids? The process apparently involves an energy-dependent step. Depletion of adenosine triphosphate (ATP) using 2-deoxyglucose and sodium azide significantly lessened the amount of fluorescent C_6-NBD-ceramide found on the inclusion [Hackstadt et al., 1996]. Incubation of cells at 20°C, which would presumably stop active vesicle fusion, also resulted in fewer C_6-NBD-ceramide molecules observed on the inclusion membrane. These data lead to the attractive hypothesis that members of the eukaryotic membrane fusion machinery (i.e. SNAREs, Rabs) are involved in lipid acquisition. This possibility is supported by the fact that Syntaxin 6, a TGN SNARE is specifically recruited on the inclusion and could potentially be involved in the hijacking of the Golgi vesicles. The extent to which SNAREs play a role in *Chlamydia* pathogenesis is unclear, but evidence is mounting that the interaction between effectors and SNAREs (or the inhibition of certain SNAREs by the bacteria) is an important hallmark of infection.

4. Multivesicular body markers are recruited to the *Chlamydia* inclusion

Multivesicular bodies (MVBs) are endosomal compartments that are involved in the sorting of surface proteins to lysosomes. They get their name from the multiple intralumenal vesicles that form as the result of invagination events at the MVB membrane. Proteins destined for destruction by lysosomal degradation are mono-ubiquitinated within the MVB and cluster at the invagination sites so that they can be exposed to degradative proteins of the lysosome for destruction.

It was traditionally thought that the *Chlamydia* inclusion did not intersect with the endosomal pathway. However, it appears that inclusions interact with MVBs and recruit MVB-associated proteins to their surface. In a series of microscopy studies, Beatty and colleagues identified three MVB markers—CD63, lysobisphosphatidic acid, and metastatic lymph node 64 (MLN64)—that trafficked to the inclusion after initial infection [Beatty, 2006]. Also observed was the absence of LAMP-1 (lysosome-associated membrane protein 1). This is in agreement with previous observations concerning the selective recruitment of vesicle-associated membrane proteins (see Introduction). CD63 actually appeared to be both on the inclusion membrane and inside the inclusion. Cryo-electron microscopy confirmed this finding [Beatty, 2006]. Lumenal CD63 seemed closely associated with the bacterial cell wall. Despite its close proximity with the bacteria, CD63 does not appear to play a significant role in the life cycle of *C. trachomatis* since the ablation of CD63 by small interfering RNA (siRNA) does not affect normal *Chalmydia* growth [Beatty, 2008].

The role of MVBs in *Chlamydia* infection is incompletely understood. One possibility is the acquisition of host lipids such as sphingomyelin [Beatty, 2008; Robertson et al., 2009]. The discovery that CD63 is transported in the inclusion lumen is important because it hints at a mechanism for acquisition of MVB components. At this point it is pure speculation as to what is being imported or how it is getting there. The most basic explanation for this phenomenon is that MVBs are fusing with the inclusion membrane and the internal vesicles are released into the lumen. Indeed, CD63 has been found on the internal vesicles of MVBs (microvesicles) [Heijnen et al., 1999]. This raises the interesting possibility that the internal vesicles of MVBs may actually be the main targets of *Chlamydia* as a source of nutrients.

MVBs are not the only way that *Chlamydia* acquire new lipids. Recently, it has been demonstrated that these bacteria were also able to hijack and fuse lipid droplets with their inclusions.

5. Corruption of host lipid droplets by *Chlamydia*

5.1 Lipid droplets play a role in intracellular homeostasis

Lipid droplets (LD) are intracellular stores of neutral lipids. LDs are found in a wide variety of eukaryotic cell types and are composed of both lipids and proteins. Once thought of as passive artifacts, LDs are now recognized as legitimate bioactive organelles. Disruption of lipid droplets (LDs) is associated with diseases such as type 2 diabetes and obesity [Farese and Walther, 2009]. It is believed that the initiation of LD formation begins with a swelling of the endoplasmic reticulum phospholipid bilayer caused by a gathering of neutral lipids. This is followed by a pinching off of the cytosol-facing leaflet to generate a cluster of neutral lipids, sterols, and sterol esters encased in a phospholipid monolayer. LDs are unique in the sense that they are the only recognized organelles to utilize a phospholipid monolayer. The exact function of LDs is unclear. Nevertheless, multiple interactions between LDs and other organelles suggest a physiologically significant role in cellular processes like metabolism.

5.2 *Chlamydia* proteins interact with host lipid droplets

A yeast genetic screen of the *Chlamydia* ORFeome uncovered three bacterial proteins (called **L**ipid **D**roplet **A**ssociated proteins, or Lda) that co-localized with yeast lipid droplets as measured by immunofluorescence: CT156 (Lda1), CT163 (Lda2), and CT473 (Lda3) [Kumar et al., 2006]. These proteins were also shown to bind to LDs in mammalian cells. Interestingly, Lda1 and Lda3 can be stably expressed in HeLa cells, but Lda2 seems to require LD biogenesis to be stable and avoid degradation *in vivo*. EGFP:Lda (enhanced green fluorescent protein) fusion proteins localized to both LDs and the inclusions themselves [Kumar et al., 2006].

Lda2 is unstable in the absence of lipid droplets. Incubation of *C. trachomatis*-infected cells with the compound triacsin C, which inhibits synthesis of cholesterol esters and triacylglycerides, resulted in the formation of smaller inclusions than those found in non-treated cells [Kumar et al., 2006]. It is not yet clear what role LD biogenesis and corruption plays in *Chlamydia* infection, but it appears to be a process critical for bacterial survival. Likewise, the exact association of Lda proteins with the membranes is unknown. Although none of the three proteins appear to contain the bi-lobed TMD structure commonly associated with inclusion proteins, it is possible that Ldas contain other as-yet-uncharacterized TMDs. It is also possible that Ldas are soluble and associate with host or *Chlamydia* proteins already present on the respective surfaces. Another compelling possibility is that post-translational modifications could lead to the addition of a lipid moiety that anchors the protein to the membrane surface. This matter is further complicated by the fact that no signal sequence specific for LDs has been identified.

Another interesting question is whether these Lda proteins are translocated through a Type 3 Secretion System. Secretion systems are a very efficient means of transporting proteins across biological membranes and are found in most, if not all, pathogenic bacteria studied to date (see section 2.1 of this chapter for more information on the *Chlamydia* T3SS). An active secretion apparatus would seem the most logical method of translocation because two lipid bi-layers separate the bacteria from the host cytosol (**Figure 2A**). The Ldas would have to traffic through these bilayers in order to gain access to lipid droplets. However, no T3SS screen has identified Lda proteins as being substrates for secretion so it is possible that Ldas are shuttled through another secretion system or by a novel method of translocation.

The lipid droplets themselves are translocated across the inclusion membrane into the lumen where they appear to physically associate with the reticulate bodies [Cocchiaro et al., 2008]. The mechanism by which LDs fuse with the inclusion membrane is unclear. LDs appear as whole, intact organelles throughout the process of translocation, providing evidence that the neutral lipids observed to be inside the inclusion are not the results of individual lipid molecules being trafficked across the membrane but rather bulk import of the entire droplet [Cocchiaro et al., 2008; Kumar et al., 2006]. A major unresolved issue is how the reticulate bodies interact with the lipid droplet once inside the inclusion lumen.

Lipid droplets are also capable of fusing with one another in a process that may resemble SNARE-mediated membrane fusion [Bostrom et al., 2007]. In this study, the authors found that SNAP23, Syntaxin 5, and VAMP4 associated with LD homogenate. In addition, NSF and α-SNAP, two proteins regulating SNARE complex dissociation, were also found to be associated with LDs via Western blot. This suggests that LD homotypic fusion might be SNARE-mediated. This conclusion is strengthened by the observation that inhibition of expression of any one SNARE (SNAP23, Syntaxin 5, or VAMP4) using siRNA constructs, significantly inhibited the rate of fusion of LDs.

6. The *Chlamydia* inclusion intersects with early and late endosomes but avoids fusion with the lysosome and acidification

6.1 *Chlamydia* does not fuse with the lysosomal compartment

Bacteria that are detected by host innate immune cells are endocytosed into phagocytic compartments that successively fuse with early and late endosomes resulting in the acidification of the phagosome and, ultimately, fusion with the lysosome where they are destroyed (**Figure 1-Left**). It has been observed that enzymes contained in the lysosome including acid phosphatase, arylsulfase, and β-acetylglucosaminidase do not enter the

Chlamydia inclusion demonstrating a lack of fusion with this compartment [Todd and Storz, 1975]. How Chlamydiae block this process is incompletely understood, although new data have been gathered showing that *Chlamydia* is able to use SNARE-like proteins to block lysosomal fusion [Paumet et al., 2009; Wesolowski and Paumet, 2010] (see section 8). It remains unclear at which step elementary (or reticulate) bodies deviate from the lysosomal pathway. The situation is further complicated by the fact that certain markers for early and late endosomes are found on inclusions [van Ooij et al., 1997]. Yet, the inclusion itself does not acidify [Schramm et al., 1996].

6.2 The transferrin receptor and CI-M6PR associate with the inclusion at distinct stages of infection

Chlamydiae have long been known to avoid lysosomal degradation (see Introduction). However, its association with other endocytic compartments has been observed. Engel and co-workers have examined the localization of early and late endocytic markers (transferrin receptor (TfR) and cation-independent mannose-6-phosphate receptor (CI-M6PR), respectively) with the inclusion as a function of time in HeLa cells infected with *C. trachomatis* [van Ooij et al., 1997]. What they observed was that, at approximately 4 hours after infection, antibodies against the TfR and CI-M6PR[3] stained brightly around the inclusion indicating possible fusion between the inclusion and early and late endosomes. These associations remained for up to 20 hours post-infection. Interestingly, the staining patterns were different for both proteins at 4 and 20 hours post-infection. At the later time point, a more defined membrane staining of the inclusion was observed as opposed to an aggregation-like pattern seen at 4 hours. Further interaction between TfR-containing endosomes and inclusions was observed when looking at the rate of transferrin recycling in *C. trachomatis*-infected cells. Recently, the association of endocytic SNAREs including VAMP3, VAMP7 and VAMP8 has been identified [Delevoye et al., 2008], supporting the interaction between the *Chlamydia* inclusion and the endocytic pathway.

Wyrick and co-workers used a pH-sensitive fluorophore attached to elementary bodies of *C. trachomatis* to measure the relative pH of compartments in which the bacteria reside. They discovered that despite intersecting with late endosomes, the inclusion does not reach a pH lower than 6 [Schramm et al., 1996]. Also, the pharmacologic inhibition of Na^+/K^+ ATPases, which oppose acidification of endosomes due to vacuolar ATPases, inhibits *Chlamydia* growth presumably due to acidification of the phagosome [Schramm et al., 1996]. Inhibition of v-ATPases had no effect on bacterial growth. This is in agreement with microscopy data showing that v-ATPases are not found on inclusion membranes and that the compounds chloroquine and ammonium chloride (which raise the endosomal pH) had no effect on *Chlamydia* growth [Heinzen et al., 1996]. In addition to v-ATPases, neither LAMP1 nor LAMP2 were found on the inclusion membrane in the study.

---

[3] It is interesting to note that the results in Van Ooij et al. (1997) regarding CI-M6PR localization are in direct contrast to those in Heinzen et al. (1996) in that the latter found no evidence for co-localization with the inclusion even though the same antibody (monoclonal anti-bovine CI-M6PR 2G11), same cell line (HeLa229), and same bacterial strain (*C. trachomatis* LGV L2) were used. Van Ooij et al. point out this discrepancy and suggest that the difference in bacterial load (multiplicity of infection, or MOI) during immunostaining could be the reason for these conflicting results.

In summary, although *Chlamydia* inclusions do interact to some extent with the endocytic pathway, they actively exclude certain endosomal markers—particularly those corresponding to lysosomes. Enzymes associated with lysosomal compartments were also apparently excluded from the inclusion lumen suggesting selective inhibition of fusion.

7. *Chlamydia* use SNARE-like proteins to block SNARE-mediated lysosomal fusion

The lack of a genetically pliable system for *Chlamydia* is a major obstacle in the study of the pathogen. However, scientists are finding new and innovative ways to study bacterial proteins *in vitro*. Inclusion-bound bacterial proteins are poorly characterized in terms of structure and function. Much research has focused on determining which proteins traffic to the inclusion, but their respective roles in infection are unknown. Inc proteins share very little sequence homology to any known eukaryotic proteins. Even within the same species of *Chlamydia*, the sequence homology of these proteins is very low. Importantly, all known members of Chlamydiae possess proteins localizing to the inclusion suggesting a critical role in survival. Recently, we have made progress in understanding how these proteins interact with host proteins. In particular, the interaction between IncA and members of the host membrane fusion machinery—namely SNARE proteins—have been indentified. The mechanism(s) uncovered in these types of studies will shed new light on the process by which Inc proteins help to subvert vesicle trafficking and establish a replicative niche inside the host.

7.1 The SNARE domain is a specialized coiled-coil domain

The defining feature of SNARE proteins is the presence of one or more SNARE domains. SNARE domains are around 70 amino acids in length and consist of tandem heptad repeats of the form *A-B-C-D-E-F-G* where *A* and *D* are hydrophobic residues and *B, C, E, F,* and *G* are polar or charged [Antonin et al., 2002; Sutton et al., 1998] (**Figure 5A**). In the SNARE domain, the *A* and *D* residues are known as *layers* and form tight hydrophobic interactions. Within the SNARE domain, there is a single polar or charged residue that resides in the *D* position towards the middle of the domain. This position is known as the *0-layer* (*zero-layer*) and is discussed in detail below. In the vast majority of SNARE proteins, this residue is either a glutamine or an arginine[4] [Fasshauer et al., 1998]. It has been proposed that the formation of the four-helix bundle begins at the N-terminus of the SNARE domain and proceeds straight through the C-terminal transmembrane domains [Melia et al., 2002; Pobbati et al., 2006]. This zipper-like motion pushes water molecules away from the hydrophobic core of the complex and brings the two membranes in close enough proximity to bring about fusion [Fasshauer, 2003; Melia et al., 2002; Stein et al., 2009]. This four-helix bundle assembles in a very organized and predictable way. The 0-layers of each SNARE domain align and interact in the final four-helix bundle as mentioned above. Likewise, each successive hydrophobic residue in the *A* and *D* positions will align with other hydrophobic residues on cognate SNAREs the same distance away from the 0-layer creating additional

[4] The presence of either glutamine (Q) or arginine (R) in the central position is so conserved that SNARE proteins are often classified as Q- or R-SNAREs, respectively. This should not be confused with the t- and v-SNARE classification.

layers of hydrophobic interactions. Layers are numbered according to their distance from the 0-layer. In order to understand whether *Chlamydia* is using SNARE-like proteins to manipulate fusion, this characteristic SNARE domain was used as a matrix to identify similar domains in the Inc proteins [Delevoye et al., 2008].

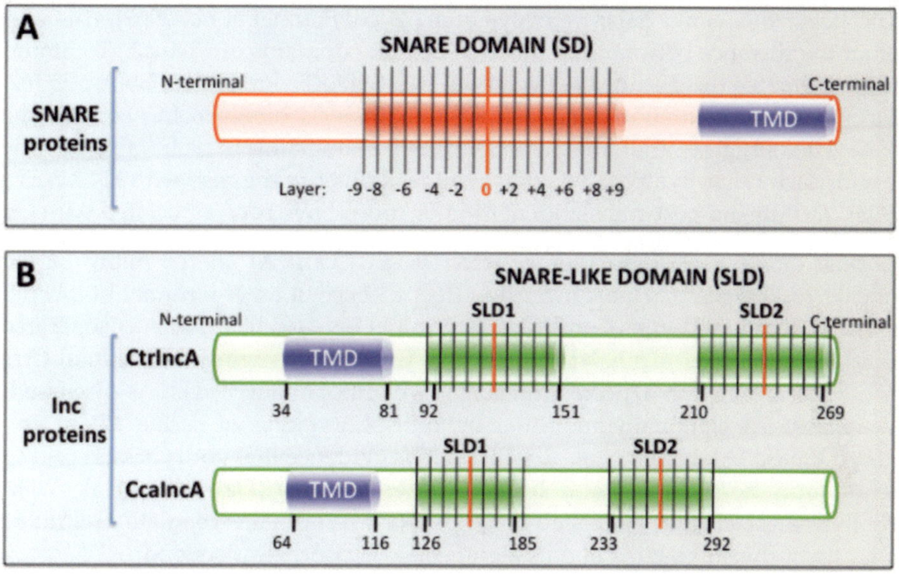

Fig. 5. The SNARE Domain is Organized into Discrete Hydrophobic Layers. **(A)** The SNARE domain is a coiled-coil domain consisting of a central polar residue and multiple hydrophobic layers. This illustration represents a typical SNARE domain. The hydrophobic residues are located in the *A* and *D* positions of the heptad repeats. The 0-layer is at position *D*, which is occupied by a polar or charged residue (usually glutamine or arginine). Layers are numbered according to their location relative to the 0-layer and are positive if counting towards the C-terminus and negative if counting towards the N-terminus. **(B)** Schematic of IncA, SNARE-like bacterial proteins found in *C. trachomatis* (CtrIncA) and *C. caviae* (CcaIncA). Residue numbers approximate the boundaries of each domain. The length of each domain is represented relative to length of the individual protein. Note that CcaIncA is actually 82 residues longer than CtrIncA. TMD=Transmembrane domain.

7.2 *IncA* from *C. trachomatis* and *C. caviae* encodes SNARE-like motifs

The severe loss of homeostatic regulation of vesicular trafficking in *Chlamydia*-infected cells and the aberrant (and *Chlamydia*-specific) translocation of proteins to the inclusion membrane suggest that bacterial effectors actively mediate this process. Two inclusion proteins of *C. trachomatis* and one protein from *C. caviae* show surprising structural homology to eukaryotic SNARE proteins. *C. trachomatis* IncA (herafter referred to as CtrIncA) is a ~34kDa protein composed of 273 amino acids. It contains the characteristic N-terminal bi-lobed transmembrane domain (TMD) altogether spanning approximately 48 amino acids (**Figure 5B and Figure 2**). Computational analysis determined that the TMD likely contains alpha helices [Dehoux et al., 2011]. It is unclear whether this hydrophobic stretch constitutes one long TMD or two shorter transmembrane domains separated by a cytosol-exposed linker region. In either case, the regions flanking the TMD are exposed to the cytoplasm. It is currently unknown what, if any, role the N-terminal cytosolic domain plays in pathogenesis since no conserved functional domains have been identified in this region. On the other hand, the C-terminal cytosolic region is significantly longer and contains two SNARE-like domains shown to be involved in corruption of host vesicle trafficking [Delevoye et al., 2004; Delevoye et al., 2008; Paumet et al., 2009]. It is interesting to note that the distance between the two SNARE-like domains of CtrIncA (59 amino acids) closely approximates the distance between the two SNARE domains of SNAP-25 (62 amino acids)—a SNARE protein containing two light chains and involved in neuronal regulated exocytosis. This suggests that the two SNARE-like domains may be able to physically interact with each other in a parallel coiled-coil fashion as is the case with SNAP-25 [Sutton et al., 1998]. To date, no post-translational modifications have been associated with CtrIncA.

Chlamydophila caviae IncA (hereafter referred to as CcaIncA) shares many of the same biochemical properties as CtrIncA including the presence of an N-terminal bi-lobed TMD, a cytoplasmic N-terminal domain, and two C-terminal SNARE-like domains separated by 48 amino acids [Delevoye et al., 2004] (**Figure 5B**). CcaIncA is slightly larger than CtrIncA at 355 amino acids and has an expected molecular weight of about 39kDa. As discussed above, CcaIncA is post-translationally modified by phosphorylation of serine 17 by an as-yet-unidentified kinase [Alzhanov et al., 2004]. There is evidence that both CtrIncA and CcaIncA are able to form homodimers and homotetramers *in vivo* [Delevoye et al., 2004]. It is currently hypothesized that the coiled-coil/SNARE-like domains regulate multimerization, but the nature of this interaction and its significance is poorly understood.

The hypothesis that IncA plays a role in regulating membrane fusion was first proposed when it was noticed that strains of *C. trachomatis* harboring mutations in their *IncA* gene developed inclusions that were smaller and more numerous than those of their wildtype counterparts [Suchland et al., 2000]. Whereas an infection with a wildtype strain results in an average of one large inclusion per infected cell, infection with an *IncA*-deficient strain results in the formation of multiple smaller inclusions that seemingly cannot fuse with one another. This homotypic fusion event seems to be important for pathogenesis because infection with strains of *C. trachomatis* that form non-fusogenic inclusions typically results in the manifestation of sub-clinical symptoms associated with *Chlamydia* [Geisler et al., 2001]. Supporting these observations, the microinjection of anti-IncA antibodies into the cytosol of infected cells replicated the non-fusogenic phenotype [Hackstadt et al., 1999] This is in agreement with a role of IncA in mediating homotypic fusion. In a yeast two-hybrid assay, CtrIncA, but not IncA from *Chlamydophila psittaci*, interacted with itself [Hackstadt et al., 1999]. This is important because *C. psittaci* infections naturally produce non-fusogenic inclusions despite having an apparently intact *IncA* gene. It is possible that *C. psittaci* IncA lacks a functional homodimerization domain.

The discovery that both CtrIncA and CcaIncA possess coiled-coil/SNARE-like domains prompted a detailed investigation of the interactions between IncA and SNARE proteins. When overexpressed in HeLa cells, CtrIncA binds to the v-SNAREs VAMP3, VAMP7, and VAMP8. This binding was confirmed *in vitro* for VAMP3 and VAMP8 [Delevoye et al., 2008]. The interaction between IncA and VAMP7 is dependent on the presence of the SNARE motif of VAMP7, since the deletion of this domain ablated inter-protein binding. If glutamine Q244 of CtrIncA is mutated to an arginine, the *in vivo* interaction with the host

SNAREs is lost. VAMP3, VAMP7, and VAMP8 are v-SNAREs that contain an arginine at their zero-layer. These observations led to the speculation that the glutamine residue of IncA coordinates with the arginines of the VAMPs to facilitate binding as was observed in typical SNARE complex formation [Delevoye et al., 2008]. It remains to be seen if this property of binding to SNAREs is conserved across Chlamydiae.

Another *C. trachomatis* protein, CT813, was found to have at least one putative coiled-coil domain in its C-terminal cytoplasmic region [Delevoye et al., 2008]. CT813 has only been shown to bind VAMP7 and, like IncA, this interaction was dependent on the presence of VAMP7 SNARE domain. No interaction between VAMP3, VAMP4, or VAMP8 was observed. CT813 has a putative length of 264 amino acids and a molecular weight of ~29kDa. Similar to CtrIncA, it is predicted to encode a heptad repeat and contains a bi-lobed TMD. Whether CT813 has the capability to inhibit SNARE-mediated membrane fusion is not yet known.

As more laboratories unravel the topology of the inclusion membrane, we can begin to learn more about the structure of the individual proteins themselves. Of the 59 putative *C. trachomatis* inclusion proteins analyzed computationally by Dehoux et al., 10 (16.9%) were noted to have significant coiled-coil potential. Likewise, about 20% of the putative inclusion proteins of *C. pneumoniae* are predicted to form coiled-coils [Dehoux et al., 2011]. Discovering binding partners for all of these proteins would greatly enhance our knowledge of *Chlamydia* infections and possibly reveal novel methods used by other intracellular bacteria to corrupt host resources for their own survival.

7.3 The *in vitro* liposome fusion assay: A biochemical approach to a biological problem

The inability to genetically manipulate Chlamydiae has proven to be a great challenge in the field. Scientists have developed novel techniques to circumvent this problem. One way to study *Chlamydia* proteins is by the directed mutagenesis of those proteins for use in *in vitro* assays. Our laboratory for example, has capitalized on a liposome fusion assay commonly used to study the biophysics of SNARE-mediated membrane fusion [Paumet et al., 2005; Varlamov et al., 2004; Weber et al., 1998].

The *in vitro* liposome fusion assay is a robust system for studying SNARE complex formation and functionality in a cell-free environment. The assay allows for the reduction of the membrane fusion machinery to its core components so that the contributions of mutations, effectors, or bioactive compounds can be studied. Although variations of this assay exist, they all follow the same basic workflow. Full-length SNARE proteins are first purified using standard protein expression and purification techniques. Next, each SNARE is reconstituted into either a t- or v-SNARE liposome population depending on the protein in question. Both liposome populations are of the same composition, except that the v-SNARE liposomes contain NBD and Rhodamine, a FRET (**F**luorescence **R**esonance **E**nergy **T**ransfer) pair in which one fluorophore (Rhodamine) quenches the other (NBD) (**Figure 6A**). After purifying and recovering the liposomes on a density gradient, both populations of liposomes are mixed at 37°C. As the liposomes fuse, the distance between the FRET pair increases, and the quenching of NBD decreases. The rate of fusion is measured as an increase in NBD fluorescence (**Figure 6B**). The main advantage of this assay comes from the fact that one can insert virtually any membrane-bound proteins into the liposome and study their effects on SNARE-mediated membrane fusion. Due to a lack of genetic tools for manipulating the *Chlamydia* inclusion, this technique may prove critical for our understanding of inclusion membrane dynamics and the function of IncA and other related bacterial effectors on membrane fusion. In fact, this assay has now been successfully used to study the function of bacterial effectors on SNARE-mediated membrane fusion [Paumet et al., 2009].

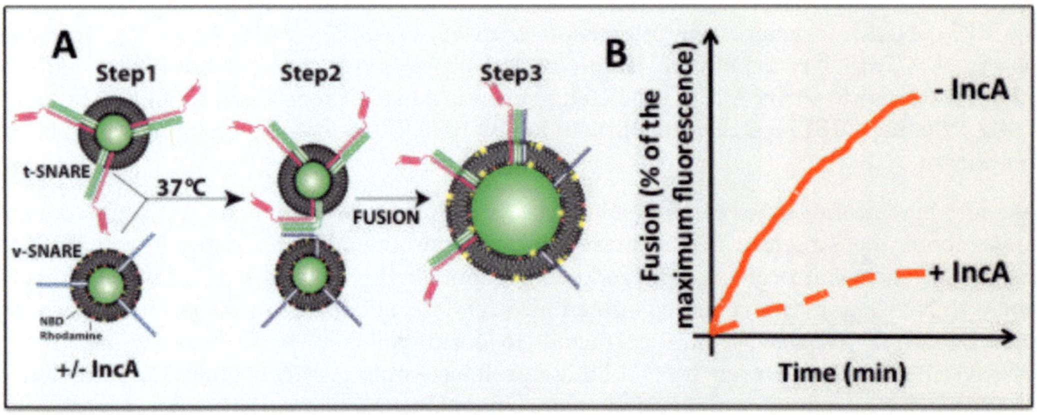

Fig. 6. Results of a Typical Liposome Fusion Assay Involving IncA. (A) t-SNARE and v-SNARE liposome populations are incubated together at 37°. To test the effect of IncA on SNARE-mediated membrane fusion, we created liposomes that contained IncA in addition to the v-SNARE. As a control, v-SNARE liposomes were created without IncA. Cognate SNARE interactions result in liposome fusion and dequenching of the FRET pair. (B) Percent of maximum fluorescence is plotted as a function of time. The t-SNARE liposomes contain Syntaxins 7 and 8 and Vti1b. v-SNARE liposomes contain either VAMP8 alone (-IncA) or VAMP8 plus IncA (+IncA). The presence of IncA on the v-SNARE liposome results in an inhibition of fusion as shown by a decrease in percent maximal fluorescence.

7.4 CtrIncA and CcaIncA inhibit SNARE-mediated endocytic fusion

The late endocytic/lysosomal SNARE complex is composed of the three t-SNAREs Syntaxin 7, Syntaxin 8 and Vti1b, and the v-SNARE VAMP8 [Antonin et al., 2000; Mullock et al., 2000]. During *Chlamydia* infection, VAMP8 has been shown to traffic to the inclusion membrane [Delevoye et al., 2008]. That IncA interacted with VAMP8 *in vitro* prompted us to investigate the role IncA played in altering endocytic membrane fusion. Using the *in vitro* liposome fusion assay described previously, our laboratory demonstrated that both CtrIncA and CcaIncA were capable of inhibiting endocytic fusion mediated by Syn7/Syn8/Vti1b (t-SNARE) and its cognate v-SNARE, VAMP8 [Paumet et al., 2009] (**Figure 6B**). The location of IncA did not alter its ability to inhibit fusion since co-incubation of IncA with either the t- or v-SNARE resulted in an inhibition of fusion. This suggests that *in vivo*, IncA may be able to inhibit lysosomal fusion before VAMP8 is recruited to the inclusion. Using truncated mutants of IncA, our group determined that the N-terminal SNARE-like domain of either CtrIncA or CcaIncA is sufficient for inhibition. The role of the C-terminal SNARE-like domain remains to be determined.

To validate the inhibitory capacity of IncA in a cellular context, RBL-2H3 (rat basophilic leukemia) cells were transfected with myc-tagged CcaIncA containing a premature stop codon before the C-terminal SNARE-like domain [Paumet et al., 2009]. We used RBL-2H3 cells because their secretory granules are lysosome-like and contain enzymes such as β-hexosaminidase. During stimulation with PMA (phorbol-12-myristate 13-acetate)/Ionomycin, β-hexosaminidase is released into the extracellular medium in a VAMP8-dependent manner [Paumet et al., 2000; Sander et al., 2008]. The amount of β-hexosaminidase present in the supernatant after stimulation can be used as a proxy for the capacity of the lysosomal granules to fuse with the plasma membrane. Myc-tagged CcaIncA co-localized with the secretory lysosomes in RBL cells. After stimulation, we observed a significant reduction in the level of β-hexosaminidase in the supernatant. This illustrates that under physiological conditions, CcaIncA is able to inhibit the fusion of intracellular membranes. **Figure 7** is a graphical representation of the proposed model for IncA-mediated membrane fusion inhibition [Wesolowski and Paumet, 2010].

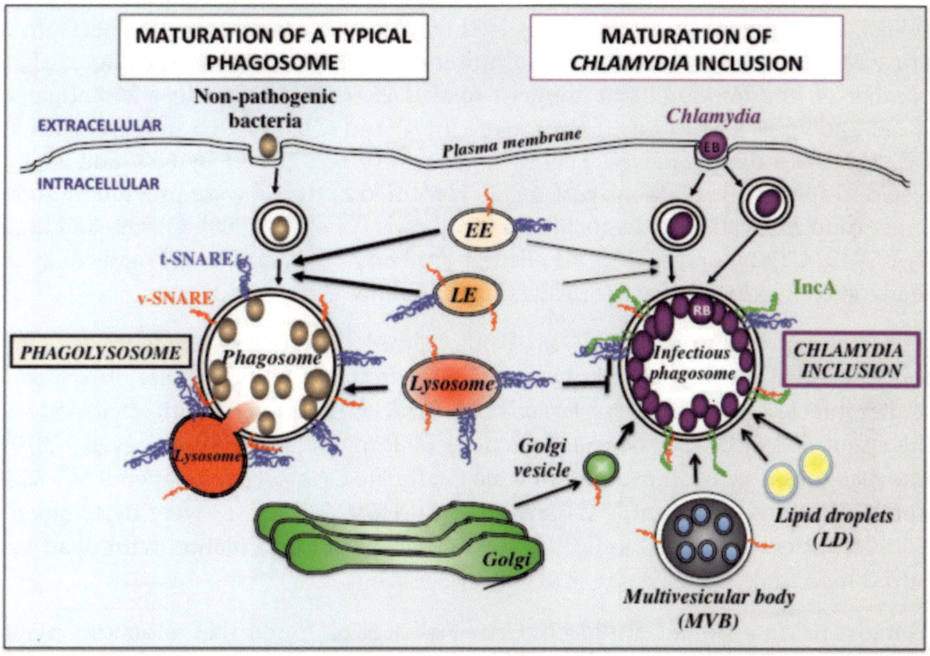

Fig. 7. Proposed Model of IncA-Mediated Inhibition of Late Endocytic Fusion with the Inclusion. (Left) The fusion of endocytic compartments (EE and LE above) leads to the acidification of the phagosome and destruction of bacteria. This process is mediated by SNARE proteins, namely Syntaxin 7, Syntaxin 8, Vti1b and VAMP8. (Right) During *Chlamydia* infection, IncA is expressed on the surface of the inclusion where it interferes with the endocytic SNAREs and blocks membrane fusion with the lysosomes. As a result, *Chlamydia* inclusion avoids the degradative pathway.

8. IncA and CT813 from *C. trachomatis* elicit antibody responses in humans

There is currently no vaccine available for *Chlamydia* infections. The challenge has been to find a phylogenetically conserved *Chlamydia* protein capable of producing a potent and prolonged immunological response. Finding the correct model organism in which to study this disease has also been a challenge. Mice are frequently used in immunology studies but are not the natural hosts of *C. trachomatis*, the causative agent of many human illnesses. Instead, mice are host to the related *C. muridarum* (also called Mouse Pneumonitis strain, or MoPn). While the use of an animal model has greatly facilitated the study of the pathogenesis of Chlamydiae infections [Brunham and Rey-Ladino, 2005], differences between the mouse and human etiologic agents of disease makes translation of results between both organisms inherently difficult to interpret. Nevertheless, progress is being made in the identification of immunogenic *Chlamydia* proteins in humans.

Array-based technologies have been utilized to scan immunized human sera for reactivity with *C. trachomatis* proteins. For example, GST-tagged *Chlamydia* proteins have been coated on a microtiter plate to scan the sera of infected women [Wang et al., 2010]. Antibodies in the sera bound to their respective antigens were visualized by horseradish peroxidase-based ELISA. Of the 933 ORFs tested, 719 were antigenic (bound to human anti-*Chlamydia* antibodies). The antigens that were recognized by 50% or greater of the patients from whom the sera were taken were designated as "immunodominant antigens" [Wang et al., 2010]. The number of immunodominant antigens totaled 26. Included in those 26 antigens were IncA (also known as CT119 for *C. trachomatis* IncA) and CT813—two proteins with known SNARE protein-binding capacity. These proteins were recognized by 65% and 79% of the sera tested, respectively. Notably, 6 of the 26 identified antigens were previously shown by the same group to localize to the inclusion membrane [Li et al., 2008]. CT089, CT119 (IncA), CT147, CT442, CT529, and CT813 all elicited antibody responses from more than 65% of infected women and localize to the inclusion membrane.

Antigens were further classified as being either infection-dependent or infection-independent based on their reactivity with serum from mice and rabbits. Briefly, animals were either infected with live *C. trachomatis* serovar D or immunized with UV-killed bacteria and their sera collected after booster infections or immunizations [Wang et al., 2010]. The antigens recognized by immunized sera were designated "infection-independent" while the rest were "infection-dependent."[5] CT089, CT442, CT529, and CT813 were determined to be infection-dependent while immunized sera produced from inoculation with dead bacteria recognized IncA and CT147 [Wang et al., 2010].

Interestingly, using a similar approach, Cruz-Fisher et al. found that antibodies against *C. muridarum* IncA (also known as TC0396) were only produced in mice infected with live elementary bodies not UV-killed organisms [Cruz-Fisher et al., 2011]. The antigenicity was not dependent on the route of infection as either intranasal or intravaginal inoculations resulted in the induction of a robust humoral response evidenced by the production of anti-IncA (anti-TC0396) antibodies. The different requirements for production of antibody by live versus dead inoculations between the two *Chlamydia* species may reflect a difference in antigen processing and presentation between mice and humans. It could also be the result of differences between the pathology of *C. muridarum* and that of *C. trachomatis*.

[5] Infection-dependent antigens were not antigenic in either mouse or rabbit but were antigenic in humans. The apparent absence of antigenicity in these animal experiments implies that antibody production is dependent on a live infection.

It is intriguing that some inclusion proteins appear to be highly immunogenic in humans, hinting at possible targets for future vaccine development[6] [Li et al., 2007]. This observation makes studying the biochemical properties of inclusion proteins all the more important. Uncovering the physiologic role(s) of these bacterial effectors could greatly advance our ability to engineer immunogenic epitopes with minimal side effects for use in vaccine studies.

Understanding more about the immunology of *Chlamydia* infections will lead to the design of novel vaccine strategies to combat the threat of sexually transmitted infections and the resulting medical complications. The discovery of highly antigenic bacterial effectors is a promising start. One challenge that remains is defining the immunogenic epitopes on each of these so-called "immunodominant antigens." By narrowing down the sites of antibody binding, it may be possible to design synthetic peptides that protect against a broad range of *C. trachomatis* serovars and elicit long-lasting cellular immunity.

9. Future research

We are still far from providing a comprehensive picture of the molecular mechanisms of *Chlamydia* infection. High-throughput functional assays could reveal a wealth of information about *Chlamydia*'s ability to corrupt host signaling and trafficking pathways. However, the lack of a genetic system has been a barrier to the development of those assays that could potentially identify novel *Chlamydia*-specific antibiotic targets. One laboratory recently reported the generation of point mutations in *C. trachomatis* after treatment with ethyl methanesulfonate [Kari et al., 2011]. This group successfully isolated a clone mutated for the *trpB* tryptophan synthase gene, but otherwise isogenic to the wildtype parent strain. The isolation and identification of mutants, however, is labor-intensive and may not be amenable to large-scale genetic screens in most laboratories. However, this represents an important step in beginning to manipulate the *Chlamydia* genome.

The function of inclusion membrane proteins needs to be explored more in depth. Their location at the host-pathogen interface makes them ideal candidates for virulence factors and also as druggable targets for novel therapeutics. Despite years of research on *Chlamydia*, little is known about the role of inclusion proteins in the etiology of infection. The best-characterized inclusion protein is IncA. Although a role for IncA in promoting homotypic inclusion fusion has been known for over ten years [Hackstadt et al., 1999], only recently has the interaction between the host endocytic SNARE complex and IncA been explored in detail. That other Inc proteins also contain putative coiled-coil domains strongly suggests that they may interact with cytosol-exposed host proteins including SNAREs. These interactions between *Chlamydia* and host proteins could potentially explain many of the observations noted by others throughout the years such as the homotypic fusion of inclusions, inhibition of fusion with late endosomes/lysosomes, or the acquisition of Golgi-associated membrane markers.

---

[6] It may seem counterintuitive that bacterial proteins expressed only within live infected host cells could have therapeutic abilities since those antibodies would most likely not bind the extracellular EB form of the organism. Recent data using mice, however, show that a vaccine consisting of recombinant CtrIncA plus murine interleukin-12 administered prior to genital challenge by *C. trachomatis* confers resistance to the pathogen beyond background levels (Li et al. 2007). This vaccine resulted in a robust humoral response correlating with reduced sequelae associated with genital infection.

Despite the lack of a tractable genetic system for studying *Chlamydia*, new and important discoveries are still being made. In particular, the cell biology of *Chlamydia* infection has revealed how intracellular infection can alter host vesicle trafficking. The availability of compartment-specific markers and fluorescent probes has greatly accelerated our understanding of the re-localization of host proteins and lipids during infection. The study regarding sphingomyelin is one example of how the use of cell biology techniques has overcome the inherent problems that come with working with a genetically recalcitrant bacterium. In order to continue to study the molecular mechanisms of *Chlamydia* infection, new techniques will have to be developed.

10. Conclusion

Despite strong efforts to combat *Chlamydia*, it continues to be the most frequently reported bacterial STD in the United States. Although *Chlamydia* is commonly associated with venereal diseases, infection also occurs in the eyes or lungs. Infection of tissues surrounding the eye can result in a form of infectious blindness known as *trachoma*—a widespread problem in regions of Africa, South America, and Asia (data from World Health Organization, Global Health Observatory). *Chlamydia pneumoniae* can colonize lung tissue and is the causative agent of a form of bacteria-induced pneumonia. Recent studies have also attributed increased risk of heart disease—including atherosclerosis—to *Chlamydia* infection [Beagley et al., 2009].

The normal course of treatment for *Chlamydia* infections involves the use of antibiotics. However, non-specific antibiotics like the ones used to treat *Chlamydia* may negatively affect the mucosal microbiome that helps to regulate essential processes like digestion, inflammation and immune responses. Additionally, some antibiotics have detrimental side effects. Therefore, finding novel and specific drug targets that protect against a wide range of *Chlamydia* serovars is of extreme importance.

As an obligate intracellular pathogen, Chlamydiae must adapt to acquire host nutrients while avoiding destruction by innate immune cells. Through the selective interactions with Golgi-derived vesicles, lipid droplets, and multivesicular bodies, Chlamydiae obtain host nutrients such as sphingomyelin that support growth and accelerate infection. While they promote fusion with these organelles, Chlamydiae simultaneously inhibit fusion with lysosomes and avoid compartment acidification and degradation by processes that are still unclear.

Evidence suggests that Chlamydiae employ a Type 3 Secretion System to translocate a special subset of effectors known as Inc proteins to the inclusion membrane surface, and that these proteins are involved in subversion of host vesicle trafficking. The identity of these Inc proteins is still unclear. This is hampered by the genetic diversity of the bacteria themselves and a lack of genetic tools for studying Chlamydiae. Incs known to localize to the inclusion membrane share little amino acid sequence homology, but may share structural or functional similarities including the presence of a bi-lobed hydrophobic transmembrane domain and, for a number of putative Incs, coiled-coil domain(s). IncA is one such inclusion protein that is transported by a T3SS and resides on the inclusion membrane. CtrIncA has been shown to interact with host SNARE proteins VAMP3, VAMP7, and VAMP8 possibly via its coiled-coils. It also inhibits endocytic SNARE-mediated fusion in a specific manner. Another *C. trachomatis* protein, CT813, localizes to the inclusion membrane [Chen et al., 2006] and may also interfere with SNARE-mediated membrane fusion [Delevoye et al.,

2008]. The biophysical studies of IncA presented in this chapter begin to reconcile our understanding of host vesicle subversion with what we know about inclusion membrane composition and could lead to the future design of novel anti-*Chlamydia* therapeutics.

11. Acknowledgement

We would like to thank the entire *Chlamydia* pathogenesis community for its work that made the review presented in this chapter possible. In particular, we are grateful to the members of the Paumet laboratory for their contributions to the *Chlamydia* SNARE-like proteins project. We would like to apologize to those authors whose work was not cited owing to space limitations. This research is supported by the National Institutes of Health grant #RO1 AI073486 (to F.P.).

12. References

Alzhanov, D., Barnes, J., Hruby, D.E., and Rockey, D.D. (2004). Chlamydial development is blocked in host cells transfected with Chlamydophila caviae incA. BMC Microbiology 4, 24 %U http://www.ncbi.nlm.nih.gov/pubmed/15230981.

Antonin, W., Fasshauer, D., Becker, S., Jahn, R., and Schneider, T.R. (2002). Crystal structure of the endosomal SNARE complex reveals common structural principles of all SNAREs. Nat Struct Mol Biol 9, 107-111 %U http://dx.doi.org/110.1038/nsb1746.

Antonin, W., Holroyd, C., Tikkanen, R., Honing, S., and Jahn, R. (2000). The R-SNARE endobrevin/VAMP-8 mediates homotypic fusion of early endosomes and late endosomes. Mol Biol Cell *11*, 3289-3298.

Bannantine, J.P., Griffiths, R.S., Viratyosin, W., Brown, W.J., and Rockey, D.D. (2000). A secondary structure motif predictive of protein localization to the chlamydial inclusion membrane. Cellular Microbiology 2, 35-47 %U http://www.ncbi.nlm.nih.gov/pubmed/11207561.

Beagley, K.W., Huston, W.M., Hansbro, P.M., and Timms, P. (2009). Chlamydial infection of immune cells: altered function and implications for disease. Crit Rev Immunol *29*, 275-305.

Beatty, W.L. (2006). Trafficking from CD63-positive late endocytic multivesicular bodies is essential for intracellular development of Chlamydia trachomatis. Journal of Cell Science *119*, 350-359 %U http://www.ncbi.nlm.nih.gov/pubmed/16410552.

Beatty, W.L. (2008). Late endocytic multivesicular bodies intersect the chlamydial inclusion in the absence of CD63. Infection and Immunity *76*, 2872-2881 %U http://www.ncbi.nlm.nih.gov/pubmed/18426873.

Bock, J.B., Klumperman, J., Davanger, S., and Scheller, R.H. (1997). Syntaxin 6 functions in trans-Golgi network vesicle trafficking. Molecular biology of the cell *8*, 1261-1271.

Bock, J.B., Matern, H.T., Peden, A.A., and Scheller, R.H. (2001). A genomic perspective on membrane compartment organization. Nature *409*, 839-841.

Bostrom, P., Andersson, L., Rutberg, M., Perman, J., Lidberg, U., Johansson, B.R., Fernandez-Rodriguez, J., Ericson, J., Nilsson, T., Boren, J., *et al.* (2007). SNARE proteins mediate fusion between cytosolic lipid droplets and are implicated in insulin sensitivity. Nature Cell Biology *9*, 1286-1293 %U http://www.ncbi.nlm.nih.gov/pubmed/17922004.

Botelho, R.J., and Grinstein, S. (2011). Phagocytosis. Curr Biol *21*, R533-538.

Brunham, R.C., and Rey-Ladino, J. (2005). Immunology of Chlamydia infection: implications for a Chlamydia trachomatis vaccine. Nat Rev Immunol *5*, 149-161.

Capmany, A., and Damiani, M.a.T. (2010). Chlamydia trachomatis intercepts Golgi-derived sphingolipids through a Rab14-mediated transport required for bacterial development and replication. PLoS One *5*, e14084 %U http://www.ncbi.nlm.nih.gov/pubmed/21124879.

Chen, C., Chen, D., Sharma, J., Cheng, W., Zhong, Y., Liu, K., Jensen, J., Shain, R., Arulanandam, B., and Zhong, G. (2006). The hypothetical protein CT813 is localized in the Chlamydia trachomatis inclusion membrane and is immunogenic in women urogenitally infected with C. trachomatis. Infection and Immunity *74*, 4826-4840.

Chen, Y.A., and Scheller, R.H. (2001). SNARE-mediated membrane fusion. Nat Rev Mol Cell Biol *2*, 98-106.

Cocchiaro, J.L., Kumar, Y., Fischer, E.R., Hackstadt, T., and Valdivia, R.H. (2008). Cytoplasmic lipid droplets are translocated into the lumen of the Chlamydia trachomatis parasitophorous vacuole. Proceedings of the National Academy of Sciences of the United States of America *105*, 9379-9384.

Conibear, E., and Stevens, T.H. (1998). Multiple sorting pathways between the late Golgi and the vacuole in yeast. Biochim Biophys Acta *1404*, 211-230.

Cruz-Fisher, M.I., Cheng, C., Sun, G., Pal, S., Teng, A., Molina, D.M., Kayala, M.A., Vigil, A., Baldi, P., Felgner, P.L., *et al.* (2011). Identification of immunodominant antigens by probing a whole Chlamydia trachomatis open reading frame proteome microarray using sera from immunized mice. Infection and Immunity *79*, 246-257.

Dehoux, P., Flores, R., Dauga, C., Zhong, G., and Subtil, A. (2011). Multi-genome identification and characterization of chlamydiae-specific type III secretion substrates: the Inc proteins. BMC Genomics *12*, 109 %U http://www.ncbi.nlm.nih.gov/pubmed/21324157.

Delevoye, C., Nilges, M., Dautry-Varsat, A., and Subtil, A. (2004). Conservation of the biochemical properties of IncA from Chlamydia trachomatis and Chlamydia caviae: oligomerization of IncA mediates interaction between facing membranes. J Biol Chem *279*, 46896-46906.

Delevoye, C.d., Nilges, M., Dehoux, P., Paumet, F., Perrinet, S.p., Dautry-Varsat, A., and Subtil, A. (2008). SNARE protein mimicry by an intracellular bacterium. PLoS Pathogens *4*, e1000022 %U http://www.ncbi.nlm.nih.gov/pubmed/18369472.

Farese, R.V., Jr., and Walther, T.C. (2009). Lipid droplets finally get a little R-E-S-P-E-C-T. Cell *139*, 855-860 %U http://www.ncbi.nlm.nih.gov/pubmed/19945371.

Fasshauer, D. (2003). Structural insights into the SNARE mechanism. Biochim Biophys Acta *1641*, 87-97.

Fasshauer, D., Sutton, R.B., Brunger, A.T., and Jahn, R. (1998). Conserved structural features of the synaptic fusion complex: SNARE proteins reclassified as Q- and R-SNAREs. Proc Natl Acad Sci U S A *95*, 15781-15786.

Fields, K.A., Fischer, E., and Hackstadt, T. (2002). Inhibition of fusion of Chlamydia trachomatis inclusions at 32 degrees C correlates with restricted export of IncA. Infection and Immunity *70*, 3816-3823 %U http://www.ncbi.nlm.nih.gov/pubmed/12065525.

Fields, K.A., and Hackstadt, T. (2002). The chlamydial inclusion: escape from the endocytic pathway. Annual Review of Cell and Developmental Biology *18*, 221-245 %U http://www.ncbi.nlm.nih.gov/pubmed/12142274.

Fukuda, R., McNew, J.A., Weber, T., Parlati, F., Engel, T., Nickel, W., Rothman, J.E., and Sollner, T.H. (2000). Functional architecture of an intracellular membrane t-SNARE. Nature *407*, 198-202.

Geisler, W.M., Suchland, R.J., Rockey, D.D., and Stamm, W.E. (2001). Epidemiology and clinical manifestations of unique Chlamydia trachomatis isolates that occupy nonfusogenic inclusions. The Journal of Infectious Diseases *184*, 879-884 %U http://www.ncbi.nlm.nih.gov/pubmed/11528595.

Hackstadt, T., Rockey, D.D., Heinzen, R.A., and Scidmore, M.A. (1996). Chlamydia trachomatis interrupts an exocytic pathway to acquire endogenously synthesized sphingomyelin in transit from the Golgi apparatus to the plasma membrane. The EMBO Journal *15*, 964-977 %U http://www.ncbi.nlm.nih.gov/pubmed/8605892.

Hackstadt, T., Scidmore, M.A., and Rockey, D.D. (1995). Lipid metabolism in Chlamydia trachomatis-infected cells: directed trafficking of Golgi-derived sphingolipids to the chlamydial inclusion. Proceedings of the National Academy of Sciences of the United States of America *92*, 4877-4881 %U http://www.ncbi.nlm.nih.gov/pubmed/7761416.

Hackstadt, T., Scidmore-Carlson, M.A., Shaw, E.I., and Fischer, E.R. (1999). The Chlamydia trachomatis IncA protein is required for homotypic vesicle fusion. Cellular Microbiology *1*, 119-130 %U http://www.ncbi.nlm.nih.gov/pubmed/11207546.

Hackstadt, T., Todd, W.J., and Caldwell, H.D. (1985). Disulfide-mediated interactions of the chlamydial major outer membrane protein: role in the differentiation of chlamydiae? Journal of Bacteriology *161*, 25-31 %U http://www.ncbi.nlm.nih.gov/pubmed/2857160.

Heijnen, H.F., Schiel, A.E., Fijnheer, R., Geuze, H.J., and Sixma, J.J. (1999). Activated platelets release two types of membrane vesicles: microvesicles by surface shedding and exosomes derived from exocytosis of multivesicular bodies and alpha-granules. Blood *94*, 3791-3799.

Heinzen, R.A., Scidmore, M.A., Rockey, D.D., and Hackstadt, T. (1996). Differential interaction with endocytic and exocytic pathways distinguish parasitophorous vacuoles of Coxiella burnetii and Chlamydia trachomatis. Infect Immun *64*, 796-809.

Hueck, C.J. (1998). Type III protein secretion systems in bacterial pathogens of animals and plants. Microbiol Mol Biol Rev *62*, 379-433.

Hutagalung, A.H., and Novick, P.J. (2011). Role of Rab GTPases in membrane traffic and cell physiology. Physiological Reviews *91*, 119-149 %U http://www.ncbi.nlm.nih.gov/pubmed/21248164.

Johnson, V.J., He, Q., Osuchowski, M.F., and Sharma, R.P. (2004). Disruption of sphingolipid homeostasis by myriocin, a mycotoxin, reduces thymic and splenic T-lymphocyte populations. Toxicology *201*, 67-75 %U http://www.ncbi.nlm.nih.gov/pubmed/15297021.

Kari, L., Goheen, M.M., Randall, L.B., Taylor, L.D., Carlson, J.H., Whitmire, W.M., Virok, D., Rajaram, K., Endresz, V., McClarty, G., *et al.* (2011). Generation of targeted Chlamydia trachomatis null mutants. Proceedings of the National Academy of Sciences of the United States of America *108*, 7189-7193.

Kumar, Y., Cocchiaro, J., and Valdivia, R.H. (2006). The obligate intracellular pathogen Chlamydia trachomatis targets host lipid droplets. Current Biology: CB *16*, 1646-1651 %U http://www.ncbi.nlm.nih.gov/pubmed/16920627.

Li, W., Guentzel, M.N., Seshu, J., Zhong, G., Murthy, A.K., and Arulanandam, B.P. (2007). Induction of cross-serovar protection against genital chlamydial infection by a targeted multisubunit vaccination approach. Clin Vaccine Immunol *14*, 1537-1544.

Li, Z., Chen, C., Chen, D., Wu, Y., Zhong, Y., and Zhong, G. (2008). Characterization of fifty putative inclusion membrane proteins encoded in the Chlamydia trachomatis genome. Infection and Immunity *76*, 2746-2757 %U http://www.ncbi.nlm.nih.gov/pubmed/18391011.

McNew, J.A., Parlati, F., Fukuda, R., Johnston, R.J., Paz, K., Paumet, F., Sollner, T.H., and Rothman, J.E. (2000). Compartmental specificity of cellular membrane fusion encoded in SNARE proteins. Nature *407*, 153-159.

Melia, T.J., Weber, T., McNew, J.A., Fisher, L.E., Johnston, R.J., Parlati, F., Mahal, L.K., Sollner, T.H., and Rothman, J.E. (2002). Regulation of membrane fusion by the membrane-proximal coil of the t-SNARE during zippering of SNAREpins. The Journal of Cell Biology *158*, 929-940.

Metchnikoff, E. (1891). Lecture on Phagocytosis and Immunity. Br Med J *1*, 213-217.

Moore, E.R., Mead, D.J., Dooley, C.A., Sager, J., and Hackstadt, T. (2011). The trans-Golgi SNARE syntaxin 6 is recruited to the chlamydial inclusion membrane. Microbiology *157*, 830-838.

Morrison, D.K. (2009). The 14-3-3 proteins: integrators of diverse signaling cues that impact cell fate and cancer development. Trends Cell Biol *19*, 16-23.

Mullock, B.M., Smith, C.W., Ihrke, G., Bright, N.A., Lindsay, M., Parkinson, E.J., Brooks, D.A., Parton, R.G., James, D.E., Luzio, J.P., *et al.* (2000). Syntaxin 7 is localized to late endosome compartments, associates with Vamp 8, and Is required for late endosome-lysosome fusion. Mol Biol Cell *11*, 3137-3153.

Muschiol, S., Bailey, L., Gylfe, A., Sundin, C., Hultenby, K., Bergstr√∂m, S., Elofsson, M., Wolf-Watz, H., Normark, S., and Henriques-Normark, B. (2006). A small-molecule inhibitor of type III secretion inhibits different stages of the infectious cycle of Chlamydia trachomatis. Proceedings of the National Academy of Sciences of the United States of America *103*, 14566-14571 %U http://www.ncbi.nlm.nih.gov/pubmed/16973741.

Paavonen, J., and Eggert-Kruse, W. (1999). Chlamydia trachomatis: impact on human reproduction. Hum Reprod Update *5*, 433-447.

Parlati, F., Varlamov, O., Paz, K., McNew, J.A., Hurtado, D., Sollner, T.H., and Rothman, J.E. (2002). Distinct SNARE complexes mediating membrane fusion in Golgi transport based on combinatorial specificity. Proceedings of the National Academy of Sciences of the United States of America *99*, 5424-5429.

Paumet, F., Brugger, B., Parlati, F., McNew, J.A., Sollner, T.H., and Rothman, J.E. (2001). A t-SNARE of the endocytic pathway must be activated for fusion. The Journal of Cell Biology *155*, 961-968.

Paumet, F., Le Mao, J., Martin, S., Galli, T., David, B., Blank, U., and Roa, M. (2000). Soluble NSF attachment protein receptors (SNAREs) in RBL-2H3 mast cells: functional role of syntaxin 4 in exocytosis and identification of a vesicle-associated membrane protein 8-containing secretory compartment. J Immunol *164*, 5850-5857.

Paumet, F., Rahimian, V., Di Liberto, M., and Rothman, J.E. (2005). Concerted auto-regulation in yeast endosomal t-SNAREs. The Journal of Biological Chemistry *280*, 21137-21143.

Paumet, F., Rahimian, V., and Rothman, J.E. (2004). The specificity of SNARE-dependent fusion is encoded in the SNARE motif. Proceedings of the National Academy of Sciences of the United States of America *101*, 3376-3380.

Paumet, F., Wesolowski, J., Garcia-Diaz, A., Delevoye, C., Aulner, N., Shuman, H.A., Subtil, A., and Rothman, J.E. (2009). Intracellular bacteria encode inhibitory SNARE-like proteins. PLoS One *4*, e7375.

Pelham, H.R. (1999). SNAREs and the secretory pathway-lessons from yeast. Exp Cell Res *247*, 1-8.

Peters, J., Wilson, D., Myers, G., Timms, P., and Bavoil, P. (2007). Type III secretion a la Chlamydia. Trends in Microbiology *15*, 241-251.

Pfeffer, S.R. (2001). Rab GTPases: specifying and deciphering organelle identity and function. Trends Cell Biol *11*, 487-491.

Pobbati, A.V., Stein, A., and Fasshauer, D. (2006). N- to C-terminal SNARE complex assembly promotes rapid membrane fusion. Science *313*, 673-676.

Robertson, D.K., Gu, L., Rowe, R.K., and Beatty, W.L. (2009). Inclusion biogenesis and reactivation of persistent Chlamydia trachomatis requires host cell sphingolipid biosynthesis. PLoS Pathogens *5*, e1000664.

Rockey, D.D., Grosenbach, D., Hruby, D.E., Peacock, M.G., Heinzen, R.A., and Hackstadt, T. (1997). Chlamydia psittaci IncA is phosphorylated by the host cell and is exposed on the cytoplasmic face of the developing inclusion. Molecular Microbiology *24*, 217-228 %U http://www.ncbi.nlm.nih.gov/pubmed/9140978.

Rockey, D.D., Heinzen, R.A., and Hackstadt, T. (1995). Cloning and characterization of a Chlamydia psittaci gene coding for a protein localized in the inclusion membrane of infected cells. Molecular Microbiology *15*, 617-626 %U http://www.ncbi.nlm.nih.gov/pubmed/7783634.

Rzomp, K.A., Scholtes, L.D., Briggs, B.J., Whittaker, G.R., and Scidmore, M.A. (2003). Rab GTPases are recruited to chlamydial inclusions in both a species-dependent and species-independent manner. Infection and Immunity *71*, 5855-5870 %U http://www.ncbi.nlm.nih.gov/pubmed/14500507.

Sander, L.E., Frank, S.P., Bolat, S., Blank, U., Galli, T., Bigalke, H., Bischoff, S.C., and Lorentz, A. (2008). Vesicle associated membrane protein (VAMP)-7 and VAMP-8, but not VAMP-2 or VAMP-3, are required for activation-induced degranulation of mature human mast cells. Eur J Immunol *38*, 855-863.

Schramm, N., Bagnell, C.R., and Wyrick, P.B. (1996). Vesicles containing Chlamydia trachomatis serovar L2 remain above pH 6 within HEC-1B cells. Infection and Immunity *64*, 1208-1214.

Schroeder, J.J., Crane, H.M., Xia, J., Liotta, D.C., and Merrill, A.H. (1994). Disruption of sphingolipid metabolism and stimulation of DNA synthesis by fumonisin B1. A molecular mechanism for carcinogenesis associated with Fusarium moniliforme. Journal of Biological Chemistry *269*, 3475 -3481 %U http://www.jbc.org/content/3269/3475/3475.abstract.

Scidmore, M.A., and Hackstadt, T. (2001). Mammalian 14-3-3beta associates with the Chlamydia trachomatis inclusion membrane via its interaction with IncG. Molecular Microbiology *39*, 1638-1650 %U http://www.ncbi.nlm.nih.gov/pubmed/11260479.

Segev, N. (2001). Ypt/rab gtpases: regulators of protein trafficking. Sci STKE *2001*, re11.

Stein, A., Weber, G., Wahl, M.C., and Jahn, R. (2009). Helical extension of the neuronal SNARE complex into the membrane. Nature *460*, 525-528 %U http://www.ncbi.nlm.nih.gov/pubmed/19571812.

Stephens, R.S., Kalman, S., Lammel, C., Fan, J., Marathe, R., Aravind, L., Mitchell, W., Olinger, L., Tatusov, R.L., Zhao, Q., *et al.* (1998). Genome sequence of an obligate

intracellular pathogen of humans: Chlamydia trachomatis. Science (New York, NY) *282*, 754-759 %U http://www.ncbi.nlm.nih.gov/pubmed/9784136.
Stewardson, A.J., Huttner, B., and Harbarth, S. (2011). At least it won't hurt: the personal risks of antibiotic exposure. Curr Opin Pharmacol.
Subtil, A., Delevoye, C., Balana, M.E., Tastevin, L., Perrinet, S., and Dautry-Varsat, A. (2005). A directed screen for chlamydial proteins secreted by a type III mechanism identifies a translocated protein and numerous other new candidates. Molecular Microbiology *56*, 1636-1647.
Subtil, A., Parsot, C., and Dautry-Varsat, A. (2001). Secretion of predicted Inc proteins of Chlamydia pneumoniae by a heterologous type III machinery. Molecular Microbiology *39*, 792-800 %U http://www.ncbi.nlm.nih.gov/pubmed/11169118.
Suchland, R.J., Rockey, D.D., Bannantine, J.P., and Stamm, W.E. (2000). Isolates of Chlamydia trachomatis that occupy nonfusogenic inclusions lack IncA, a protein localized to the inclusion membrane. Infection and Immunity *68*, 360-367 %U http://www.ncbi.nlm.nih.gov/pubmed/10603409.
Sutton, R.B., Fasshauer, D., Jahn, R., and Brunger, A.T. (1998). Crystal structure of a SNARE complex involved in synaptic exocytosis at 2.4 A resolution. Nature *395*, 347-353 %U http://www.ncbi.nlm.nih.gov/pubmed/9759724.
Tamura, A., Matsumoto, A., Manire, G.P., and Higashi, N. (1971). Electron microscopic observations on the structure of the envelopes of mature elementary bodies and developmental reticulate forms of Chlamydia psittaci. Journal of Bacteriology *105*, 355-360.
Todd, W.J., and Storz, J. (1975). Ultrastructural cytochemical evidence for the activation of lysosomes in the cytocidal effect of Chlamydia psittaci. Infect Immun *12*, 638-646.
van Ooij, C., Apodaca, G., and Engel, J. (1997). Characterization of the Chlamydia trachomatis vacuole and its interaction with the host endocytic pathway in HeLa cells. Infect Immun *65*, 758-766.
Varlamov, O., Volchuk, A., Rahimian, V., Doege, C.A., Paumet, F., Eng, W.S., Arango, N., Parlati, F., Ravazzola, M., Orci, L., *et al.* (2004). i-SNAREs: inhibitory SNAREs that fine-tune the specificity of membrane fusion. The Journal of Cell Biology *164*, 79-88 %U http://www.ncbi.nlm.nih.gov/pubmed/14699088.
Wang, J., Zhang, Y., Lu, C., Lei, L., Yu, P., and Zhong, G. (2010). A genome-wide profiling of the humoral immune response to Chlamydia trachomatis infection reveals vaccine candidate antigens expressed in humans. Journal of immunology *185*, 1670-1680.
Watson, R.T., and Pessin, J.E. (2000). Functional cooperation of two independent targeting domains in syntaxin 6 is required for its efficient localization in the trans-golgi network of 3T3L1 adipocytes. The Journal of Biological Chemistry *275*, 1261-1268.
Weber, T., Zemelman, B.V., McNew, J.A., Westermann, B., Gmachl, M., Parlati, F., Sollner, T.H., and Rothman, J.E. (1998). SNAREpins: minimal machinery for membrane fusion. Cell *92*, 759-772.
Wesolowski, J., and Paumet, F. (2010). SNARE motif: a common motif used by pathogens to manipulate membrane fusion. Virulence *1*, 319-324.
Worrall, L.J., Lameignere, E., and Strynadka, N.C. (2011). Structural overview of the bacterial injectisome. Curr Opin Microbiol *14*, 3-8.
Yeung, T., Heit, B., Dubuisson, J.F., Fairn, G.D., Chiu, B., Inman, R., Kapus, A., Swanson, M., and Grinstein, S. (2009). Contribution of phosphatidylserine to membrane surface charge and protein targeting during phagosome maturation. The Journal of Cell Biology *185*, 917-928.

4

Host Immune Response to Chlamydia Infection

Chifiriuc Mariana Carmen[1], Socolov Demetra[2], Moshin Veaceslav[3],
Lazăr Veronica[1], Mihăescu Grigore[1] and Bleotu Coralia[1,4]
[1]*University of Bucharest, Bucharest*
[2]*Grigore T. Popa University of Medicine and Pharmacy, Iassy*
[3]*National Center of Reproductive Health and Medical Genetics, Chisinau,*
[4]*Stefan S. Nicolau Institute of Virology, Bucharest,*
[1,2,4]*Romania*
[3]*Republic of Moldavia*

1. Introduction

From the immunological point of view, the infections produced by intracellular bacteria have several particular features:

1. protection against intracellular bacteria is mediated by T cells, which are interacting, not directly with the pathogen, but with the infected cell surface; antibodies exhibit a minor effect on the immune protection against intracellular infections;
2. infections by intracellular bacteria is accompanied by delayed hypersensitivity reactions that occur after the local administration of soluble antigens, mediated by T cells, whose effectors are macrophages;
3. tissular reactions to anti- intracellular bacteria are granulomatous in nature, both the protective responses and pathology being caused by them. Breaking granuloma favors pathogen dissemination and extension of lesions;
4. intracellular bacteria are expressing little or no toxic effects to the host cell, and pathology results from the activation of the immune response, mediated primarily by T lymphocytes. In contrast, extracellular bacteria secrete extracellular toxins, some of them being extremely potent and producing direct tissue damage;
5. intracellular bacteria are well adapted for coexisting with the host cell for long periods, by maintaining a balance between the persistent infection and the protective immunity mechanisms, resulting in a long incubation period and the development of a chronic infectious process. The infection *per se* is distinct from the pathological process. In contrast, extracellular bacteria cause acute infections, which are triggered soon after infection and ending after the immune response reaches an optimal intensity.

Some pathogenic bacteria such *M. tuberculosis, M. bovis, M. leprae, S. enterica, Brucella sp., L. monocytogenes, Francisella tularensis*, are facultatively intracellular, passing through a intracellular phase during their infectious cycle, without being strictly dependent on the cellular environment. They could infect primarily monocytes, but also other cells. In contrast, strictly intracellular parasitic bacteria (*Chlamydia, Rickettsia*) do not survive in the extracellular environment of the host. They infect endothelial and epithelial cells, and monocytes.

2. Life cycle of clamydiales

Chlamydiae are Gram-negative intracellular bacteria found in a wide variety of hosts. *Chlamydia* species infectious to humans are: *Chlamydophila psittaci, Chlamydia trachomatis* (biovar lymphogranuloma venereum - LGV and trachoma) and *Chlamydia pneumoniae.* Differentiation is based on their antigenic composition, susceptibility to sulfonamides and pathogenesis. *Chlamydia pecorum* is infectious to animals, but not to humans. *Chlamydophila psittaci* is parasitic on birds and mammals, and much more rarely to cold-blood vertebrates and humans. *Chlamydia trachomatis* is parasitic for mice and humans. In mammals and birds, both species produce eye conjunctiva, urogenital, respiratory and digestive tract infections and possibly at other sites (Barnes, 1990).

Chlamydia species have similar morphology and a common development cycle. By adapting to the intracellular compartment, chlamydiae lost a lot of the energy producing metabolic ways and the ability to produce ATP, but preserved some major metabolic activities, such are: glycolysis, respiration, pentoses biosynthesis. Development of intracellular chlamydiae depends on ATP and other high energy compounds derived from the host cell. *Chlamydiae* possess the enzymatic systems required for DNA, RNA and proteins synthesis, but they use many of the host cell precursors (nucleotides, amino acids, nutrients, vitamins, various cofactors) (Madigan et al., 1997).

In terms of structure, there were identified two chlamydia types: the infectious, nonreplicating elementary body (EB) and the noninfectious, but actively replicating reticulate body (RB), which are alternating in the development of the infectious cycle. The two morphologically distinct forms - the EBs and RBs - are representing adaptations to the extracellular environment and respectively to the intracellular one. The infectious particle, stable in the extracellular environment is a small cell, called the elementary body. They enter the host cell, multiply and disseminate in the extracellular environment. To complete these steps, chlamydiae undergo a developmental cycle that includes forms with alternating morphology and function.

Chlamydia cell wall is similar to the Gram-negative bacteria, with increased lipid content, but does not contain peptidoglycan (Hatch, 1996) (Fig. 1). Pentapeptidic similar components may be present, because their growth and division is altered in the presence of β-lactam antibiotics.

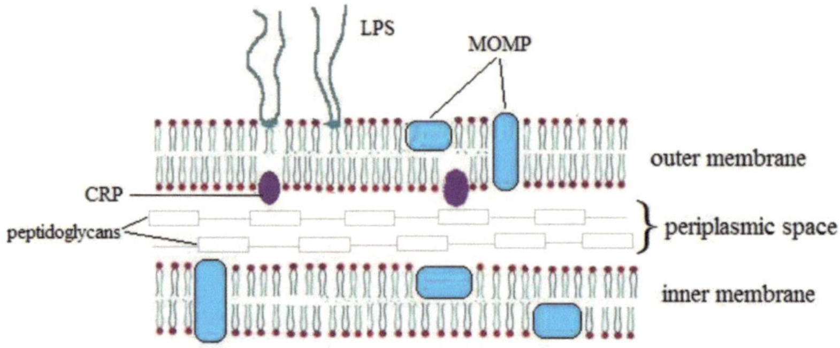

Fig. 1. Structure of the *Chlamydia* cell wall (membrane Momp major out membrane protein, CRP, cysteine-rich protein)

The outer membrane of *Chlamydia pneumoniae* is composed of lipopolysaccharides (LPS) and heat-shock proteins (HSP) that are genus specific (Matsumoto et al., 1991, Shirai et al., 2000). The bacterial family of *Chlamydiaceae* comprises a group of obligate intracellular pathogens which harbour a highly truncated LPS, being composed of KDO (2-keto-3-deoxyoctonate) units only. In all chlamydial species, the linear trisaccharide a-KDO-(2 - 8)-a-KDO-(2 - 4)-a-Kdo has been found, thereby constituting a family specific antigen. Antibodies raised against these neoglycoconjugates displayed a wide range of specificities and affinities.

Several major outer membrane proteins (MOMP) identified are detectable by monoclonal antibodies and are species specific (Matsumoto et al., 1991, Shirai et al., 2000). Under these persistence-inducing conditions, the chlamydial Hsp60 appears to be highly upregulated. Chlamydial Hsp60 has proinflammatory effects by directly activating mononuclear leukocytes, which are mediating the inflammatory response. Chlamydial persistence is characterized by morphologically aberrant RBs that do not undergo cytokinesis, considered a third chlamydial type, called the noninfectious, nonreplicating persistent body (PB). Persistent *Chlamydia*, however, re-enter the productive life cycle upon removal of the stress factor.

The infectious chlamydial form is the EB, which is adhering to the target cell membrane and initiates penetration. Elementary body is small, dense, with a rigid cell wall, given by the multiple SS bonds and to two other major outer membrane proteins (CRPs): a wall protein of 60 kDa and the outer membrane lipoprotein of 12 kDa. EB is resistant to environmental factors favouring survival in the extracellular environment after cell lysis and switching from one cell or one host to another. EB is not dividing, is metabolically inert, but has high affinity for epithelial cells. Its role is to spread the infection from one cell to another. Its membrane contains heparan-sulphate (proteoglycan), a ligand, through which they are attached to the microvilli and subsequently embedded in clatrin vesicles by receptors mediated endocytosis. Chlamydiae remain in the intracellular vacuole with non acid pH and avoid the fusion of the phagocytic vesicle with the lysosomes by unknown mechanisms. Inside the large vacuole, chlamydiae are redistributed from the cell periphery to the nucleus periphery by a mechanism dependent on actin F. The EB undergoes morphological changes and reorganization in the RB which is larger, metabolically active, and divides repeatedly by binary fission and becomes visible as a microcolony known as chlamydial inclusion. RB contains 4 times more RNA than DNA and RNA, while the EB contains equal proportions of RNA and DNA.

The EB - RB conversion requires the alteration of the outer membrane structure by the cleavage of SS bonds. Reduction of SS bonds leads to increased membrane fluidity, increased permeability, favours the nutrients transport from the host cell and the intiation of metabolic activity. After a period of growth and division, EB is reorganized; it condenses and forms numerous EBs. Development cycle is complete, with the host cell lysis and subsequent release of EB which are initiating a new infection cycle (fig. 2). The complete development cycles, when studied in cell cultures, is taking 47-72 hours and vary depending on the strain, the host cell and the environmental conditions (Campbell & Kuo, 2004).

The pathological processes due to chlamydial infection appear to be mediated by the immune reactivity. The host immune response stimulated by repeated episodes of infection increases the pathological lesions. Reinfection or persistence state causes pathological changes. Persistence of infection has been shown in different cell cultures being associated with PBs, which remain viable but not replicating, suggesting an innate ability of chlamydiae to persist intracellularly, and the mechanism by which they induce a pathological process. The factors favouring the persistence are unknown.

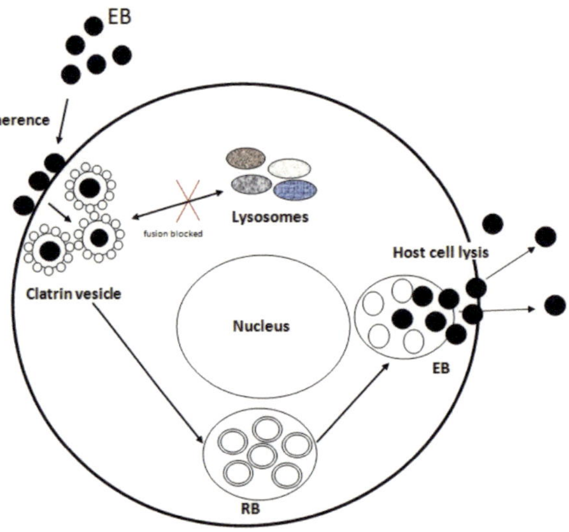

Fig. 2. Life cycle to *Chlamydia pneumoniae*

Chlamydiae, and other intracellular pathogens, are circumventing the normal mechanisms of host cell defences. Endocitated chlamydiae are sequestered in the host cell membrane derived phagosome. The key event that allows the survival of the infectious agent in the host cell is the inhibition of phagosome–lisosome fusion. Persistently infected cultures are less sensitive to rifampicin and clortetracycline, which suggests that chlamydiae DNA transcription and translation continues in the persistent forms.

In vitro, chlamydia can invade host cells deficient in nutrients and after the entry they adopt a dormant, non-infectious, but viable state. The persistence of the non-replicative stage is reversible. By adding for example, L-isoleucine, an essential aminoacid for chlamydiae and host cells is sufficient to enable development of chlamydiae. It is believed that the persistence of chlamydiae is the result of competition between host and parasitic cells for L-isoleucine. The treatment with cicloheximide, an inhibitor of host cell protein synthesis - stops the competition between the host cell and chlamydiae for L-isoleucine that remains available for bacterial protein synthesis. Chlamydiae induce synthesis of interferon that has been shown to inhibit pathogen growth in cell culture.

3. Immunological aspects of acute and chronic *Chlamydia* infection

The protective immunity for *Chlamydia pneumoniae* and *Chlamydia trachomatis* infections is quite similar. Innate immunity is of key importance in primary recognition of invading pathogens. Infected epithelial cells respond in similar, but not identical ways to different invading pathogens and the pathogens are capable of modifying the host cell response (Severin & Ossevarde, 2006).

Cell-mediated immunity and especially participation of type 1 Th cells are crucial for eradication or limitation of the infection at a culture negative stage. Primary infection induces development of antigen-specific immunity. *Chlamydia pneumoniae* is generally transmitted from person to person via the respiratory route (Kuo et al., 1995, Grayston, 2002), where mechanical barriers and innate immune mechanisms comprise the first defense systems of the host. Epithelial cells lining the trachea and nasopharynx are the first cellular barriers against inhaled pathogens. Infection of airway epithelial cells can trigger a preliminary cascade of pro- and antiinflammatory immune reactions (secretion of IL-8, and expression of the epithelial adhesion molecule-1) that initiate drifting of polymorphonuclear neutrophils (PMN) and acute inflammation. Trachoma is the leading infectious cause of blindness. Eighty-five million children have active (inflammatory) trachoma, and about 7 million people, mainly adults, are blind from late scarring sequelae (Thylefors et al., 1995).

In trachoma, ocular *Chlamydia trachomatis* infection causes inflammatory changes in the conjunctiva, and repeated infections sometimes lead to fibrosis and scarring of the sub tarsal conjunctiva. The reasons for the heterogeneity in susceptibility to chlamydial infection and disease progression following a rather uniform bacterial exposure remain incompletely understood, but however, it has been postulated that the early secretion of pro-inflammatory cytokines and chemokines by epithelial cells following *Chlamydia trachomatis* infection may initiate and sustain a chronic inflammatory process associated with pathology (Stephens, 2003).

Natividad et al. (2009) tried to investigate how genetic variation detected in IL8 and CSF2 (colony stimulating factor) could affect risk of trachoma: IL8, CSF2 and MMP9 (matrix-metallo proteinase) are co-expressed in the *Chlamydia trachomatis* infected conjunctiva and these gene products could interact at the site of infection to augment and sustain inflammatory processes. MMP9 enhance the activity of IL8, whereas activation of neutrophils by IL-8 may trigger the release of pro-MMP9, creating a potential for a positive feedback loop. Similarly, CSF2 release by the infected epithelial cells may mediate the influx and activation of inflammatory cells at the site of infection. Secreted CSF2 may trigger MMP9 production by monocytes, which could act to enhance and sustain the pro-inflammatory cascade initiated by CSF2.

The onset of acquired antigen-specific immune responses depends on the speed of microbial dissemination from the initial site to local lymph nodes (Lipscomb et al., 1995). A preliminary pulmonary infection occurs in the alveoli, where the invading *Chlamydia* undergoes phagocytosis by dendritic cells (Prebeck et al., 2001) or alveolar macrophages (Nakajo et al., 1990; Redecke et al., 1998). The destruction of intracellular bacteria is dependent on the macrophage activation and mediated by reactive oxygen and nitrogen intermediates.

Chlamydia can protect against the microbicidal systems of the activated macrophages by inhibiting the phagolysosomal fusion and replicating in a special nonacidic chlamydial inclusion (Mihaescu et al., 2009). The migration of some infected macrophages and dendritic cells to regional lymph nodes contributes significantly to the initiation of the antigen-specific immune response (Lipcomb et al., 1995)

The acquired immune response, both humoral and cell-mediated in *Chlamydia pneumoniae* and *Chlamydia trachomatis* infection is detectable from 1 to 2 weeks after the primary infection. Monocytes/macrophages and dendritic cells participate in the development of antigen-specific cell-mediated immunity by: (1) acting as antigen presenting cells (APC) and by (2) secretion of pro- IL-6, IL-1, IL-12) and antiinflammatory (IL-10, IL-13, cytokines, which activate other immune cells. In particular, the balance of IL-12 and IL-10 is crucial in regulating the development and functional characteristics of T cell responses (Surcel et al., 2005).

Chlamydial peptides processed by professional APC are further presented by MHC class II molecule to T CD4+ cells, although some chlamydial peptides are available also for MHC class I presentation. Activation of type 1 Th cell responses by IL-12 and IL-18 is considered the most important cytokine controlling chlamydiae infections, by regulating the cytotoxic T cells and by direct induction of nitric oxide synthase and the nitric oxide production in the macrophages as well as tryptophan depletion that inhibit chlamydial growth (Surcel et al., 2005). Activation of a type 2 cytokine response is associated with increased susceptibility to *Chlamydia trachomatis* and *Chlamydia pneumoniae* infection in experimental animal models.

Protective impact of T cells involves promotion of type 1 responses by activating other inflammatory cells, monocytes and macrophages, and cytotoxic T cells and B cells via cytokine secretion. CD4+ T cell activation generally dominates over CD8+ in *in vitro* and *in vivo* studies (Halme et al., 2000) especially in later stages of infection.

In primary infection in healthy people, circulating lymphocytes respond equally to *Chlamydia pneumoniae* and *Chlamydia trachomatis* antigens, suggesting that conservative chlamydial structures dominate over the species-specific ones as targets for the cell-mediated responses (Halme et al., 1997). The immune escape of chlamydiae within the host includes mechanisms for evasion of T cell recognition by interfering with the expression of MHC molecules. *Chlamydia pneumoniae* can suppress MHC class II expression on human monocytes (Airenne et al., 2002) or MHC class I expression on a monocytic cell line (Caspar-Baughil et al., 2000). In this process, *Chlamydia pneumoniae* secretes a proteolytically active molecule (Fan et al., 2002) a homologue of chlamydial protease-like activity factor of *Chlamydia trachomatis,* which can degrade constitutive transcription factors RFX5 and USF-1 molecules needed for antigen transcription during microbial infection (Zhong et al., 2001) . IL-10 by infected macrophages seems to inhibit the expression of MHC molecules (Caspar-Banguil et al., 2000).

Concerning the antibodies responses in chlamydiae infection, IgM response appears 2–3 weeks after the first symptoms of the illness and IgG response after 6–8 weeks. IgA antibodies are only occasionally found during the primary infection but appear frequently in the reinfection. The main antigens triggering an antibody mediated response are LPS and HSP-60. The protective value of these antibodies is still to be established.

Most of the times, especially in the infectious processes, immune responses are beneficial, having a role in eliminating pathogens. Sometimes, however, after the contact with some antigens (in particular molecular ones), activation of immune function is damaging and unfavorable for the host, causing two types of clinical manifestations: hypersensitivity and autoimmune diseases. Decreased immune system activity, generates a particular type of clinical manifestations generically known as immunodeficiencies. They can be congenital (primary) or acquired (secondary).

The state of hypersensitivity (HS) is a consequence of the fact that the primary immunization after the contact with the antigen and generation of immune effectors (antibodies and effector lymphocytes) do not give always a positive state, i.e. the resistance of the organism to an infection. Primary contact with the antigen creates sometimes a state of alert to the respective antigen, and at the second contact with the respective antigen, the human body responds by pathological hypersensitivity states, characterized by too high intensity or inappropriate immune response, which are the origin of tissue damage. The equivalent term commonly used for hypersensitivity is the allergy (allos, ergon, greek = other energy).

Autoimmunity is essentially an immune response against self antigens, which initiates the autoimmune conflict. One of the axioms of Immunology, that the host normal immune reactivity, does not produce antibodies against the body's own constituents, is frequently violated because the immune system turns against its own tissue components, disrupting the state of tolerance. Especially in the elderly, there are synthesized autoantibodies or autoreactive lymphocytes could occur (Lazar et al., 2005; Mihaescu et al., 2009).

By extending its effects, the autoimmune conflict can lead to autoimmune diseases characterized by the proliferative expansion of lymphocytes reactive against self components and generated effectors (autoreactive cells and antibodies) (Mihaescu and Chifiriuc, 2009). There are diseases with autoimmune phenomena well expressed, but their primary etiology is unknown. Among the variate range of acute infections caused by *Chlamydia pneumoniae* (pharyngitis, bronchitis, pneoumonia), late complications (asthma, allergic rhinitis, heart disease, multiple sclerosis, Alzheimer's) could occur (Friedman et al., 2004).

Chlamydia could induce a local T cell immunosuppression and inflammatory response revealing a possible host-pathogen scenario that would support both persistence and inflammation. For example, *Chlamydia pneumoniae* could inhibit activated, but not nonactivated human T cell proliferation in a pathogen specific maner, heat sensitive, and multiplicity of infection dependent. The *Chlamydia pneumoniae* antiproliferative effect is linked to T cell death associated with caspase 1, 8, 9, and IL-1β production, indicating that both apoptotic and proapoptotic cellular death pathways is activated after pathogen-T cell interactions (Olivares-Zavaleta et al., 2011).

Although T-cell activation during acute *Chlamydia pneumoniae* infections has been described, little is known about the frequency or the role of the *Chlamydia pneumoniae*-specific memory T cells that reside in the human body after the resolution of the infection. The analysis of *Chlamydia pneumoniae*-induced T-cell responses in peripheral blood mononuclear cells showed that following short-term stimulation with *Chlamydia pneumoniae,* both gamma interferon (IFN-γ)- and interleukin-2 (IL-2)-producing CD4 (+) T-cell responses could be detected in some PBMC culture from healthy individuals. *Chlamydia pneumoniae*-activated CD4(+) T cells expressed CD154, a marker for T-cell receptor-dependent activation, and displayed a phenotype of central memory T cells showing dominant IL-2 production but also IFN-gamma production.

Interestingly, individuals with both IFNγ and IL-2-producing responses showed significantly decreased immunoglobulin G reactivity toward *Chlamydia pneumoniae* RpoA and DnaK, antigens known to be strongly upregulated during chlamydial persistence, compared to IgG reactivity of seropositive individuals with no T-cell response or CD4(+) T-cell responses involving the production of a single cytokine (IFN-γ or IL-2). Among seropositive individuals, the presence or the absence of dual IFN-γ and IL-2-producing T-cell responses was associated with distinct patterns of antibody responses toward persistence-associated *Chlamydia pneumoniae* antigens.

4. *Chlamydia pneumoniae* infection and chronic diseases with immunopathological background

There are many seroepidemiological, pathological, animal, immunological and antibiotic treatment studies demonstrating the role of chlamydial infection in atherosclerosis. EBs of *Chlamydia pneumoniae* is internalized by endocytosis in the alveolar macrophages, and differentiates in RBs, which are multiplying. Circulating monocytes are infected and the appearance of chlamydial inclusions in the vascular endothelium modulates their adhesion. The adhered macrophages migrate later in the intimate of blood vessels, where they cause infection of other cell types, including arterial macrophages, which will start to accumulate LDL (low density lipoproteins), getting a "foamy" aspect because of the stored cholesterol. Under nonatherogenic conditions, LDL uptake causes the transcriptional downregulation of its receptor. Scavenger receptors, however, may bypass this control by allowing the endocytosis of modified LDL. *Chlamydia pneumoniae* heat shock protein–60 (cHsp60) was found to induce cellular oxidation of LDL cholesterol, while *Chlamydia pneumoniae* LPS as the antigen that could enhance LDL cholesterol uptake and downregulate cholesterol efflux in monocytes and macrophages (Kalayoglu et al., 2002; Higgins, 2003).

Smooth muscle fibers will also be infected by the EBs and will proliferate, and infected endothelial cells will secrete a number of cytokines, which will ultimately lead to the destabilization of the ateromatous plaque and thrombus formation, with an increased risk of myocardial infarction.

Currently, serological methods could fail in detecting chronic or persistent *Chlamydia pneumoniae* infection and other blood markers such as *Chlamydia pneumoniae* immune complexes and circulating leukocytes, e.g. macrophages with detectable *Chlamydia pneumoniae* DNA and mRNA as markers of underlying infection are needed (Ngeh et al., 2002; Ngeh & Gupta, 2002). The association of some inflammatory markers such as C-reactive protein (CRP) with *Chlamydia pneumoniae* serology has indicated the existence of some correlations between "infectious" and "inflammatory" burdens and atherosclerosis (Leinonen & Saikku, 2002). Cytokines released by these immune cells, such as IL-6, induce acute phase response proteins, and elevated CRP levels, (a marker for atherosclerosis) are an indication of chronic inflammation. The inflammatory nature of the early atheroma causes modifications to LDL, which allow the molecule to bypass the usual regulatory mechanisms for entry into cells, thus facilitating foamy cell formation. Furthermore, the effect of inflammation on endothelial cells allows for greater arterial permeability to LDL and increased adhesion molecule expression and diapedesis of leukocytes.

The presence of *Chlamydia pneumoniae* was evidenced by different methods including immunocytochemistry, PCR, *in situ* hybridization and electron microscopy not only in coronary arteries, but also in cerebral, carotid, internal mammary, pulmonary, aorta, renal, iliac, femoral, and popliteal arteries, and occluded bypass grafts, obtained from postmortem and surgical atheromatous tissues (Leinonen & Saikku, 2002; Ngeh et al., 2002, Ngeh & Gupta, 2002, Rassu et al., 2001). However, it must be taken into account that *Chlamydia pneumoniae* can also be detected in about 10% of noncardiovascular and granulomatous tissues, showing a nonspecific, ubiquitous distribution in the human body (Ngeh et al., 2002, Ngeh & Gupta, 2002).

Animal models have shown that *Chlamydia pneumoniae* infection could initiate and accelerate atherosclerotic process. Repeated *Chlamydia pneumoniae* infection in genetically modified mouse such as ApoE-deficient mouse known to develop atherosclerosis in the absence of a fatty diet in has been shown to accelerate atherosclerotic lesion progression by specifically increasing the T lymphocyte influx in the atherosclerotic plaques and accelerating the formation of more advanced atherosclerotic lesions (Ezzahiri et al., 2002).

The exact pathogenesis of multiple sclerosis (MS), the most common demyelinating disease of the central nervous system (CNS) (Noseworthy, 1999; Nosewrothy et al., 2002) remains unknown, but current hypothesis are reffering to an autoimmune background that may be influenced by an infectious process. *Chlamydia pneumoniae* has been found to be associated with the rapidly progressive multiple sclerosis (Sriram et al., 1998), or relapsing multiple sclerosis, markedly improved after targeted antimicrobial therapy (Sriram et al., 1999)

The association between *Chlamydia pneumoniae* and multiple sclerosis was demonstrated in experimental pathogenesis, showing that after intraperitoneal inoculation of mice with *Chlamydia pneumoniae,* following immunization with neural antigens, an increased severity of experimental allergic encephalitis (EAE), an animal model of multiple sclerosis was observed. An attenuation of EAE following therapy with the antimicrobial agent fluorphenicol (Du et al., 2002) was observed. Persistence of *Chlamydia pneumoniae* in the CNS is likely to provide an environment that can lead to the activation of autoreactive T cells and contribute to the pathogenesis of a chronic disease such as multiple sclerosis (Stratton & Sriram, 2004).

Alzheimer's disease (AD) is a progressive neurodegenerative condition that accounts for the most common and severe form of dementia in the elderly The pathology observed in the brain includes neuritic senile plaques, neurofibrillary tangles, neuropil threads and deposits of cerebrovascular amyloid (Balin et al., 2005).

Balin et al. (1998) demonstrated by polymerase chain reaction (PCR) that the DNA of *Chlamydia pneumoniae* was present in 90% of postmortem brain samples examined from sporadic AD.). Immunohistochemistry revealed the presence of *Chlamydia pneumoniae* antigens *in* perivascular macrophages, microglia, and astroglial cells in areas of the temporal cortices, hippocampus, parietal cortex, and prefrontal cortex in AD patients, but not in control samples. Electron microscopy revealed chlamydial inclusions that contained elementary (EB) and reticulate (RB) bodies. Microglia responds to insult with the production of proinflammatory cytokines, and the generation of reactive oxygen species and other products (Simpson et al., 1998). Monocytes acutely or chronically *in vitro* infected with *Chlamydia pneumoniae* appeared to increase the expression of amyloid precursor protein as well as the increased breakdown of the precursor into fragments that contained 1-40 immunoreactive epitopes, generating the initial focal points for amyloid deposition (Balin et al., 2004).

The way by which *Chlamydia pneumoniae* croos the blood–brain barrier to reach the central nervous system is probably represented by the circulating monocytes infected with *Chlamydia pneumoniae* (Boman et al., 1998; Airenne et al., 1999). The transmigration is facilitated by the increased surface expression of the surface adhesins on the endothelial cells and the integrins on the monocytes. *Chlamydia pneumoniae* may reach into the central nervous system through the the olfactory neuroepithelium of the nasal olfactory system, in direct contact with the infected epithelial cells.

Reactive arthritis is a sterile immune-mediated pathogenesis process of the joint that follows bacterial infection of either the gastrointestinal or urogenital system (Whittum-Hudson et al., 2004). Chronic reactive arthritis associated with chlamydial infection is manifested with activation of TH1/TH2 CD4+ cells and macrophages at sites of inflammation (Carter & Dutton, 1996). In addition, at sites of chlamydial infections, proinflammatory cytokines IL-6, and TH1-associated cytokines and IL-12 have been identified (Mosmann & Coffman, 1989).

It is not clear whether chlamydial infection elicits an inflammatory response because of upregulated cytokine production in infected or neighbouring cells, or if the immune response to infected cells drives the inflammatory response via influx of cytokine-producing lymphocytes and macrophages. Nonetheless, synovial materials have been studied for the panel of cytokines present in *Chlamydia trachomatis*- and *Chlamydia pneumoniae*-induced inflammatory arthritis. After development of inflammation, Th1/Th2 CD4+ cells, as well as CD8+ cells and macrophages, have been detected in synovial fluid (Simon et al., 1993). Many studies have indicated that, in patient materials from individuals with early disease, proinflammatory cytokines such as IL-12 and are prominent (Kotake et al., 1999; Simon et al., 1993). In *Chlamydia trachomatis*-infected joint tissues from chronic reactive arthritis patients, IL-10, IL-8, IL-15 and MCP-1t (Gérard et al., 2002) have been identified. In the same study, it was shown that in synovial tissue samples from arthritis patients chronically infected at that site with *Chlamydia pneumoniae,* essentially only mRNA encoding IL-8, and RANTES were present.

Acute *Chlamydia pneumoniae* infection can cause acute bronchitis and pneumonia, and lower respiratory tract illnesses can develop into asthma and chronic bronchitis. Chronic *Chlamydia pneumoniae* infection has also been associated with a wide variety of chronic upper-airway illnesses, as well as with acute and chronic lower-airway conditions including acute bronchitis, asthma and COPD.

Chlamydia pneumoniae infection could have three distinguishable causal effects: acute asthma *exacerbations* (Allegra et al., 1994, Clementsen et al., 2002); *promoting* asthma severity (von Hertzen, 2002); or *initiate* asthma (Hahn et al., 2005).

A significant association between asthma and *Chlamydia pneumoniae*-specific IgA (Hahn et al., 2000, Genkay et al., 2001, Falk et al., 2002) and also with chlamydial heat shock protein-60 (Hsp60) antibodies (Roblin et al., 2000, Huttinen et al., 2001) has been reported by different authors.

It is already established that the inflammatory processes of chlamydial pathogenesis are elicited by infected host cells and are necessary and sufficient to account for chronic and intense inflammation and the promotion of cellular proliferation, tissue remodelling and scarring, the ultimate cause of disease sequelae (Stephens, 2003).

One mechanism by which infection can initiate autoimmune disease is molecular mimicry, the phenomenon of protein products from dissimilar genes sharing similar structures that elicit an immune response to both self and microbial proteins. The strongest cases for molecular mimicry seem to have been made for chlamydial heat shock proteins 60, the DNA primase of *Chlamydia trachomatis*, and chlamydial OmcB proteins (Bachmaier & Penninger, 2005). So, the HSPs are expressed by cells within atherosclerotic plaques, and anti-HSP antibodies serum titres have been reported to be positively related to future risk of coronary heart disease. On the other hand, purified anti-HSP antibodies recognise and mediate the lysis of stressed human endothelial cells and macrophages *in vitro* and future immunisation with HSP exacerbates atherosclerosis in experimental animal models. Taking into account that some human vaccines, such as BCG, contain HSPs, hence although vaccination programmes are vital for maintaining 'herd' immunity and the prevention of serious infectious disease, they may leave a legacy of increased susceptibility to atherosclerosis (Lamb et al., 2003).

To investigate the conditions under which autoimmune responses can be generated against self hsp60, Yi et al., (1997) demonstrated that autoimmune responses characterized by strong T-cell proliferation and high titers of antibody to self hsp60 are induced only by concurrent immunization with mouse and chlamydial hsp60. They observed that switches in cytokine production patterns may mediate the pathogenesis of hsp60-associated *Chlamydia trachomatis* immunopathology. Immunization with mouse hsp60 alone induced lymphocytes that secreted high levels of interleukin-10 (IL-10) but did not proliferate in response to *in vitro* stimulation with mouse hsp60. On the other hand, co-immunization with mouse and chlamydial hsp60s induced lymphocytes that proliferated strongly in response to mouse hsp60, secreted 6-fold less IL-10, and exhibited a 12-fold increase in the ratio of IFNγ /IL-10 production (Yi et al., 1997). The development of infertility is reported due to enhanced immune responses to *Chlamydia trachomatis* (Debattista et al., 2003), and cHSP60 and cHSP10 antibodies seem to perform well in predicting tubal factor infertility (Spandorfer et al., 1999; LaVerda et al., 2000; den Hartog et al., 2005; Dadamessi et al., 2005; Linhares & Witkin, 2010). During *Chlamydia* infection a crucial for controlling the duration of infection and subsequent tubal pathology have Th1/Th2 responses: Th1 cells produce IFN-γ that promotes the destruction of *Chlamydia* (Beatty et al., 1993), but can also promote inflammatory damage and fibrosis (Rottenberg et al., 2002) whereas Th2 cells produce IL-4, IL-5, and IL-13 believed to be critical for defense against extracellular pathogens. The production of TNF-α and IL-10 was examined because their levels have been reported to be high in cervical secretions of *Chlamydia trachomatis* infected infertile women (Reddy et al., 2004). In order to elucidate the actual role in the cause of infertility, Srivastava et al., (2008) studied the specific cytokine responses of mononuclear cells from the infectious site to cHSP60 and cHSP10. Exposure to chlamydial heat shock proteins (cHSP60 and cHSP10) could significantly affect mucosal immune function by increasing the release of IFN-γ, IL-10 and TNF-alpha by cervical mononuclear cells, much more in infertile group as compared to fertile group.

5. Conclusion

Chlamydia infection has excited considerable attention in the last time research, not only as a genital or respiratory pathogen but because of its association with a number of acute and chronic diseases. The true significance of *Chlamydia* infection in the development of chronic manifestations still remains puzzling. The factors that drive immune responses to pathogenic species, the role of host genetic background, HLA molecules and cytokine gene polymorphism, environmental and epidemiological factors, mixed infections, and species or dose of the infecting agent probably all interact in a final balance of the immune defense mechanisms. Chlamydial infections *in vivo* typically result in chronic inflammation characterized cellularly by the presence of activated monocytes and macrophages and by the secretion of Th-1/Th-2 cytokines, which could lead to the dysregulation of the immune response resulting in autoimmune diseases. Understanding the mechanisms by which chlamydial infections, especially chronic and persistent ones interfere with the host immune defence system is necessary to develop better therapies to treat and possibly even prevent *Chlamydia* associated diseases. However, the early identification and treatment of genital chlamydial infection of women, of eye infection in children and of *Chlamydia pneumoniae* in chronic airways disease will be important to prevent the development of chronic sequelae, with immunological basis.

6. Acknowledgment

Acknowledgement: to the ANCS bilateral project Romania -Republic of Moldavia, no 423/04.06.2010 and National Project PN2 42119/2008 and PN2 42150/2008.

7. References

Airenne, S.; Kinnunen, A.; Leinonen, M.; Saikku, P. & Surcel, H.M. (2002). Secretion of IL-10 and IL-12 in *Chlamydia pneumoniae* infected human monocytes, presented at *Chlamydial Infections Proceedings of the Tenth International Symposium on Human Chlamydial Infections,* Antalya, Turkey.

Allegra, L.; Blasi, F.; Centanni, S.; Cosentini, R.; Denti, F.; Raccanelli, R.; Tarsia, P. & Valenti, V. (1994). Acute exacerbations of asthma in adults: Role of *Chlamydia pneumoniae* infection, *Eur. Respir.J.* Vol. 7, pp. 2165–2168.

Airenne, S.; Surcel, H.M.; Alakarppa, H.; Laitinen, K.; Paavonen, J.; Saikku, P. & Laurila, A. (1999). *Chlamydia pneumoniae* infection in human monocytes, *Infect. Immun.* Vol. 67, pp. 1445–1449. [published erratum appears in *Infect. Immun.* (1999) 67:6716].

Bachmaier, K. & Penninger, J.M. (2005). Chlamydia and antigenic mimicry. Curr Top Microbiol Immunol. Vol. 296, pp.153-63.

Balin, B.J.; Hammond, C.J.; Little, C.S.; Macintyre, A. & Appelt, D.M. (2005). Chlamydia pneumoniae in the Pathogenesis of Alzheimer's Disease, In: Chlamydia pneumoniae: Infection and disease. Friedman H., Yamamoto Y, Bendinelli M. pp. 211-226, Ed. Kluwer Academic Publishers, ISBN 0-306-48487-0, New York.

Balin, B.J.; Gerard, H.C.; Arking, E.J.; Appelt, D.M.; Branigan, P.J.; Abrams, J.T.; Whittum-Hudson, J.A. & Hudson, A.P. (1998). Identification and localization of *Chlamydia pneumoniae* in the Alzheimer's brain, *Med. Microbiol. Immunol.* Vol. 187, pp. 23–42.

Barnes, R.C. (1990). Infections Caused by *Chlamydia trachomatis,* In *Sexually Transmitted Diseases.* Morse. SA, Moreland AA, Thompson SE, eds, J.B. Lippincott. Philadelphia

Beatty, W.L.; Byrne, G.I. & Morrison, R.P. (1993). Morphologic and antigenic characterization of interferon gamma-mediated persistent *Chlamydia trachomatis* infection in vitro. *Proc Natl Acad Sci USA,* Vol. 90, pp. 3998-4002.

Boman, J.; Soderberg, S.; Forsberg, J.; Birgander, L.S.; Allard, A.; Persson, K.; Jidell, E.; Kumlin, U.; Juto, P.; Waldenstrom, A. & Wadell, G. (1998). High prevalence of *Chlamydia pneumoniae* DNA in peripheral blood mononuclear cells in patients with cardiovascular disease and in middle-aged blood donors, *J. Infect. Dis. Vol.* 178, pp. 274–277.

Campbell, L.A. & Kuo, C.C. (2004). *Chlamydia pneumoniae* – an infectious risk factor for atherosclerosis? *Nature Reviews Microbiology*, Vol. 2, pp. 23-32.

Carter, L.L. & Dutton, R. W. (1996). Type 1 and Type 2: A fundamental dichotomy for all T-cell subsets, *Curr. Opin. Immunol.*, Vol. 8, pp. 336–342.

Caspar-Bauguil, S.; Puissant, B.; Nazzal, D.; Lefevre, J.C.; Thomsen, M.; Salvayre, R. & Benoist, H. (2000). *Chlamydia pneumoniae* induces interleukin-10 production that downregulates major histocompatibility complex class I expression, *J. Infect. Dis.* Vol. 182, No. 5, pp. 1394-1401.

Clementsen, P.; Permin, H. & Norn, S. (2002). *Chlamydia pneumoniae* infection and its role in asthma and chronic obstructive pulmonary disease, *J. Invest. Allergol. Clin. Immunol.* Vol. 12, pp. 73–79.

Dadamessi, I.; Eb, F. & Betsou. F. (2005). Combined detection of *Chlamydia trachomatis* specific-antibodies against the 10 and 60-kDa heat shock proteins as a diagnostic tool for tubal factor infertility: Results from a case-control study in Cameroon. *FEMS Immunol Med Microbiol*, Vol. 45, pp. 31-35.

Debattista, J.; Timms, P.; Allan, J. & Allan, J. (2003). Immunopathogenesis of chlamydia trachomatis infections in women. Fertil Steril. Vol. 79, No. 6, pp. 1273-1287.

den Hartog JE, Land JA, Stassen FR, Kessels AG, Bruggeman CA: Serological markers of persistent *Chlamydia trachomatis* infections in women with tubal factor subfertility. *Hum Reprod* 2005, 20:986-990.Debattista, J.; Timms, P.; Allan, J. & Allan, J. (2003). Immunopathogenesis of *Chlamydia trachomatis* infections in women. *Fertil Steril.* Vol. 79, pp. 1273-1287.

Du, C.; Yi-Yao, S.; Rose, A. & Sriram, S. (2002). *Chlamydia pneumoniae* infection of the central nervous system worsens EAE, *J. Exp. Med.*, Vol. 196, pp. 1639–1644.

Ezzahiri, R.; Nelissen-Vrancken, H.J.M.G.; Kurvers, H.A.J.M.; Stassen, F.R.M.; Vliegen, I.; Grauls, G.E.L.M.; van Pul, M.M.L.; Kitslaar, P.J.E.H.M. & Bruggeman, C.A. (2002). Chlamydophila pneumoniae (*Chlamydia pneumoniae*) accelerates the formation of complex atherosclerotic lesions in Apo E3-Leiden mice, *Cardiovasc. Res.* Vol. 56, pp. 269–276.

Falck, G.; Gnarpe, J.; Hansson, L.O.; Svärdsudd, K. & Gnarpe, H. (2002). Comparison of individuals with and without specific IgA antibodies to *Chlamydia pneumoniae.* Respiratory morbidity and the metabolic syndrome, *Chest*, Vol. 122, pp. 1587–1593.

Fan, P.; Dong, F.; Huang, Y. & Zhong, G. (2002). *Chlamydia pneumoniae* secretion of a protease-like activity factor for degrading host cell transcription factors is required for major histocompatibility complex antigen expression, *Infect. Immun.* Vol. 70, No. 3, pp. 345-349.

Gencay, M.; Rüdiger, J.J.; Tamm, M.; Solér, M.; Perruchoud, A.P. & Roth, M. (2001). Increased frequency of *Chlamydia pneumoniae* antibodies in patients with asthma, *Am.J.Respir. Crit. Care Med.* Vol. 163, pp. 1097–1100.

Gérard, H.C.; Wang, Z.; Whittum-Hudson, J.A.; El-Gabalawy, H.; Goldbach-Mansky, R.; Bardin, T.; Schumacher, H.R. & Hudson, A.P. (2002). Cytokine and chemokine mRNA produced in synovial tissue chronically infected with Chlamydia trachomatis and Chlamydia pneumoniae, J. Rheumatol. Vol. 29, pp. 1827–1835.

Grayston, J.T. (2002) Background and current knowledge *of Chlamydia pneumoniae* and atherosclerosis, *J. Infect. Dis.* Vol. 181, S3, pp. S402-S410.

Hahn, D.L.; Peeling, R.W.; Dillon, E.; McDonald, R. & Saikku, P. (2000). Serologic markers for *Chlamydia pneumoniae* in asthma, *Ann. Allergy Asthma Immunol.* Vol. 84, No. 2, 227–233.

Hahn D.L. (2005). Role of *Chlamydia pneumonia* as an Inducer of Asthma. *In* Friedman H., Yamamoto Y, Bendinelli *M. ed. Infectious agents and pathogenesis.* Kluwer Academic/Plenum Publishers, pp. 1-10.

Halme, S.; Latvala, J.; Karttunen, R.; Palatsi, I.; Saikku, P. & Surcel, H.M. (2000). Cell-mediated immune response during primary *Chlamydia pneumoniae* infection, *Infect. Immun.* Vol. 68, No. 12, pp. 7156-7158.

Halme, S.; Syrjälä, H.; Bloigu, A.; Saikku, P.; Leinonen, M.; Airaksinen,J. & Surcel, H.M. (1997). Lymphocyte responses to *Chlamydia antigens* in patients with coronary heart disease, *Eur. Heart J.* Vol. 18, No. 7, pp. 1095-1101.

Hatch, T.P. (1996). Disulfide Cross-Linked Envelope Proteins: the Functional Equivalent of Peptidoglycan in Chlamydia? J. Bacteriol., Vol. 178, No. 1, pp. 1-5.

Higgins, J.P. (2003). *Chlamydia pneumoniae* and coronary artery disease: The antibiotic trials, *Mayo Clin. Proc.* Vol. 78, No. 3, pp. 321–332.

Kalayoglu, M.V.; Libby, P. & Byrne, G.I. (2002). *Chlamydia pneumoniae* as an emerging risk factor in cardiovascular disease, *JAMA* Vol. 288, pp. 2724–2731.

Kotake, S.; Schumacher, H.R.; Arayssi, T.K.; Gérard, H.C.; Branigan, P.J.; Hudson, A.P.; Yarboro, C.H.; Klippel, J.H. & Wilder, R.L. (1999). IL-10, and IL-12 p40 gene expression in synovial tissues from patients with recent-onset *Chlamydia*-associated arthritis, *Infect. Immun.* Vol. 67, pp. 2682–2686.

Kuo, C.C.; Jackson, L.A.; Campbell, L.A. & Grayston, J.T. (1995). *Chlamydia pneumoniae* (TWAR), *Clin. Microbiol. Rev.* Vol. 8, No. 4, pp. 451-461.

LaVerda, D.; Albanese, L.N.; Ruther, P.E.; Morrison, S.G.; Morrison, R.P.; Ault, K.A. & Byrne, G.I. (2000). Seroreactivity to *Chlamydia trachomatis* Hsp10 correlates with severity of human genital tract disease. *Infect Immun*, Vol. 68, No. 1, pp. 303-309.

Lamb DJ, El-Sankary W, Ferns GA. 2003 Molecular mimicry in atherosclerosis: a role for heat shock proteins in immunisation. Atherosclerosis. Vol. 167, No. 2, pp. 177-85.

Lazar, V.; Balotescu, M.C.; Cernat, R.; Bulai, D. & Stewart-Tull, D. (2005). *Imunobiologie*, Ed. Univ. din Bucuresti, Bucharest, 250 p. ISBN-973-73-7124-0

Leinonen, M. & Saikku, P. (2002). Evidence for infectious agents in cardiovascular disease and atherosclerosis, *Lancet Infect. Dis.* Vol. 2, No. 2, pp. 11–17.

Linhares, I.M. & Witkin, S.S. (2010). Immunopathogenic consequences of Chlamydia trachomatis 60 kDa heat shock protein expression in the female reproductive tract. *Cell Stress Chaperones.* Vol. 15, No. 5, pp. 467-473.

Lipscomb, M.F.; Bice, D.E.; Lyons, C.R.; Schuyler, M.R. & Wilkes, D. (1995). The regulation of pulmonary immunity, *Adv. Immunol.* Vol. 59, pp. 369-455.

Madigan, M.; Martinko, J.; Parker, J. (2008). In *Brock's Biology of Microorganisms.* (12th Edition), ISBN 0132324601, New Jersey: Prentice Hall.

Matsumoto, A.; Bessho, H.; Uehira, K. & Suda, T. (1991). Morphological studies of the association of mitochondria with chlamydial inclusions and the fusion of chlamydial inclusions, *J. Electron Microsc.* Vol. 40, No. 5, pp. 356–363.

Mihăescu, G. & Chifiriuc, M.C. (2009). Organizarea sistemului imunitar la vertebrate, 2009, in vol. *Imunogenetică şi Oncogenetică*, Ed. Academia Român .

Mihăescu, G.; Chifiriuc, C.; Ditu, L.M. (2009) *Imunobiologie,* Ed. Univ. din Bucuresti, 572 p., 978-973-737-734-0.

Mosmann, T. R. & Coffman, R. L., (1989). TH1 and TH2 cells: Different patterns of lymphokine secretion lead to different functional properties, *Annu. Rev. Immunol.* Vol. 7, pp. 145–173.

Nakajo, M.N.; Roblin, P.M.; Hammerschlag, M.R.; Smith, P. & Nowakowski, M. (1990). Chlamydicidal activity of human alveolar macrophages, *Infect. Immun.* Vol. 58, No. 11, pp. 3640-3644.

Natividad, A.; Hull, J.; Luoni, G.; Holland, M.; Rockett, K.; Joof, H.; Burton, M.; Mabey, D.; Kwiatkowski, D.& Bailey, R. (2009). Innate immunity in ocular Chlamydia trachomatis infection: contribution of IL8 and CSF2 gene variants to risk of trachomatous scarring in Gambians. *MC Med Genet.* Vol. 10, pp.138. doi:10.1186/1471-2350-10-138

Ngeh.J.; Anand, V. & Gupta, S. (2002). *Chlamydia pneumoniae* and atherosclerosis-what we know and what we don't, *Clin. Microbiol. Infect.* Vol. 8, No. 1, pp. 2–13.

Ngeh, J. & Gupta, S. (2002). Inflammation and infection in coronary artery disease, in: *Cardiology: Current Perspectives* (G.Jackson, ed.), Martin Dunitz Ltd., London., 125–144.

Noseworthy, J.H. (1999). Progress in determining the causes and treatment of multiple sclerosis, *Nature,* Vol. 399, 6738 Suppl., pp. A40–A47.

Noseworthy, J.H.; Lucchinetti, C.; Rodriguez, M. & Weinshenker, B.G. (2000). Multiple Sclerosis, *New. Eng.J. Med.,* Vol. 343, No. 13, pp. 938–946.

Olivares-Zavaleta, N.; Carmody, A.; Messer, R.; Whitmire, W.M. & Caldwell, H.D. (2011). Chlamydia pneumoniae inhibits activated human T lymphocyte proliferation by the induction of apoptotic and pyroptotic pathways. *J Immunol.* Vol. 186, No. 12, pp. 7120-7126.

Prebeck, S.; Kirschning, C.; Durr, S.; da Costa, C.; Donath, B.; Brand, K.; Redecke, V.; Wagner, H. & Miethke, T. (2001). Predominant role of toll-like receptor 2 versus 4 in *Chlamydia pneumoniae*–induced activation of dendritic cells, *J. Immunol.* Vol. 167, No. 6, 3316-3323.

Rassu, M.; Cazzavillan, S.; Scagnelli, M.; Peron, A.; Bevilacqua, P. A.; Facco, M.; Bertoloni, G.; Lauro, F. M.; Zambello, R. & Bonoldi, E. (2001). Demonstration of *Chlamydia pneumoniae* in atherosclerotic arteries from various vascular regions, *Atherosclerosis,* Vol. 158, No. 1, pp.73–79.

Reddy, B.S.; Rastogi, S.; Das, B.; Salhan, S.; Verma, S. & Mittal, A. (2004). Cytokine expression pattern in the genital tract of *Chlamydia trachomatis* positive infertile women - implication for T-cell responses. *Clin Exp Immunol,* Vol. 137, No. 3, pp. 552-558.

Redecke, V.; Dalhoff, K.; Bohnet, S.; Braun, J. & Maass, M. (1998). Interaction of *Chlamydia pneumoniae* and human alveolar macrophages: Infection and inflammatory response, *Am. J. Resp. Cell. Mol. Biol.* Vol. 19, No. 5, pp. 721-727.

Rottenberg, M.E.; Gigliotti-Rothfuchs, A. & Wigzell, H. (2002). The role of IFN-gamma in the outcome of chlamydial infection. *Curr Opin Immunol,* Vol. 14, pp. 444-451.

Roblin, P.M.; Witkin, S.S.; Weiss, S.M.; Gelling, M. & Hammerschlag, M.R. (2000). Immune response to *Chlamydia pneumoniae* in patients with asthma: Role of heat shock proteins (HSPs), in: *Proceedings: Fourth Meeting of the European Society for Chlamydia Research,* Helsinki, Finland, Esculapio, Bologna, Italy, p. 209.

Severin, J.A. & Ossewaarde J.M. (2006) Innate immunity in defense against Chlamydia trachomatis infections. Drugs Today (Barc). Vo. 42, Suppl A:75-81.

Shirai, M.; Hirakawa, H.; Kimoto, M.; Tabuchi, M.; Kishi, F.; Ouchi, K.; Shiba, T.; Ishii, K.; Hattori, S.; Kuhara, S. & Nakazawa, T. (2000). Comparison of whole genome sequencesof *Chlamydia pneumoniae* J 138 from Japan and CWL 029 from USA, *Nucleic Acid Res.* Vol. 28, No. 12, pp. 2311–2314.

Simon, A.K.; Seipelt, E.; Wu, P.; Wenzel, B.; Braun, J. & Sieper, J. (1993). Analysis of cytokine profiles in synovial T cell clones from chlamydial reactive arthritis patients: Predominance of the Th1 subset, Clin. Exp. Immunol. Vol. 94, pp. 122–126.

Simpson, J.E.; Newcombe, J.; Cuzner, M.L. & Woodroofe, M.N. (1998). Expression of monocyte chemoattractant protein-1 and other beta-chemokines by resident glia and inflammatory cells in multiple sclerosis lesions, *J. Neuroimmunol.*Vol. 84, pp. 238–249.

Spandorfer, S.D.; Neuer, A.; LaVerda, D.; Byrne, G.; Liu, H.C.; Rosenwaks, Z. & Witkin, S.S. (1999). Previously undetected *Chlamydia trachomatis* infection, immunity to heat shock proteins and tubal occlusion in women undergoing in-vitro fertilization. *Hum Reprod,* Vol. 14, No. 1, pp. 60-64.

Sriram, S.; Mitchell, W. & Stratton, C. (1998). Multiple sclerosis associated with *Chlamydia pneumoniae* infection of the CNS, *Neurology,* Vol. 50, No. 2, pp. 571–572.

Sriram, S.; Stratton, C.W.; Yao, S.; Tharp, A.; Ding, L.; Bannan, J.D. & Mitchell, W.M. (1999). *C. pneumoniae* infection of the CNS in MS, *Ann. Neurol.* Vol. 46, No. 1, pp. 6–14.

Srivastava, P.; Jha, R.; Bas, S.; Salhan, S. & Mittal, A. (2008). In infertile women, cells from Chlamydia trachomatis infected sites release higher levels of interferon-gamma, interleukin-10 and tumor necrosis factor-alpha upon heat-shock-protein stimulation than fertile women. Reprod Biol Endocrinol. Vol. 6, pp. 20, doi:10.1186/1477-7827-6-20.

Stephens RS. (2003). The cellular paradigm of chlamydial pathogenesis. *Trends Microbiol.* Vol. 11, No. 1, pp. 44-51.

Stratton, C.W. & Sriram, S. (2005). *Chlamydia pneumoniae* as a candidate pathogen in multiple sclerosis. Chlamydia pneumoniae*: Infection and disease.* In: Chlamydia pneumoniae: Infection and disease. Friedman H., Yamamoto Y, Bendinelli M. pp. 199-210, Ed. Kluwer Academic Publishers, ISBN 0-306-48487-0, New York.

Surcel H.M. (2005). *Chlamydia pneumoniae* Infection and Diseases: Immunity to *Chlamydia Pneumoniae,* In: Chlamydia pneumoniae: Infection and disease. Friedman H., Yamamoto Y, Bendinelli M. pp. 81-98, Ed. Kluwer Academic Publishers, ISBN 0-306-48487-0, New York.

Thylefors, B.; Negrel, A.D.; Pararajasegaram, R. & Dadzie K.Y. (1995). Global data on blindness. *Bull World Health Organ,* Vol. 73, No. 1, pp. 115-121.

Yi, Y.; Yang, X. & Brunham, R.C. (1997). Autoimmunity to heat shock protein 60 and antigen-specific production of interleukin-10. Infect Immun. Vol. 65, No. 5, pp. 1669-74.

von Hertzen, L., Vasankari, T., Liippo, K., Wahlström, E. & Puolakkainen, M. (2002). *Chlamydia pneumoniae* and severity of asthma, *Scand. J. Infect. Dis.* Vol. 34, No. 1, pp. 22–27.

Whittum-Hudson, J.A.; Schumacher, H.R. & Hudson A.P. (2005). *Chlamydia pneumoniae* and Inflammatory Arthritis, In: Chlamydia pneumoniae: Infection and disease. Friedman H., Yamamoto Y, Bendinelli M. pp. 227-238, Ed. Kluwer Academic Publishers, ISBN 0-306-48487-0, New York.

Zhong, G.; Fan, P.; Ji, H.; Dong, F. & Huang, Y. (2001). Identification of a chlamydial protease-like activity factor responsible for the degradation of host transcription factors, *J. Exp. Med.* Vol. 193, No. 8, pp. 935-942.

5

The Role of T Regulatory Cells in *Chlamydia trachomatis* Genital Infection

Kathleen A. Kelly, Cheryl I. Champion and Janina Jiang
Department of Pathology and Laboratory Medicine, David Geffen School of Medicine at UCLA, University of California, Los Angeles
USA

1. Introduction

T cell-mediated immune suppression of adaptive immune responses is important for the homeostatic function of tissues. Compelling evidence has found that the normal immune system produces T cells with a specialized function in immune suppression and this type of T cell is called a regulatory T cell (TRC). There are various types of TRCs with suppressive function. The majority of TRCs express the transcription factor called forkhead box p3 or Foxp3, and play a pivotal role in the maintenance of immune tolerance by preventing autoimmunity and rejection of transplanted tissue [Grazia Roncarolo et al., 2006; Sakaguchi et al., 2008]. Recently TRCs have also been implicated in preventing inflammatory diseases. Extensive evidence has shown that TRCs exacerbate and suppress inflammatory responses in various diseases, including the human multiple sclerosis model, experimental autoimmune encephalomyelitis (EAE) [Farias et al., 2011] and chronic inflammatory bowel disease [Veltkamp et al., 2011]. TRCs also play major roles in regulating immunity to infections of viral, bacterial or parasitic pathogens. TRCs dampen immune response which control pathogen replication. In many instances, these responses increase pathogen survival. Alternatively, TRCs can also limit collateral tissue damage caused by powerful immune responses directed toward microbes [Belkaid & Tarbell, 2009]. However, tumors and microbes commandeer the immune suppressive properties of TRCs to evade host immunity and cause disease. This is especially prominent at mucosal tissues since they are exposed to a plethora of pathogens. In this review, we will introduce the broad category of TRCs with focus on their phenotype, function and role in maintaining mucosal tissues, especially of the genital tract.

2. Characterization of T regulatory cells in mice and humans

Control of immune responses is critical to host survival and there are many mechanisms that can mediate control. Intrinsic control mechanisms exist which are programmed as the immune system develops. However, control also exists at the cellular level and involves interaction with specialized TRCs. TRCs are categorized into two general compartments based on their origin, mechanism of action, and generation; natural TRCs (nTRCs) or induced TRCs (iTRCs). The distinction between the two has been blurred by showing that regulatory function can be induced in previously non-regulatory T cells. T regulatory functions can be induced by signals received in the environment such as; regulatory cytokines, immunosuppressive drugs and antigen presenting cells (APC) modified by infectious agents [Belkaid & Tarbell, 2009]. Thus, iTRCs can be further divided into Tr1 cells which secrete IL-10, TRCs which secrete TGF-β and TRCs which express Foxp3. However, all of these markers of T regulatory function, with the exception of Foxp3, do not always correlate with suppressive function. The finding that loss of function mutations in the Foxp3 gene of humans lead to a severe multi-organ autoimmune and inflammatory syndrome called immunodysregulation polyendocrinopathy enteropathy X-linked syndrome (IPEX) and a similar disorder in scurfy mice allowed the definitive identification of TRC [Bennett et al., 2001; Brunkow et al., 2001; Chatila et al., 2000; Wildin et al., 2001].

Subsequent studies focused on the ability of Foxp3$^+$ cells to cause various tissue pathologies. Foxp3 is primarily expressed in CD4 cells. The first approach was in knock-in mice which showed that cell-intrinsic regulatory functions did not rely on Foxp3 but it was indispensible for lack of expression and was responsible for disease in humans and mice

[Chen et al., 2005; Fontenot et al., 2003; Fontenot et al., 2005; Hsieh et al., 2006; Wan & Flavell, 2005]. Further studies using anti-Foxp3 antibodies or conditional knock-out mice in the Cre-lox system to target various epithelial cells, proved without a doubt, that the suppressive function of Foxp3-dependent T cells was important for immune homeostatsis and tissue integrity [Kim et al., 2009; Liston et al., 2007; Rudensky, 2011].

The balance of TRCs with other immune cells has a bearing on immunity and immunopathology after infection. Evidence has been reported for two functions of TRCs in immunity against infection. In the first, increasing the number of TRCs interferes with pathogen elimination and supports survival and persistence in humans and mice. Examples are *Leishmania* [Belkaid et al., 2006; Belkaid et al., 2002; Campanelli et al., 2006], *Plasmodium*, [Amante et al., 2007; Hisaeda et al., 2004; Torcia et al., 2008; Walther et al., 2005] and *Mycobacteria* [Chen et al., 2007; Kursar et al., 2007; Scott-Browne et al., 2007]. The pathogen exploits TRCs to its advantage to persist in the host. Secondly, while decreasing the number of TRCs leads to better pathogen control, it also increases the immunopathology formed. Examples of this type of effect of TRCs include infection with herpes simplex virus (HSV) [Suvas et al., 2004] and *C. albicans* [Montagnoli et al., 2002].

A few studies have examined the involvement of TRCs in chlamydial infections. As described below, TRCs are found in a number of mucosal surfaces of which *Chlamydia* cause infection. The first study focused on *C. trachomatis* infection of the ocular mucosa. *C. trachomatis* infects the conjunctiva of the eye and eventually facilitates accumulation of inflammatory cells and organized follicle formation or clinical signs of progression to trachoma. The authors, Faal, N. et al. [Faal et al., 2006] divided individuals into three groups: Group 1: those with acute infection as defined as chlamydial PCR positive; Group 2: those with serological evidence of past chlamydial infection plus clinical disease signs of trachoma; and Group 3: those with serological evidence of past chlamydial infection and no signs of clinical disease. The authors showed that *FOXP3* mRNA was found in Group 1 (only acute infection) and Group 2 (past infection and clinical disease) but not in Group 3 or those with past chlamydial infection but no signs of developing trachoma. The data clearly showed that during acute infection, *FOXP3* mRNA was present. However, it was intriguing that Foxp3 transcripts continued to be elevated despite the fact that acute infection had resolved in the group that presented with clinical signs of trachoma development. The authors speculated that since the presence of Foxp3 transcripts correlated with acute infection, Foxp3 was present to protect conjunctival tissue from immune damage during acute infection. However, its continued presence in the group which had resolved the disease but also showed signs of clinical disease, suggested that Foxp3 was unable to prevent tissue damage in certain individuals [Faal et al., 2006]. The mechanism of tissue protection has not been determined and one must exercise caution when interpreting data based on FOXP3 transcript levels as opposed to expression of protein in cells since these do not directly correlate [Probst-Kepper, 2006].

TRCs cells have also been identified in the lungs of mice infected with *C. pneumoniae* using Foxp3 protein expression in cells identified by flow cytometry. *C. pneumoniae* infection of the lung regulates the degree of T cell activation and can exacerbate development of asthma. In this model, depletion of TRCs increases T cell activation and lung tissue damage [Crother et al., 2011; Schröder et al., 2008]. These data further supported the hypothesis that TRCs prevent tissue from damaging immune responses.

TRCs are also present in the genital mucosa during chlamydial infection. Marks, E. *et. al.* [Marks et al., 2010] found Foxp3 expression in the upper genital tracts of mice following chlamydial genital infection. The expression of Foxp3 also corresponded to the number of Th1 cells in that site. These authors further noted that depleting TRCs increased immunopathology in the upper genital tract [Marks et al., 2007]. Similar to the trachoma study above, only transcripts of *FOXP3* were followed in tissue as evidence of the presence of TRCs. Recently; we have shown that Foxp3+ TRCs are present in the genital tract after infection with the murine model of *C. trachomatis* infection, *C. muridarum*. TRCs were identified by expression of Foxp3 protein on the cell surface and quantitiated by flow cytometry. We found that Foxp3$^+$ TRCs peaked during early infection and correlated with the disappearance of Th1 cells in the genital tract [Moniz et al., 2010]. We have further investigated the role of TRCs during genital infection using Foxp3-EGFP-DTR mice (gift from T. Chatila). The Foxp3$^+$ TRCs can be depleted by administration of diphtheria toxin and followed by monitoring green fluorescent TRCs [Haribhai et al., 2011]. Our preliminary studies show that Th1 cell numbers inversely correlate with the number of TRCs. Further, the depletion of TRCs before and during early infection, at a time when TRCs peak in the genital tract, resulted in a decrease in tissue pathology in the oviducts (unpublished data). This suggests that TRCs do not protect upper genital tract tissue from pathology but instead contribute to tissue pathology by interfering with the eradicating function of Th1 cells in the genital tract.

The few studies reported in chlamydial infections have provided evidence that TRCs can both protect tissue and contribute to tissue damage as described above. These reports differ in the means TRCs were defined, by FOXP3 mRNA transcripts or cellular protein expression. In addition, they differ in the type of mucosal surface studied, such as conjunctiva, lung and genital tract. Although the mechanisms by which TRCs influence immune responses have been identified, none have been thoroughly examined in chlamydial infection. However, the data reported are consistent in that they all implicate TRCs with tissue pathology, either by prevention or exacerbation. Therefore, one can conclude that TRCs play a role in tissue pathology following chlamydial infection and additional studies are needed for a complete understanding of the mechanism(s). We would propose that TRCs form a third type of function in chlamydial infection; TRCs interfere with the elimination of organism but do not enhance chronic persistence of the organism and instead contribute to tissue pathology by prolonging organism elimination from tissues.

2.1 Defining T regulatory cells by expression of phenotypic markers

Complex human biological systems require immune regulatory mechanisms which are effective at containing immune responses to self and foreign antigens, as well as to commensal microorganisms. Presently, TRCs are classified into two subsets: "natural" $CD4^+Foxp3^+$ TRCs (nTRCs) which emerge from the thymus as a distinct lineage [Fontenot et al., 2005; Sakaguchi et al., 1995]; and "induced" $CD4^+CD25^+$ TRCs (iTRCs). iTRCs have a different developmental program compared to nTRCs and develop outside the thymus from $CD4^+CD25^-$ T cell precursors. They are then converted to TRCs by antigenic stimulation and the surrounding cytokine milieu [Chen et al., 2003; Curotto de Lafaille et al., 2004].

Experiments have found that CD25, the high-affinity subunit of the IL-2 receptor, is an important marker of thymic-derived TRCs. $CD4^+CD25^+$ TRCs were capable of preventing autoimmunity not only in neonatal thymectomized mice [Asano et al., 1996], but also in the lymphopenic animal infused with pathogenic effector T cells [Sakaguchi et al., 1995]. Adoptive transfer of $CD25^+$ T cell-depleted splenocytes into lymphopenic hosts induced a multi-organ autoimmunity syndrome with similar characteristics of neonatal thymectomized mice [Sakaguchi et al., 1995]. Later on, the transcription factor, Foxp3, was found by three independent laboratories to be expressed constitutively by $CD25^+$ TRCs [Fontenot et al., 2003; Hori et al., 2003; Wildin et al., 2002]. Foxp3 is a forkhead transcription factor family member and mutations in the Foxp3 coding gene were identified as responsible for the immune dysregulation [Brunkow et al., 2001]. It was concluded that Foxp3 was mandatory for the development of nTRCs in the thymus and its expression constituted a valuable marker for this independent lineage of T cells [Kim & Rudensky, 2006]. Data has shown that adoptive transfer of nTRCs isolated from normal wild type mice significantly prevented disease and related mortality in the Foxp3 mutant mice [Kim & Rudensky, 2006].

Even though iTRCs may be phenotypically similar to nTRCs, they differ in their developmental requirements and function. iTRCs differentiate outside of the thymus under more varied conditions. During induction of oral tolerance, iTRCs first are induced in mesenteric lymph nodes (MLN) in response to microbial and food antigens [Mucida et al., 2005]. iTRCs also continuously differentiate in peripheral tissues such as the lamina propria of the gut [Coombes et al., 2007], tumors [Liu et al., 2007], chronically inflamed tissues [Curotto de Lafaille et al., 2008] and transplanted tissues [Cobbold et al., 2004]. The microenvironments that support the development of iTRCs are not yet completely understood. However, it was determined that TCR stimulation and the cytokines TGF-β and IL-2 are required [Chen et al., 2003; Davidson et al., 2007; Zheng et al., 2007]. Studies on the gene expression of Foxp3 between the two subtypes of TRCs identified that the Foxp3 locus of nTRCs show complete demethylation within an evolutionary conserved region and maintain Foxp3 expression and suppressive functions in the absence of TGF-β stimulation. In contrast, iTRCs lose both Foxp3 expression and suppressive functions without TGF-β re-stimulation [Floess et al., 2007; Huehn et al., 2009]. Thus, iTRCs can be viewed as "transient" suppressive cells.

2.2 Types of T regulatory cells

There are multiple subsets of Foxp3$^+$TRCs that exist within an individual [Stephens et al., 2007]. The majority is CD4$^+$ but small number of CD8$^+$, CD4$^+$CD8$^+$ and CD4$^-$CD8$^-$ αβTCR^{hi} thymocytes and peripheral T cells are also found. Not all Foxp3$^+$TRCs are MHC class I or II restricted [Stephens et al., 2007]. In addition, Foxp3$^+$TRCs can be categorized as "natural". This subset is constitutively present and prevents development of immune responses against self-tissues. In contrast, subsets of Foxp3$^+$TRCs are also induced by inflammation or infection and are call "inducible or adaptive" Foxp3$^+$TRCs. It has been debated whether nTRCs and iTRCs are separate types of TRCs with differing function. [Bluestone & Abbas, 2003]. Both iTRCs and nTRCs have suppressive function as shown by their ability to prevent T cell activation [Fantini et al., 2006; Huter et al., 2008; Mottet et al., 2003]. However, the contribution of each cell type to peripheral tolerance is dependent on the model studied [Curotto de Lafaille et al., 2008; Haribhai et al., 2009]. Recent data has disclosed that each subset of TRCs have distinct functions; nTRCs prevent lethal disease while iTRCs prevent chronic inflammation and mostly have distinct TCR repertoires [Haribhai et al., 2011]. The TRCs that participate in chlamydial infection appear to be members of iTRCs and we will discuss them in depth.

2.2.1 Inducible or transient tregs

Naïve CD4$^+$Foxp3$^-$ cells can be converted to functional regulatory CD4$^+$CD25$^+$ by cytokines in the environment and are called iTRCs. In general, there are two types of iTRCs that have been described based on the cytokines which are responsible for their conversion to iTRCs: TGF-β$^+$ iTRCs and IL-10$^+$ iTRCs. Both types of iTRCs have suppressive properties *in vitro* and *in vivo* [Chen et al., 2003; Grazia Roncarolo et al., 2006; Groux et al., 1997]. However, they are quite distinctive on molecular level. TGF-β$^+$ iTRCs express Foxp3 and secrete mainly TGF-β whereas IL-10 iTRCs do not express Foxp3 after conversion and secrete IL-10.

T cells that are exposed to TGF-β, IL-2 and are stimulated by co-stimulation through the TCR are converted to TGF-β+ iTRCs. Chen et al. has shown that addition of TGF-β to TCR-stimulated naïve CD4 T cells induced the transcription of Foxp3, acquisition of anergic and suppressive activities *in vitro*, and the ability to suppress inflammation in an experimental asthma model [Chen et al., 2003]. Further it has been disclosed that TGF-β induces transcription of *FOXP3* and involves cooperation of the transcription factors STAT3 and NFTA at a Foxp3 gene enhancer element [Josefowicz & Rudensky, 2009]. Consistently, *in vivo* neutralization of TGF-β inhibited the differentiation of antigen-specific Foxp3+ iTRCs [Mucida et al., 2005] and also blocked iTRCs cell-dependent tolerance to tissue grafts in an experimental model [Cobbold et al., 2004]. The ability of cells to be converted to iTRCs occurs in a finite time frame and depends on the presence of TGF-β. Conversion takes place only when TGF-β is added within a 2-3 day window of TCR stimulation, and withdrawal of TGF-β results in the loss of Foxp3 within 4 days [Selvaraj & Geiger, 2007]. Thus, microenvironments commonly found to contain TGF-β, such as the genital tract, have the propensity to produce iTRCs.

IL-2 appears to be essential for the generation and/or homeostasis of iTRCs. *In vitro,* stimulation of naïve CD4 T cells with anti-CD3 and TGF-β found that IL-2 was required to release the TGF-β-mediated inhibition of proliferation [Chen et al., 2003]. By neutralizing IL-

2 and using IL-2 deficient T cells, Zheng et al. has shown that IL-2 is required for *in vitro* TGF-β induction of Foxp3 transcription and suppressor activity [Zheng et al., 2007]. Unlike TGF-β, IL-2 is not required to maintain Foxp3 expression, since iTRCs transferred into RAG-deficient recipient mice did not lose their suppressive functions [Davidson et al., 2007].

2.2.2 Antigen specificity

Recent findings have shifted attention to other types of TRCs which do not fit into the traditional classification scheme described above. One of them is IL-35 induced TRCs found in both human and animal models [Belkaid & Chen, 2010; Collison et al., 2010; Collison et al., 2007]. IL-35 belongs to the IL-12 cytokine family, including IL-12, IL-23 and IL-27. IL-35 is a heterodimeric cytokine composed of an alpha chain (p19, p28 or p35) and a beta chain (p40 or Ebi3). IL-35 signals through any of five receptor chains (IL-12Rβ1, IL-12β2, IL-23R, gp130 and WSX-1)[Collison & Vignali, 2008]. Although IL-12, IL-23, IL-27 and IL-35 belong to one family, their tissue source, activity, function and kinetics of expression are quite different. IL-12, IL-23 and IL-27 share the common feature of inducing IFN-γ, promoting Th1 differentiation and proliferation. In contrast, the function of IL-35 is solely suppressive [Collison et al., 2007]. It has been shown in humans, that IL-35 is required for maximal suppressive capacity of TRCs by upregulating Epstein-Barr-virus-induced gene 3 (EB13) and IL-12A. This was not found to occur with TGF-β or IL-10 exposure. Thus, IL-35 secreting TRCs mediate contact-independent suppression which is IL-35 dependent [Chaturvedi et al., 2011].

Accumulating evidence demonstrates that TRCs are not only defined by markers but also more precisely by their ability to regulate immune responses. $CD8^{+}$TRCs can exercise non-contact dependent regulatory function by secreting IL-10 or increasing IL-4 mRNA to generate more IL-4 [Gilliet & Liu, 2002; Zhou et al., 2001]. In addition, our group and others have shown that natural killer T (NKT) cells can regulate immune responses and prevent extensive tissue damage [Seino et al., 2001; Jiang, J. et al., submitted]. Seino, et al. reported that NKT cells expressing the invariant chain, Valpha 14, were necessary to produce cardiac allograft acceptance and prevent graft rejection [Seino et al., 2001]. We have found that CD1d-restricted NKT cells, activated by antigens contained in chlamydial elementary bodies, can regulate the number of effector T cells during inflammatory responses by inducing the production of multiple inflammatory cytokines and chemokines. The prolonged induction of chemokines results in the accumulation of T cells dominated by Th1 cells in a murine model of chlamydial genital infection [Jiang, J. et al., submitted]. Thus, there are numerous examples of non-Foxp3 expressing T cells with regulatory functions that are important for controlling immune responses against microbial and alloantigens which prevent excessive inflammation in peripheral tissues.

3. Understanding mechanisms of T regulatory cell function

Regulatory T cells play a crucial role in self-antigen tolerance, tissue grafts, and suppression of autoimmune reactions. These cells modulate the intensity and quality of immune responses through attenuation of the activities of reactive immune cells. They modulate immunity by 1) secreting inhibitory cytokines, 2) direct killing cytolysis, 3) metabolic disruption of T cells and 4) modulation of dendritic cell maturation or function.

3.1 Suppression by inhibitory cytokines

TRCs cells produce immunoregulatory cytokines at the site of inflammation. Those regulatory cytokines, including IL-10, IL-35, TGF-β, directly affect the activity of cytotoxic T cells and antigen presenting cells (APCs).

3.1.1 IL-10

IL-10 released by TRCs down regulates the ability of APCs to produce IL-12 and further inhibits the differentiation and responses of Th1-type cells [Moore et al., 2001]. Interaction of T cells with APCs triggers IL-2 production, which acts to enhance reactive T cell proliferation. Thus IL-10 reduces the activity of APCs and indirectly lowers the intensity of entire immune reaction through inhibition of IL-2 production.

3.1.2 IL-35

IL-35 is a newest member of the IL-12 family. In the CD4 T cell population, IL-35 is expressed by resting and activated TRCs but not effector cells [Collison et al., 2007]. In addition, it has been suggested that IL-35 can suppress Th17 development *in vivo* and improve collagen-induced arthritis [Niedbala et al., 2007]. More studies are needed to define the mechanism.

3.1.3 TGF-β

TGF-β reduces cytokine secretion by activated CD4 T cells [Zheng et al., 2004], without limiting their capacity to expand and without inducing their apoptosis [Cottrez & Groux, 2001]. TGF-β also induces IL-10 production in Th1 cells, which further inhibits cytokine production and directly attenuates effector T cell function [Annacker et al., 2001]. In a correlative interaction, IL-10 also enhances the response of activated T cells to TGF-β [Cottrez & Groux, 2001]. Therefore, the combined effects of TGF-β and IL-10 inhibit the activity of effector T cells with minor changes on their expansion

3.2 Suppression by cytolysis

One other potential mechanism for regulatory T cell mediated suppression would be cytolysis of target cells. Many human $CD4^+$ cells display the ability to lyse other cells via cytotoxic mechanisms. Together, TRCs in certain contexts can differentiate and function as cytotoxic suppressor cells.

3.2.1 Granzyme A

It has been reported that human $CD4^+CD25^+Foxp3^+$ TRCs can be activated and lyse target cells which requires granzyme A and perforin [Grossman et al., 2004]. The authors further showed that granzyme A and perforin mediated target cell lysis through adhesion of CD18.

3.2.2 Granzyme B

Activation of mouse TRCs cells also lead to up-regulation of granzyme B expression [Gondek et al., 2005]. The up-regulation of granzyme B induced a reduction in contact mediated suppression by TRCs *in vivo* [Gondek et al., 2005].

3.2.3 Perforin

Although other cell types required granzyme B and perforin to mediate cytoxicity, it is not true for cytotoxicity mediated by TRCs. This is shown by the independent suppression of contact sensitivity by TRCs using perforin-/- mice [Gondek et al., 2005].

3.3 Suppression by metabolic disruption

There are several examples of TRCs mediating suppression by metabolic disruption. These include IL-2 cytokine deprivation and intracellular or extracellular release of adenosine nucleosides [Vignali et al., 2008a].

3.3.1 IL-2 cytokine deprivation

T effector cells require IL-2 for growth but TRCs do not and instead use IL-7. The hypothesis of IL-2 mediated suppression is that CD25 expression could cause the consumption of IL-2 and "starve" T effector cells [de la Rosa et al., 2004; Thornton & Shevach, 1998]. One study has reported this occurs by inducing apoptosis [Pandiyan et al., 2007].

3.3.2 Cyclic AMP-mediated inhibition

TRCs have been reported to transfer the ability of cyclic AMP (cAMP) to mediate suppression by passing on the cAMP to T effector cells through gap junctions [Bopp et al., 2007]. However, this is the only study which reports this mechanism and further reports are needed as confirmation that this is a general mechanism of suppression.

3.3.3 Adenosine receptor-2A

TRCs have been shown to express the ectoenzymes, CD39 and CD73 and generate adenosine secretion [Deaglio et al., 2007; Kobie et al., 2006]. Development of TRCs does not occur in the presence of IL-6 and also requires the presence of TGF-β. The binding of adenosine to the adenosine receptor-2A, not only suppresses T effector cell function but also produces additional TRCs by inhibiting IL-6 production and favoring TGF-β secretion [Zarek et al., 2008].

3.4 Suppression by modulation of dendritic cell maturation or function

There is evidence to support a function of TRCs which act directly on dendritic cells to influence the ability of dendritic cells to activate effector T cells [Bluestone & Tang, 2005; Tang et al., 2006].

3.4.1 Modulation of co-stimulatory molecules

Many studies have reported that TRCs reduce effector T cell function by acting on dendritic cells to influence their maturation [Lewkowich et al., 2005; Misra et al., 2004; Serra et al., 2003]. One of the prominent means for a dendritic cell to influence effector T cell function is modulation of co-stimulatory molecules. Studies have disclosed this function by showing that the use of antibodies which block the function of T-lymphocyte antigen-4 (CTLA4) or CLTA4-deficient T cells have a reduction in the suppression of effector T cells [Oderup et al.,

2006; Serra et al., 2003]. Alternatively, TRCs can also act on dendritic cells to decrease the expression of CD80 and CD86 [Cederbom et al., 2000].

3.4.2 Indoleamine 2,3-dioxygenase

TRCs have also been shown to alter effector T cell function by causing the dendritic cells to produce indoleamine 2,3-dioxygenase (IDO). IDO has the ability to regulate cellular function by encouraging apoptosis by producing precursors from the catabolism of tryptophan. This also results in the down-regulation of CTLA4, CD80 and CD86 [Fallarino et al., 2003; Mellor & Munn, 2004].

3.4.3 LAG/MHC class II

TRCs have also been reported to mediate suppression through the expression of lymphocyte activation gene-3 (LAG3). LAG3 molecules on murine [Liang et al., 2008)] TRCs bind to MHC II molecules on immature dendritic cells and suppress maturation by transducing an inhibitory signaling pathway. Alternatively, human TRCs have been shown to express a greater amount of LAG3 and potentially could interact directly with effector T cells [Baecher-Allan et al., 2006].

4. Induction of T regulatory cells

As described above, although many types of TRCs have been identified, two major subsets have emerge; nTRCs and iTRCs. The nTRCs mature in the thymus [Fontenot et al., 2005; Sakaguchi et al., 1995]. On the other hand, iTRCs have a different developmental program compared to nTRCs and develop outside the thymus from $CD4^{+}CD25^{-}$ T cell precursors. They are then converted to TRCs by antigenic stimulation and the surrounding cytokine milieu [Chen et al., 2003; Curotto de Lafaille et al., 2004]. However, both subsets are identified by the expression of Foxp3.

4.1 Expression of Foxp3

Foxp3 is a forkhead transcription factor family member and mutations in the Foxp3 coding gene were identified as responsible for the immune dysregulation [Brunkow et al., 2001]. The FOXP3 gene is essential for the ability of nTRCs to mature in the thymus and this subset always expressed Foxp3 [Kim & Rudensky, 2006]. This subset of TRCs is important throughout the life of the individual for preventing lethal autoimmune diseases [Kim & Rudensky, 2006]. Conversely, iTRCs only transiently express Foxp3 and Foxp3 expression correlates with suppressive function [Floess et al., 2007; Huehn et al., 2009]. Thus, expression of Foxp3 is necessary for TRCs to suppress immune responses.

4.2 Infections associated with T regulatory cell function

Pathogens are not the only culprits of tissue inflammation. Adaptive immune responses against host-antigens which have escaped deletion or control in the periphery provoke tissue inflammation [Rudensky et al., 2006]. This has been demonstrated during transplantation rejection and autoimmune diseases. Pathogens associated with chronic infections are hypothesized to encourage immune responses against host antigens.

Alternatively, microbial infections may simultaneously recruit regulatory cells to tissues to prevent inflammation while anti-microbial immune responses eliminate the pathogen [Sinclair, 2004]. The inability of a host to mount and recruit a sufficient regulatory response in tissues appears to result in tissue inflammation [Sather et al., 2007].

4.3 Dendritic cell populations

There have been many reports that TRCs target dendritic cells to mediate immune suppression. The interaction of TRCs with immature or activated myeloid dendritic cells or marrow-derived dendritic cells results in the down-regulation of co-stimulatory molecules CD80, CD86 and CD40 and MHC on dendritic cells [Tadokoro et al., 2006] as well as up-regulation of inhibitory factors [Mahnke et al., 2007], leading to impaired T cell stimulatory function of dendritic cells. Consistent with *in vitro* data, *in vivo* evidence in experiment models show that TRCs inhibit T cell immune response mediated by dendritic cells at various locations [Mahnke et al., 2007]. TRCs exert an early effect on immune responses by attenuating the establishment of stable contacts during priming of naïve T cells and dendritic cells and by forming synapses and aggregation with dendritic cells more frequently than with naïve T cells. Moreover, visualization of adoptively transferred TRCs in the lymph nodes of mice revealed that TRCs form stable associations with dendritic cells that in turn prevents subsequent strong interactions between dendritic cells and autoreactive effector T cells [Tang & Bluestone, 2006]. Together, strong evidence implies that dendritic cells are the primary targets of TRCs *in vivo* [Tadokoro et al., 2006; Tang et al., 2006].

Dendritic cells are needed to influence the development of adaptive TRCs. Production of Foxp3$^+$TRCs can be induced by plasmacytoid dendritic cells (pDC) by causing expression of Foxp3 in non-regulatory T cells within peripheral tissues. However, the precise dendritic cell subset is under debate and actively investigated [Tang & Bluestone, 2006]. The current consensus states that immature conventional dendritic cells and pDC can induce expression of Foxp3 in non-regulatory T cells within peripheral tissues. Although little is known regarding the interaction of pDCs and TRCs, recent evidence shows that this interaction occurs in draining lymph nodes and not spleen, and is specific for foreign antigens [Ochando et al., 2006]. Evidence suggests that newly activated Foxp3$^+$TRCs may act on conventional dendritic cells to limit production of T effector cells [Kim et al., 2007]. Plasmacytoid dendritic cells induce Foxp3 expression by interacting with T cells via certain co-stimulatory molecules such as ICOS-L [Akbari et al., 2002].

5. Migration of T regulatory cells

TRCs also influence the composition of immune cells in the genital tract as TRCs were shown to regulate the trafficking of cells between vaginal tissue and the lymph node inductive site in a murine herpes simplex model. Specifically, Lund, et al. has found that TRCs influence chemokine secretion in secondary lymphoid organs which interferes with the trafficking of immune cells to the vaginal mucosa and viral clearance in herpes simplex infected mice [Lund et al., 2008]. This implies that microbes activate TRCs which orchestrate immune responses.

5.1 Chemokine receptor expression

As mentioned above, TRCs can also perform immunosuppressive functions at inductive sites within draining lymph nodes. Homing properties of dendritic cells are very important for their ability to induce iTRCs. Production of retinoic acid occurs through $CD103^+$ dendritic cells. The activated $CD103^+$ dendritic cells must first be able to induce expression of CCR7 and travel to a MLN in order to promote the production of iTRCs during T cell activation. It was shown that the lack of *ccr7* gene in knockout mice prevents development of oral tolerance in CCR7-/- mice [Mora et al., 2003]. During activation of T cells, retinoic acid also induces the homing receptor, $\alpha4\beta7$, and the chemokine which attracts cells to the intestinal mucosa, CCR9 [Iwata et al., 2004; Mora et al., 2003; Papadakis et al., 2003; Svensson et al., 2002]. The ability of TRCs to express tissue-specific homing properties appears to follow the same rules as effector T cells [Siewert et al., 2007].

5.2 Control of migration of CD8+ cells

An additional function of TRCs that requires further investigation is their ability to migrate into tissue to prevent or control the activation of effector T cells. In a $CD8^+$ model of type I diabetes, transgenic expression of TNF-α was shown to be necessary for the TRCs to enter the pancreas, accumulate and prevent destruction and development of $CD8^+$ cells specific for islet cells [Green et al., 2003]. In support of this, a subset of TRCs has been shown to express CCR6 and accumulate in the CNS of mice which have EAE [Kleinewietfeld et al., 2005]. Taken together, these data suggest that a subset of TRCs may prevent the continued activation of effector T cells within peripheral tissues.

6. Suppression of specific cell populations by T regulatory cells

The majority of studies show that TRCs inhibit functions of effector T cells. However, TRCs have been reported to control B cells [Zhao et al., 2006]. In addition, TRCs have also been shown to prevent the killing of tumor cells [Cao et al., 2007]. It is anticipated that other types of cells will also be regulated by TRCs since they are important for controlling a plethora of diseases.

6.1 Targeting dendritic cells

Several reports have demonstrated that TRCs modulate the maturation, activation and function of various subsets of human and murine dendritic cells both *in vitro* and *in vivo*. This gives further evidence that TRCs "educate" dendritic cells and impact outcomes of immune responses [Mahnke et al., 2007; Tadokoro et al., 2006; Tang et al., 2006]. *In vitro*, the interaction of TRCs with immature or activated myeloid dendritic cells or marrow-derived dendritic cells results in the down-regulation of co-stimulatory molecules CD80, CD86 and CD40 and MHC [Tadokoro et al., 2006] and up-regulates inhibitory factors [Mahnke et al., 2007]. TRCs also target dendritic cells and form stable interactions preventing naïve T cell activation [Tang & Bluestone, 2006]. Since TRCs regulate many types of immune responses it is plausible that dendritic cells are a major target of TRCs [Tadokoro et al., 2006; Tang et al., 2006].

6.2 CD4 effector T cells

A major target of TRCs is CD4 effector T cells. TRCs have been reported to prevent activation by directly acting on effector T cells to prevent clonal expansion and proliferation by limiting access to IL-2 [Thornton & Shevach, 1998], modulating T cell activation through exposure by suppressive cytokines such as IL-10 [Annacker et al., 2001] and TGF-β [Zarek et al., 2008]. These diverse ways to prevent T cell activation suggest that there are either multiple subsets of TRCs or one type of TRC with plastic development. This has been debated in recent review and likely will be the subject of ongoing research [Vignali et al., 2008b].

6.3 Innate immune cells

There are a few reports of TRCs modulating the functions of innate immune cells, particularly monocytes and macrophages [Taams et al., 2005; Tiemessen et al., 2007]. These reports use human cells and may be specific to humans.

7. Implications (implications) for vaccines and therapies to prevent reproductive tract inflammation

The primary function of TRCs is to suppress immune responses which are harmful for the individual and maintain survival. As we have reviewed, TRCs are important for numerous diseases and mediate suppression thorough a number of mechanisms. This suggests that certain TRCs as defined by function or phenotype can be exploited as therapeutics to prevent autoimmune disease. This has been accomplished in mice to prevent joint inflammation using two approaches; genetic transfer of TCRs from TRCs and the transfer of Foxp3 cells [Wright et al., 2009]. TRCs have also been proposed to prevent allergy and may replace tolerating injections which are effective for preventing allergic reactions [Robinson et al., 2004]. However, TRCs may also interfere with beneficial immune responses and inhibit tumor or pathogen eradication as described above. In the specific case of developing a vaccine for chlamydial infection, speculation on TRCs is premature, and will likely depend on the tissue site of infection as shown in the few studies to date. The ability of TRCs to prevent asthma may encourage preventative therapeutics. Chlamydial infection is widespread across the world and 92 million cases of genital infection and near 40 million cases of blindness due to chlamydial infection was reported around the beginning of the decade [Resnikoff et al., 2004; WHO, 2004]. This number of infections suggests that harnessing of TRCs could greatly reduce morbidity following infection.

8. Conclusion

T regulatory cells (TRCs) play a central role in adaptive and innate immunity by controlling immune responses and affecting the outcome of tissue inflammation. They initially comprised a phenotypic group of thymic-derived natural TRCs (nTRCs), which also expressed Foxp3. Currently, the group has been expanded to include a number of T cells ($CD4^+CD25^+Foxp3^+$, IL-35 secreting TRCs, CD8+ and NKT cells) which can be induced to acquire immune suppressive function especially at mucosal surfaces. They have been shown to mediate immune suppression by a number of mechanisms, both contact-dependent and through secretion of cytokines. In addition, TRCs influence immunity at mucosal surfaces by orchestrating the composition of immune cells in response to microbial infection. The combination of phenotype, mechanism of suppression, influence on immune cell migration and type of microbial infection, impart TRCs with a crucial function in mucosal tissues.

9. Acknowledgment

The published reports and unpublished studies of Foxp3 were supported by a grant from the National Institutes of Health, AI026328 (K.K.), sponsored research award from Abraxis Bioscience, Inc (K.K.) and special funds from the Dept. of Pathology and Laboratory Medicine, UCLA. We are also grateful for the helpful discussions of the function of T regulatory cells in chlamydial infections with Toni Darville and Moshe Arditi.

10. References

Akbari, O., Freeman, G.J., Meyer, E.H., Greenfield, E.A., Chang, T.T., Sharpe, A.H., Berry, G., DeKruyff, R.H., & Umetsu, D.T. (2002). Antigen-specific regulatory T cells develop via the ICOS-ICOS-ligand pathway and inhibit allergen-induced airway hyperreactivity. *Nat Med* 8, 1024-1032.

Amante, F.H., Stanley, A.C., Randall, L.M., Zhou, Y., Haque, A., McSweeney, K., Waters, A.P., Janse, C.J., Good, M.F., Hill, G.R., & Engwerda, C.R. (2007). A role for natural regulatory T cells in the pathogenesis of experimental cerebral malaria. *Am J Pathol* 171, 548-559, 0002-9440.

Annacker, O., Pimenta-Araujo, R., Burlen-Defranoux, O., Barbosa, T.C., Cumano, A., &Bandeira, A. (2001). CD25+ CD4+ T cells regulate the expansion of peripheral CD4 T cells through the production of IL-10. *J Immunol* 166, 3008-3018.

Asano, M., Toda, M., Sakaguchi, N., & Sakaguchi, S. (1996). Autoimmune disease as a consequence of developmental abnormality of a T cell subpopulation. *J. Exp. Med.* 184, 387-396, 0022-1007. (Print) 0022-1007 (Linking).

Baecher-Allan, C., Wolf, E., & Hafler, D.A. (2006). MHC class II expression identifies functionally distinct human regulatory T cells. *J Immunol* 176, 4622-4631.

Belkaid, Y., Blank, R.B., & Suffia, I. (2006). Natural regulatory T cells and parasites: a common quest for host homeostasis. *Immunol Rev* 212, 287-300, 1600-065X.

Belkaid, Y., & Chen, W. (2010). Regulatory ripples. *Nat. Immunol.* 11, 1077-1078, 1529-2908.

Belkaid, Y., Piccirillo, C.A., Mendez, S., Shevach, E.M., & Sacks, D.L. (2002). CD4+CD25+ regulatory T cells control *Leishmania* major persistence and immunity. *Nature* 420, 502-507, 0028-0836.

Belkaid, Y., & Tarbell, K. (2009). Regulatory T Cells in the Control of Host-Microorganism Interactions. *Ann Rev Immunol* 27, 551-589.

Bennett, C.L., Christie, J., Ramsdell, F., Brunkow, M.E., Ferguson, P.J., Whitesell, L., Kelly, T.E., Saulsbury, F.T., Chance, P.F., & Ochs, H.D. (2001). The immune dysregulation, polyendocrinopathy, enteropathy, X-linked syndrome (IPEX) is caused by mutations of FOXP3. *Nat Genet* 27, 20-21, 1061-4036.

Bluestone, J.A., & Abbas, A.K. (2003). Natural versus adaptive regulatory T cells. *Nat Rev Immunol* 3, 253-257.

Bluestone, J.A., & Tang, Q. (2005). How do CD4+CD25+ regulatory T cells control autoimmunity? *Curr Opin Immunol* 17, 638-642, 0952-7915.

Bopp, T., Becker, C., Klein, M., Klein-Heßling, S., Palmetshofer, A., Serfling, E., Heib, V., Becker, M., Kubach, J., Schmitt, S., *et al.* (2007). Cyclic adenosine monophosphate is a key component of regulatory T cell-mediated suppression. *J Exp Med* 204, 1303-1310.

Brunkow, M.E., Jeffery, E.W., Hjerrild, K.A., Paeper, B., Clark, L.B., Yasayko, S.-A., Wilkinson, J.E., Galas, D., Ziegler, S.F., & Ramsdell, F. (2001). Disruption of a new forkhead/winged-helix protein, scurfin, results in the fatal lymphoproliferative disorder of the scurfy mouse. *Nat. Genet.* 27, 68-73, 1061-4036.

Campanelli, A.P., Roselino, A.M., Cavassani, K.A., Pereira, M.S.F., Mortara, R.A., Brodskyn, C.I., Gonçalves, H.S., Belkaid, Y., Barral-Netto, M., Barral, A., & Silva, J.S. (2006). CD4+CD25+ T cells in skin lesions of patients with cutaneous leishmaniasis exhibit phenotypic and functional characteristics of natural regulatory T cells. *J Infect Dis* 193, 1313-1322.

Cao, X., Cai, S.F., Fehniger, T.A., Song, J., Collins, L.I., Piwnica-Worms, D.R., & Ley, T.J. (2007). Granzyme B and perforin are important for regulatory T cell-mediated suppression of tumor clearance. *Immunity* 27, 635-646, 1074-7613.

Cederbom, L., Hall, H., & Ivars, F. (2000). CD4+CD25+ regulatory T cells down-regulate co-stimulatory molecules on antigen-presenting cells. *Eur J Immunol* 30, 1538-1543, 1521-4141.

Chatila, T.A., Blaeser, F., Ho, N., Lederman, H.M., Voulgaropoulos, C., Helms, C., &Bowcock, A.M. (2000). JM2, encoding a fork head–related protein, is mutated in X-linked autoimmunity–allergic disregulation syndrome. *J Clin Invest* 106, 0-0, 0021-9738.

Chaturvedi, V., Collison, L.W., Guy, C.S., Workman, C.J., & Vignali, D.A. (2011). Cutting edge: Human regulatory T cells require IL-35 to mediate suppression and infectious tolerance. *J. Immunol.* 186, 6661-6666, 1550-6606 (Electronic), 0022-1767 (Linking).

Chen, W., Jin, W., Hardegen, N., Lei, K.-j., Li, L., Marinos, N., McGrady, G., & Wahl, S.M. (2003). Conversion of peripheral CD4+CD25− naive T cells to CD4+CD25+ regulatory T cells by TGF-β induction of transcription factor Foxp3. *J. Exp. Med.* 198, 1875-1886.

Chen, X., Zhou, B., Li, M., Deng, Q., Wu, X., Le, X., Wu, C., Larmonier, N., Zhang, W., Zhang, H., & *et al.* (2007). CD4+CD25+FoxP3+ regulatory T cells suppress *Mycobacterium tuberculosis* immunity in patients with active disease. *Clin Immunol* 123, 50-59, 1521-6616.

Chen, Z., Benoist, C., & Mathis, D. (2005). How defects in central tolerance impinge on a deficiency in regulatory T cells. *Proc Natl Acad Sci USA* 102, 14735-14740.

Cobbold, S.P., Castejon, R., Adams, E., Zelenika, D., Graca, L., Humm, S., & Waldmann, H. (2004). Induction of Foxp3+ regulatory T cells in the periphery of T cell receptor transgenic mice tolerized to transplants. *J. Immunol.* 172, 6003-6010, 0022-1767 (Print), 0022-1767 (Linking).

Collison, L.W., Chaturvedi, V., Henderson, A.L., Giacomin, P.R., Guy, C., Bankoti, J., Finkelstein, D., Forbes, K., Workman, C.J., Brown, S.A., & *et al.* (2010). IL-35-mediated induction of a potent regulatory T cell population. *Nat. Immunol.* 11, 1093-1101, 1529-2908.

Collison, L.W., & Vignali, D.A.A. (2008). Interleukin-35: odd one out or part of the family? *Immunol Rev* 226, 248-262, 1600-065X.

Collison, L.W., Workman, C.J., Kuo, T.T., Boyd, K., Wang, Y., Vignali, K.M., Cross, R., Sehy, D., Blumberg, R.S., & Vignali, D.A.A. (2007). The inhibitory cytokine IL-35 contributes to regulatory T-cell function. *Nature* 450, 566-569, 0028-0836.

Coombes, J.L., Siddiqui, K.R.R., Arancibia-Cárcamo, C.V., Hall, J., Sun, C.-M., Belkaid, Y., &Powrie, F. (2007). A functionally specialized population of mucosal CD103+ DCs induces Foxp3+ regulatory T cells via a TGF-β– and retinoic acid–dependent mechanism. *J. Exp. Med.* 204, 1757-1764,

Cottrez, F., & Groux, H. (2001). Regulation of TGF-β Response During T Cell Activation Is Modulated by IL-10. *J Immunol* 167, 773-778,

Crother, T.R., Schröder, N.W.J., Karlin, J., Chen, S., Shimada, K., Slepenkin, A., Alsabeh, R., Peterson, E., & Arditi, M. (2011). *Chlamydia pneumoniae* infection induced allergic airway sensitization is controlled by regulatory T-cells and plasmacytoid dendritic cells. *PLoS One* 6, e20784,

Curotto de Lafaille, M.A., Kutchukhidze, N., Shen, S., Ding, Y., Yee, H., & Lafaille, J.J. (2008). Adaptive Foxp3+ regulatory T cell-dependent and -independent control of allergic inflammation. *Immunity* 29, 114-126, 1097-4180 (Electronic), 1074-7613 (Linking).

Curotto de Lafaille, M.A., Lino, A.C., Kutchukhidze, N., & Lafaille, J.J. (2004). CD25- T cells generate CD25+Foxp3+ regulatory T cells by peripheral expansion. *J. Immunol.* 173, 7259-7268, 0022-1767 (Print), 0022-1767 (Linking).

Davidson, T.S., DiPaolo, R.J., Andersson, J., & Shevach, E.M. (2007). Cutting edge: IL-2 is essential for TGF-beta-mediated induction of Foxp3+ T regulatory cells. *J. Immunol.* 178, 4022-4026, 0022-1767 (Print), 0022-1767 (Linking).

de la Rosa, M., Rutz, S., Dorninger, H., & Scheffold, A. (2004). Interleukin-2 is essential for CD4+CD25+ regulatory T cell function. *Eur J Immunol* 34, 2480-2488, 1521-4141.

Deaglio, S., Dwyer, K.M., Gao, W., Friedman, D., Usheva, A., Erat, A., Chen, J.-F., Enjyoji, K., Linden, J., Oukka, M., *et al.* (2007). Adenosine generation catalyzed by CD39 and CD73 expressed on regulatory T cells mediates immune suppression. *J. Exp. Med.* 204, 1257-1265.

Faal, N., Bailey, R.L., Jeffries, D., Joof, H., Sarr, I., Laye, M., Mabey, D.C., & Holland, M.J. (2006). Conjunctival FOXP3 expression in trachoma: do regulatory T cells have a role in human ocular *Chlamydia trachomatis* infection? *PLoS Med* 3, e266.

Fallarino, F., Grohmann, U., Hwang, K.W., Orabona, C., Vacca, C., Bianchi, R., Belladonna, M.L., Fioretti, M.C., Alegre, M.-L., & Puccetti, P. (2003). Modulation of tryptophan catabolism by regulatory T cells. *Nat Immunol* 4, 1206-1212, 1529-2908.

Fantini, M.C., Becker, C., Tubbe, I., Nikolaev, A., Lehr, H.A., Galle, P., & Neurath, M.F. (2006). Transforming growth factor β induced FoxP3+ regulatory T cells suppress Th1 mediated experimental colitis. *Gut* 55, 671-680.

Farias, A.S., Talaisys, R.L., Blanco, Y.C., Lopes, S.C., Longhini, A.L., Pradella, F., Santos, L.M., & Costa, F.T. (2011). Regulatory T cell induction during *Plasmodium chabaudi* infection modifies the clinical course of experimental autoimmune encephalomyelitis. *PLoS One* 6, e17849, 1932-6203 (Electronic), 1932-6203 (Linking).

Floess, S., Freyer, J., Siewert, C., Baron, U., Olek, S., Polansky, J., Schlawe, K., Chang, H.D., Bopp, T., Schmitt, E., *et al.* (2007). Epigenetic control of the foxp3 locus in regulatory T cells. *PLoS Biol.* 5, e38, 1545-7885 (Electronic), 1544-9173 (Linking).

Fontenot, J.D., Gavin, M.A., & Rudensky, A.Y. (2003). Foxp3 programs the development and function of CD4+CD25+ regulatory T cells. *Nat Immunol* 4, 330-336, 1529-2908 (Print), 1529-2908 (Linking).

Fontenot, J.D., Rasmussen, J.P., Williams, L.M., Dooley, J.L., Farr, A.G., & Rudensky, A.Y. (2005). Regulatory T cell lineage specification by the forkhead transcription factor foxp3. *Immunity* 22, 329-341, 1074-7613 (Print). 1074-7613 (Linking).

Gilliet, M., & Liu, Y.J. (2002). Generation of human CD8 T regulatory cells by CD40 ligand-activated plasmacytoid dendritic cells. *J. Exp. Med.* 195, 695-704, 0022-1007 (Print), 0022-1007 (Linking).

Gondek, D.C., Lu, L.-F., Quezada, S.A., Sakaguchi, S., & Noelle, R.J. (2005). Cutting ddge: contact-mediated suppression by CD4+CD25+ regulatory cells involves a granzyme B-dependent, perforin-independent mechanism. *J Immunol* 174, 1783-1786.

Grazia Roncarolo, M., Gregori, S., Battaglia, M., Bacchetta, R., Fleischhauer, K., & Levings, M.K. (2006). Interleukin-10-secreting type 1 regulatory T cells in rodents and humans. *Immunol Rev* 212, 28-50, 1600-065X.

Green, E.A., Gorelik, L., McGregor, C.M., Tran, E.H., &Flavell, R.A. (2003). CD4+CD25+ T regulatory cells control anti-islet CD8+ T cells through TGF-β–TGF-β receptor interactions in type 1 diabetes. *Proc Natl Acad Sci U S A* 100, 10878-10883.

Grossman, W.J., Verbsky, J.W., Barchet, W., Colonna, M., Atkinson, J.P., & Ley, T.J. (2004). Human T regulatory cells can use the perforin pathway to cause autologous target cell death. *Immunity* 21, 589-601, 1074-7613.

Groux, H., O'Garra, A., Bigler, M., Rouleau, M., Antonenko, S., de Vries, J.E., & Roncarolo, M.G. (1997). A CD4+ T-cell subset inhibits antigen-specific T-cell responses and prevents colitis. *Nature* 389, 737-742, 0028-0836 (Print), 0028-0836 (Linking).

Haribhai, D., Lin, W., Edwards, B., Ziegelbauer, J., Salzman, N.H., Carlson, M.R., Li, S.-H., Simpson, P.M., Chatila, T.A., & Williams, C.B. (2009). A central role for induced regulatory T cells in tolerance induction in experimental colitis. *J Immunol* 182, 3461-3468.

Haribhai, D., Williams, Jason B., Jia, S., Nickerson, D., Schmitt, Erica G., Edwards, B., Ziegelbauer, J., Yassai, M., Li, S.-H., Relland, Lance M., *et al.* (2011). A requisite role for induced regulatory T cells in tolerance based on expanding antigen receptor diversity. *Immunity* 35, 109-122, 1074-7613.

Hisaeda, H., Maekawa, Y., Iwakawa, D., Okada, H., Himeno, K., Kishihara, K., Tsukumo, S.-i., & Yasutomo, K. (2004). Escape of malaria parasites from host immunity requires CD4+CD25+ regulatory T cells. *Nat Med* 10, 29-30, 1078-8956.

Hori, S., Nomura, T., & Sakaguchi, S. (2003). Control of regulatory T cell development by the transcription factor Foxp3. *Science* 299, 1057-1061, 1095-9203 (Electronic), 0036-8075 (Linking).

Hsieh, C.-S., Zheng, Y., Liang, Y., Fontenot, J.D., & Rudensky, A.Y. (2006). An intersection between the self-reactive regulatory and nonregulatory T cell receptor repertoires. *Nat Immunol* 7, 401-410, 1529-2908.

Huehn, J., Polansky, J.K., & Hamann, A. (2009). Epigenetic control of FOXP3 expression: the key to a stable regulatory T-cell lineage? *Nat Rev Immunol* 9, 83-89, 1474-1741 (Electronic), 1474-1733 (Linking).

Huter, E.N., Stummvoll, G.H., DiPaolo, R.J., Glass, D.D., &Shevach, E.M. (2008). Cutting edge: Antigen-specific TGFβ-induced regulatory T cells suppress Th17-mediated autoimmune disease. *J Immunol* 181, 8209-8213,

Iwata, M., Hirakiyama, A., Eshima, Y., Kagechika, H., Kato, C., & Song, S.-Y. (2004). Retinoic acid imprints gut-homing specificity on T cells. *Immunity* 21, 527-538, 1074-7613.

Josefowicz, S.Z., & Rudensky, A. (2009). Control of regulatory T cell lineage commitment and maintenance. *Immunity* 30, 616-625, 1097-4180 (Electronic), 1074-7613 (Linking).

Kim, J., Lahl, K., Hori, S., Loddenkemper, C., Chaudhry, A., deRoos, P., Rudensky, A., & Sparwasser, T. (2009). Cutting edge: Depletion of Foxp3+ cells leads to induction of autoimmunity by specific ablation of regulatory T cells in genetically targeted mice. *J mmunol* 183, 7631-7634.

Kim, J.M., Rasmussen, J.P., & Rudensky, A.Y. (2007). Regulatory T cells prevent catastrophic autoimmunity throughout the lifespan of mice. *Nat Immunol* 8, 191-197.

Kim, J.M., & Rudensky, A. (2006). The role of the transcription factor Foxp3 in the development of regulatory T cells. *Immunol Rev* 212, 86-98, 0105-2896 (Print), 0105-2896 (Linking).

Kleinewietfeld, M., Puentes, F., Borsellino, G., Battistini, L., Rötzschke, O., & Falk, K. (2005). CCR6 expression defines regulatory effector/memory-like cells within the CD25+CD4+ T-cell subset. *Blood* 105, 2877-2886.

Kobie, J.J., Shah, P.R., Yang, L., Rebhahn, J.A., Fowell, D.J., & Mosmann, T.R. (2006). T regulatory and primed uncommitted CD4 T cells express CD73, which suppresses effector CD4 T cells by converting 5'-adenosine monophosphate to adenosine. *J Immunol* 177, 6780-6786.

Kursar, M., Koch, M., Mittrücker, H.-W., Nouailles, G., Bonhagen, K., Kamradt, T., & Kaufmann, S.H.E. (2007). Cutting ddge: Regulatory T cells prevent efficient clearance of *Mycobacterium tuberculosis*. *J Immunol* 178, 2661-2665.

Lewkowich, I.P., Herman, N.S., Schleifer, K.W., Dance, M.P., Chen, B.L., Dienger, K.M., Sproles, A.A., Shah, J.S., Köhl, J., Belkaid, Y., &Wills-Karp, M. (2005). CD4+CD25+ T cells protect against experimentally induced asthma and alter pulmonary dendritic cell phenotype and function. *J Exp Med* 202, 1549-1561.

Liang, B., Workman, C., Lee, J., Chew, C., Dale, B.M., Colonna, L., Flores, M., Li, N., Schweighoffer, E., Greenberg, S., *et al.* (2008). Regulatory T cells inhibit dendritic cells by lymphocyte activation gene-3 engagement of MHC class II. *J Immunol* 180, 5916-5926.

Liston, A., Farr, A.G., Chen, Z., Benoist, C., Mathis, D., Manley, N.R., & Rudensky, A.Y. (2007). Lack of Foxp3 function and expression in the thymic epithelium. *J Exp Med* 204, 475-480.

Liu, V.C., Wong, L.Y., Jang, T., Shah, A.H., Park, I., Yang, X., Zhang, Q., Lonning, S., Teicher, B.A., & Lee, C. (2007). Tumor evasion of the immune system by converting CD4+CD25- T cells into CD4+CD25+ T regulatory cells: role of tumor-derived TGF-beta. *J. Immunol.* 178, 2883-2892, 0022-1767 (Print), 0022-1767 (Linking).

Lund, J.M., Hsing, L., Pham, T.T., & Rudensky, A.Y. (2008). Coordination of Early Protective Immunity to Viral Infection by Regulatory T Cells. *Science* 320, 1220-1224.

Mahnke, K., Ring, S., Johnson, T.S., Schallenberg, S., Schönfeld, K., Storn, V., Bedke, T., & Enk, A.H. (2007). Induction of immunosuppressive functions of dendritic cells *in vivo* by CD4+CD25+ regulatory T cells: Role of B7-H3 expression and antigen presentation. *Eur J Immunol* 37, 2117-2126, 1521-4141.

Marks, E., Tam, M.A., & Lycke, N.Y. (2010). The female lower genital tract is a privileged compartment with IL-10 producing dendritic cells and poor Th1 immunity following *Chlamydia trachomatis* infection. *PLoS Pathog* 6, e1001179.

Marks, E., Verolin, M., Stensson, A., & Lycke, N. (2007). Differential CD28 and ICOS signaling requirements for protective CD4+ T cell mediated immunity against genital tract *Chlamydia trachomatis* infection. *Infect Immun*, IAI.00465-00407.

Mellor, A.L., & Munn, D.H. (2004). IDO expression by dendritic cells: tolerance and tryptophan catabolism. *Nat Rev Immunol* 4, 762-774, 1474-1733.

Misra, N., Bayry, J., Lacroix-Desmazes, S., Kazatchkine, M.D., & Kaveri, S.V. (2004). Cutting edge: Human CD4+CD25+ T cells restrain the maturation and antigen-presenting function of dendritic cells. *J Immunol* 172, 4676-4680.

Moniz, R.J., Chan, A.M., Gordon, L.K., Braun, J., Arditi, M., & Kelly, K.A. (2010). Plasmacytoid DC regulate the number of Foxp3+ cells and target tissue damage during a *Chlamydia* genital infection *FEMS Immunol Med Microbiol* 58, 397-404.

Montagnoli, C., Bacci, A., Bozza, S., Gaziano, R., Mosci, P., Sharpe, A.H., & Romani, L. (2002). B7/CD28-dependent CD4+CD25+ regulatory T cells are essential components of the memory-protective immunity to *Candida albicans*. *J Immunol* 169, 6298-6308,

Moore, K.W., de Waal Malefyt, R., Coffman, R.L., & O'Garra, A. (2001). Interleukin-10 and the interleukin-10 receptor. *Annu Rev Immunol* 19, 683-765.

Mora, J.R., Bono, M.R., Manjunath, N., Weninger, W., Cavanagh, L.L., Rosemblatt, M., & von Andrian, U.H. (2003). Selective imprinting of gut-homing T cells by Peyer's patch dendritic cells. *Nature* 424, 88-93, 0028-0836.

Mottet, C., Uhlig, H.H., & Powrie, F. (2003). Cutting edge: Cure of colitis by CD4+CD25+ regulatory T cells. *J Immunol* 170, 3939-3943.

Mucida, D., Kutchukhidze, N., Erazo, A., Russo, M., Lafaille, J.J., & Curotto de Lafaille, M.A. (2005). Oral tolerance in the absence of naturally occurring Tregs. *J.Clin. Invest.* 115, 1923-1933, 0021-9738 (Print), 0021-9738 (Linking).

Niedbala, W., Wei, X.-q., Cai, B., Hueber, A.J., Leung, B.P., McInnes, I.B., & Liew, F.Y. (2007). IL-35 is a novel cytokine with therapeutic effects against collagen-induced arthritis through the expansion of regulatory T cells and suppression of Th17 cells. *Eur J Immunol* 37, 3021-3029, 1521-4141.

Ochando, J.C., Homma, C., Yang, Y., Hidalgo, A., Garin, A., Tacke, F., Angeli, V., Li, Y., Boros, P., Ding, Y., & *et al.* (2006). Alloantigen-presenting plasmacytoid dendritic cells mediate tolerance to vascularized grafts. *Nat Immunol* 7, 652-662.

Oderup, C., Cederbom, L., Makowska, A., Cilio, C.M., & Ivars, F. (2006). Cytotoxic T lymphocyte antigen-4-dependent down-modulation of costimulatory molecules on dendritic cells in CD4+ CD25+ regulatory T-cell-mediated suppression. *Immunology* 118, 240-249, 1365-2567.

Pandiyan, P., Zheng, L., Ishihara, S., Reed, J., & Lenardo, M.J. (2007). CD4+CD25+Foxp3+ regulatory T cells induce cytokine deprivation-mediated apoptosis of effector CD4+ T cells. *Nat Immunol* 8, 1353-1362, 1529-2908.

Papadakis, K.A., Landers, C., Prehn, J., Kouroumalis, E.A., Moreno, S.T., Gutierrez-Ramos, J.-C., Hodge, M.R., & Targan, S.R. (2003). CC chemokine receptor 9 expression defines a subset of peripheral blood lymphocytes with mucosal T cell phenotype and Th1 or T-regulatory 1 cytokine profile. *J. Immuno.* 171, 159-165.

Probst-Kepper, M. (2006). Conjunctival *FOXP3* in Trachoma: T Cells not specified. *PLoS Med* 3, e506.

Resnikoff, S., Pascolini, D., Etya'ale, D., Kocur, I., Pararajasegaram, R., Pokharel, G.P., &Mariotti, S.P. (2004). Global data on visual impairment in the year 2002. *Bulletin Of The World Health Organization* 82, 844-851.

Robinson, D.S., Larché, M., &Durham, S.R. (2004). Tregs and allergic disease. *J Clin Invest* 114, 1389-1397, 0021-9738.

Rudensky, A.Y. (2011). Regulatory T cells and Foxp3. *Immunol Rev* 241, 260-268, 1600-065X.

Rudensky, A.Y., Gavin, M., & Zheng, Y. (2006). FOXP3 and NFAT: Partners in tolerance. *Cell* 126, 253-256, 0092-8674.

Sakaguchi, S., Sakaguchi, N., Asano, M., Itoh, M., &Toda, M. (1995). Immunologic self-tolerance maintained by activated T cells expressing IL-2 receptor alpha-chains (CD25). Breakdown of a single mechanism of self-tolerance causes various autoimmune diseases. *J. Immunol.* 155, 1151-1164, 0022-1767 (Print), 0022-1767 (Linking).

Sakaguchi, S., Yamaguchi, T., Nomura, T., & Ono, M. (2008). Regulatory T cells and immune tolerance. *Cell* 133, 775-787, 0092-8674.

Sather, B.D., Treuting, P., Perdue, N., Miazgowicz, M., Fontenot, J.D., Rudensky, A.Y., & Campbell, D.J. (2007). Altering the distribution of Foxp3+ regulatory T cells results in tissue-specific inflammatory disease. *J. Exp. Med.* 204, 1335-1347.

Schröder, N.W.J., Crother, T.R., Naiki, Y., Chen, S., Wong, M.H., Yilmaz, A., Slepenkin, A., Schulte, D., Alsabeh, R., Doherty, T.M., & *et al.* (2008). Innate immune responses during respiratory tract infection with a bacterial pathogen induce allergic airway sensitization. *J Allergy Clin Immunol* 122, 595-602.e595, 0091-6749.

Scott-Browne, J.P., Shafiani, S., Tucker-Heard, G.s., Ishida-Tsubota, K., Fontenot, J.D., Rudensky, A.Y., Bevan, M.J., & Urdahl, K.B. (2007). Expansion and function of Foxp3-expressing T regulatory cells during tuberculosis. *J Exp Med* 204, 2159-2169.

Seino, K.I., Fukao, K., Muramoto, K., Yanagisawa, K., Takada, Y., Kakuta, S., Iwakura, Y., Van Kaer, L., Takeda, K., Nakayama, T., & *et al.* (2001). Requirement for natural killer T (NKT) cells in the induction of allograft tolerance. *Proc Natl Acad Sci USA* 98, 2577-2581, 0027-8424 (Print), 0027-8424 (Linking).

Selvaraj, R.K., & Geiger, T.L. (2007). A kinetic and dynamic analysis of Foxp3 induced in T cells by TGF-beta. *J. Immunol.* 179, 11 p following 1390, 0022-1767 (Print), 0022-1767 (Linking).

Serra, P., Amrani, A., Yamanouchi, J., Han, B., Thiessen, S., Utsugi, T., Verdaguer, J., & Santamaria, P. (2003). CD40 ligation releases immature dendritic cells from the control of regulatory CD4+CD25+ T cells. *Immunity* 19, 877-889, 1074-7613.

Siewert, C., Menning, A., Dudda, J., Siegmund, K., Lauer, U., Floess, S., Campbell, D.J., Hamann, A., & Huehn, J. (2007). Induction of organ-selective CD4+ regulatory T cell homing. *Eur J Immunol.* 37, 978-989, 1521-4141.

Sinclair, N.R. (2004). B cell/antibody tolerance to our own antigens. *Front Biosci* 1, 3019-3028.

Stephens, G.L., Andersson, J., & Shevach, E.M. (2007). Distinct subsets of Foxp3+ regulatory T cells participate in the control of immune responses. *J Immunol* 178, 6901-6911.

Suvas, S., Azkur, A.K., Kim, B.S., Kumaraguru, U., & Rouse, B.T. (2004). CD4+CD25+ regulatory T cells control the severity of viral immunoinflammatory lesions. *J Immunol* 172, 4123-4132.

Svensson, M., Marsal, J., Ericsson, A., Carramolino, L., Brodén, T., Márquez, G., & Agace, W.W. (2002). CCL25 mediates the localization of recently activated CD8αβ+ lymphocytes to the small-intestinal mucosa. *J. Clin. Invest.* 110, 1113-1121, 0021-9738.

Taams, L.S., van Amelsfort, J.M.R., Tiemessen, M.M., Jacobs, K.M.G., de Jong, E.C., Akbar, A.N., Bijlsma, J.W.J., & Lafeber, F.P.J.G. (2005). Modulation of monocyte/macrophage function by human CD4+CD25+ regulatory T cells. *Hum Immunol* 66, 222-230, 0198-8859.

Tadokoro, C.E., Shakhar, G., Shen, S., Ding, Y., Lino, A.C., Maraver, A., Lafaille, J.J., & Dustin, M.L. (2006). Regulatory T cells inhibit stable contacts between CD4+ T cells and dendritic cells in vivo. *J Exp Med* 203, 505-511.

Tang, Q., Adams, J.Y., Tooley, A.J., Bi, M., Fife, B.T., Serra, P., Santamaria, P., Locksley, R.M., Krummel, M.F., & Bluestone, J.A. (2006). Visualizing regulatory T cell control of autoimmune responses in nonobese diabetic mice. *Nat Immunol* 7, 83-92, 1529-2908.

Tang, Q., & Bluestone, J.A. (2006). Plasmacytoid DCs and Treg cells: casual acquaintance or monogamous relationship? *Nat Immunol* 7, 551-553,

Tang, Q., & Bluestone, J.A. (2006). Plasmacytoid DCs and T(reg) cells: casual acquaintance or monogamous relationship? *Nat Immunol* 7, 551-553.

Thornton, A.M., & Shevach, E.M. (1998). CD4+CD25+ immunoregulatory T cells suppress polyclonal T cell activation in vitro by inhibiting interleukin 2 production. *J Exp Med* 188, 287-296.

Tiemessen, M.M., Jagger, A.L., Evans, H.G., van Herwijnen, M.J.C., John, S., & Taams, L.S. (2007). CD4+CD25+Foxp3+ regulatory T cells induce alternative activation of human monocytes/macrophages. *Proc Natl Acad Sci U S A* 104, 19446-19451.

Torcia, M.G., Santarlasci, V., Cosmi, L., Clemente, A., Maggi, L., Mangano, V.D., Verra, F., Bancone, G., Nebie, I., Sirima, B.S., & *et al.* (2008). Functional deficit of T regulatory cells in Fulani, an ethnic group with low susceptibility to *Plasmodium falciparum* malaria. *Proc Natl Acad Sci USA* 105, 646-651.

Veltkamp, C., Anstaett, M., Wahl, K., Moller, S., Gangl, S., Bachmann, O., Hardtke-Wolenski, M., Langer, F., Stremmel, W., Manns, M.P., & *al.* (2011). Apoptosis of regulatory T lymphocytes is increased in chronic inflammatory bowel disease and reversed by anti-TNF-apha treatment. *Gut*, 1468-3288 (Electronic), 017-5749 (Linking).

Vignali, D.A., Collison, L.W., & Workman, C.J. (2008a). How regulatory T cells work. *Nat Rev Immunol* 8, 523-532, 1474-1741 (Electronic).

Vignali, D.A.A., Collison, L.W., &Workman, C.J. (2008b). How regulatory T cells work. *Nat Rev Immunol* 8, 523-532, 1474-1733.

Walther, M., Tongren, J.E., Andrews, L., Korbel, D., King, E., Fletcher, H., Andersen, R.F., Bejon, P., Thompson, F., Dunachie, S.J., *et al.* (2005). Upregulation of TGF-beta, FOXP3, and CD4+CD25+ regulatory T cells correlates with more rapid parasite growth in human malaria infection. *Immunity* 23, 287-296, 1074-7613.

Wan, Y.Y., & Flavell, R.A. (2005). Identifying Foxp3-expressing suppressor T cells with a bicistronic reporter. *Proc Natl Acad Sci USA* 102, 5126-5131.

WHO (2004). Global prevalence and incidence of selected curable sexually transmitted infections overview and estimates.

Wildin, R.S., Ramsdell, F., Peake, J., Faravelli, F., Casanova, J.-L., Buist, N., Levy-Lahad, E., Mazzella, M., Goulet, O., Perroni, L., & *et al.* (2001). X-linked neonatal diabetes mellitus, enteropathy and endocrinopathy syndrome is the human equivalent of mouse scurfy. *Nat Genet* 27, 18-20, 1061-4036.

Wildin, R.S., Smyk-Pearson, S., & Filipovich, A.H. (2002). Clinical and molecular features of the immunodysregulation, polyendocrinopathy, enteropathy, X linked (IPEX) syndrome. *J. Med. Genet.* 39, 537-545, 1468-6244 (Electronic), 0022-2593 (Linking).

Wright, G.P., Notley, C.A., Xue, S.-A., Bendle, G.M., Holler, A., Schumacher, T.N., Ehrenstein, M.R., & Stauss, H.J. (2009). Adoptive therapy with redirected primary regulatory T cells results in antigen-specific suppression of arthritis. *Proc Natl Acad Sci U S A* 106, 19078-19083.

Zarek, P.E., Huang, C.-T., Lutz, E.R., Kowalski, J., Horton, M.R., Linden, J., Drake, C.G., & Powell, J.D. (2008). A2A receptor signaling promotes peripheral tolerance by inducing T-cell anergy and the generation of adaptive regulatory T cells. *Blood* 111, 251-259.

Zhao, D.-M., Thornton, A.M., DiPaolo, R.J., & Shevach, E.M. (2006). Activated CD4+CD25+ T cells selectively kill B lymphocytes. *Blood* 107, 3925-3932,

Zheng, S.G., Wang, J., Wang, P., Gray, J.D., & Horwitz, D.A. (2007). IL-2 is essential for TGF-beta to convert naive CD4+CD25- cells to CD25+Foxp3+ regulatory T cells and for expansion of these cells. *J. Immunol.* 178, 2018-2027, 0022-1767 (Print), 0022-1767 (Linking).

Zheng, S.G., Wang, J.H., Gray, J.D., Soucier, H., & Horwitz, D.A. (2004). Natural and induced CD4+CD25+ cells educate CD4+CD25- cells to develop suppressive activity: The role of IL-2, TGF-β, and IL-10. *J Immunol* 172, 5213-5221.

Zhou, J., Carr, R.I., Liwski, R.S., Stadnyk, A.W., & Lee, T.D. (2001). Oral exposure to alloantigen generates intragraft CD8+ regulatory cells. *J. Immunol.* 167, 107-113, 0022-1767 (Print), 0022-1767 (Linking).

Part 2

Overview on Clinical Involvement of Chlamydia

6

Insights into the Biology, Infections and Laboratory Diagnosis of *Chlamydia*

H.N. Madhavan, J. Malathi and R. Bagyalakshmi
Larsen and Toubro Microbiology Research Centre, Kamal Nayan Bajaj Institute for Research in Vision and Ophthalmology, Vision Research Foundation, College Road, Sankara Nethralaya, Chennai
India

1. Introduction

Chlamydia are Gram negative obligate intracellular bacteria of eukaryotic cells and have a unique developmental cycle consisting of formation of infectious particle called elementary body and non-infectious particle called reticulate body. They are included in the order *Chlamydiales* and the order *Chlamydiales* belongs to the class *Chlamydiae*, phylum *Chlamydiae*, domain bacteria. The genus *Chlamydia* consists of important species *C. muridarum*, (affects only mice and hamsters) *C. suis* (affects only swine) *and C. trachomatis* (a human pathogen). *Chlamydia* are Gram-negative obligate intracellular eubacteria. Originally, they were taxonomically categorized into their own order *Chlamydiales*, with one family, *Chlamydiaceae*, and a single genus, *Chlamydia*.[1] The genus included four species: *C. trachomatis*, *C. psittaci* ,*C. pneumoniae* and *C. pecorum* .In 1999, it was proposed by Everett et al [2] that *Chlamydia* should be divided in two genera, *Chlamydia and Chlamydophila,* containing altogether nine species (Table 1) in addition to the five new species and three new families (*Parachlamydiaceae,*

Species	Host	Route of entry
	CHLAMYDIA	
Chlamydia trachomatis	Humans	Pharyngeal, ocular, genital, rectal
Chlamydia suis	Pigs	Pharyngeal
Chlamydia muridarum	Mouse, hamster	Pharyngeal, genital
	CHLAMYDOPHILA	
Chlamydophila abortus	Mammals	Oral, genital
Chlamydophila caviae	Guinea pig	Pharyngeal, ocular, genital, urethral
Chlamydophila felis	Cats	Pharyngeal, ocular, genital
Chlamydophila pecorum	Mammals	Oral
Chlamydophila pneumoniae	Humans ,frog, koala, horse	Pharyngeal, ocular
Chlamydophila psittaci	Birds	Pharyngeal, ocular, genital

Table 1. The family *Chlamydiaceae* as proposed by Everett et al (1999)

Simniaceae and *Waddliaceae*).The molecular characteristics distinguishing *Chlamydia* and *Chlamydiales* is shown in Table 2. However, the proposal to change the taxonomic nomenclature for the *Chlamyadiaceae* family has not been generally accepted in the field. [3] Two of the species, *C. trachomatis* and *C. pneumoniae*, are common pathogens in humans, whereas the other species occur mainly in animals.

Genus	Approximate Genome Size (million DNA base pairs)	Detectable Glycogen	Number of Ribosomal Operons
Chlamydophila	1.2	Absent	1
Chlamydia	1.0	Present	2

Table 2. Molecular Criteria Distinguishing *Chlamydiaceae*

2. Life cycle

Chlamydia trachomatis exhibits an affinity for the epithelial cells of mucous membranes such as those found on the surfaces of the cervix, urethra, rectum, nasopharynx and conjunctiva, and enter these cells by a phagocytic process. [4] Within infected cells, *Chlamydiae* occur in intra cytoplasmic vesicles, or inclusion bodies. Within these inclusion bodies, morphological development takes place and two distinct particles are observed: a small, dense infective particle, the elementary body which is transformed in the host cell into the larger less dense form, the reticulate body. These non-infective but metabolically active reticulate bodies synthesize proteins and their own DNA and RNA, then replicate by binary fission to form micro colonies within the inclusion bodies. Between 18-24 hours post infection, the reticulate bodies divide and then ultimately some of the reticulate bodies reorganize into large numbers of elementary bodies. Between 48 and 72 hours post infection, the host cells ruptures releasing elementary bodies which can infect new host cells.[5] The life cycle of *C. trachomatis* is shown in Figure 1. The species of *Chalmydia* causing infections is shown in Table 3.

Species of Chlamydia	Serovars	Infection caused by the serovars
Chlamydia trachomatis	A, B ,Ba, C	Blinding trachoma
	D - K	Genital infections and infant pneumonia, Inclusion conjunctivitis
	L1,L2,L3	Lymphogranuloma venereum (LGV)
Chlamyophila psitacii	-	Psittacosis
Chlamydophila pneumoniae	-	Acute respiratory disease

Table 3. *Chalmydia* causing different infections

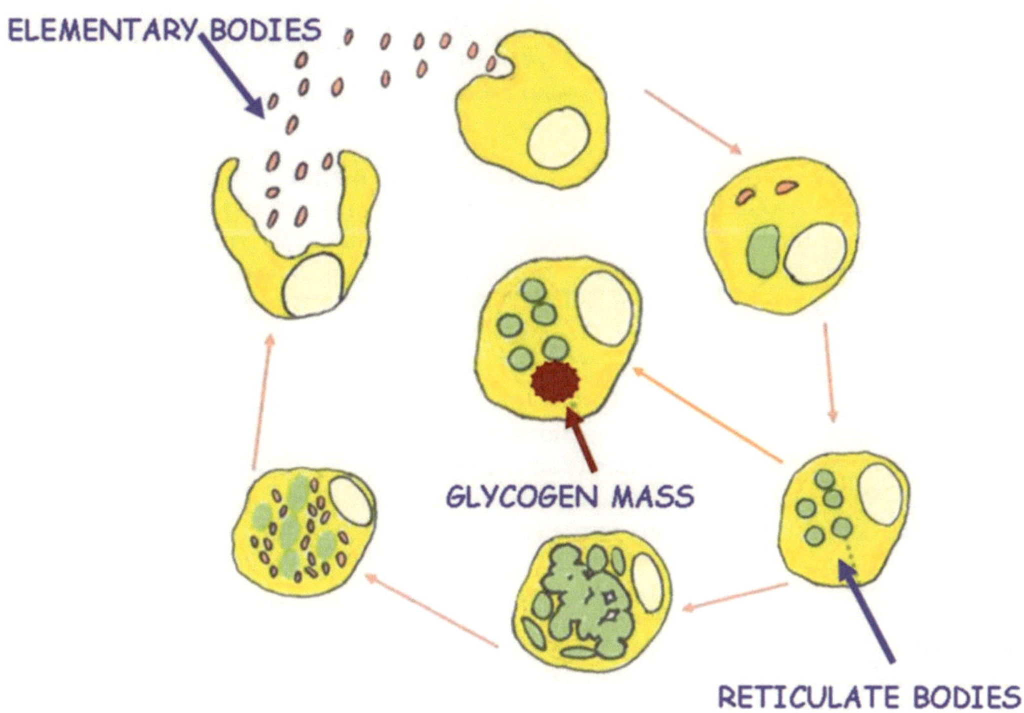

Fig. 1. Life Cycle of *Chlamydia*

3. Clinical manifestations

C. trachomatis causes trachoma, infant pneumonia, LGV and nongonococcal urethritis.

Although most infections caused by *C. trachomatis* in women are asymptomatic, clinical manifestations include cervicitis, urethritis, endometritis, Pelvic Inflammatory Disease (PID) or abscess of the Bartholin glands.[6] Although the initial site of infection is usually the cervix, the urethra and rectum may also be infected. [7] The prevalence of *C. trachomatis* infection in pregnant women ranges from 2 to 35%.[8] Pregnant women with chlamydial infections are at increased risk for adverse outcomes of pregnancy, and postpartum PID.

C. trachomatis is the most common cause of neonatal conjunctivitis and pneumonia in early infancy .[9] Fifteen to 25% of treated infants who were exposed at birth develop conjunctivitis, and 3 to 16% develop pneumonia . Symptoms of conjunctivitis usually develop within 2 weeks of delivery, and if the infection is untreated, chlamydial pneumonia can develop at 4 to 17 weeks after delivery .[10] These conditions are occasionally difficult to treat, and prolonged hospitalization may be necessary . Infants with chlamydial pneumonia are at increased risk for later pulmonary dysfunction and possibly for chronic respiratory disease .[11]

Trachoma. Endemic trachoma is a chronic disease caused by repeated infections of the conjunctiva and cornea by *C. trachomatis.* Trachoma is probably the most common cause of preventable blindness worldwide. Epidemiologic studies of trachoma in developing countries have shown that this disease is most often due to infection by *C. trachomatis* serotypes A to C. Scarring of the conjunctiva with resultant trauma to the cornea appears to be due to repeated exposure to the chlamydial agent, which is transmitted primarily by nonsexual mechanisms. The ability to identify *C. trachomatis* from the conjunctivae of trachoma patients may vary greatly depending on the duration and clinical stage of the disease.[12]

Lymphogranuloma venereum (LGV) LGV is a systemic disease caused by *C. trachomatis* serovars L1 to L3. The LGV serovars of *C.trachomatis* are more invasive than other genital serovars, resulting in infection of the epithelial layers and underlying soft tissue.[13] The primary symptom is a painless genital ulcer or papule. The most common manifestation of the secondary stage of LGV in men, and the reason most men seek treatment, is inflammation and swelling of the inguinal lymph nodes .Women tend to be less symptomatic at this stage: only 20 to 30% of women present with inguinal lymphadenopathy and approximately one-third of women without proctocolitis present with lower abdominal and back pain.[14] The secondary stage of infection is characterized by systemic symptoms including fever, malaise, chills, anorexia, myalgia, and arthralgia .[15] Untreated infections can lead to late complications including ulceration and hypertrophy of the genitalia, arthritis, and fistula formation involving the rectum, bladder, vagina, or vulva .[14]

Nongonococcal urethritis. *C. trachomatis* serotypes D to K are the organisms most frequently associated with nongonococcal urethritis in men As many as one-third of men who harbor urethral *Chlamydia* may be asymptomatic In 1 to 2% of chlamydial urethral infections, infection can evolve to epididymitis. *C. trachomatis* is the most commonly isolated microorganism in young heterosexual men with epididymitis in whom there is no structural abnormality of the genitourinary disease. *C. trachomatis* infects the endocervix of women and may cause mucopurulent cervicitis.[8]

This infection frequently spreads to the urethra and urinary bladder and may result in the "acute urethral syndrome"of abacteriuric pyuria .[12]

Pneumonia Pneumonia and bronchitis are the most frequently recognized illnesses associated with *C. pneumoniae*, although asymptomatic infection or unrecognized, mildly symptomatic illnesses are the most common result of infection. In a series of studies 10% of cases of pneumonia and approximately 5% of bronchitis and sinusitis cases in adults have been attributed to the organism [16].No set of symptoms or signs is unique to pulmonary infections with *C. pneumoniae*; however, several characteristics of the clinical presentation may help distinguish it from other causes .[17] A subacute onset is common. Pharyngitis, sometimes with hoarseness, is often present early in the course of the illness. There may be a biphasic pattern to the illness, with resolution of pharyngitis prior to development of a more typical bronchitis or pneumonia syndrome. Cough is very common and is often prolonged.[18,19]

Psittacosis. Reiter's classic description of respiratory disease associated with avian exposure (ornithosis, formerly "psittacosis") was the first modern recognition of *C. psittaci* disease . Both psittacine and nonpsittacine birds can harbor the infectious agent, and avian *C. psittaci* strains cause illness in bird handlers and poultry workers. Because of the antigenic diversity of *C. psittaci*, serologic methods based on detection of antibody responses to genus-specific antigens of chlamydiae are used for the presumptive diagnosis of ornithosis. Although *C. psittaci* can be isolated in cell culture or by animal inoculation with clinical specimens, the low sensitivity of these methods and the biohazard of *C. psittaci* in the laboratory have made serologic diagnosis the indicated laboratory method for diagnosis of ornithosis.

Mammalian. In spite of the broad range of non human hosts, zoonotic *C. psittaci* strains other than avian strains have infrequently been reported to cause human infection. A few cases of human infection resulting in abortion have been reported following infection by ovine *C. psittaci* strains .Rare cases of infective endocarditis presumed to be due to *C. psittaci* from avian and nonavian sources have also been reported. *C. psittaci* strains TWAR infections a novel group of chlamydial organisms has been associated with acute respiratory disease in humans. The acronym TWAR is derived from Taiwan-acute respiratory, the designations given to the first University of Washington studies that produced these strains. TWAR organisms have morphologic, antigenic, and developmental similarities to *C. psittaci* and are not inhibited *in vitro* by sulfonamides. Molecular studies of deoxyribonucleic acid relatedness suggest that TWAR agents are genetically homogeneous and differ from both *C .psittaci* and *C. trachomatis.* [20]

4. Epidemiology

Although *C. trachomatis* infection did not become a fully reportable disease in the United States until 1996, it is known to be the most common bacterial sexually transmitted disease (STD). The actual incidence of chlamydial infection is not yet known due to lack of reporting in all 50 states up to 1996; however, national trends have been estimated by using data from states that reported cases prior to 1996, sentinel surveillance, surveys, and models based on proxies of infection .[21,22] Worldwide, it is estimated that there are more than 50 million new cases of *C. trachomatis* infection annually.[23] Although the major impact of disease caused by *C. trachomatis* is on the female reproductive tract, this agent also causes infections in men and children. [24] The prevalence of *C. trachomatis* infection in sexually active adolescent women, the population considered most at risk, generally exceeds 10%, and in some adolescent and STD clinic populations of women, the prevalence can reach 40%. [25] The prevalence of *C.trachomatis* infection ranges from 4 to 10% in asymptomatic men and from 15 to 20% in men attending STD clinics. [26, 27] Chlamydial infections in newborns occur as a result of perinatal exposure; approximately 65% of babies born from infected mothers become infected during vaginal delivery.[28]

4.1 Clinical sequelae of *C. trachomatis* infections in infants

C. trachomatis is the most common cause of neonatal conjunctivitis and one of the most common causes of pneumonia in early infancy. Prophylactic treatment of the eyes with silver nitrate does not prevent chlamydial infection; 15 to 25% of treated infants who were exposed at birth develop conjunctivitis, and 3 to 16% develop pneumonia.[29] Symptoms of conjunctivitis usually develop within 2 weeks of delivery and if the infection is untreated, chlamydial pneumonia can develop at 4 to 17 weeks after delivery. These conditions are occasionally difficult to treat, and prolonged hospitalization may be necessary. Infants with chlamydial pneumonia are at increased risk to develop pulmonary dysfunction and possibly chronic respiratory disease.[30]

4.2 Clinical sequelae of *C. trachomatis* infections in men

Among heterosexual men, chlamydial infections are usually urethral and up to 50% are asymptomatic [31]. When symptoms do occur, usually 1 to 3 weeks following exposure, they are indistinguishable from those of gonorrhea (urethral discharge and/or pyuria). However, compared with gonococcal urethritis, chlamydial urethritis is more likely to be asymptomatic. In older men, epididymitis is more often due to other etiologies associated with urinary tract abnormalities or instrumentation rather than sexually transmitted origins.[32] Unilateral scrotal pain is the primary symptom, and common clinical signs of this infection include scrotal swelling, tenderness, and fever. If urethral symptoms are also present, a sexually transmitted bacterial etiology is likely .[33]

4.3 Reitter's syndrome

Reitter's syndrome is caused by *Chlamydia trachomatis* The manifestations of reactive arthritis include the following triad of symptoms: an inflammatory arthritis of large joints including commonly the knee and the back (due to involvement of the sacroiliac joint), inflammation of the eyes in the form of conjunctivitis or uveitis, and urethritis in men or cervicitis in women. Patients can also present with mucocutaneous lesions, as well as psoriasis-like skin lesions such as circinate balanitis, and keratoderma blennorrhagica. Not all affected persons have all the manifestations, and the formal definition of the disease is the occurrence of otherwise unexplained non-infectious inflammatory arthritis combined with urethritis in men, or cervicitis in women.[34] Symptoms generally appear within 1-3 weeks but can range from 4 to 35 days from the onset of the inciting episode of the disease. The classical presentation is that the first symptom experienced is a urinary symptom such as burning pain on urination (dysuria) or an increased frequency of urination. Other urogenital problems may arise such as prostatitis in men and cervicitis, salpingitis and/or vulvovaginitis in women. [35] The arthritis that follows usually affects the large joints such as the knees causing pain and swelling with relative sparing of small joints such as the wrist and hand. Eye involvement occurs in about 50% of men with urogenital reactive arthritis and about 75% of men with enteric reactive arthritis. Conjunctivitis and uveitis can include redness of the eyes, eye pain and irritation, or blurred vision. [36]

4.4 Laboratory diagnosis of chlamydial infections

Specimens used for detecting *Chlamydiae* must be handled cautiously following universal precautions. Handling of specimens for the detection of *C. psittaci* requires type III containment facility. The organism is air-borne and is highly virulent. [20] The most common anatomic site used to obtain specimens for the isolation of *C. trachomatis* from women is the endocervix, which is sampled with a swab (endocervix, Dacron and calcium alginate) or cytologic brush. The swab should be inserted into the cervical os past the squamocolumnar junction, about 1 to 2 cm deep, rotated for 15 to 30 s, and removed without touching the vaginal mucosa. [13] The transport medium may contain fetal calf serum up to 10% to preserve the viability of the organisms. The transport media may contain gentamycin or vancomycin , nystatin/ amphotericin B at a concentration of 10 microgram /ml to prevent the growth of other bacteria and fungi respectively while transport. Specimen upon receipt in the laboratory should be processed as early as possible. In case of delay the specimen can be stored for a maximum period of 48 hours in the refrigerator. If further delay is expected the specimen should be stored at -70⁰C until further processed. [37,38] The earlier methods used for the direct detection include iodine staining which stains the glycogen present in the cell lines. Giemsa staining is applied to detect the inclusion bodies of the organism. Later mononclonal antibodies raised against the major outer membrane protein gene of the organism tagged with a Fluorecein Iso thiocyanate (FITC) dye· was widely used for the rapid detection of the agent from direct clinical specimens.[39]

4.5 Cultivation

Until recently, culture was considered the gold standard for detection of *Chlamydia in* specimens because it has a specificity that approaches 100% . The usual cell lines in use are HeLa 229, L434 mouse fibroblasts or McCoy cells in the case of *C. trachomatis* and *C. psittaci;* Buffalo green monkey kidney cells for *C. psittaci* and *C. pecorum* , HeLa or Hep2 cells for *C. pneumoniae.* The disadvantages of using culture as a gold standard include its relative insensitivity compared with DNA amplification techniques. [40] With the exception of 'fast growing' strains like the LGV biovar of *C. trachomatis,* it was usually necessary to assist the process of infection by centrifugation of the clinical material onto monolayers of the appropriate cells in tissue culture. Growth of the organisms was also facilitated by the use of anti-metabolites directed against the host cell (cycloheximide; emetine or mitomycin C) or, for the *C. trachomatis* TRIC: Trcahoma Inclusion conjunctivitis biovar, by the use of charged anionic polymers such as Poly - L - lysine or DEAE dextran. Compounds like polyethylene glycol or high energy glucose 6 phosphate also aided the growth of some chlamydiae. [41]

4.6 Rapid shell vial technique for cultivation

Modified culture technique where the cells are grown over cover slips placed inside a glass shell vial is used for the rapid cultivation of Chlamydia. Here the cells are grown over the

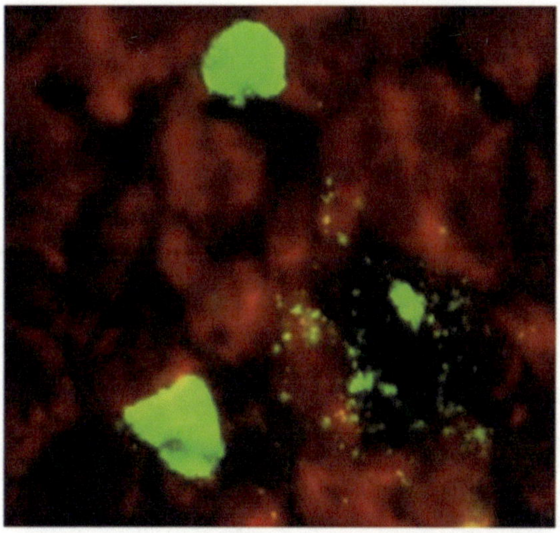

Fig. 2. Immunofluorescence staining showing Reticulate and Elementary bodies of *Chlamydia trachomatis* isolated from a case of ophthalmia neonatorum in McCoy cell culture (40 X)

cover slips and treated with cycloheximide (1microgram/ml) containing medium for 24 hours. [42]After the medium is aspirated out 200 micro liters of clinical specimen is added and the culture is centrifuged centrifuged at 3000 rpm for 1 hour. At the end of 1 hour, Dulbecco's minium essential medium with 10% fetal calf serum and 1-3 microgram cycloheximide is added and incubated at 37 ^{o}C (10 % CO_2 atmosphere) for 48-72 hours. At the end of incubation period the medium is aspirated out, the cover slip is fixed and stained with the antisera (Figure 2). This method is rapid and more sensitive in isolation of *Chlamyida.* [43]

Since susceptibility of a cell line is an important factor for cultivation of *C. trachomatis*, Malathi et al [44] have compared McCoy, HeLa, BHK-21, HEp-2, Vero and A549 cell lines for growth characteristics of *C. trachomatis.* These were inoculated with 150 infection-forming units (IFU) of *C. trachomatis* A, B, Ba and C serovars. Growth was graded according to the number of IFUs per microscopic field (100X). A549-cell line was not susceptible to infection by any of the serovars. The growth of *C. trachomatis* was good to very good in McCoy and HeLa cell lines. Vero, BHK-21 and HEp-2 cell lines varied considerably in the susceptibility to infection.[44]

4.7 Polymerase chain reaction (PCR) and Ligase chain reaction (LCR)

Plasmids of *Chlamydia* are known to exist in 7 copy numbers. Due to the rapidity, increased sensitivity and specificity PCR, LCR methods have widely replaced the conventional culture methods. [42,43] The major target for amplification based tests against *C. trachomatis* are generally multiple-copy gene products, such as the cryptic chlamydial plasmid (Figure 3) or ribosomal RNA, Major outer membrane protein gene. Starting with a multiple copy gene offers a clear starting advantage with respect to sensitivity. The application of initial nucleic acid amplification based tests had increased the clinical sensitivity of detection of chlamydial DNA in clinical samples. [42,45] The major advantage of nucleic acid based amplification technique is the combined sensitivity and specificity. Automation is possible and a large volume of sample can be handled at a time. The technique was helpful to establish the etiology of the *C. pneumoniae* in optic neuritis[46] where cultivation of the organism was not possible

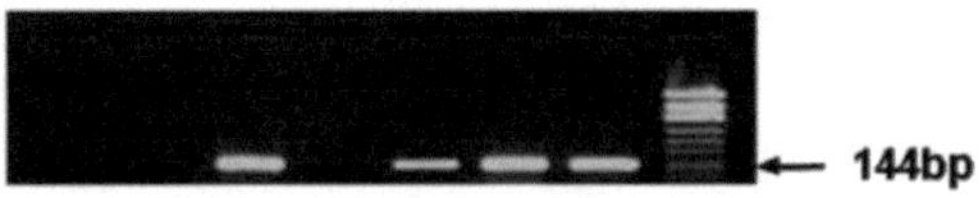

1 : Negative control

2 : Extraction control

3, 5 & 6 : conjunctival swabs positive for PCR

4 : specimen negative for PCR

p : positive control : *C. trachomatis* Ba DNA

M : PHI X 174 DNA/ *Hinf* I digest

Fig. 3. Agarose electrophoretogam showing the MOMP amplified products of *C. trachomatis* from conjunctival swabs

5. Screening tests for chlamydia

C. trachomatis infection is asymptomatic in 80% of women making diagnosis and detection difficult. Chlamydia has its high prevalence amongst young men and women and more than 13.5% of women < 25 years old have lower genital tract infections.[47] Screening women for lower genital tract infection with *C. trachomatis* is important in the prevention of PID, ectopic pregnancy and infertility.[48] The screening tests available for *C. trachomatis* include nucleic acid based amplification assays, PCR and LCR, gene probe and enzyme immuno assay. The sensitivity and specificity of Chlamydia trachomatis screening tests is provided in Table 4.

Test	Sensitivity	Specificity	Detection limit (no of organisms)
NAAT[a]	90-95	>99	1-10
DFA[b]	80-85	>99	10-500
EIA[c]	60-85	99	500-1000
DNA Probe[d]	75-85	> 99	500 -1000
Cell culture	50-85	100	5-100
POC[e]	20-55	>90	>10,000

NOTE:

[a] DNA based amplicor assay (Roche diagnostic, Basel Switzerland), LCR (Abbott Lab, Abbott Park IL, USA)

[b] DFA Expansion: Direct fluorescence assay - Syva MicroTrak (Syva Co, Palo, Alto, CA, USA)

[c] EIA - Vidas (BioMerieux, Craporre France)

[d] DNA probe based hybrid capture assay (QIAGEN, Hilden Germany), Ampliprobe system (Imclone systems, NY, USA) RNA Based (Gen probe San Diego CA, USA)

[e] Point of care test : Handilab C (Zonda incorporated Dallas TX, USA), Biorapid *Chlamydia* antigen test (Biokit, Barcelona, Spain) Quick Vue Chlamydia test (Quidel Corporation, San Diego CA, USA)

Table 4. Sensitivity and specificity of *Chlamydia trachomatis* detection assays and most widely used commercially available tests [49]

Screening programmes are promoted to control transmission and prevention of female reproductive tract morbidity caused by genital *Chlamydia*. Offering an annual screening test to men and women aged under 20 years may be the most cost effective strategy if PID progression is 10% or higher. Screening is essential to reduce the propagation of the disease. Annual testing is recommended for women at high risk for Chlamydial infection. According to Centre for Disease Control (CDC), the following patients population should be screened for *Chlamydia* infection.

- Sexually active female adolescents
- Women undergoing induced abortion
- Women attending STD clinic
- Women with mucopurulent cervicitis
- Women with new / multiple sexual partners within 3 months of presentation[50]

5.1 Chlamydial infection in chronic ill patients

C. pneumoniae infection can cause acute respiratory illnesses (including sinusitis, bronchitis, and pneumonia) that are sometimes associated with wheezing. Little is known about whether acute infection in a previously unexposed, non asthmatic individual can produce persistent wheezing leading to a diagnosis of chronic asthma. Hahn et al [51] conducted a study on 163 primary outpatient adults (average age 43, 45% male) who had acute wheezing illnesses or chronic asthma to evaluate *C. pneumoniae* infection by serologic testing. *C. pneumoniae* infection was diagnosed if the organism was detected one or more times by culture, or if a patient met accepted serologic criteria for acute infection: an IgM antibody titer of 1:16 or greater, a fourfold or greater rise in IgM, IgG or total Ig titer between acute and convalescent sera, or a single IgG or total Ig titer of 1:512 or greater.[11] Criteria for an acute primary (first exposure) *C. pneumoniae* infection include the presence of IgM antibody in a titer of 1:16 or greater whereas IgM is absent in acute secondary infection (re-exposure).In the setting of acute bronchitis or pneumonia, a single IgG titer of 1:512 or greater correlates with organism identification and is also indicative of acute infection.

Acute *C. pneumoniae* respiratory tract infections in previously unexposed, non asthmatic individuals can result in chronic asthma. Patients previously diagnosed with chronic asthma should be evaluated for possible chronic *C. pneumoniae* infection.

5.2 Chlamydial infections in pregnancy

Prematurity is one of the leading causes of perinatal mortality. Uterine contractions may be induced by cytokines, proteolytic enzymes or prostaglandins released or induced by microorganisms. Some studies [52,53] suggest that maternal *C. trachomatis* infection in pregnancy is associated with premature delivery. Termination of pregnancy (i.e. induced abortion) is one of the most commonly performed gynecological procedures. Post-abortal PID is a well recognized complication of termination of pregnancy, with its attendant risks of tubal dysfunction and either infertility or subsequent ectopic pregnancy.

6. Prevention

Chlamydia prevention programs have been implemented to reduce the burden of reproductive sequelae resulting from chlamydial infection. Because most reproductive complications of *Chlamydia* occur in females and most infections are asymptomatic, the cornerstone of *Chlamydia* prevention is screening young females for infection. Nucleic acid amplification tests are the preferred diagnostic tests because of their superior sensitivity, and they can be performed on easily collected specimens, such as urine or vaginal swabs.[53] Highly efficacious treatment options include single-dose oral azithromycin or a 1-week course of doxycycline. National chlamydia screening recommendations were first released in 1993. Currently, CDC, the U.S. Preventive Services Task Force (USPSTF), and numerous professional medical associations recommend annual chlamydia screening for all sexually active females aged < 25 years and for females aged ≥ 25 years if they are at increased risk for infection (e.g., if they have new or multiple sex partners.[54]

C. pneumoniae is difficult to prevent because it is spread by respiratory droplets from other sick people.Because people with this type of pneumonia do not always feel very sick, they often continue to attend school, go to work, and go to other public places. They then spread the bacteria in the tiny droplets that are released into the air during coughing. Therefore, this pneumonia is very difficult to prevent and often occurs in outbreaks within communities.[20] Prevention of *C. trachomatis* pneumonia involves recognizing the symptoms of genital infection in the mother and treating her prior to delivery of her baby.[53]

6.1 Prognosis of *Chlamydia* infection

The 'prognosis' of *Chlamydia* usually refers to the likely outcome of *Chlamydia.* The prognosis of Chlamydial infection may include the duration, chances of complications of *Chlamydia* infection , probable outcomes, prospects for recovery, recovery period for *Chlamydia,* survival rates, death rates, and other outcome possibilities in the overall prognosis of Chlamydia. Naturally, such forecast issues are by their nature unpredictable

The following are statistics from various sources about deaths related to Chlamydia:

Chlamydia death statistics for various regions worldwide:

- About 1,000 deaths from Chlamydia in Africa 2002
- About 8,000 deaths from Chlamydia in South East Asia 2002
- About 1,000 deaths from Chlamydia in Eastern Mediterranean 2002[55]
- Treated with antibiotics, chlamydial infections can be cured 95% of the time.

6.2 Chlamydial infection in children

Exposure to *C. trachomatis* during delivery can cause ophthalmia neonatorum (conjunctivitis) in neonates or chlamydial pneumonia at one to three months of age.

6.3 Ophthalmia neonatorum

Ophthalmia neonatorum usually occurs within five to 12 days of birth but can develop at any time up to one month of age. It may cause swelling in one or both eyes with mucopurulent drainage. Prophylaxis with silver nitrate or antimicrobial ointment, which reduces the risk of gonococcal infection in neonates, does not reduce the risk of chlamydial infection. Testing for chlamydial infection in neonates can be done by culture or nonculture techniques. The eyelid should be everted and the sample obtained from the inner aspect of the eyelid. Sampling the exudates is not adequate because this technique increases the risk of a false-negative test. Ophthalmia neonatorum can be treated with erythromycin base or ethylsuccinate at a dosage of 50 mg per kg per day orally, divided into four doses per day for 14 days. The cure rate for both options is only 80 percent, so a second course of therapy may be necessary. Topical treatment is ineffective for ophthalmia neonatorum and should not be used even in conjunction with systemic treatment.[53]

6.4 Chlamydial pneumonia

Acute lower respiratory tract infection (ALRTI) is the major cause of morbidity and mortality in young children world wide.*Chlamydia pneumoniae* is a common respiratory pathogen which is responsible for about 10% of community acquired pneumonia (CAP). The best method of microbiological diagnosis at the acute stage of Chlamydial infection is undecided, because the organism grows poorly on cell culture.[20] Testing can be performed on a sample obtained from the nasopharynx. Nonculture techniques may be used, but they are less sensitive and specific for nasopharyngeal specimens than for ocular specimens. If tracheal aspirates or lung biopsies are being collected for pneumonia in infants one to three months of age, the samples should be tested for *C. trachomatis*.

Like ophthalmia neonatorum, pneumonia secondary to *C. trachomatis* is treated with erythromycin base or ethylsuccinate at a dosage of 50 mg per kg per day orally, divided into four doses per day for 14 days. As with ophthalmic infection, a second course of therapy may be necessary.[53]

7. Advanced research

7.1 Polymorphisms associated with ocular and genital isolates of *C. trachomatis*

Genome sequence of several diverse strains has revealed a remarkable level of genomic synteny suggesting that minor genetic differences determine the pathogen host and tissue specific infection characteristics. To better understand the genetic basis of Chalmydial pathobiologic diversity, Carlson et al [56] performed a comparative DNA -DNA microarray genomic hybridization and reported with all 15 *Chlamydia trachomatis* serovariants and reported only a few major genetic differences. An exception was the cytotoxin locus located in the plasticity zone, a region that exhibited significant polymorphisms among serovars. The cytotoxin gene was interrupted by extensive mutants and deletions among different serovars however 3 basic open reading frames (ORF) were discovered that correlated with non invasive genitotropic serovars which possess an intact N terminal portion of the putative toxin gene. This region contains the UDP Glucose binding domain and the glycosyl transferase domain required for enzymatic activity of *Clostridium* toxin homologues suggesting a role in urogenital infection/ pathogenesis.[57]

C. trachomatis exists as multiple serovariants that exhibit distinct organo tropism for the eye or urogenital tract. The genome of an oculotropic trachoma isolate (A/HAR-13) was sequenced and compared to the genome of a genitotropic (D/UW-3) isolate. Remarkably, the genomes share 99.6% identity, supporting the conclusion that a functional tryptophan synthase enzyme and toxin might be the principal virulence factors underlying disease organotropism. Tarp (translocated actin-recruiting phosphoprotein) was identified to have variable numbers of repeat units within the N and C portions of the protein. A correlation exists between lymphogranuloma venereum serovars and the number of N-terminal repeats. Single-nucleotide polymorphism (SNP) analysis between the two genomes highlighted the minimal genetic variation. A disproportionate number of SNPs were observed within some members of the polymorphic membrane protein (pmp) autotransporter gene family that corresponded to predicted T-cell epitopes that bind HLA class I and II alleles. These results implicate Pmps as novel immune targets, which could advance future chlamydial vaccine strategies. Lastly, a novel target CTA0934 for PCR diagnostics was discovered that can discriminate between ocular and genital strains. This discovery will enhance epidemiological investigations in nations where both trachoma and chlamydial STD are endemic. The results suggest that Tarp is among the few genes to play a role in adaptations to specific niches in the host.[58]

7.2 Chlamydial L,L – diaminopimelate aminotransferase

Recent phylogenetic studies have revealed that chlamydia shares a common ancestor with modern plants and retains unusual plant-like traits (both genetically and physiologically). In particular, the enzyme L,L-diaminopimelate aminotransferase, which is related to lysine production in plants, is also linked with the construction of chlamydia's cell wall. The genetic encoding for the enzymes is remarkably similar in plants and chlamydia, demonstrating a close common ancestry.[59] This unexpected discovery may help scientists develop new treatment avenues: if scientists could find a safe and effective inhibitor of L,L-diaminopimelate aminotransferase, they might have a highly effective and extremely specific new antibiotic against chlamydia.

7.3 Emerging Chlamydial infections

Several Chlamydial like bacteria have recently been identified as potential emerging public threats or pathogenic agents in animals. *Parachlamydia acanthamoebae, Parachalmydia naegelerophila and Simkania negerensis* have been reported as possible aetiological agents of pneumonia in humans. To define further the possible pathogenetic potential of these *Chlamydia* like bacteria new diagnostic tools are needed to demonstrate the agent within tissue lesions.[60] Borel et al [60] have used tissue microarray technology to establish the immuno histochemistry protocols and to determine the specificity of new antisera against various Chlamydia like bacteria for future use on formalin fixed and paraffin embedded tissues. The antisera exhibited strong reactivity against autologous antigen and closely related heterologous antigen but no cross reactivity with distantly related species.

8. References

[1] Moulder, J.W., Hatch, J.P., Kuo, C.C., Schachter, J.T. , Storz, J.(1984) Genus *Chlamydia.* In: Krieg NR & Holt JG (eds) Bergey's Manual of Systematic Bacteriology, vol 1. Williams & Wilkins, Baltimore, MD, 729–739.

[2] Everett, K.D., Bush, R.M, Andersen, A.A, (1999) Emended description of the order *Chlamydiales,* proposal of *Parachlamydiaceae fam. nov.* and *Simkaniaceae fam. nov.,* each containing one monotypic genus, revised taxonomy of the family *Chlamydiaceae,* including a new genus and five new species, and standards for the identification of organisms. *International Journal of Systematic Bacteriology,* 49 (2), 415–440.

[3] Schachter, J., Stephens, R.S., Timms, P., Kuo, C., Bavoil ,P.M., Birkelund, S., Boman, J., Caldwell, H., Campbell, L.A., Chernesky, M., Christiansen, G., Clarke, I.N., Gaydos, C., Grayston, J.T., Hackstadt, T., Hsia, R., Kaltenboeck, B., Leinonnen, M., Ocjius, D., McClarty, G., Orfila, J., Peeling, R., Puolakkainen, M., Quinn, T.C., Rank, R.G,, Raulston, J., Ridgeway, G.L., Saikku, P., Stamm, W.E., Taylor-Robinson, D.T., Wang, S.P. , Wyrick, P.B., (2001) .Radical changes to chlamydial taxonomy are not necessary just yet. *International Journal of Systematic Evolutionary Microbiology,* 51 (249), 251–243.

[4] Barbour, A.G., Amano, K., Hackstadt, T., Perry, L., Caldwell, H.D., (1982).*Chlamydia trachomatis* has penicillin-binding proteins but not detectable muramic acid. *Journal of Bacteriology* , 151, 420–428.

[5] Fox. A, Rogers. J.C., Gilbart, J., Morgan, S., Davis, C.H., Knight, S. ,Wyrick, P.B.,(1990). Muramic acid is not detectable in *Chlamydia psittaci* or *Chlamydia trachomatis* by gas chromatography-mass spectrometry. *Infection and Immunity*, 58, 835–837.

[6] Stephens, R.S. Chlamydial evolution: a billion years and counting. In: Schachter J et al. (eds) Chlamydial Infections. *Proceedings of the Tenth International Symposium on Human Chlamydial Infections. Antalya, Turkey,* June 2002, 3–12.

[7] Bleker, O.P., Smalbraak, D.J., Shutte, M.F., (1990) .Bartholin's abscess: the role of *Chlamydia trachomatis. Genitourinary. Medicine,* 66,24–25.

[8] Dunlop, E.M.C.,Goh,B.T., Darougar, S., Woodland, R., (1985). Triple culture tests for the diagnosis of Chlamydial infection of the female genital tract. *Sexually Transmitted. Diseases* 12 ,68–71.

[9] Sweet, R.L., Landers, D.V., Walker ,C., Schachter, J., (1987). *Chlamydia trachomatis* infection and pregnancy outcome. *American Journal of Obstetetrics and Gynecology,* 156, 824–833.

[10] Hammerschlag, M.R., Cummings, C., Roblin, P.M,, Williams, T.H, Delkem, I.(1989) Efficacy of neonatal ocular prophylaxis for the prevention of chlamydial and gonococcal conjunctivitis. New England Journal of Medicine, 320,769-772

[11] Claesson, B.A., Trollfors, B., Brolin, I.,Granstrom, M., Henrichsen, J., Jodal, U., Juto,P., Kallings, I., Kanclerski, K.,Lagergard, T.,(1989). Etiology of community-acquired pneumonia in children based on antibody responses to bacterial and viral antigens. *Pediatric Infectious Diseases Journal*, 8, 856–862.

[12] Saikku,P. *Chlamydia pneumoniae* - an update on clinical disease. In: Schachter J et al. (eds) Chlamydial Infections. Proceedings of the Tenth International Symposium on Human Chlamydial Infections. Antalya, Turkey, June 2002, 443–453.

[13] Black,C.N., (1997).Current methods of laboratory diagnosis of *Chlamydia trachomatis* infections. *Clinical Microbiology Reviews,* 10 (1),160-184

[14] Pearlman, M.D., McNeeley, S.G.,(1992). A review of the microbiology,immunology, and clinical implications of *Chlamydia trachomatis* infections. *Obstetrics Gynecology. Survey*, 47, 448–461.

[15] Perine, P.L., Osoba, A.O., (1990). Lymphogranuloma venereum, p 195–204. *In* K. K. Holmes, P.-A. Mårdh, P. F. Sparling, and P. J. Wiesner (ed.), Sexually transmitted diseases. McGraw Hill Book Co., New York,N.Y.

[16] Grayston, J.T., (1992). Infections caused by *Chlamydia pneumoniae* strain TWAR. *Clinical Infectious Disease*,15,757–763.

[17] Grayston, J.T., Aldous, M.B., Easton, A., Wang, S.P., Kuo, C.C., Campbell, L.A., Altman, J., (1993). Evidence that *Chlamydia pneumoniae* causes pneumonia and bronchitis. *Journal of Infectious Diseases;* 168,1231–1235.

[18] Grayston, J.T., Kuo, C.C., Wang, S.P., Altman, J, (1986).A new *Chlamydia psittaci* strain, TWAR, isolated in acute respiratory tract infection.*New. England Journal of Medicine* 315,161–168.

[19] Thom, D.H., Grayston, J.T., Wang, S.P., Kuo, C.C., Altman, J., (1990). *Chlamydia pneumoniae* strain TWAR, *Mycoplasma pneumoniae* and viral infections in acute respiratory disease in a university student health clinic population. *American Journal of Epidemiology*, 132, 248–256.

[20] Kuo, C.C., Jackson, L.A, Campbell, L.A, Grayston, J.T.,(1995) *Chlamydia pneumoniae* (TWAR) *Clinical Microbiology Reviews* ; 4: 451-461

[21] Washington, A.E., Johnson, R..E, Sanders, L.L,(1987). *Chlamydia trachomatis* infections in the United States. What are they costing us? *Journal of Amercian Medical Association* 257:2070–2072.

[22] Washington, A.E., Johnson, R.E., Sanders, L.L., Barnes, R.C., Alexander, E.R. Incidence of *Chlamydia trachomatis* infections in the United States using reported Neisseria gonorrhoeae as a surrogate, 1986 ;p. 487–490. In D. Oriel, G. Ridgway, J. Schachter, et al. (ed.), Chlamydia infections.Proceedings of the Sixth International Symposium on Human Chlamydial Infections. Cambridge University Press, Cambridge, England.

[23] Krul , K.G, (1995) Closing in on Chlamydia. *CAP Today*, 9:1–20.

[24] Batteiger B. E., Jones, R.B,(1987).Chlamydial infections. *Infectious Diseases in Clinical North America,* 1:55–81.

[25] Centres for disease control and prevention recommendations for the prevention and management of Chlamydia trachomatis infections 1993; MorbidMortal. Weekly Rep. 42(No. RR-12):1–39

[26] Rietmeijer, C.A.M, Judson, F.N., van Hensbroek, M.B., Ehret, J.M., Douglas, J.M., Jr ,(1991). Unsuspected *Chlamydia trachomatis* infection in heterosexual men attending a sexually transmitted diseases clinic: evaluation of risk factors and screening methods. *Sexually Transmitted. Disease,* 18:28–35.

[27] Stamm, W.E., Koutsky, L.A., Benedetti, J.K., Jourden, J.L., Brunham, R.C., Holmes, K.K.,(1984) Chlamydia trachomatis urethral infections in men. Prevalence, risk factors, and clinical manifestations.*Annals of Internal Medicine,* 100:47–51.

[28] Schachter, J., Grossman, M., Sweet, R.L., Holt, J., Jordan, C., Bishop, E, (1986). Prospective study of perinatal transmission of *Chlamydia trachomatis* . *Journal of American Medical Association* , 255: 3374–3377.

[29] Thompson, S., B. Lopez, K..H., Wong, R.,(1982). A prospective study of chlamydial and mycoplasmal infections during pregnancy, p. 155–158. In P.-A. Mårdh, K. K. Holmes, J. D. Oriel, J. Schachter, and P. Piot (ed.),Chlamydial infections. Fernstrom Foundation Series. Elsevier Biomedical Press, Amsterdam, The Netherlands.

[30] Preece, P.M., Anderson, J.M., Thompson, R.G.,(1989) *Chlamydia trachomatis* infection in infants: a prospective study. *Archives of Diseases in Children* , 64: 525-529.

[31] Claesson, B. A., Trollfors, B., Brolin, I.,Granstrom, M., Henrichsen, J., Jodal, U., Juto, P., Kallings, I., Kanclerski, K., Lagergard, T,(1989), Etiology of community-acquired pneumonia in children based on antibody responses to bacterial and viral antigens. *Pediatrics. Infectious Diseases. Journal,*; 8:856–862.

[32] Weiss, S.G., Newcomb, R.W., Beem, M.O., (1986). Pulmonary assessment of children after Chlamydia pneumonia of infancy. *Journal of Paediatrics,*108: 659-664

[33] Zelin, J.M., Robinson, A.J., Ridgway, G.L., Allason-Jones, E., .Williams, P. (1995). Chlamydial urethritis in heterosexual men attending a genitourinary medicine clinic: prevalence, symptoms, condom usage and partner change. *International Journal of Sexually Transmitted Diseases AIDS* 6:27–30.

[34] Wallace, D.J., Weisman, M, (2000). "Should a war criminal be rewarded with eponymous distinction? The double life of Hans Reiter (1881–1969)". *Journal of Clinical Rheumatology,* 6 : 49–54.

[35] Kvien ,T., Glennas, A., Melby, K., Granfors, K.(1994) "Reactive arthritis: Incidence, triggering agents and clinical presentation". *Journal of Rheumatology* , 21 : 115–22.

[36] Pearlman, M. D., McNeeley, S.G. (1992). A review of the microbiology immunology, and clinical implications of *Chlamydia trachomatis* infections. *Obsteterics Gynecology Survey,*.47:448–461

[37] Madhavan, H.N., (1999). Laboratory investigations on viral and *Chlamydia trachomatis* infections of the eye: Sankara Nethralaya experiences. Indian Journal of Ophthalmology. , 47:241-6

[38] Rao, S.K., Madhavan, H.N., Padmanabhan, P., Lakshmi, G.S., Natarajan, K., Garg, D, (1996) Ocular chlamydial infections. Clinicomicrobiological correlation. Cornea, 15:62-5.

[39] Madhavan, H.N., Rao, S.K., Natarajan, K., Sitalakshmi, G., Jayanthi, I., Roy, S., (1994). Evaluation of laboratory tests for diagnosis of chlamydial infections in conjunctival specimens. *Indian Journal of Medical Research.* 100:5-9.

[40] Claas, H.C., Melchers, W.J., de Bruijn, I.H., De Graaf, M., van Dijk ,W.C., Lindeman, J., Quint ,W.G. (1990) Detection of *Chlamydia trachomatis* in clinical specimens by the polymerase chain reaction. *European Journal of Clinical Microbiology and Infectious Diseases;*9:864–868

[41] Dutilh, B., Bebear, C., Rodriguez, P., Vekris, A., Bonnet, J., Garret, M,.(1989).Specific amplification of a DNA sequence common to all *Chlamydia trachomatis* serovars using the polymerase chain reaction. *Research in. Microbiology,* 140:7–16

[42] Malathi, J., Madhavan ,H.N., Therese, K.L., Rinku, J.P., Narender, K.P.. (2002) Prevalence of *Chlamydia trachomatis* and herpes simplex virus in males with urethritis & females with cervicitis attending STD clinic. Indian *Journal of Medical Research,*116:58-63

[43] Malathi, J., Madhavan, H.N., Therese, K.L., Joseph, P.R.,(2003). A hospital based study on the prevalence of conjunctivitis due to *Chlamydia trachomatis .Indian Journal of Medical Research* , 117: 71-5

[44] Malathi, J., Shyamala, G., Madhavan, H.N.,(2004) Relative susceptibility of six continuous cell lines for cultivation of *Chlamydia trachomatis.* Indian *Journal of Medical Microbiology* ,22: 169-71

[45] Malathi, J., Madhavan, H.N., Therese, K.L., Shyamala, G. ,(2004) Polymerase chain reaction to detect Chlamydia trachomatis and adenovirus in the nasopharyngeal aspirates from paediatric patients with lower respiratory infections *.Indian Journal of Pathology and Microbiology.* 47:302-5.

[46] Malathi, J., Shyamala, G., Feeba, V., Therese, K.L., Madhavan, H.N. (2007).Optimization of a polymerase chain reaction (PCR) for increasing its sensitivity to detect

Chlamydia pneumoniae specific genome. *Indian Journal of Pathology and Microbiology* 2007,50 : 104-106

[47] Andrea ,S.B., Chapin ,K.C. (2011). "Comparison of Aptima Trichomonas vaginalis Transcription-Mediated Amplification Assay and BD Affirm VPIII for Detection of T. vaginalis in Symptomatic Women: Performance Parameters and Epidemiological Implications.". *Journal of Clinical Microbiology* , 49 : 866–9.

[48] Svensson, L.O., Mares, I., Olsson, S.E., Nordstrom, M.L. (1991).Screening for *Chlamydia trachomatis* infectionin women and aspects of the laboratory diagnostics. *Acta Obstetrics Gynaecology Scandinavia*, 70: 587-590

[49] Watson, E.J., Templeton, A., Russell, I., Paavonen, J., Mardh, P., Sracy, A., Pederson, B.S, (2002). The accuracy and efficacy of screening tests for *Chlamydia trachomatis*: a systematic review. *Journal of Medical Microbiology*,154 : 1021-1031

[50] Land, J.A., Van Bergen, J.E.A.M., Morne, S.A., Postma, M.J. (2010) Epidemiology of *Chlamydia trachomatis* infection in women and the cost effectiveness of screening. *Human reproduction Update* , 16 : 189-204

[51] Hahn ,D.L., McDonald, R., (1998) Can acute Chlamydia pneumoniae respiratory tract infection initiate chronic asthma. *Annals of Allergy Asthma and Immunology,* 81: 339-344

[52] French, J. I., McGregor, J. A., Draper, D., Parker, R. & McFee, J. (1999). Gestational bleeding, bacterial vaginosis, and common reproductive tract infections: risk for preterm birth and benefit of treatment. *Obstetrics & Gynecology* 93, 715 - 724.

[53] Gencay, M., Koskiniemi, M., Saikku, P., Puolakkainen, M., Raivio, K., Koskela, P. & Vaheri, A. (1995). *Chlamydia trachomatis* seropositivity during pregnancy is associated with perinatal complications. *Clinical Infectious Diseases* 21, 424 - 426.

[54] US Preventive Services Task Force. Screening for chlamydial infection: U.S. Preventive Services Task Force recommendation statement.(2007) Annals of Internal Medicine,147:128--34

[55] Grayston, J. T., Kuo, C.C., Wang, S.P. Altman J.,(1986).A new Chlamydia psittaci strain called TWAR from acute respiratory infections. *New England. Journal of Medicine,* 315:161-168.

[56] World Health Organization (WHO) Report on the prevention of Chlamydia trachomatis infection 2004

[57] Carlson, J.H,, Hughes, S., Hogan, D., Cieplak, G., Sturdevant, D.E., McClarty, G., Caldwell, H.D., Belland, R.J,(2004) Polymorphisms in *Chlamydia trachomatis* cytotoxin locus associated with ocular and genital isolates *Infection and Immunity,* 72: 7063-7072

[58] Lulter, E.I., Bonner, C., Holland ,M.T., Suchland, R., Stamm, W.E., Jewett, T.J., McClarty, G., Hackstadt, T,(2010). Phylogenetic analysis of *Chlamydia trachomatis* Tarp and correlation with clinical phenotype. Infection and Immunity , 78: 3678-3688

[59] McCoy, A.J., Adams, N.E., Hudson, A.O, Gilvarg, C., Leustek, T., Maurelli, A.T. (2006). "L,L-diaminopimelate aminotransferase, a trans-kingdom enzyme shared by *Chlamydia* and plants for synthesis of diaminopimelate/lysine". Proceedings of . National. Academy and Sciences. U.S.A. ,103 : 17909–14.

[60] Borel ,N., Casson, N., Entenza, J.M., Kaiser, C., Pospischil, A., Greub, G. (2009).Tissue microarray and immunohistochemistry as tools for evaluation of antibodies against *Chlamydia* like bacteria Journal of Medical Microbiology, 58: 863-866

7

Chlamydia trachomatis Infections in Neonates

Eszter Balla and Fruzsina Petrovay
National Center for Epidemiology
Hungary

1. Introduction

Chlamydia trachomatis is the most commonly reported agent among sexually transmitted bacteria in Europe and in the US (CDC, 2011; ECDC, 2011). In 2009 the constantly growing number of notified cases in Europe exceeded 340 000. This is presumably far below the true figure due to the asymptomatic nature of infections, which often remains undiagnosed. Genital *C. trachomatis* infections (serotype D-K) are especially common among sexually active young people (between 15 and 25 years of age), who represent as many as 75% of all reported infections across Europe (ECDC, 2011). Adolescents are threatened by acute urogenital manifestations (*urethritis, epididymitis, cervicitis*, etc.), that may turn into chronic complications (PID, infertility, ectopic pregnancy, etc.). The wide range of infections of the female genital tract poses a major reproductive health problem both on an individual and a community level.

Neonates of infected mothers form another important risk-group as women may transfer chlamydia not only to their sexual partners but if pregnant, to their infants as well. This vertical type of transmission is a well known phenomenon, which may result in ocular or in respiratory tract infection. Neonatal *C. trachomatis* infections include descending types of manifestation of syndromes, beginning with inclusion *conjunctivitis*, and/or nasopharyngal colonisation, which may be followed by neonatal *pneumonia*. These infections are generally mild-moderate in the case of an early and adequate treatment. The definitive diagnosis is hampered by the common phenomenon of asymptomatic, therefore often undiagnosed maternal infection, as well as by the need for adequate sample-collection and targeted screening techniques.

Neonatal infections due to vertical transmission have a so called "indicator" function too, namely, that they point to the infected mother and her sexual partner/s. It means that this kind of infections has a great epidemiological importance so the diagnostic and therapeutic efforts should be extended to cover all the exposed persons. Several specialists may be involved in this process, among them neonatologists, gynaecologists, urologists too. Unfortunately this seems to be a neglected area of neonatal infectology and there is only estimated data regarding the incidence of neonatal *C. trachomatis* infection, although all the necessary diagnostic means are available to identify the affected neonates. Focused screening efforts should be made to reduce the number of infected pregnant women and thereby the rate of vertical transmission.

2. Microbiology - Pathogenesis

Chlamydia trachomatis is an obligate intracellular pathogen. This species is currently divided into 19 serovars based on the antigenic difference between the major outer membrane proteins (MOMP) and numerous serovariants differentiated with genotyping by restriction fragment length polymorphism (RFLP) analysis of the PCR-amplified *omp1* gene. Urogenital, thereby neonatal infections are predominantly related to the D-K serotypes, while the A-C and L serotypes are not significantly associated with the latter group. Main target sites of the pathogen are the uro-anogenital organs of adults, the respiratory tract of neonates and the conjunctivae in both age groups. These local, non-invasive infections are typically limited to the epithelial surface of the mucous membranes.

The main transmission route involves sexual contact where due to the infected genital secretion a direct transfer of the pathogen occurs, which leads to the common clinical manifestations of uro-anogenital infection, however auto- or heteroinoculation may seldom result in *conjunctivitis*. Untreated maternal *C. trachomatis* carriage represents a special case of multiple risks threatening pregnant women themselves, their sexual partners as well as their infants.

Infants commonly acquire the pathogen by vertical transmission, typically during transit through the infected birth channel at delivery, however there are many reports suggesting intrauterine *C. trachomatis* infection. Besides the indirect evidence of a heightened risk of adverse pregnancy outcomes associated with *C. trachomatis,* the presence of *C. trachomatis* DNA in the fetal membranes detected by PCR confirms the intrauterine infection theory. A suspected choriodecidual inflammation and histological *chorioamnionitis* can give a possible explanation for the mechanism that may lead to the premature rupture of amniotic membranes. *Chorioamnionitis* is frequently seen in the case of premature babies, but the role of chlamydial infection in subsequent respiratory insufficiency is yet to be determined (Blas et al, 2007; Givner et al, 1981; Mårdh, 2002; Numazaki, 2004; Rastogi et al, 1999, 2003; Yoshida et al, 2000).

3. Epidemiology – Transmission rates

Due to the clinically unapparent nature of *C. trachomatis* infection in adults the reported cases allow only an estimation of its true prevalence. High risk groups may serve as a hidden reservoir of the pathogen, where the infection can easily spread through untreated carriers. A complex STI surveillance and screening programmes are required to gain more accurate information. Epidemiological studies may help to assess the role of this agent in various clinical pictures. Genital chlamydia infection rates among sexually active women in Europe are predominantly in the range of 4-10%, which varies by age, socio-economic background and geographical location (Pellowe & Pratt, 2006; Wilson et al., 2002).

In the United States the overall *C. trachomatis* prevalence among sexually active females aged 14-19 years was found to be 6,8%, which is nearly three times the rate among those aged 25-39 years. There are significant differences between the various socioeconomic, ethnic and racial groups as well (CDC, 2011). It is a proven fact that young age (<25 years) and an improvident sexual behavior (new or multiple partners; unsafe sex, infection with another sexually transmitted disease, etc.) are associated with an increased risk of infection, which may also be attributable to other physiological/hormonal factors, such as an immature cervix, cervical friability/ectopy, or alteration in the cervical mucus (Peipert, 2003).

In a recent, population-based study *C. trachomatis* prevalence was found 3,9% among more than 4,000 pregnant women, while during a previous, five-year period study 4,7% of 5531 pregnant women proved to be infected (Rours et al, 2011; Schachter et al, 1986). The rate of occurrence among infants is directly related to the maternal carriage of the pathogen, and strongly depends on the perinatal prevention strategies. The estimated data of neonatal prevalence rates range from 4 to 60 per 1000 live births depending on the population tested (Zar, 2005), which makes this microorganism the most frequent sexually transmitted pathogen in the industrialised countries, although detailed surveillance reports are nowadays still lacking. In a prospective study focusing on asymptomatic neonatal chlamydial colonisation and on symptomatic infection, the incidence per 1000 live birth was found to be 6,5 and 8,2 respectively, a summarised value of those represents a 14,7‰ prevalence of all chlamydia-positive infants (Preece et al, 1989).

The direct contact transmitting the pathogen derives sometimes from the infected nursing persons, mainly from family members or hospital staff or other care-takers, whose contaminated fingers or towels, etc. may spread chlamydiae to the infants. However rare this route of the infection may be, it should always be considered when investigating the source of neonatal infection (Mårdh, 2002).

Vertical transmission rates are relatively high as 50-75% of infants born vaginally acquire *C. trachomatis* directly from their infected mothers (Chen et al, 2007; Rours et al, 2008). One or more organs of neonates may be colonised, including the *nasopharynx* as the leading target site. *Conjunctivae* and the lower *anogenital tract* are less frequently involved, however the *rectal* and *vaginal* persistance may last as long as 3 years (Schachter et al, 1979). Chronic infection of the conjunctivae due to an untreated neonatal condition was also described, while the isolation of the pathogen was successful even at age of six years (Thompson et al, 2001). Most of these latter cases remain symptomless, but that fact may have medico-legal importance and must be carefully explored. From a clinical point of view only 20-50% of colonisations will result in acute *conjunctivitis,* and approximately 5-20% in neonatal *pneumonia,* respectively (Darville, 2005; Numazaki et al, 1989; Schachter et al, 1986).

Recent studies suggest that prenatal transmission rates due to an ascending intrauterine infection seem to be significantly lower than those with vaginal delivery. Chorionic villus sampling completed with PCR technique can reveal *C. trachomatis* infection even in early pregnancy, when the incidence of *chorioamnionitis* related to the pathogen proved to be 5,1% (Dong et al, 1998). Another sampling possibility targets the amniotic fluid, which may be investigated by serology, antigen- or DNA detecting methods too. There is data about the presence of a specific *C. trachomatis* antigen in 3,8% of the amniotic samples (Djukić et al, 1996). There are documented cases of neonatal chlamydial infections after caesarean deliveries with ruptured membranes, and more rarely with intact membranes (Mohile et al, 2002). The prevalence of *C. trachomatis* infection among newborns after a caesarean section was found to be 8,3% (Bell et al, 1994; Preece et al, 1989; Yu et al, 2009). These data indicate that intrauterine *C. trachomatis* infections can occur in any phase of the pregnancy, however at a relatively low risk.

4. Antenatal complications of maternal *C. trachomatis* infection

Infected pregnant women and their fetuses are threatened by various complications resulting from ascension of pathogens into the upper genital tract and invasion of the amniotic cavity. Bacterial exposition can lead to infection at any time during pregnancy. Adverse pregnancy outcomes related to *C. trachomatis* include spontaneous abortion, premature rupture of membranes (PROM), preterm delivery and postpartum *endometritis* (Baud et al, 2008; Brocklehurst & Rooney, 2007; Ostaszewska-Puchalska et al, 2005).

The actual cause of **spontaneous abortion** often remains unexplained. Besides chromosomal, immunologic or hormonal abnormalities, organic or functional disorders, an infective etiology may also be presumed. Controversial data is available regarding the role of *C. trachomatis* but recent studies seem to confirm it. In a prospective study investigating the presence of specific DNA in aborted tissues prevalence of *C. trachomatis* was found to be a surprisingly high 32% (Magoń et al, 2005).

Prenatal infection is thought to be a relevant cause of **preterm deliveries** in up to 40-48% of all cases, that may occur either spontaneously or in form of a **premature rupture of membranes (PROM)** (Baud et al, 2008; Lamont et al, 1987; Locksmith & Duff, 2001; Maxwell, 1993). Ascending microbial invasion of placenta, fetal membranes, and amniotic fluid is associated with an intense maternal inflammatory response that may eventually trigger a fetal inflammatory response. This pathological process is histologically characterised by *funisitis* and/or *chorioamnionitis*, caused by the same microbes as those isolated from the lower genital tract of pregnant women (Rezeberga et al., 2008). *Chorioamnionitis* is found in overall 30-70% of preterm births, while only in 4-18% of full term deliveries (Locksmith & Duff, 2001). Despite often being a subclinical condition, *chorioamnionitis* may facilitate the weakening and rupture of membranes. The main problem with histologic diagnosis comes from the fact that the sampling of the placenta and fetal membranes can be carried out only after delivery. The unfavourable consequences of placental inflammation are not yet completely understood, but direct impact of pathogens or organ damage due to inflammatory cytokines and proteolytic enzymes may both serve as an explanation. Several surveys indicate that among other bacteria deriving from urogenital reservoir *C. trachomatis* carriage also increases the risk of the premature rupture of membranes (PROM), as well as that of **preterm uterine activity** in infected women, which may contribute to fetal morbidity and mortality (Blas et al, 2007; Mårdh, 2002, Yu et al; 2009). Much of the harmful complications of *C. trachomatis* infection are supposed to occur via immunopathological damage (Baud et al, 2008).

C. trachomatis infection was found to be responsible for several perinatal complications, such as **low-birth-weight** and **prematurity**, defined as being born before 37 completed gestational weeks (Gencay et al, 2001; Rastogi et al, 1999). Chlamydial etiology was proven in preterm infants suffering from severe **acute respiratory distress** within the first day of life, requiring mechanical ventillation and supplemental oxygen (Colarizi et al, 1996). It was documented being associated with **chronic respiratory disease** in premature infants as well, while the presence of specific IgM suggested intrauterine infections during late pregnancy (Mårdh, 2002; Numazaki et al, 1986, 2003). Since it occasionally has a serious impact on the fetus, prenatal *C. trachomatis* infection should be prevented by comprehensive screening programs during pregnancy.

5. Postnatal clinical manifestations in *C. trachomatis* infected neonates

There are two main target sites of the pathogen in affected neonates, which are responsible for the principal clinical manifestations of infection, accordingly ocular and respiratory tract infections are among the commonest neonatal complications. The possible association between inclusion *conjunctivitis* and subsequent infantile *pneumonitis* was first documented in a case report in 1975 (Schachter et al, 1975). Due to direct exposure to the infected maternal genital secretion, conjunctivae may be easily colonized by *C. trachomatis*, followed by an early onset of ocular symptoms, while respiratory tract infections due to aspiration of the bacteria generally show a descending pattern, deriving from an acute/subacute *nasopharyngitis* and resulting later in a clinical condition of *pneumonia*. The relatively frequent **conjunctivitis, nasopharyngitis** and the less common **pneumonia**, as the most serious complication often may combine, and these associated symptoms refer to the stepwise progression of the infection. A retrospective study analysing the occurrence rate of various clinical appearances found that *conjunctivitis* was present in 73%, *pneumonia* in 20% and both diseases in 7% of affected newborns. Hospitalisation was needed in 20% of infants (Jain, 1999). Other, less frequent clinical findings include **rhinitis**, **otitis media**, while **myocarditis** and **encephalitis** have been documented as rare, unusual manifestations of the infection.

5.1 Conjunctivitis, or ophthalmia neonatorum

Neonatal *conjunctivitis* is one of the most common types of infections in the first 30 days of life. It is defined as an inflammation of the conjunctivae that may be caused by various toxic or infectious agents. Chlamydiae as obligate intracellular agents can intensely replicate in conjunctival cells, which leads to epithelial damage. In case of acquiring *C. trachomatis* (serotypes D-K) the ocular infection manifests as a so called **inclusion conjunctivitis**, when during intracellular development cycles of chlamydiae infectious elementary bodies of the pathogen differentiate into large, metabolically active reticulate bodies. The latter accumulate in the endosomes of host cells turning them into cytoplasmic inclusions, which can be detected after Giemsa staining even by a conventional light microscope. During the inflammatory response, granulocytes invade the site of infection, which appears clinically in the form of a mucopurulent exudate. The untreated infection resolves spontaneously in most patients during a couple of months, however, a formation of a *micropannus* (granulation tissue-membrane) or of a *pannus* (corneal neovascularizaton) may sometimes occur. Infrequently persistent *conjunctivitis* and trachoma-like corneal/conjunctival scarring have been documented too (Darville, 2005; Quirke & Cullinane, 2008).

C. trachomatis has been regularly reported as a leading agent for neonatal *conjunctivitis*, or *ophthtalmia neonatorum* in several studies analysing bacterial etiology. There are some surveys which still support that prominent position by investigating certain populations (Rours et al, 2008; Salpietro et al, 1999; Schaller & Klauss 2001). It is an interesting fact that the pathogen itself was first isolated precisely from a neonatal *conjunctivitis* in 1959 (Jones et al, 1959). In the 1980's *C. trachomatis* was detected in as many as 14-46% of neonatal *conjunctivitis*, however, the latest studies estimate the descending prevalence of *C. trachomatis* as being approximately 8% in this condition. Its significant role moreover seems to be recently extinguished by some classical pyogenic bacteria, such as *Staphylococcus aureus, Haemophilus influenzae* and *Streptococcus pneumoniae* (Di Bartolomeo et al, 2001; Persson et al, 1983; Valencia et al, 2000).

The results of studies implemented in various countries clearly reflect that the distribution of major etiological agents of neonatal conjunctivitis is in accordance with the actual prevalence of STI pathogens among pregnant women. In examination of newborns in the United Arabic Emirates less than 5% of all cases were attributable to *C. trachomatis* and *Neisseria gonorrhoeae. C. trachomatis* alone was responsible in Norway for only 6%, while in India and in Kenya for 24% and 28,7% of all neonatal *conjunctivitis* respectively (Dannevig et al, 1992; Mohile et al, 2002; Nsanze et al, 1996; Schaller & Klauss, 2001). In the Netherlands chlamydial screening of pregnant women is not a routine practice, which may play a significant role in high rates of *C. trachomatis* detection, which was calculated over 60% of studied infants presenting *conjunctivitis* (Rours et al, 2008). In the 1980's the incidence of chlamydial *ophthalmia neonatorum* was found 3 - 250 cases per 1,000 live births, which has radically declined to 0,65 per 1,000 live births in Europe during the last three decades. This decreasing trend can be particularly observed in developed countries, where screening and treatment during pregnancy is a regular part of *C. trachomatis* surveillance (Darville, 2005; Di Bartolomeo et al, 2001; Krohn et al, 1993; Persson et al, 1983; Preece et al, 1989; Quirke & Cullinane, 2008).

In contrast with classical trachoma caused by A-C serotypes, those responsible for neonatal eye infection belong to the D-K serotypes and correlate with the actual distribution of urogenital maternal carriage of the pathogen (Di Bartolomeo et al, 2001; Isobe et al, 1996). Some data suggest that certain genotypes may be strongly asssociated with *ophthtalmia neonatorum*, as an epidemiological link was recently found between genotype E and the ocular symptoms (Gallo Vaulet et al, 2010). The perinatal transmission rate of infection resulting in *conjunctivitis* is relatively high, as the risk of a newborn acquiring *C. trachomatis* in case of maternal carriage varies between 8-44%. Based on pooled results of previous studies, the point estimate of incidence of *ophthalmia neonatorum* proved to be 15% among infants exposed to *C. trachomatis* perinatally (Rosenman et al, 2003). The incubation period usually lasts between 5-14 days after delivery, which may be shorter in the case of an intrauterine infection due to PROM. The median age of onset of the ocular symptoms is typically 1-2 weeks after birth. That means that the signs of infection acquired intrapartum will usually develop after leaving hospital, generally up to one month of age (Miller, 2006; Persson et al, 1983). Affected newborns would have most often been seen and treated by two or more physicians before establishing the definitive diagnosis of *C. trachomatis* infection. In case it is recognised promptly and treated adequately, a complete recovery can be expected without any late complications (Preece et a, 1989). Misdiagnosis or mistreatment with topical and/or inadequate medications will just facilitate the persistence of the disease. Due to the slowly progressive nature of the untreated condition, it can be only occasionally diagnosed in infants after two months of age (Mårdh, 2002; Rours et al, 2008).

Neonatal chlamydial *conjunctivitis* generally starts mono-ocularly, but after 2-7 days the progressive involvement of the other eye can be observed in 75% of the newborns. Clinical signs can widely vary and range from mild conjunctival injection to serious exsudative *ophthalmitis*. Classifying the severity of the symptoms, more than half of the detected cases proved to be moderate, while a serious condition was found in almost 37% of the patients in an extended survey (Stenberg & Mårdh, 1990). Conjunctival erythema, palpebral edema, chemosis and scanty discharge are typical in this condition. The triad of hyperemia, swelling and discharge should always be evaluated as a warning sign, however, there are some infected newborns who do not show this complete clinical picture. Initially the exudate may be watery, turning later mucoid, or pucopurulent. In the case of an intense inflammation, the massive exudate adheres to the conjunctivae and so evolves a characteristic pseudomembrane. Everted conjunctivae may bleed at examination or at sampling procedure. Bloody discharge may occasionally develop, which has a particular diagnostic value being highly specific for *C. trachomatis*. *Rhinitis*, as a frequently associated sign was observed in 60% of newborns suffering from chlamydial ophthalmia (Dannevig et al, 1992). Most untreated cases tend to spontaneous recovery and do not threaten the vision of the affected babies, but may occasionally persist for a longer period accompanied by superficial corneal vascularisation and conjunctival scarring. Despite the prescribed treatment the persistance of ocular infection was observed in 12% of patients, confirmed by the reisolation of *C. trachomatis*, which may refer to an inadeqaute therapy or lack of compliance. The most serious late complication manifests as visual loss due to trachoma-like tarsal scarring and pannus formation. Blindness develops in this chronic condition much slower than compared to gonococcal *conjunctivitis* (Darville, 2005; Mårdh, 2002; Persson et al, 1983; Rees et al, 1981; Quirke & Cullinane, 2008; Zar, 2005).

The differential diagnosis of chlamydial *ophthtalmia neonatorum* is assisted by the knowledge of potential etiological agents, however, in the majority of patients the actual cause remains obscure. „Red eye" as an early symptom often develops at newborns, and besides infection it may be evoked by trauma or by chemical irritation due to some topical medications. Redness and purulent discharge related to silver-nitrate instillation usually starts on the first day of life, but lasts only for a few days. However, this clinical condition may be associated with several microorganisms, and the significance of those has varied over time. Infectious origin pertains predominantly to bacteria apart from the easily recognizable but rare herpes simplex virus infection. Based on etiology studies neither other viruses, nor genital mycoplasmas play any significant role in the pathogenesis (Krohn et al, 1993; Prentice et al, 1977). When the *conjunctivitis* persists beyond three days and is not healed by the use of a frequent normal saline irrigation, then one should immediately start empiric treatment before getting laboratory results indicating some kind of infection.

Main bacterial pathogens including *C. trachomatis*, *Neisseria gonorrhoeae* and other pyogenic species can be identified only in 35-60% of the cases (Di Bartolomeo et al, 2001; Jarvis et al, 1987; Krohn et al, 1993; Pierce et al, 1982). In a well-designed study in the Netherlands an uncommonly high detection rate was documented with 84% of identified pathogens (Rours et al, 2008). Chlamydial *ophthalmia* may be occasionally superinfected with other agents, which may make the accurate diagnosis more difficult. In complicated, therapy-resistant cases one should consider the presence of *N. gonorrhoeae* or of other nosocomial pathogens as well (Winceslaus et al, 1987). The elimination of the disease may be interfered not only by secondary infections, but by the recurrence of the original agent as well. In a follow-up study the recurrence rate of chlamydial neonatal *conjunctivitis* was found as much as 35%, which raises questions about therapeutic efficacy and compliance (Mohile et al, 2002).

N. gonorrhoeae was once the commonest cause of *ophthtalmia neonatorum* leading to irreversible corneal damage and subsequent blindness in several cases, which had caused major health problems in many countries for centuries before Credé's prophylaxis was introduced in 1881. Since Credé's time the prevalence of sight-threatening gonorrhoeal *conjunctivitis* among newborns has radically decreased due to comprehensive prevention efforts. As a result, *N. gonorrhoeae* now counts as a rare ocular isolate. Some surveys could detect not a single case of gonococcal *ophthalmia* among newborns (Dannevig et al, 1992; Prentice et al, 1977; Solberg et al, 1991). Clinically the symptoms of a *N. gonorrhoeae* infection would begin much earlier than those of *C. trachomatis* infection, as the former usually starts 2-5 days after birth with a severe purulent discharge that tends to rapid progression leading occasionally to corneal penetration and *endophthalmitis* (Quirke & Cullinane, 2008). Just as in case of other pyogenic bacteria, the definitive laboratory diagnosis is based on traditional culture of the exudate, however the examination of a Gram-stained smear may be very informative and allows a presumptive, rapid detection of pathogens (Winceslaus et al, 1987).

Common expected pathogens further include *Staphylococcus aureus, Streptococcus pneumoniae, Haemophilus influenzae, Pseudomonas aeruginosa,* members of the *Enterobacteriaceae* family and other Gram-negative bacteria. The altered distribution pattern of pathogens indicates that *S. aureus* took over the leading role of previous agents in purulent *conjunctivitis* since it can be isolated in approximately 50% of this condition (Dannevig et al, 1992; Nsanze et al, 1996; Sandström, 1978; Solberg et al, 1991). Being a nosocomial infection, staphylococcal *conjunctivitis* usually derives from the hospital environment and it is characterised by a more massive purulent discharge and a milder injection than chlamydial *conjunctivitis* (Darville, 2005; Prentice et al, 1977; Schaller & Klauss, 2001). Nonchlamydial, nongonorrhoeal bacterial pathogens seem to account for a considerable proportion of neonatal *conjunctivitis* that can not be fully prevented by usual ocular prophylaxis. As the spectrum of potential pathogens is not completely determined yet more research is needed in this field.

Partly pre-, partly postnatal managements can be used to prevent *ophthalmia neonatorum*. The targeted screening of pregnant women will be discussed later, as this clinical condition cannot be handled as a separate syndrome. Postnatal prophylaxis regarding neonatal *conjunctivitis* however still remains an important issue. The introduction of Credé's silver-nitrate solution dramatically changed the prevalence, and subsequently the distribution of major ocular pathogens, as it was highly active against *N. gonorrhoeae* strains. Due to the systematic and extended application of 1% silver-nitrate ophthalmic drops, gonococcal *ophthalmia neonatorum* has become uncommon by now in the industrialised part of the world where its incidence decreased to 0,04 per 1,000 live births. However its toxic and irritating side-effect, which may induce a chemical *conjunctivitis*, did not make it an optimal medicament.

In comparison, the topical application of a 0,5% erythromycin- or 1,0% tetracycline ointment was just as effective as silver-nitrate in preventing gonococcal *conjunctivitis*, except for the emerging resistant strains, but none of them proved to reduce the incidence of *ophthalmia neonatorum* due to *C. trachomatis*. The failure rate of antichlamydial prophylaxis in the case of erythromycin was calculated to be 7-19,5% (Black-Payne et al, 1989). Other antibiotics, such as chloramphenicol, neomycin or gentamicin have been widely applied too, but there is no convincing data about their efficacy (Assadian et al, 2002). A widespread use of topical antibiotics furthermore may always carry the risk of increasing antimicrobial resistance.

Accordingly, the local administration of any of these drugs does not offer an adequate protection against chlamydial *conjunctivitis*, and cannot either eliminate the accompanying nasopharyngeal chlamydial colonisation (Dannevig et al, 1992; Miller, 2006; Quirke & Cullinane, 2008; Salpietro et al, 1999; Zar, 2005). The failure of the complete eradication of chlamydiae may result in long-term ocular complications, such as recurrent or persistent *conjunctivitis* (Rees et al, 1981).

The application of a less toxic, antiseptic 2,5% povidone-iodine solution, which has a special antichlamydial effect as well, may offer a reasonable and cheap alternative in the developing countries with a high prevalence rate of *N. gonorrhoeae* (Isenberg et al, 2003; Schaller & Klauss, 2001; Zar, 2005). Another relatively new, promising agent may be fusidic acid, but there is insufficient data supporting its prophylactic value (Zuppa, 2011). In the industrialised areas though, depending on the actual prevalence values, Credé's classic prophylactic method seemes to be unnecessary any more, so its value should be reconsidered (Darling & McDonald, 2010; Silva et al, 2008). As it happens, it was the same idea that has resulted in the discontinuation of general prophylaxis against *ophthalmia neonatorum* in some countries (Schaller & Klauss, 2001). The main problem with postnatal prophylaxis regarding *C. trachomatis conjunctivitis* lies in that there are no topical medications which would be able to eradicate chlamydiae from all colonised sites, including the inner respiratory organs of a newborn's organism (Ratelle et al, 1997). Focusing on newborns who are threatened by proven maternal chlamydial carriage the benefits of oral erythromycin prophylaxis were weighed against the risk of *pyloric stenosis,* which is a potential, recently confirmed adverse effect of the treatment. Until the recognition of this association The Committee on Infectious Diseases of the American Academy of Pediatrics had recommended a 14-day course of oral erythromycin for all neonates exposed to *C. trachomatis* at delivery. Based on analysis of the results of this selective prevention programme only a close observation of these infants was suggested. Oral erythromycin treatment is recommended now exclusively for those newborns who develop symptoms of infection (Rosenman et al, 2003). In the absence of a harmless, even systematically effective ideal drug, prevention depends on the prenatal screening and/or on the early treatment of a manifestating *C. trachomatis* infection.

5.2 Respiratory tract infections

Based on the actual age of the patient **neonatal pneumonia** can be classified as early or late onset. Some authors suggest the first week of life for separating the two main groups associated with different etiology, while intrauterine acquired *pneumonia* can be ranged as a special subgroup among early onset conditions (Duke, 2005). This type of classification can be applied to respiratory tract infections caused by *C. trachomatis* too, because this pathogen can affect either the fetus or the newborn characterised by a distinct clinical presentation due to different pathogenesis. Ascending chlamydial infections in pregnant women may result in intrauterine complications, such as *chorioamnionitis* and *PROM*. Subsequent transplacental infections occur predominantly in cases with ruptured membranes, and less frequently with intact membranes (Mohile et al, 2002; Preece et al, 1989). Affected fetuses are at a higher risk of being born preterm and of developing respiratory distress symptoms early after birth, though this is a rare kind of vertical transmission and an uncommon congenital condition due to *C. trachomatis* (Boo, 2008; Colarizi et al, 1996; López-Hurtado et al, 1999; Sollecito et al, 1992; Zar, 2005).

The pathogenesis of most neonatal pulmonary cases rather involves the aspiration either of the infectious genital secret of the mother or that of the ocular discharge, draining from the lacrimal duct as a kind of extension of a concomitant *conjunctivitis*. These may be the direct or indirect colonisation routes leading to the pharyngeal presence of *C. trachomatis,* which is the most frequent target site detected in about 70-77% of the infected neonates (Darville, 2005; Stenberg & Mårdh, 1990) and that serves as an infectious focus giving rise to recurrent *conjunctivitis* or *pneumonia*. *Pharyngitis* occasionally may persist up to 2 years of age or beyond (Bell et al, 1992; Mårdh, 2002; Rees et al, 1981, Zar et al, 1999). Fortunately, this type of colonisation remains often subclinical, as its progression to *pneumonia* is observed only in 30% of the cases (Chen et al, 2007). Based on pooled published data point estimate of incidence of *pneumonia* was calculated 7% among infants exposed to *C. trachomatis* perinatally. The estimated rate of hospitalisation is 20% among newborns suffering from *pneumonia,* which makes it the most significant complication of *C. trachomatis* infection (Rosenman et al, 2003).

The **early onset** type of the chlamydial respiratory distress syndrome in very preterm infants was characterised by a biphasic clinical manifestation showing a transient improvement, but followed by a significant worsening of the respiratory status, when also apneic spells were noted. All the affected patients needed assisted ventilation with oxygen therapy. In this second phase chest X-rays showed hypoexpansion and the reticular pattern of the lungs, while conjunctival and respiratory tract's samples proved to be positive for *C. trachomatis* (Sollecito et al, 1992). Severe congenital *pneumonia* due to *C. trachomatis* may even lead to fatal consequences in very preterm babies (25-32 weeks of gestation) (Attenburrow & Barker, 1986). **Respiratory failure** may affect primarily very preterm, low birth-weight infants, but there are documented cases of these also among near term babies or in untreated neonatal *pneumonia* (Herieka & Dhar, 2001, Zar et al, 1999). *C. trachomatis* infection has been associated with seriously chronic, occasionally lethal forms of pulmonary disorders of ventilated preterm neonates. Despite the occasional presence and specific antibody response its etiologic role in **bronchopulmonary dysplasia (BPD)** has however not yet been confirmed (Attenburrow & Barker, 1986; López-Hurtado et al, 1999; Numazaki et al, 1986; Zar, 2005).

The "classical" chlamydial *pneumonia* belongs to **late onset**, mild to moderate neonatal diseases, as in full-term babies the symptoms of a *C. trachomatis* infection acquired intranatally usually onset between 2 and 19 weeks, typically around 6 weeks of age (Duke, 2005; Marín Gabriel et al, 2004; Pellowe & Pratt, 2006). That relative delay may be explained by the time that is needed for the newborns to develop cellular immunity (Mårdh, 2002). Concomitant *conjunctivitis* can be detected in as many as half of the cases and may act as an important diagnostic clue (Darville, 2005). Tympanic membrane involvement seemes to be an infrequent accompanying symptom in about only 6% of the patients, however, even recurrent episodes of *otitis media* have been described among infants under 6 months exposed to *C. trachomatis* (Numazaki, 1984; Schaefer et al, 1985). Generally minor and aspecific clinical signs are present, such as subfebrility and slight *tachypnoea,* which cause a difficulty in recognising the condition. More than 95% of the infected newborns are afebrile. *Rhinitis* may be present in 20-67% of infected neonates, predominantly associated with *conjunctivitis*. *Rhinorrhoea* as a prodromal symptom with a duration of one-two weeks often precedes the lower respiratory tract signs, such as *tachypnoea* and persistent cough (Chen et al, 2007; Iskandar & Naguib, 1998; Numazaki et al, 1989). Staccato-like coughing and congestion may however point to the possibility of a respiratory tract infection, while expiratory wheezes are uncommon (Klein & Barnett, 1998). Persistent cough may interfere with feeding, moreover the nutrition problems have been significantly linked to the respiratory complication (Pellowe & Pratt, 2006; Rours 2008; Zar, 2005).

The diagnosis is supported by crepitant inspiratory rales on auscultation and chest X-rays showing *hyperinflation* and diffuse bilateral, usually *interstitial infiltrates*. Generalised nodular shadowing has also been documented (Herieka & Dhar, 2001). The radiographic image may show a more serious condition than suggested by the physical examination (Darville, 2005; Miller, 2006). *Retraction* and *cyanosis* have also been described among the conspicuous clinical signs of respiratory distress as well, observed primarily in the youngest newborns under one month of age (Numazaki, 1984; Preece et al, 1989). In the majority of the patients peripheral *eosinophilia* contributes to abnormal, but nonspecific laboratory results, suggesting that it has a significant diagnostic value (Chen et al, 2007; Darville, 2005; Mårdh, 2002; Numazaki, 1984).

Recognising and differentiating a chlamydial neonatal *pneumonia* is hampered by multiple difficulties, such as aspecific symptoms, the high number of potential other pathogens, the possibility of a superinfection and the various transmission routes. The infectious source of the neonatal *pneumonia* can be present in the maternal birth canal, in the hospital/nursery environment or at home. That means that the broad etiologic spectrum of infant *pneumonitis* extends from perinatally colonising agents via nosocomial pathogens to community acquired microbes (Klein & Barnett, 1998). Several viruses, such as human respiratory syncytial virus (RSV), adenovirus, cytomegalovirus and bacteria, such as *Streptococcus agalactiae, Staphylococcus aureus, Streptococcus pneumoniae, Bordetella pertussis*, Ureaplasma species etc., and a parasite (*Pneumocystis carinii*) have been documented to be responsible for the condition. However, in most studies the actual cause of pediatric *pneumonia* could not be established in 40-60% of the cases, while mixed infections may contribute to further diagnostic problems (Jadavji, 1997). Multiple pathogens were generally identified in 24-27% of the patients. Concurrent infections are typically characterised by more severe clinical signs, measured by the occurrence of *apnea* and the need for oxygen therapy and mechanical ventilation (Chen et al, 2007; Ejzenberg et al, 1996; Mårdh, 2002; Numazaki et al, 1989; Stagno et al, 1981).

In the developing countries *C. trachomatis* is accepted as one of the leading causes of late neonatal *pneumonia*, where approximately half of the cases were attributable to this pathogen (Were et al, 2002). The clinical significance of *C. trachomatis* is supported by the fact that recently it has still been detected as the second most frequent respiratory pathogen of infants aged less than 6 months after the human respiratory syncytial virus in the Netherlands (Rours et al, 2009). Also in another study RSV proved to be the most prevalent agent in as many as 44% of the patients suffering from lower respiratory tract infections (Vieira et al, 2003). The clinical manifestation of *C. trachomatis* infection may be indistinguishable from RSV infection, however, the latter usually follows a seasonal pattern, and is more often associated with fever and characteristic wheezing due to airway obstruction (Darville, 2005; Duke, 2005; Preece et al, 1989). Cytomegalovirus tends to affect other organs as well, while adenovirus or parainfluenzavirus infections are not linked with eosinophilia and staccato cough. Pyogenic bacteria, like *Streptococcus agalactiae, Staphylococcus aureus, Streptococcus pneumoniae* or *Enterobacteriaceae* species etc. typically cause more severe, febrile, occasionally septic symptoms with distinctive radiologic signs. *Bordetella pertussis* is a rare respiratory pathogen of newborns known to develop characteristic signs of an intense paroxysmal cough with an inspiratory whoop, often followed by emesis. In its most serious form it may affect the unvaccinated, vulnerable age groups, especially the infants born prematurely (de Greeff et al, 2010). *Ureaplasma urealyticum* far more frequently colonises the airways of preterm premature infants than *C. trachomatis,* as Ureaplasma strains could be detected by PCR in 45%, while less than 2% of those proved to be infected by *C. trachomatis*. The long-term sequelae however may not differ from each other because Ureaplasma carriage has been reported to correlate significantly with the development of *bronchopulmonary dysplasia* (BPD) (Da Silva et al, 1997; Garland & Bowman, 1996).

5.3 Rare organ manifestations and complications of *C. trachomatis* infection

Neonatal **encephalitis** due to *C. trachomatis* was described in an immunodeficient infant, where the presence of the pathogen was confirmed in the tracheal aspirate and in the cerebrospinal fluid as well. Neurological symptoms followed the onset of neonatal *pneumonia* and may be associated with the defect of the alternative complement pathway (Bertsche et al, 2008). Infectious **myocarditis** was reported in an infant suffering from chlamydial *pneumonitis*. There have been only a few reported cases of childhood *myocarditis* in the literature associated with *C. trachomatis* infection, so heart muscle cells act as an especially rare target site (Odeh & Oliven, 1992; Ringel et al, 1983).

Uro-anogenital colonisation occurs usually at birth though the carriage of the pathogen may asymptomatically persist for a long time. However the presence of *C. trachomatis* in the rectal or the genital area in a child over 3 years of age should always be evaluated as a potential warning sign of sexual abuse (Darville, 2005; Schachter et al, 1986). Without evidence of child sexual abuse other transmission routes should be considered, as it is reported in a case of a family cluster of *C. trachomatis* infection (Thompson et al, 2001).

Extragenital persistance of untreated neonatal *C. trachomatis* infections may last even longer, occasionally up to 6 years. The *nasopharynx*, the *oropharynx* and the *conjunctivae* are described to possible sites of such an enormous duration of colonisation. The cumulative proportion of untreated or mistreated infants still colonised at the age of 1 year was reported as many as 35% (Bell 1992; Mårdh, 2002), which may serve as explanation when sexual assaults of the affected child can be definitely excluded.

A recent study confirmed the presence of both *C. trachomatis* and *C. pneumoniae* organisms in the lungs of patients suffering from **chronic pulmonary disease, including asthma** and other inflammatory airway disease. Corticosteroids have also been confirmed to reactivate persisting chlamydiae, so the combination of both inhaled and oral steroid treatment might act as a triggering factor of increased reactivation of chlamydiae contributing to asthmatic or other symptoms. Due to that phenomenon the latent respiratory carriage of these pathogens may turn into symptomatic disorder. The exact role of the *Chlamydiaceae* family is not fully understood yet so further research is needed concerning the etiology and exacerbation of paediatric *asthma* and other chronic respiratory diseases (Webley et al, 2009).

6. Laboratory diagnosis

According to its clinical and epidemiological relevance targeted diagnostic tests should include *C. trachomatis* for all infants aged less than 6 months who have suspicious clinical signs of *ophthalmia neonatorum* and/or *pneumonia* or other organ manifestations. The potential etiological role of *C. trachomatis* should be especially considered in countries with a high prevalence of the pathogen among young women and/or in the absence of an adequate screening programme in pregnancy. The topical use of antibiotics should be judged as an unreliable, insufficient mode of prevention. The correct laboratory results depend on the collection of relevant samples done by clinicians and on the use of the proper diagnostic test chosen by the microbiologists.

6.1 Sample collection

Conjunctivitis: Specimens for direct detection tests should be obtained from the everted eyelid using a Dacron-tipped swab or an equivalent recommended by the test kit manufacturer. As chlamydiae are obligate intracellular bacteria, it is important to collect some conjunctival cells from the inner surface of the eyelid, instead of sampling only the ophthalmic exudate. The latter procedure otherwise may lead to false-negative laboratory results. Serology is not informative because in the absence of a systemic immune response there are no detectable IgM levels in this localised type of infection (Mahony et al, 1986; Miller, 2006).

Pneumonia and other respiratory tract infections: In case of *rhinitis* or *pharyngitis*, specimen rich in mucosal cells should be collected from the affected upper air ways. In suspected *otitis media* the middle ear effusion is the optimal sample for confirming the presence of pathogen. From patients suffering from *pneumonia* respiratory tract samples should be collected, preferably from the nasopharyngeal area, acting as a common infectious source. However, the more relevant lower respiratory tract samples such as tracheal aspirates, lavage fluid, pleural fluid, bronchoscopic or lung biopsy specimens should also be definitely tested if they are available. Native blood or serum samples should be **always** enclosed, as one may expect a specific immune response in these conditions. According to some previous studies, the testing of cord blood samples may also be informative (Gencay et al, 2001).

Additional source tracking: Proven neonatal infections always indicate a human reservoir in the close environment, as *C. trachomatis* is a relatively sensitive micoorganism transferred by infectious secretions predominantly from urogenital or some other mucosal focus. Supposing vertical transmission, the maternal urogenital screening for *C. trachomatis* is suggested. Possible positive results represent a diagnosed infection, being often asymptomatic in adults, moreover it may confirm the infectious source of the neonatal condition. In the event that the maternal tests are negative, but there are verified positive neonatal laboratory results, other routes of transmission should be considered, and the screening efforts should be extended to other persons from the family or the nursing environment. Serology is unnecessary, because only the direct detection methods can be informative about acute urogenital infections.

6.2 Laboratory methods

6.2.1 Direct detection techniques

Direct detection techniques historically were limited to **tissue culture**, as conventional culture methods do not enable the isolation of this obligate intracellular pathogen. For optimal results tissue culture requires the presence of viable microorganisms, so the clinical specimen should contain not only exsudate but epithelial cells as well from the infected area. Besides appropriate sampling technique adequte transport media are also needed for maintaining the cultivability of the bacteria. Culture testing for *C. trachomatis* has always been the reference standard against which all the laboratory tests developed later have been compared. However, it can not be used for routine diagnostic purposes because of being difficult to standardize, technically demanding, time-consuming and expensive. This relatively insensitive method (its sensitivity ranges between 70-85%) is available only in specialized laboratories but maintains its advantage in forensic cases of suspected sexul abuse, where it may provide conclusive evidence of a sexually transmitted infection (Johnson et al, 2002; Schachter & Stamm, 1995).

Newer, non-viability dependent tests place less demands on specimen transport. The antigen detection tests applied most frequently rely either on the identification of chlamydial elementary bodies using fluorochrome-labelled, specific monoclonal antibodies (direct fluorescent antibody, or **DFA** test) or on the capture and detection of chlamydial antigen using enzyme immunoassay based techniques (enzyme immunoassay, or **EIA**). These two basic methods are widely used, being quite simple to perform and evaluate. However they are not considered „gold standard" diagnostic procedures any more, because in the meantime nucleic acid-based methods (hybridization-probes and amplification techniques) have been developed, which generally have more advantages.

Although at a greater cost and with a greater requirement for trained staff and technical conditions, the nucleic acid-based methods generally offer superior sensitivity and specificity, while non-invasively taken urogenital samples (urine for example) may count as adequate specimen as well. Nucleic acid amplification techniques (NAAT) include polymerase chain reaction (**PCR**), ligase chain reaction (**LCR**), strand displacement amplification (**SDA**) and transcription mediated amplification (**TMA**). The key advantage of multiplex molecular method is that they have the ability to detect other coinfecting pathogens (eg. *Neisseria gonorrhoeae*) in a single specimen as well. They also give rise to further typization tests such as restriction fragment length polymorphism (**RFLP**) analysis of the PCR-amplified *omp1* gene used for differentiating the genotypes, that may have epidemiological importance contributing to surveillance studies (Petrovay et al, 2009).

6.2.2 Serology

The demonstration of specific antibodies in adults is rarely indicative for an acute urogenital infection of *C. trachomatis*, its use may be rather limited to only chronic, ascending infections.

Other superficial mucosal infections, such as chlamydial *conjunctivitis* of patients of any age will not develop a systemic immune response either. However, when investigating neonates with pneumonia, the special circumstances of the condition (high probability of the actual presence of the pathogen in the upper respiratory tract, and the simultaneously detectable immune response) allow the completion of the laboratory tests with serological assays. Due to the high number of circulating B cells, plasma cells and large amounts of secreted antibodies, **serology** has become a crucial tool of laboratory tests in neonatal pneumonia. Sera of Japanese infants proved to be posivite for IgM antibodies to *C. trachomatis* in 29% of patients with *pneumonia*, furthermore in 66% of this subgroup even the direct detection technique could confirm the presence of the pathogen from nasopharyngeal samples. All the positive laboratory results corresponded with the clinical signs of neonatal *pneumonia* (Numazaki, 1984).

The results of several studies suggest that neonatal *pneumonia* may be accurately diagnosed by the detection of high IgM antibody titers in serum. The maternal IgM do not pass across the placenta, so the presence of *C. trachomatis* IgM antibody on newborns' blood samples unambiguously refers to neonatal infection, which proves to be a quite reliable sign of a systemic *C. trachomatis* infection, moreover, it may already be present at birth. In such cases as these IgM antibody titers in serum generally rise quickly after birth and approach maximal titers approximately by the second week of life and may persist for up to 3 months (Mahony et al, 1986). The intrauterin transmission of the pathogen has revealed that not only common serum samples taken postnatally but even cord blood samples of infected infants may contain specific IgM (Gencay et al, 2001; Numazaki et al, 1986).

Due to the antigenic relationship between various chlamydia species the cross reaction may frequently result in unreliable results while using tests of low-medium grade specificity. The highest specificity can be achieved by choosing a **micro-immunofluorescence test (MIF)** and the diagnostic criteria are adapted to elevated levels of *C. trachomatis* IgM detected by MIF. The cut-off value was defined as a titer **≥ 1:16** which is strongly suggestive of *C. trachomatis* infection (Numazaki, 1984). The use of other serological methods, such as ELISA tests are not recommended for that purpose. Due to the high occurance rates, the routine testing for *C. trachomatis* is needed in hospitalised infants having pneumonia.

6.3 Results and evaluation

Between January 2004 and June 2011 we examined the serum samples of **282** infants suffering from respiratory tract infection by *C. trachomatis* MIF (FOCUS) test in our laboratory (Second Department of Bacteriology, National Centre for Epidemiology, Budapest). The majority of the samples (92,6%) were taken from infants younger than 20 weeks, which corresponds to the fact that this condition develops mainly in the first five months. The detailed results indicate that newborns aged **0-4** months represent more than **84**% of all patients with a proven *C. trachomatis* infection. Positive IgM results were found altogether in **95** patients (**33,7%**) in ≥1:16 titers. The positivity rate of our survey provided similar data to other reported findings, where the *C. trachomatis* infection was detected in approximately 30% of patients (Chen et al, 2007; Numazaki, 1984). That means that *C. trachomatis* still may be responsible for neonatal *pneumonia* in about one third of patients with manifest symptoms where the chlamydial etiology was presumed.

Age (weeks)	Female Positive/Studied (prevalence %)	Male Positive/Studied (prevalence %)	Total Positive/Studied (prevalence %)
≤ 4	8/16 (50.0%)	10/22 (45.5%)	18/38 (47.4%)
5 - 8	10/27 (37.0%)	14/51 (27.5%)	24/78 (30.8%)
9 - 12	3/29 (10.3%)	15/52 (28.8%)	18/81 (22.2%)
13 - 16	8/17 (47.1%)	12/20 (60.0%)	20/37 (54.1%)
17 - 20	5/14 (35.7%)	7/13 (53.8%)	12/27 (44.4%)
21 - 24	1/1 (100.0%)	0/8 (0.0%)	1/9 (11.1%)
25 - 28	0/2 (0.0%)	0/3 (0.0%)	0/5 (0.0%)
28 <	0/2 (0.0%)	2/5 (40.0%)	2/7 (28.6%)
Total	35/108 (32.4%)	60/174 (34.5%)	95/282 (33.7%)

Table 1. Prevalence of *C. trachomatis* IgM serum antibodies in newborns with pneumonia

7. Therapy

Topical treatments, like silver nitrate eye drops (Credé-prophylaxis), antibiotics, povidone-iodine solution or others are ineffective in neonatal *conjunctivitis* and are unnecessary when a systemic treatment is administered. As chlamydial *conjunctivitis* is considered a local manifestation of a systemic colonisation, a systemic treatment is required. The drug of choice for the treatment of **neonatal conjunctivitis and pneumonia is** erythromycin 50 mg/kg/day orally divided into 4 doses for 14 and for 21 days, respectively (Mårdh, 2002). The most serious complication of oral erythromycin treatment may be the development of *hypertrophic pyloric stenosis*. Another disadvantage of this regimen is a relatively high failure rate that was found 20% in cases of *opthtalmia neonatorum* or *pneumonia*. Therapeutic efficacy could be reliably controlled only by culture as nucleic acid detection techniques may give positive results detecting non-viable microbes up to 3 weeks after an adequate therapy, so the latter ones are inadequate for that purpose. A poor recovery rate was observed especially in too short (10 days or less) or too low-dose regimens. In recurring or persistent infections a second or even a third course of erythromycin may be needed (Miller, 2006; Quirke & Cullinane, 2008; Zar, 2005).

Newer macrolide drugs, such as clarithromycin, roxithromycin or azithromycin may be effective therapeutic alternatives as well. The latter can have several advantages of use, such as a lower incidence of adverse effects, better tolerability and easier dosage regimen, however there is little data available about experiences in neonates. The specific diagnosis of *C. trachomatis* infection assists not only in the management of an infant's illness but also confirms the need for treating the mother and her sexual partner(s).

8. Prevention

Preventing neonatal morbidity caused by *C. trachomatis* can be achieved by different levels of probability of infection, but none of the interventions target the newborns directly. As detailed above, neither local nor systemic administration of drugs on neonates proved to be reliable and efficient means of prevention. Related to the vertical nature of transmission, chlamydiae should be eradicated from female organisms before and/or during pregnancy. Currently the CDC, the US Preventive Services Task Force (USPSTF), and numerous other professional medical associations recommend an annual chlamydia screening for all sexually active females aged <25 years and for females aged ≥25 years if they are at increased risk for infection (CDC, 2011).

The maternal testing for *C. trachomatis* and the treatment of infections is invaluable in reducing perinatal transmission. The newest STD Treatment Guidelines (CDC, 2010) suggest that a test for *C. trachomatis* should be routinely performed at the first prenatal visit on **all pregnant women**. Women aged less than 25 years and those at increased risk (i.e., having a new sexual partner or multiple sexual partners) should be retested during the third trimester to prevent maternal postnatal complications and to reduce infant morbidity. Women with chlamydial infection diagnosed during the first trimester should be controlled for chlamydial eradication (preferably by NAAT) 3 weeks after the completion of the therapy **AND** they should be retested 3 months after the treatment, preferably before the third trimester.

In the absence of a comprehensive screening during pregnancy, clinicians should have a higher index of suspicion for neonatal and maternal chlamydial infections when the possibility of infection cannot be excluded. Infants born to mothers with untreated chlamydiae are at an even higher risk of infection but instead of a prophylactic therapy, a long-term observation is indicated as the efficacy of such prophylaxis is not confirmed yet. In the case of developing suspicious symptoms, children should be examined and given an adequate treatment (Darville, 2005).

Routine antenatal screening is the optimal solution not only for preventing neonatal chlamydial infections but also postpartum/chronic maternal complications. Maternal carriage always indicates the screening and treatment of sexual partner(s) as reinfection may occur at any time. Treatment should be given for the improvement of the pregnancy outcome as *C. trachomatis* may be related to perinatal complications, premature labor, and respiratory insufficiency of preterm infants too. As a first-line antichlamydial drug, azithromycin is recommended for treating urogenital infection in pregnancy, while amoxicillin may be a safe and well tolerable alternative regimen (Miller, 2006). The eradication of the pathogen may result in a decreasing rate of adverse pregnancy outcomes as reported by several studies (Allaire et al, 1995; Rastogi, 2003; Zar, 2005). The end of the second trimester is likely to be the most optimal time for screening pregnant women, if it is limited to only one occasion. In recognised infections an adequate therapy may still prevent the adverse pregnancy outcomes, while there is only 3 months left to potentially acquire the pathogen (Mårdh, 2002).

9. Conclusion

C. trachomatis represents an important STI pathogen among adults having also the ability to cause frequent neonatal infections. Neonatal inclusion *conjunctivitis* and infantile *pneumonia* may give rise to diagnostic and therapeutic difficulties. The aspecific, often mild-moderate symptoms may delay the definitive diagnosis while the complete eradication of the pathogen can be achieved only by a repeated therapy in several documented cases.

Our aim was to demonstrate the significant morbidity in infancy associated with *C. trachomatis* infection. Maternal *C. trachomatis* infection may cause various fetal or neonatal complications, and also indicates the urogenital presence of the pathogen of the mother and of her sexual partner(s). As 70-80% of the infected women are asymptomatic, the definitive diagnosis of neonatal infections may be occasionally the only epidemiologic clue that points to the infection of untreated mothers. The impact of this microorganism requires focused diagnostic approaches and an adequate antibiotic therapy not only applied to the affected infant but to both the mother and her partner(s) too.

Primary STI prevention should include the education and counselling of people about the risks of unsafe sexual behaviours, while secondary prevention consists of screening programs of asymptomatic persons at risk as well as the diagnosis and treatment of the infected patients. A national screening programme of pregnant women should also be established in Hungary, which concentrates on early diagnosis, effective treatment and close follow-up. The incidence of reinfection also needs to be investigated in further studies. Clinicians and neonatal nurses will need to be aware of the possibility of *C. trachomatis* infection, as early treatment rather than prevention seems to remain the best strategy for now, which will eventually lead to a decline in the incidence of perinatal chlamydial infection. The objective of this chapter has been to draw the attention to these infantile infections, which especially when overlooked, may still manifest as a severe condition that needs hospitalisation.

10. Acknowledgements

We express thanks to the laboratory staff: Ms. Éva Kelemen and Ms. Zsuzsa Kertész for their precise technical assistance, and to István Németh, PhD for ensuring an excellent, rapid analysis of our laboratory results.

11. References

Assadian, O. et al. (2002). Prophylaxis of ophthalmia neonatorum--a nationwide survey of the current practice in Austria. *Wiener Klinische Wochenschrift,* Vol. 114, No. 5-6, pp. 194-199

Attenburrow, A. A. & Barker, C. M. (1986). Chlamydial pneumonia in the low birthweight neonate. *Archives of Disease in Childhood,* Vol. 60, No. 12, pp. 1169-1172

Baud, D.; Regan, L. & Greub, G. (2008). Emerging role of Chlamydia and Chlamydia-like organisms in adverse pregnancy outcomes. *Current Opinion in Infectious Diseases,* Vol. 21, No. 1, pp. 70-76

Bell, T.A. et al (1992). Chronic *Chlamydia trachomatis* infections in infants. *JAMA: The Journal of the American Medical Association,* Vol. 267. No. 3, pp. 400-402

Bell, T.A. et al. (1994). Risk of perinatal transmission of *Chlamydia trachomatis* by mode of delivery. *The Journal of Infection,* Vol. 29, No. 2, pp. 165-169

Bertsche, A. et al. (2008). An unusual manifestation of a neonatal *Chlamydia trachomatis* infection. *Journal of Child Neurology,* Vol. 23, No. 8, pp. 948-949

Black-Payne, C., Bocchini J.A. Jr. & Cedotal, C. (1989). Failure of erythromycin ointment for postnatal ocular prophylaxis of chlamydial conjunctivitis. *The Pediatric Infectious Disease Journal,* Vol. 8, No. 8, pp. 491-495

Blas, M.M. et al. (2007). Pregnancy outcomes in women infected with *Chlamydia trachomatis*: a population-based cohort study in Washington State. *Sexually Transmitted Infections*,Vol. 83, No. 4, pp. 314-318

Boo, N.Y. (2008). Current understanding of congenital pneumonia. *Pediatric Health*, Vol. 2, No. 5, pp. 563-569

Brocklehurst, P. & Rooney, G. (2007). Interventions for treating genital *Chlamydia trachomatis* infection in pregnancy. *Cochrane Database of Systematic Reviews*, Issue 4. Art. No.: CD000054. DOI: 10.1002/14651858.CD000054.

Chen, C. J. et al. (2007). Characteristics of *Chlamydia trachomatis* infection in hospitalized infants with lower respiratory tract infection. *Journal of Microbiology, Immunology, and Infection*, Vol.40, No.3, pp.255-259.

Centers for Disease Control and Prevention. (2010). Sexually Transmitted Diseases Treatment Guidelines. *Morbidity and Mortality Weekly Report, Recommendations and Reports*, No. 59, No. 12, pp. 1-114

Centers for Disease Control and Prevention. (2011). CDC Grand Rounds: Chlamydia Prevention: Challenges and Strategies for Reducing Disease Burden and Sequelae. *Morbidity and Mortality Weekly Report, Recommendations and Reports*, Vol. 60, No. 12, pp. 370-373

Colarizi, P. et al. (1996). *Chlamydia trachomatis*-associated respiratory disease in very early neonatal period. *Acta Paediatrica*, Vol. 85, No. 8, pp. 991-994

Dannevig, L.; Straume B. & Melby, K. (1992). Ophthalmia neonatorum in northern Norway. II. Microbiology with emphasis on *Chlamydia trachomatis. Acta Ophthalmologica,* Vol. 70, No. 1, pp. 19-25

Darling, E.K. & McDonald, H. (2010). A meta-analysis of the efficacy of ocular prophylactic agets used for the prevention of gonococcal and chlamydial opthhalmia neoatorum. *Journal of Midwifery & Women's Health,* Vol. 55, No. 4, pp. 319-327

Darville, T. (2005). *Chlamydia trachomatis* infections in neonates and young children. *Seminars in Pediatric Infectious Diseases.* Vol. 16, No. 4, pp. 235-244.

Da Silva, O.; Gregson, D. & Hammerberg, O. (1997). Role of *Ureaplasma urealyticum* and *Chlamydia trachomatis* in development of bronchopulmonary dysplasia in very low birth weight infants. *The Pediatric Infectious Disease Journal,* Vol. 16, No. 4, pp. 364-369

De Greeff, S.C. et al. (2010). Pertussis Disease Burden in the Household: How to Protect Young Infants. *Clinical Infectious Diseases,* Vol. 50, No. 10, pp. 1339-1345

Di Bartolomeo, S. et al. (2001). Incidence of *Chlamydia trachomatis* and other potential pathogens in neonatal conjunctivitis. *International Journal of Infectious Diseases*,Vol. 5, No. 3, pp. 139-143

Djukić, S. et al. (1996). Intra-amniotic *Chlamydia trachomatis* infection. *Gynecologic and Obstetric Investigation,* Vol. 42, No. 2, pp. 109-112

Dong, Z.W. et al. (1998). Detection of *Chlamydia trachomatis* intrauterine infection using polymerase chain reaction on chorionic villi. *International Journal of Gynecology & Obstetrics,* Vol. 61, No. 1, pp. 29-32.

Duke, T. (2005). Neonatal pneumonia in developing countries. *Archives of Disease in Childhood. Fetal and Neonatal Edition,* Vol. 90, No. 3, pp. 211-219

Ejzenberg, B. et al. (1996). Aerobic bacteria, *Chlamydia trachomatis, Pneumocystis carinii* and Cytomegalovirus as agents of severe pneumonia in small infants. *Revista do Instituto de Medicina Tropical de São Paul,* Vol. 38, No. 1, pp. 9-14

European Centre for Disease Prevention and Control (2011). Sexually transmitted infections in Europe, 1990-2009. Stockholm: ECDC

Gallo Vaulet, L. et al. (2010). Distribution study of *Chlamydia trachomatis* genotypes in symptomatic patients in Buenos Aires, Argentina: association between genotype E and neonatal conjunctivitis. *BMC Research Notes*, Vol. 3, No. 34, pp. 1-6

Garland, S.M. & Bowman, E.D. (1996). Role of *Ureaplasma urealyticum* and *Chlamydia trachomatis* in lung disease in low birth weight infants, *Pathology,* Vol. 28, No. 3, pp. 266-269

Gencay, M. et al. (2001). *Chlamydia trachomatis* infection in mothers with preterm delivery and in their newborn infants. *APMIS: Acta Pathologica, Microbiologica, et Immunologica Scandinavica,* Vol. 109, No. 9, pp. 636-640

Givner, L.B. et al. (1981). *Chlamydia trachomatis* infection in infant delivered by caesarean section. *Pediatrics,* Vol. 68, No. 3, pp. 420-421.

Herieka, E. & Dhar, J. (2001). Acute neonatal respiratory failure and *Chlamydia trachomatis. Sexually Transmitted Infections,*Vol. 77, No. 2,pp. 135-136

Isobe, K. et al. (1996). Serotyping *Chlamydia trachomatis* from inclusion conjunctivitis by polymerase chain reaction and restriction length polymorphism analysis. *Japanese Journal of Ophthamology,* Vol. 40, No. 2, pp. 279-285

Iskandar, N.M. & Naguib, M.B. (1998). *Chlamydia trachomatis*: An underestimated cause for rhinitis in neonates. *International Journal of Pediatric Otorhinolaryngology,* Vol. 42, No. 3, pp. 233-237

Jadavji, T. et al. (1997). A practical guide for the diagnosis and treatment of pediatric pneumonia. *Canadian Medical Association Journal,* Vol. 156, No. 5, pp. 703-711.

Jain, S. (1999). Perinatally aquired *Chlamydia trachomatis* associated morbidity in young infants. *Journal of Maternal-Fetal Medicine,* Vol. 8, No. 3, pp. 130-133

Jarvis, V. N.; Levine, R. & Asbell P.A. (1987). Ophthalmia neonatorum: study of a decade of experience at the Mount Sinai Hospital. *British Journal of Ophtalmology,* Vol. 71, No. 4, pp. 295-300

Johnson, R. E. et al. (2002). Screening Tests To Detect *Chlamydia trachomatis* and *Neisseria gonorrhoeae* Infections. *Morbidity and Mortality Weekly Report, Recommendations and Reports,* Vol. 51, No. 15, pp. 1-37

Jones, B.R.; Collier, L.H. & Smith, C.H. (1959). Isolation of virus from inclusion blennorrhoea. *Lancet* Vol. 1, No. 7079, pp. 902-905.

Klein, J.O. & Barnett, E.D. (1998). Neonatal pneumonia. *Seminars in Pediatric Infectious Diseases,* Vol. 9, No. 3, pp. 212-216

Krohn, M. A. et al. (1993). The bacterial etiology of conjunctivitis in early infancy. *American Journal of Epidemiology,* Vol. 138, No. 5, pp. 326-332

Lamont, R.F. et al. (1987). The role of mycoplasmas, ureaplasmas and chlamydiae in the genital tract of women presenting in spontaneous early preterm labour. *Journal of Medical Microbiology,* Vol. 24, No. 3, pp. 253-257

Locksmith, G. & Duff, P. (2001). Infection, antibiotics, and preterm delivery. *Seminars in Perinatology,*Vol. 25, No. 5, pp. 295-309

López-Hurtado, M. et al. (1999). Prevalence of *Chlamydia trachomatis* in newborn infants with respiratory problems. *Revista latinoamericana de microbiología,* Vol. 41, No. 4, pp. 267-272

Magoń, T. et al. (2005). The PCR assessed prevalence of *Chlamydia trachomatis* in aborted tissues. *Medycyna wieku rozwojowego,* Vol. 9, No. 1, pp. 43-48.

Mahony, J.B. et al. (1986). Accuracy of immunoglobulin M immunoassay for diagnosis of chlamydial infections in infants and adults. *Journal of Clinical Microbiology,* Vol. 24, No. 5, pp. 731-735

Mårdh, P.A. (2002). Influence of infection with *Chlamydia trachomatis* on pregnancy outcome, infant health and life-long sequelae in infected offspring. *Best Practice & Research Clinical Obstetrics & Gynaecology,* Vol. 16, No. 6, pp. 847-864.

Marín Gabriel, M.A. et al (2004). Respiratory infection due to *Chlamydia trachomatis* in infants. Clinical presentation and outcome in 18 patients. *Anales de pediatría (Barcelona, Spain : 2003),* Vol. 60, No. 4, pp. 349-353

Maxwell, G.L. (1993). Preterm premature rupture of membranes. *Obstetrical & Gynecological Survey,* Vol. 48, No. 8, pp. 576-583.

Miller, K. E. (2006). Diagnosis and treatment of *Chlamydia trachomatis* infection. *American Family Physician,* Vol. 73, No. 8, pp. 1411-1416

Mohile, M. et al. (2002). Microbiological study of neonatal conjunctivitis with special reference to *Chlamydia trachomatis. Indian Journal of Ophthalmology,* Vol. 50, No. 4, pp. 295-299

Nsanze, H. et al. (1996). Ophthalmia neonatorum in the United Arab Emirates. *Annals of Tropical Paediatrics,* Vol. 16, No. 1, pp. 27-32.

Numazaki, K. et al. (1984). Pneumonia due to *Chlamydia trachomatis* in Japanese Infants. *The Tohoku Journal of Experimental Medicine,* Vol. 143, No. 4, pp. 413-420

Numazaki, K. et al. (1986). Chronic respiratory disease in premature infants caused by *Chlamydia trachomatis. Journal of Clinical Pathology,* Vol.39, No.1, pp.84-88

Numazaki, K.; Wainberg, M.A. & McDonald, J. (1989). *Chlamydia trachomatis* infections in infants. *Canadian Medical Association Journal,* Vol. 140, No.6, pp.615-622.

Numazaki, K.; Asanuma, H. & Niida, Y. (2003). *Chlamydia trachomatis* infection in early neonatal period. *BMC Infectious Diseases,* Vol. 3, No. 2, pp. 1-5

Numazaki, K. (2004). Current problems of perinatal *Chlamydia trachomatis* infections. *Journal of Immune Based Therapies and Vaccines,* Vol. 2, No. 1, pp. 1-7

Odeh, M. & Oliven, A. (1992). Chlamydial Infections of the Heart. *European Journal of Clinical Microbiology & Infectious Diseases,* Vol. 11, No. 10, pp. 885-893

Ostaszewska-Puchalska, I. et al. (2005). *Chlamydia trachomatis* infections in women with adverse pregnancy outcome. *Medycyna wieku rozwojowego,* Vol. 9, No. 1, pp. 49-56

Peipert, J.F. (2003). Clinical practice. Genital chlamydial infections. *The New England Journal of Medicine,* Vol. 349, No. 25, pp. 2424-2430.

Pellowe, C. & Pratt, R.J. (2006). Neonatal conjunctivitis and pneumonia due to chlamydia infection. *Infant,* Vol. 2, No. 1, pp. 16-17

Persson, K. et al. (1983). Neonatal chlamydial eye infection: an epidemiological and clinical study. *British Journal of Ophtalmology,* Vol. 67, No. 10, pp. 700-704

Petrovay, F. et al. (2009). Genotyping of *Chlamydia trachomatis* from the endocervical specimens of high-risk women in Hungary. *Journal of Medical Microbiology,* Vol. 58, No. 6, pp. 760-764

Pierce, J.M.; Ward, M.E. & Seal, D.V. (1982). Ophthalmia neonatorum in the 1980's: incidence, aetiology and treatment. *British Journal of Ophthalmology*, Vol. 66, No. 11, pp. 728-731

Preece, P.M.; Anderson, J.M. & Thompson, R.G. (1989). *Chlamydia trachomatis* infection in infants: a prospective study. *Archives of Disease in Childhood,* Vol. 64, No. 4, pp. 525-529.

Prentice, J.M.; Hutchinson, G. R. & Taylor-Robinson, D. (1977). A microbiological study of neonatal conjunctivae and conjunctivitis. *British Journal of Ophthalmology*, Vol. 61, No. 9, pp. 601-607

Quirke, M. & Cullinane, A. (2008). Recent trends in chlamydial and gonococcal conjunctivitis among neonates and adults in an Irish hospital. *International Journal of Infectious Diseases*, Vol. 12, No. 4, pp. 371-373

Rastogi, S. et al. (1999). *Chlamydia trachomatis* infection in pregnancy: risk factor for an adverse outcome. *British Journal of Biomedical Science*. Vol. 56, No. 2, pp. 94-98

Rastogi, S. et al. (2003). Effect of treatment for *Chlamydia trachomatis* during pregnancy. *International Journal of Gynecology & Obstetrics,* Vol. 80, No. 2, pp. 129-37

Ratelle, S. et al. (1997). Neonatal chlamydial infections in Massachusetts, 1992-1993. *American Journal of Preventive Medicine,* Vol. 13, No. 3, pp. 221-224

Rees, E. et al. (1981). Persistence of chlamydial infection after treatment of neonatal conjunctivitis. *Archives of Diseases in Childhood,* Vol. 56, No. 3, pp. 193-198

Rezeberga, D. et al. (2008). Placental histological inflammation and reproductive tract infections in a low risk pregnant population in Latvia. *Acta Obstetricia et Gynecologica,* Vol. 87, No. 3, pp. 360-365

Ringel, R.E. et al. (1983). Myocarditis as a complication of infantile *Chlamydia trachomatis* pneumonitis. *Clinical Pediatrics,*Vol. 22, No. 9, pp. 631-633

Rosenman, M. B. et al (2003). Oral erythromycin prophylaxis vs watchful waiting in caring for newborns exposed to *Chlamydia trachomatis*. *Archives of Pediatrics and Adolescent Medicine,* Vol. 157, No. 6, pp. 565-571

Rours, G.I. et al. (2008). *Chlamydia trachomatis* as a cause of neonatal conjunctivitis in Dutch infants. *Pediatrics,* Vol. 121, No. 2, pp. 321-326

Rours, G.I. et al. (2009). *Chlamydia trachomatis* respiratory infection in Dutch infants. *Archives of Diseases in Childhood,* Vol. 94, No. 9, pp. 705-707

Rours, G.I. et al. (2011). *Chlamydia trachomatis* infection during pregnancy associated with preterm delivery: a population-based prospective cohort study. *European Journal of Epidemiology,* Vol. 26, No. 6, pp. 493-502

Salpietro, C.D. et al. (1999). *Chlamydia trachomatis* conjunctivitis in the newborn. *Archives de pédiatrie,* Vol. 6, No. 3, pp. 317-320

Sandström, I. (1987). Etiology and diagnosis of neonatal conjunctivitis. *Acta Paediatrica Scandinavica,* Vol. 76, No. 2, pp. 221-227

Schachter, J. et al. (1975). Pneumonitis following inclusion blennorrhoea. *The Journal of Pediatrics,* Vol. 87, No. 5, pp. 779-780

Schachter, J. et al. (1979). Infection with *Chlamydia trachomatis*: involvement of multiple anatomic sites in neonates. *The Journal of Infectious Diseases,* Vol. 139, No. 2, pp. 232-234.

Schachter, J. et al. (1986). Prospective study of perinatal transmission of *Chlamydia trachomatis*. *JAMA: The Journal of the American Medical Association*, Vol. 255. No. 24, pp. 3374-3377

Schachter, J. & Stamm, W.E. (1995). Chlamydia, In: *Manual of clinical microbiology*, Murray, P.R. et al, pp. 669–677, American Society for Microbiology, Washington, D.C.

Schaefer, C. et al. (1985). Illnesses in infants born to women with *Chlamydia trachomatis* infection. A prospective study. *American journal of diseases of children*, Vol. 139, No. 2, pp. 127-133

Schaller, U. & Klauss, V. (2001). Is Crede's prophylaxis for ophthalmia neonatorum still valid? *Bulletin of the World Health Organisation*, Vol. 79, No. 3, pp. 262-263

Silva, L. R. et al. (2008). Current usefulness of Credé's method of preventing neonatal ophthalmia. *Annals of Tropical Paediatrics*, Vol. 28, No. 1, pp. 45-48

Solberg, R.; Meberg, A. & Schøyen, R. (1991). Neonatal conjunctivitis in a nursery and a neonatal unit. *Tidsskrift for den Norske lægeforening*, Vol. 111, No. 10, pp. 1230-1232

Sollecito, D. et al. (1992). *Chlamydia trachomatis* in neonatal respiratory distress of very preterm babies; biphasic clinical picture. *Acta Paediatrica*, Vol. 81, No. 10, pp. 788-791

Stagno, B. et al. (1981). Infant pneumonitis associated with cytomegalovirus, Chlamydia, Pneumocystis and Ureaplasma: a prospective study. *Pediatrics*, Vol. 68, No. 3, pp. 322-329

Stenberg, K. & Mårdh, P.A. (1990). Chlamydial conjunctivitis in neonates and adults. History, clinical findings and follow-up. *Acta Ophthalmologica*, Vol. 68, No. 6, pp. 651-657

Thompson, C; Macdonald, M. & Sutherland, A. (2001). A family cluster of *Chlamydia trachomatis* infection, *British Medical Journal*, Vol. 322, No. 7300, pp. 1472-1474

Valencia, C. et al. (2000). Prevalence of the *Chlamydia trachomatis* in neonatal conjunctivitis determination by indirect fluorescence and gene amplification. *Revista médica de Chile*, Vol. 128, No. 7, pp. 758-765

Vieira, R.A. et al. (2003). Clinical and laboratoty study of newborns with lower respiratory tract infection due to respiratory viruses. *The Journal of Maternal-Fetal and Neonatal Medicine*, Vol. 13, No. 5, pp. 341-350

Were, F.N. et al. (2002). Chlamydia as a cause of late neonatal pneumonia at Kenyatta National Hospital, Nairobi. *East African Medical Journal*, Vol. 79, No. 9, pp. 476-479

Webley, W.C. et al. (2009). Occurrence of *Chlamydia trachomatis* and *Chlamydia pneumoniae* in paediatric respiratory infections. *The European Respiratory Journal*, Vol. 33, No. 2, pp. 360-367

Wilson, J. S. et al. (2002). A systematic review of the prevalence of *Chlamydia trachomatis* among European women. *European Society of Human Reproduction and Embryology*,Vol. 8, No. 4, pp. 385-894.

Winceslaus, J. et al. (1987). Diagnosis of ophthalmia neonatorum. *British Medical Journal*, Vol. 295, No. 6610, pp. 1377-1379

Yoshida, H. et al. (2000). Reversal of intra-amniotic *Chlamydia trachomatis* antigen status. *Gynecologic and Obstetric Investigation*, Vol. 50, No. 4, pp. 278-280.

Yu, J. et al. (2009). Vertical transmission of *Chlamydia trachomatis* in Chongqing China. *Current Microbiology*, Vol. 58, No. 4, pp. 315-320

Zar, H.J. et al. (1999). *Chlamydia trachomatis* lower respiratory tract infection in infants. *Annals of Tropical Paediatrics*, Vol. 19, No.1, pp. 9-13

Zar, H.J. (2005). Neonatal chlamydial infections: prevention and treatment. *Pediatric Drugs*, Vol. 7, No. 2, pp. 103-110

Zuppa, A.A. et al. (2011). Ophthalmia neonatorum: what kind of prophylaxis? *The Journal of Maternal-Fetal and Neonatal Medicine*, Vol. 24, No. 6, pp. 769-773

8

The Role of Chlamydophila (Chlamydia) Pneumoniae in the Pathogenesis of Coronary Artery Disease

Mirosław Brykczynski
Cardiac Surgery Department, Pomeranian Medical University, Szczecin Poland

1. Introduction

Atherosclerosis is a leading cause of death and disability in the modern world. Generations of researchers have worked to establish the risk factors of this disease. It was Rudolf Virchow who identified inflammation as one of those risk factors in his fundamental dissertation entitled Cellular Pathology, which was published in 1858. From this time onwards more that 250 risk factors of atherosclerosis have been found. Atherosclerosis is chronic progressive disease. Inflammation, similarly to atherosclerosis, activates endothelial cell damage, leucocyte migration and monocytes activation or smooth muscle proliferation. The discovery made at the end of the 20th century concerning the role that infection with Helicobacter pylori in the pathogenesis of peptic ulcer disease, has drawn much attention. Interest has been focused on the potential role of this and indeed other bacteria in pathogenesis of various chronic diseases. Epidemiological studies have revealed that the risk of such an infection increases in tandem with the age of the studied population (Veldhuyzen van Zanten et al., 1994). The role that Helicobacter pylori as well as other bacteria and viruses play in the pathogenesis of atherosclerosis was extensively studied at the end of the previous century in the nineteen nineties. These studies concluded that the connection between infection and atherosclerosis is much stronger for Chlamydophila pneumoniae (C. pneumoniae) than for Helicobacter pylori or any other organism (Blasi et al., 1996, Wald et al., 1997). A large numbers of studies reported on association between C. pneumoniae and symptoms of atherosclerosis such as coronary artery disease (Saikku et al., 1988. Jackson et al., 1997), carotid artery stenosis (Cochrane et al., 2003), lower extremities artery obstruction (Kuo et al., 1997) or aneurysms (Blasi et al., 1996. Lindholt et al., 1998)

2. History and taxonomy

Chlamydophila pneumoniae is a Gram-negative, obligate intracellular, bacterium that infects humans as a respiratory pathogen. This bacterium is responsible for many of cases of mild pneumonia, bronchitis and sinusitis in all parts of the world (Kuo et al., 1995). It was first named Chlamydia TWAR (for Taiwan Acute Respiratory), when close resemblance was found between bacteria isolated in patients from Taiwan and those treated for acute respiratory failure in the USA (Grayston et al., 1986). The new strain was later found to be significantly different from the already known Chlamydia trachomatis and Chlamydia pisttaci, and was named Chlamydia pneumoniae (Grayston et al., 1989). The name was later officially changed to the one used at present, namely Chlamydophila pneumoniae.

3. Developmental cycle

C. Pneumoniae has a biphasic life cycle, existing as either an EB (elementary body) or a RB (reticulate body). The EB is the extracellular infectious non-replicating form which, when internalized by a susceptible cell in the human respiratory tract, differentiates into the metabolically active RB. The RB replicates thus forming an intracellular microcolony and then re-differentiates back into EB forms, which are released from the infected cell to begin next infection cycle. Although this explains why it can be found in the lungs it was nonetheless a surprise to discover that it can also be found in atherosclerotic vessels (Blasi et al., 1996). This fact had to be confirmed by means of the polymerase chain reaction method (PCR). Despite the fact that bacteria specific DNA was found in the diseased arteries no trace of the RNA was seen at the same time (Valassima et al., 2001). This suggests that what may be found in the arteries is not a metabolically active organism. The authors of this study conclude that the DNA remains only as a result of macrophages migration. But others have proved that in vitro C. pneumoniae can infect vascular endothelial cells, initiating lesion formation (Selzman et al., 2003). Animals infected with C. pneumoniae develop atherosclerosis lesion in arteries and several studies in man suggested an association between persistent infection and ischaemic heart disease.

4. Diagnosis of the C. pneumoniae infection

Culturing of the organism is the gold standard in the diagnosis of the infection, but sensitivity of this technique in the C. pneumoniae infection is only 60%. Compared the sensitivity of serological examination is close to 100%. This makes it most common method of diagnosing C. pneumoniae is to examine patient's serum for species-specific IgM, IgG and IgA class antibodies. Determining the dynamics of appearance and disappearance of particular immunoglobulin classes allows one to diagnose what kind of infections the patient suffers from: primary, chronic, or reinfection. In an acute primary infection, IgM class antibodies appear first and their levels remain increased for about 2 months, to gradually subside later. Next, the IgG class antibody titer levels increase, and then the same elevation is noticed in the IgA class. In case of successful treatment and no reinfection, the antibody levels slowly decrease, despite the fact that elevation in IgG class antibody levels is usually observed proportionally to the patient's age. Increased, but remaining stable, the level of IgG class antibodies, and, in particular, IgA class antibodies may indicate a chronic infection and/or frequently reoccurring infections. Persistent production of IgA class antibodies compared to long-lasting IgG antibodies, seems to be a good marker of chronic infection (Saikku et al 1999). C. pneumoniae primary infection is more common in children et persons at middle age. Approximately 50% of young adults have serological evidence of previous C. pneumoniae infection. Reinfection or persistent infection is more common in elderly persons and evidence of past infection have 75% of them. This disease is reported more common in males (60-90%) that in females. The evidence of previous C. pneumoniae infection is higher in smokers end ex-smokers. The higher prevalence of smoking in men does not explain the C. pneumoniae antibody prevalence in men compared with women (Karvonen et al. 1994). After controlling for the effect of smoking, the risk of C. pneumoniae seropositivity remained 1.4 times higher in men than in women. In men, the estimated risk for C. pneumoniae seropositivity was significant only for smokers (1.5) and (1.7) for ex-smokers. C pneumoniae infection is more common in smokers. Smoking predisposes for the development of a chronic C pneumoniae infection. The synergistic negative effect of smoking and C pneumoniae chronic infection may be one mechanism in the pathogenesis of airway obstruction and atherosclerosis progression (von Hertzen et al., 1996).

5. Coronary artery diseases et C. pneumonia infection

C. pneumoniae usually causes acute upper respiratory tract infections, which range in severity from asymptomatic disease to severe pneumonia. It has been estimated to account for up to 20% of community-acquired pneumonia and, because it can maintain a chronic or latent infection, recurrence of the disease is frequent, despite treatment with antibiotics (Ewing et al., 2003). Such infections most frequently occur in elderly male smokers and such patients are naturally predisposed to atherosclerosis. However, there are other features to these infections, such as for example the periodical occurrence of epidemics every four years does not to seem to have much in common with atherosclerosis. Saikku was the first man to show that coronary artery diseases were more likely to have detectable in patients with higher anti - C. pneumoniae antibodies (Saikku et al., 1988). The conclusion reached was to start trials with antibiotics in such patients (Gurfinkel et al., 1997, 1999, Gupta et al., 1997, Muhlestein et al., 1998, Anderson et al., 1999, Grayston et al., 1999). Gurfinkel's group tested roxitromycin in patients with acute coronary syndromes. Gupta's group used azithromycin in patients with stable angina. A significant reduction in incidences of combined events including the recurrence of angina, myocardial infarction and death was noted in the early phase of the ROXIS trial (Gurfinkel et al., 1997). The following studies in the same patients did not show any long-term benefits of such therapy (Gurfinkel et al., 1999). Other groups have not been found to benefit from the use of antibiotics for the treatment of chronic or unstable angina (Zahn et al., 2003, O'Connor et al., 2005, Cannon et al., 2005). Indeed any evidence gathered from many trials performed to date does not demonstrate an overall benefit of antibiotic therapy in reducing mortality or cardiovascular events in patients with coronary artery disease (Andraws et al., 2005). The authors of the paper believe that the treatment with antichlamydial antibiotics failed to improve the clinical outcomes of acute coronary events and chronic disorders. One must accept that the problem is a difficult case to study. For example although the presence of C. pneumoniae in the arterial wall may be confirmed by laboratory tests such as PCR or IHC testing, a positive culture from such a specimen should not be expected. Published studies have detected C. pneumoniae in atherosclerosis arterial tissue using two different techniques such as polymerase chain reaction (PSR) and immunohistochemistry (IHC) but results are often difficult to interpret. (Cambell et al., 1995, Davidson et al., 1998) None of these techniques nowadays is perfect to detect the C. pneumoniae infection. There are long terms studies needed if we want to determine a potential role of C. Pneumoniae infection in the start of atherosclerosis plaque or only in arteriosclerosis progression Coronary artery disease being a specific form of atherosclerosis, is a very difficult case for studying. Despite technical progress of visualisation of coronary artery, currently there are no examinations giving a possibility of observation in progressing of the atherosclerosis in these arteries. Diagnosis stated on classical coronarography do not give any information about the coexistence of coronary artery disease et chronic infection caused by C. Pneumoniae. In this situation we have not data on the infection anticipates in coronary artery. On the base of observation we know that laboratory inducted infection may lead to lowering of the HDL level and the increasing CRP if this examination at company high cholesterol diet. (Birck et al., 2011). Many states of the disease make this comparison difficult because in absolutely divergences illness early study od changes in artery or acute coronary syndrome and end stage circulatory insufficiency cause by coronary disease. Multiple sampling from the coronary artery is in practice impossible. That is why most researchers take species from the aortic wall. (Brykczyński 2000, Kribis et al., 2005). Frequently cited work of Kuo saying about C. Pneumonia founded directly in coronary artery wall was based only on 36 autopsies hearts (Kuo et al., 1993). In this paper the presents of C. Pneumoniae was confirmed during DNE study in 13 cases and 15 during immunochemistry examination. In total positive results was achieved in 20 cased. This says that positives results are not gained by different methods in all cases. The big advantage of this work is a confirmation of the presence of the metabolically active EB form of C. Pneumonia. Muhlestein presented positive results examining specimen of atherosclerotic plaque taking during coronary artery ednarteriectomy in immunochemistry examination in 73% of cases (Muhlestein et al., 1995). In many papers in diagnoses it is accepted to take into account the positive results in PCR and negative IHC or the other way round. It happens that positive results in patients without antibodies against C. pneumoniae take place. Researchers have always debated issues concerning the changing titers of antibodies against C. pneumoniae. It goes without saying that it is very important which antibodies are taken into account. It seems that the presence of IgA class antibodies is more important to diagnose a chronic C. pneumoniae infection than the more commonly present IgG antibody. The association between high titers of IgA antibodies and the subsequent risk of death from coronary artery disease was noted by Caerphilly prospective study (Strachan et al., 1999). Interestingly he did not show any relation between IgG antibodies and mortality. Lidholt described the presence of anti- C. pneumoniae IgA in patients with chronic abdominal aortic aneurysm (Lindholt et al., 1999). Others note the association between high titers of anti- C. pneumoniae IgA with the levels of fibrinogen and C-reactive protein (Toss et al., 1999, Zairis et al., 2003). It is interesting to note that although Saikku (1988) analyzed both IgA and IgG class antibodies, the other groups following him in this field limited their interest to only the IgG isotype (Zahn et al., 2003, O'Connor et al., 2005, Cannon et al., 2005). In my own research I have demonstrated the presence of antibodies against C. pneumoniae in 150 patients accepted for coronary surgery (Brykczynski 2001). Patients with coronary artery disease confirmed angiographic and qualified for coronary artery bypass grafting were enrolled. This study showed specific antibodies against C. pneumoniae in IgG class in 110 patients, and in IgA class in 90 patients. In 81 patients antibodies in both IgA class and IgG class were found. In 36 surgery patients no antibodies in either of those classes were found. Group consisting of 50 patients with high levels of antibodies against C. pneumoniae qualified for heart surgery and treated with antibiotic

(Rulid 2 x 150 mg) for 30 days prior to surgery. A monthly treatment with roxytromycin before the operation in those patients resulted in bringing down their levels of: fibrinogen, von Willebrand factor, complement component 3, prealbumin, acid α1-glycoprotein, homocysteine as well as total cholesterol levels. However the negative effect of this therapy was a fall in the level of HDL cholesterol. Other studies with azithromycin resulted in a similar reduction of inflammatory markers (Gupta et al., 1997, Anderson et al., 1999, Grayston et al., 1999). Despite the fact that these results may be encouraging it is nevertheless doubtful if one could base the diagnosis of infection only on the grounds of increased levels of antibodies. Furthermore no one has as yet described the result of antimicrobial treatment over a long time span. It may well be the case that any promising short-term result may not be necessarily related to the specific treatment of the C.

pneumoniae infection. The beneficial influence of antibiotics on mortality observed in the Roxis trial was very limited. The lack of any clear results may be due to the fact that no established criteria of C. pneumoniae infection were given. The study was based on a single test of antibody titers, which may well only be a sign of a past but not necessarily an ongoing infection. Although all these doubts call for further research there exist very few studies in this area. It is for this reason that I have decided to follow my own patients, in which an examination of the presence of antibodies and the evaluation of the progress of coronary disease were performed 6 years after the operation (Brykczynski et al., 2010). The data were completed for all 150 patients in the first study 6 years after 82,5% patients were still alive, 17,4% patients died, and 6.45% living patients did not consent to participate in the control study. The objective of this study was 118 patients. The group consisted of 20% women, mean age 61.7 years, and 80% men, mean age 56.4 years In this study we also tried to evaluate the influence of C. pneumoniae infection on the late results of surgical treatment of coronary artery disease. In the first study IgA and IgG class antibodies were found in 53,4% patients, but in the control 83,9% patients had those antibodies. The number of patients with IgA class antibodies increased from 58,5% to 86,4% patients. In 30,5% patient's antibodies were found for the first time, and in 51,7% patients an significant increase of their titer occurred. Similarly, the number of patients with a positive test result for IgG class antibodies increased from 72.0% to 94,1% patients. In 22% patients IgG class antibodies were found for the first time, while in 39,8% patients an increase of their titer occurred. Only in 3,4% patients were no antibodies in either IgA or IgG class found - compared to 22,9% patients from the first study. Their preoperative coronary complaints were evaluated according to the Canadian Cardiovascular Score (CCS) scale. The average degree on the CCS score before operation was 3,8. Six years after the average CCS degree decreases to 1,65. These results show no connection between the increased serological symptoms of chronic infection caused by C. pneumoniae and coronary complaints. A steady increase of antibodies titers with the rise in the age of patients was observed. However this increase did not correspond with the intensity of the coronary artery disease symptoms. Many authors describe the link between the C. pneumoniae infection and pathogenesis of aortic aneurysms or with the progression of the atherosclerotic plaque in carotid arteries. Despite there being many published articles concerning this matter there remained to be found a universally accepted explanation of such an influence. Nonetheless a few hypotheses are proposed. One is the hypothesis which assumes that the C. pneumoniae infection spreads through the monocytes which get into the bloodstream via the lungs and then infiltrate the arterial walls as foam cells forming fatty streaks. The second theory is the plasma theory, which explains the role of C. pneumoniae infection by its influence on the increasing plasma concentration of other independent factors related to atherosclerosis progression like fibrinogen, von Willebrand factor or C-reactive protein. Third theory links this infection with an autoimmunological reaction. At present the most popular theory is the one that assumes a crossover reaction with the heat shock proteins (HSP). C. pneumoniae contains heat shock protein like HSP 10, HSP 60 and HSP 70. All three of them can be found in the membrane complexes EB and RB. The human and bacterial proteins of this kind are very much alike. The expression of such proteins rises under stress, with high blood pressure or during infection. C. pneumoniae may produce large quantities of HSP. Another way may base on the synergistic negative effect of linked with advanced age, male sex, smoking habit, or higher level of fibrinogen et CRP. All of them are characteristic for chronic C. pneumoniae infection et atherosclerosis progression. Most researchers have been discouraged by lack of any clear proof that the C. pneumoniae infection is important in the pathogenesis of atherosclerosis. The fact that there is a multitude of independent risk factors predisposing to atherosclerosis may be changing due to the infection. This is because it makes it possible that a large number of these influences may not always be present in some patients, while in others may only be important In the presence of very specific circumstances. Without prospective studies based on large populations we may never learn whether the C. pneumoniae infection is an important risk factor for coronary artery disease or only an "innocent bystander " as suggested by West in his commentary (West, 1999). Patients with coronary artery disease represent a heterogeneous group, the same applies to patients with C. pneumoniae infections. Antibiotic treatment in acute or chronic infection may produce different results. One large study analyses the results of such treatment in atypical pulmonary infections (Arnold et al., 2007). These infections were caused by Legionella pneumophila, Mycoplasma pneumoniae and C. pneumoniae. The incidence of such infections is as high as 22% in the USA and 28% in Europe. In South America, Africa and Asia it is much lower. The diagnosis of pneumonia caused by the C. pneumoniae was arrived at in this study on the very strict basis with high IgG titer (1:512). Most of the patients were male and their mean age was over 65 years. The study retrospectively compares the group of patients treated with antibiotics covering the atypical infections with the group of patients who did not receive such treatment. Patients in the second group spend more time in hospital and had a higher mortality. Mortality in the second group was more than 10%. Perhaps this may be the explanation why there was a good short-term result of using antibiotics in the ROXIS study population of patients who had been treated for acute coronary syndromes.

6. Summary

In conclusion we have to state categorically that a high level of anti- C. pneumoniae antibodies is present in the majority of patients with diagnosed coronary artery disease. It seems that we may need to depend more on the IgA class antibodies examination in any future research because the IgG class antibodies are almost universally present in the population.

Additionally we need to establish a strict criteria to differentiate the acute and the latent C. pneumoniae infection. We still do not know what effect a C. pneumoniae infection has on the progression of coronary artery disease. Certainly a rise in the levels of the fibrinogen or the CRP during such infections is a sign that it may have some kind of influence. This suggests that an atypical pneumonia caused by C. pneumoniae in patients with the coronary artery disease is not so "innocent".

7. References[1]

Anderson JL, Muhlestein JB, Carlquist J, Allen A, Trehan S, Nielson C, Hall S, Brady J, Egger M, Horne B, Lim T.: Randomized secondary prevention trial of azithromycin in patients with coronary artery disease and serological evidence for Chlamydia pneumoniae infection: the Azithromycin in Coronary Artery Disease: Elimination of Myocardial Infection with Chlamydia (ACADEMIC) study. Circulation. 1999; 99:1540–1547

Andraws R, Berger JS, Brown DL,: Effects of antibiotic therapy on outcomes of patients with coronary artery disease. JAMA. 2005; 21: 2641-2647

Arnold FW, Summersgill JT, Lajoie AS, Peyrani P, Marrie TJ, Rossi P, Blasi F, Fernandez P, File TM, Rello J, Mendez R., Marzoratti L, Luna C, Ramirez JA, and CAPO investigators.: A worldwide perspective of atypical pathogens in community-acquired pneumonia. Am J Respir Crit Care Med 2007; 10: 1086-1093

Birck MM, Pesonen E, Odermarsky M, Hansen A, Persson K, Frikke-Schmidt H, Heegaard PMH,Liuba P.; Infection-induced coronary dysfunction and systemic inflammation in piglets are dampened in hypercholesterolemic milieu. AJP - Heart Published online 2011

Blasi F, Denti F, Erba M, Cosentini R, Raccanelli R, Rinaldi A, Fagetti L, Esposito G, Ruberti U, Allegra L.: Detection of Chlamydia pneumoniae but not Helicobacter pylori in atherosclerotic plaques of aortic aneurysm. J Clin Microbiol 1996; 34: 2766-2769

Brykczyński M.: Evaluation of roxithromycin therapy in patients with chronic Chlamydia pneumoniae infection operated for ischaemic heart disease. Annales Academiae Medicae Stetinensis. 2001. Sup 64

Brykczyński M, Żych A, Gorący I, Mączyńska I, Wojciechowska-Koszko I, Mokrzycki K, Giedrys-Kalemba S, Sielicki P.: Evaluation of the level of antibodies against Chlamydophila (Chlamydia) pneumoniae in post-surgery heart ischaemia patients and their clinical conditions - six-year study. Arch Med Sci 2010;6 (2):214-220

Cambell LA, O'Brien ER, Cappuccio AL, Kuo CC, Wang SP, Stewart D, Patton DL, Cummings PK, Grayston JT.: Detection of Chlamydia pneumoniae TWAR in human coronary atherectomy tissues. J Infect Dis 1995; 172: 585-588

Cannon CP, Braunwald E, McCabe CH, Grayston JT, Muhlestein B, Giugliano RP, Cairns R, Skene AM.: Pravastatin or Atorvastatin Evaluation and Infection Therapy-Thrombolysis in Myocardial Infarction 22 Investigators. Antibiotic treatment of Chlamydia pneumoniae after acute coronary syndrome. N Engl J Med. 2005; 16: 1646-1654

[1] PS. Preparing this publication I found very sad information that Dr Enrique Gurfinkel (ROXIS study) died of lung cancer 2 May 2011. www.theheart.org/article/1219603

Cochrane M, Pospschil A, Walker P, Gibbs H, Timmps P.: Distribution of Chlamydia pneumoniae DNA in atherosclerosis carotid arteries: significance for sampling procedures. J Clin Microbiol 2003; 41: 1454-1457

Davidson M, Kuo CC, Middaugh JP, Wang SP, Newman WP, Finley JC, Grayston JT.: Confirmed previous infection with Chlamydia pneumoniae (TWAR) and presence in early coronary atherosclerosis. Circulation 1998; 98: 628-633

Ewig S, Torres A.: Is Chlamydia pneumoniae an important pathogen in patients with community-acquired pneumonia? Eur Respir J 2003; 5: 741-742

Grayston JT, Kuo CC, Wang SP, Altman J.: A new Chlamydia psittaci strain, TWAR, isolated in acute respiratory infections. N Engl J Med 1986; 315: 161-168

Grayston JT, Kuo CC, Cambell LA, Wang SP.: Chlamydia pneumoniae sp. nov. For Chlamydia sp. Strain TWAR. Int J Syst Bacteriol. 1989; 39: 88-90

Grayston JT.: Antibiotic treatment trials for secondary prevention of coronary artery disease events. Circulation. 1999; 99: 1538–1539

Gurfinkel E, Bozovich G, Darooca A, Beck E, Mautner B, for the ROXIS Study Group.: Randomized trial of roxithromycin in non-Q-wave coronary syndromes: ROXIS pilot study. Lancet. 1997; 350: 404–407

Gurfinkel E, Bozovich G, Beck E, Testa E, Livellara B, Mautner B and ROXIS Study Group.: Treatment with the antibiotic roxytromycin in patients with acute non-Q-wave coronary syndromes. The final report of the ROXIS study. Eur Heart J. 1999; 2: 121-127

Gupta S, Leatham EW, Carrington D, Mendall MA, Kaski JC, Camm AJ.: Elevated Chlamydia pneumoniae antibodies, cardiovascular events and azithromycin in male survivors of myocardial infarction. Circulation. 1997; 96: 404–407

Jackson L, Campbell L, Schmidt R, Kuo C, Cappuccio A, Grayston J.: Specificity of detection of Chlamydia pneumoniae in cardiovascular and non-cardiovascular tissues: evaluation of the innocent bystander hypothesis. Am J Pathol 1997; 150: 1785-1790

Karvonen M, Tuomilehto J, Pitkaniemi J, Naukkarinen A, Saikku P.: Importance of Smoking for Chlamydia pneumoniae Seropositivity. Int. J. Epidemiol. 1994: 23 (6): 1315-1321.

Kirbis J, Kese D, Petrovic D.: Presence of Presence of Chlamydia pneumoniae DNA in the artery wall-biomarker of coronary artery disease. Folia Biol (Praha) 2005; 51(5): 145-14

Kuo CC, Shor A, Campbell LA, Fukushi H, Patton DL, Grayston JT.: Demonstration of Chlamydia pneumionae in atrerosclerosis lesions of coronary arteries. J Infect Dis 1993; 167: 841-849

Kuo CC, Jackson LA, Cambell LA, Grayston JT.: Chlamydia pneumoniae (TWAR). Clin Microbiol Rev. 1995; 8: 451-461

Kuo C, Coulson A, Cambell L, Cappuccio A, Lawrence R, Wang S, Grayston J.: Detection of Chlamydia pneumoniae in atherosclerotic plaques in walls of arteries of lower extremities from patients undergoing bypass operation for arterial obstruction J Vasc Surg 1997; 26: 29-31

Lindholt JS, Juul S, Vammen S, Lind I, Fasting H, Henneberg EW.: Immunoglobulin A antibodies against Chlamydia pneumoniae are associated with expansion of abdominal aortic aneurysm. Br J Surg. 1999; 86: 634–638

Muhlestein JB, Hammond EH, Carlquist JF, Radicke E, Thomson MT, Karagounis LA, Woods ML, Anderson JL.: Increased incidence of Chlamydia species within the coronary arteries of patients with symptomatic atherosclerotic versus other forms of cardiovascular disease. J Am Coll Cardiol 1996; 27: 1555-1561

Muhlestein JB, Anderson JL, Hammond EH, Zhao L, Trehan S, Schwobe EP, Carlquist JF.: Infection with Chlamydia pneumonia accelerates the development of atherosclerosis and treatment with azithromycin prevents it in a rabbit model. Circulation. 1998; 97: 633–636O'Connor CM, Dunne MW, Pfeffer MA, Muhlestein JB, Yao L, Gupta S, Benner RJ, Fisher MR, Cook TD; Investigators in the WIZARD Study.: Azithromycin for the secondary prevention of coronary heart disease events: the WIZARD study: a randomized controlled trial. JAMA. 2003; 11: 1459-66

Saikku P, Leinonen M, Mattila M.: Serological evidence of an association of a novel chlamydia, TWAR, with chronic coronary heart disease and acute myocardial infarction. Lancet. 1988; 2: 983–985

Saikku P.: Chronic Chlamydia pneumoniae infections. In: Allegra L, Blasi F (eds) Chlamydia pneumoniae. The Lung and the Heart. Springer-Verlag, Milan: 96-113.

Selzman CH, Netea MG, Zimmerman MA, Weinberg A, Reznikow LL, Grover FL, Dinarello CA.: Atherogenic effects of Chlamydia pneumoniae: refuting the Innocent bystander hypothesis. J Thorac Cardiovasc Surg. 2003; 3: 688-693

Strachan DP, Carrington D, Mendall MA, Ballam L, Morris J, Butland BK, Sweetnam PM, Elwood PC.: Relation of Chlamydia pneumoniae serology to mortality and incidence of ischaemic heart disease over 13 years in the Caerphilly prospective heart disease study. BMJ 1999; 318: 1035-1039

Toss H, Gnarpe J, Gnarpe H, Siegbahn A, Wallentin L.: Increased fibrinogen levels are associated with persistent Chlamydia pneumoniae infection in unstable coronary artery disease. Eur Heart J 1999; 19: 570-577.

Valassina M, Migliorini L, Sansoni A, Sani G, Corasaro D, Cusi MG, Valensin PE, Cellesi C.: Serch for Chlamydia pneumoniae genes and their expression in atheroscleroslerotic plaques of carotid arteries. J Med. Microbiol. 2001; 50: 228-232

Veldhuyzen van Zanten SJO, Pollak PT, Best LM, Bezanson GS, Marrie T.: Increasing prevalence of Helicobacter pylori infection with age. The Journal of Infectious Diseases 1994; 2: 434-437

von Hertzen L, Isoaho R, Leinonen M, Koskinen R, Laipala P, Toyryla M. Kivela SL, Saikku P.: Chlamydia pneumoniae antibodies in chronic obstructive pulmonary diseases. Int J Epidemiol 1996; 25:658–664

Wald NJ, Law MR, Morris JK, Bagnall AM.: Helicobacter pylori infection and mortality form ischaemic heart disease: negative result from a large, prospective study. BMJ. 1997; 315: 1199-1201

West RR.: Chlamydia pneumoniae infection and ischaemic heart disease. BMJ 1999; 318: 1039-1040

Zahn R, Schneider S, Frilling B, Seidl K, Tebbe U, Weber M, Gottwik M, Altmann E, Seidel F, Rox J, Hoffler U, Neuhaus KL, Senges J; Working Group of Leading Hospital

Cardiologists.: Antibiotic therapy after acute myocardial infarction: a prospective randomized study. Circulation. 2003; 9: 1253-1259

Zairis MN, Papadaki OA, Psarogianni PK, Thoma MA, Andrikopoulos GK, Batika PC, Poulopoulou CG, Trifinopoulou KG, Olympios CD, Foussas SG.: Serologic markers of persistent Chlamydia pneumoniae infection and long-therm prognosis after successful coronary stenting. Am Heart J. 2003; 146: 1082-1089

9

Chlamydiae in Gastrointestinal Disease

Aldona Dlugosz and Greger Lindberg
Karolinska Institutet, Department of Medicine
Sweden

1. Introduction

Disorders of gut function are among the most prevalent problems presented to physicians practicing in gastroenterology as well as primary care physicians and irritable bowel syndrome (IBS) is the most common functional gastrointestinal disorder. There is no biomarker of IBS. Instead, the diagnosis is based on symptom criteria and the absence of an organic cause for symptoms (Longstreth et al., 2006). Patients with IBS complain of recurrent abdominal pain, bloating after meals, and disturbed bowel habits. The population prevalence of IBS shows considerable variation between countries. In Asian countries the prevalence varies between 4.0%-22.1% (Makharia et al., 2011), in Europe 6.2%-12% (Hungin et al., 2003) and in North America 11.6%-12.1% (Thompson et al., 2002). In most studies females dominate over males with a factor of 1.4-1.9.

An intriguing finding is that 6%-17% of patients with IBS report that the onset of their disease followed from an acute infection (Spiller, 2007). So called post-infectious IBS (PI-IBS) has mainly been reported after bacterial gastroenteritis but over the years PI-IBS has been reported also after infection with viruses, worms, and protozoa. A study from our group showed that the infectious agent *per se* was not a risk factor for PI-IBS (Törnblom et al., 2007) and this led to the hypothesis that a host factor could be the determinant of PI-IBS.

Although IBS is not a life-threatening disease, the chronic nature of IBS tends to interfere with the normal daily life and IBS can have a strong impact on patients' quality of life (Amouretti et al., 2006; Drossman et al., 2009). IBS has been associated with fibromyalgia, chronic fatigue syndrome, temporo-mandibular joint disorder and chronic pelvic pain (Williams et al., 2004). Despite its abundance the cause of IBS has remained unclear. It has long been considered a psychosomatic disorder but a number of studies have reported signs of immune activation with increased numbers of lymphocytes, activated macrophages or mast cells in mucosa biopsies from the small bowel or the large bowel (Akiho et al., 2011). We investigated full-thickness biopsies from the jejunum of 10 patients with IBS and found increased numbers of mucosal lymphocytes in 4/10 patients (Törnblom et al., 2002). We also found low-grade inflammation of myenteric plexa in 9/10 patients and neuron degeneration in 7 patients. These findings were confirmed in a larger series of patients with severe IBS and the concomitant finding of enteric dysmotility (Lindberg et al., 2009). The driving force behind observed immune activation is not known but both innate and adaptive immune responses seem to be involved in IBS pathogenesis (Öhman & Simrén, 2010).

The gastrointestinal tract is also the largest endocrine organ in the body. Enteroendocrine cells (EEC), which are present in the mucosa of the stomach, small intestine, colon, and rectum, are highly specialized cells that produce hormones and other signalling substances that are vital to the normal function of the gut. Due to their diffuse localisation EEC are difficult to study and so far, their role in the pathogenesis of bowel disorders has been only little explored. A well-characterised subset of EEC are the enterochromaffin cells, which are the main source of the biogenic amine serotonin (5-hydroxytryptamine, 5-HT) in the GI tract (Kim & Camilleri, 2000). The aminoacid tryptophan serves as a precursor for the production of serotonin, which is transported from the cytosol to large dense-core secretory vesicles (LDCV) by the vesicular monoamine transporter (VMAT1) in the membrane of LDCV (Jakobsen et al., 2001). Serotonin influences the intestinal homeostasis by altering gut motor activity and secretion and has been implicated in the pathophysiology of various GI disorders, including inflammatory bowel disease (IBD) and IBS (Sikander et al., 2009).

2. Hypothesis and aim of studies

Life style, genetic risk factors and the individual's microbiome can all act as host factors for disease. The latter includes the microbial flora of skin, airways, uro-genital organs and the gastrointestinal tract. Over the years we also become populated by a number of viruses, intracellular bacteria and parasites that have the ability to remain in our own cells. One typical example is *Varicella zoster* virus (VZV), which causes chickenpox in children or adults when first infected. After healing of the acute infection virus will remain in a persistent state in nerve cells and can later become reactivated causing shingles. Several bacteria including *Myocbacterium tuberculosis*, *Salmonella enterica* serovar Typhi, and *Chlamydia spp.* also have the ability to survive in a persistent state (Monack et al., 2004).

We hypothesized that a pre-existing persistent infection could be an important host factor for the development of IBS, most evident in so called post-infectious IBS. A candidate agent should be compatible with an asymptomatic carrier-ship, have a preference for female gender, and have the ability to become persistent and to live in bowel epithelium. There were several observations to support the idea that a persistent infection with *Chlamydia trachomatis* might constitute such a host factor. Trachoma related blindness is 2-4 times more likely to affect females compared to males (Courtright & West, 2004). It is known that IBS occurs in a high proportion (35-38 %) of females with chronic pelvic pain syndrome, which is often caused by a chronic infection with *C. trachomatis* (Williams et al., 2004; Zondervan et al., 2001). Previous experience from veterinary medicine has shown that *Chlamydia spp.* can infect the intestines of calves and sheep and also lead to persistent infections (Storz & Spears, 1979).

The aim of our studies was to find out if a persistent infection of the gut with the obligate intracellular pathogen *C. trachomatis* might have a role in the pathogenesis of IBS. At the beginning of our studies it was unknown whether *Chlamydia spp.* could reside in the human gut or not. It was also unknown if *Chlamydia* had any particular cell tropism that would be compatible with a long-term persistence in the gut.

The thought that *C. trachomatis* could be involved in IBS was not unique. Based on the frequent concomitance of IBS and pelvic inflammatory disease an attempt was made to link *C. trachomatis* to IBS using serum IgG antibodies but the study showed no significant difference between control subjects and patients with IBS (Francis et al., 1998). However, we think that IgG antibody patterns may be insufficient to rule out persistence of *Chlamydia* due to a dominating cellular immune response to infection (Witkin, 2002).

3. Chlamydial antigens in small bowel mucosa of patients with IBS

We investigated archived biopsies from the small bowel of 65 patients (61 females) with IBS (Dlugosz et al., 2010). IBS was defined according to the Rome-II criteria (Thompson et al., 1999). Full-thickness biopsies of the jejunum were available in 60 patients and mucosa biopsies from the jejunum or the duodenum in 24 patients. We recruited 32 (22 females) healthy controls, which underwent mucosa biopsy of the jejunum and we utilized archived full-thickness small bowel biopsies from another 10 (7 females) obese but otherwise healthy control subjects. In order to detect chlamydial antigens we used a genus-specific mouse monoclonal antibody to *Chlamydia* lipopolysaccharide (LPS) that was FITC conjugated with Evans blue (RDI-PROAC1FT, Fitzgerald Industries International, Concord, USA). We also used a mouse monoclonal antibody to *C. trachomatis* major outer membrane protein (MOMP) (Gene-Tex, San Antonio, USA) and a species-specific mouse monoclonal antibody to *C. pneumoniae* as primary antibodies with a polyclonal rabbit anti-mouse antibody-FITC conjugated (Dako, Glostrup, Denmark) as secondary antibody. In addition we used a number of cell-specific antibodies to identify different cell types. Enteroendocrine cells were identified using antibodies to chromogranin-A, mast cells using antibodies to CD117, macrophages using antibodies to CD68, and dendritic cells using antibodies to CD11c.

From each biopsy 6 new sections were taken up for immunofluorescence staining. Sections were investigated using a fluorescent microscope (Leica DMRXA, Leica Microsystems, Wetzlar, Germany). Positive staining for *Chlamydia* LPS was seen in triangular cells mainly at the crypt level (Figure 1A) but also in irregularly shaped cells in *lamina propria* (Figure 1B). Staining for *Chlamydia* LPS was positive in 58/65 patients with IBS and only 6/42 controls. The odds ratio ratio, corrected for differences in age and gender distributions, for mucosal *Chlamydia* LPS being indicative for presence of IBS was 43.1 (95% CI: 13.2-140.7).

No LPS-positive cells were found in the deeper levels of the bowel wall, i.e. submucosa, muscle layers and the enteric nervous system. Staining for *C. trachomatis* MOMP (Figure 1C) was positive in 69% of LPS-positive biopsies, including 2/6 LPS-positive biopsies from control subjects, but none was positive in staining for *C. pneumoniae.*

Further characterization of LPS-positive cells was done using double staining with antibodies to LPS and cell specific markers. Double staining with antibodies to LPS and chromogranin-A showed that *Chlamydia* LPS was present in enteroendocrine cells of the epithelium (Figure 1D-F). Similarly, double staining with antibodies to LPS and CD117, CD11c and CD68 showed that in *lamina propria* the LPS-positive cells were macrophages (Figure 1G-I). In order to validate our findings of *Chlamydia* LPS we examined 20 slides (10 LPS-positive and 10 LPS-negative) using a different antibody to *Chlamydia* LPS, a polyclonal rabbit antibody (Fitzgerald Industries International, Concord, USA) and an immuno-enzymatic assay with Streptavidin-Biotin Complex (Dako, Glostrup, Danmark). All 10 biopsies that were positive for *Chlamydia* LPS remained positive also in this experiment, whereas all LPS-negative biopsies remained negative. We took new biopsies from 4 patients in whom a previous biopsy had been positive for *Chlamydia* LPS. The new biopsies were also positive for *Chlamydia* LPS in immunofluorescence and the presence of LPS was confirmed using Western blot analysis. However, an attempt to confirm the presence of bacteria using real-time PCR after amplification of 23S ribosomal DNA (Everett et al., 1999) was negative in all 4 biopsies.

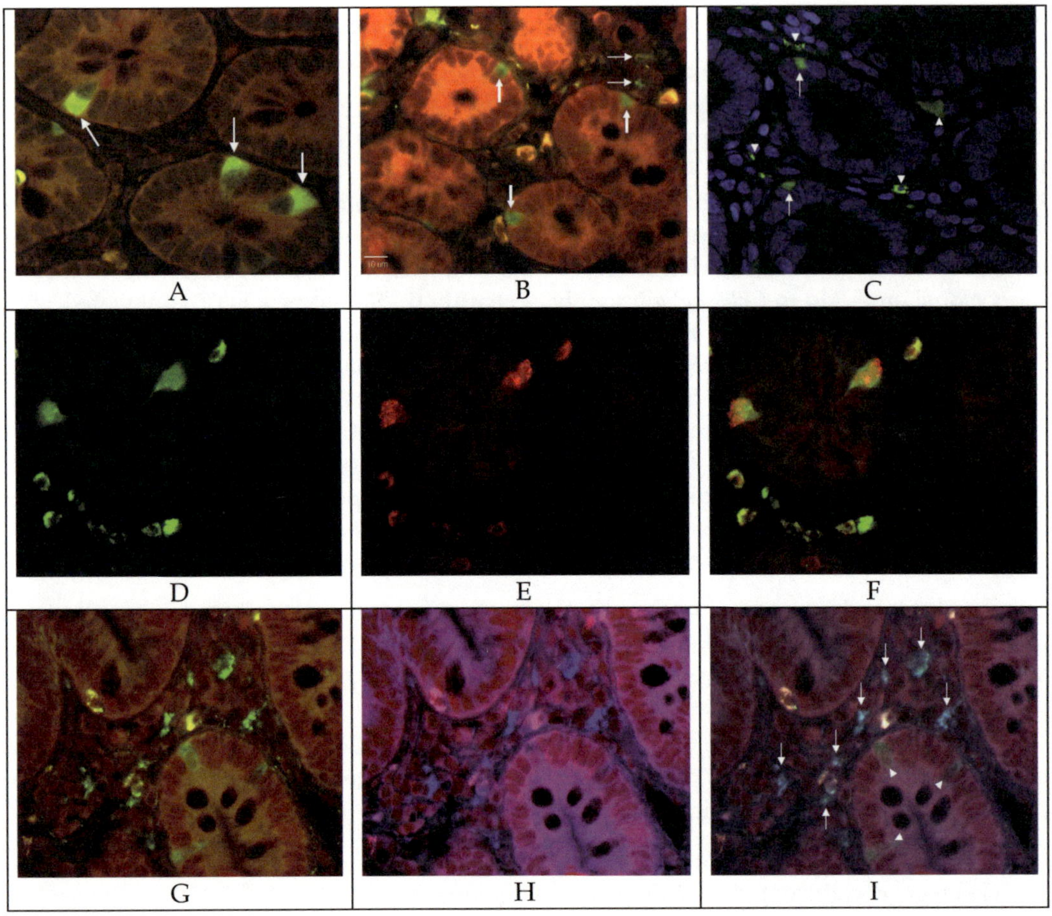

Fig. 1. Fluorescent microscope images of small bowel preparations from patients with IBS. A: *Chlamydia* LPS in EEC-like cells with apical nuclei and strong basal immunofluorescence (arrows); (Monoclonal FITC-conjugated antibody with Evans blue; original magnification × 63). B: *Chlamydia* LPS in a few cells within the epithelium (thick arrows) and *lamina propria* (thin arrows); (Monoclonal FITC-conjugated antibody with Evans blue; original magnification × 63). C: *Chlamydia trachomatis* MOMP-positive immunofluorescence within 2 EEC-like cells (arrows) and 4 cells within *l. propria* (arrowheads); Mouse MOMP-antibody and FITC-conjugated rabbit anti-mouse antibody; original magnification × 63; Hoechst (DAPI conjugated) for nuclear staining. D-F: Immunostainings for (D) *Chlamydia* LPS (FITC, green); (E) chromogranin A (Alexia 568, red); and (F) merged showing co-localisation of chromogranin A and *Chlamydia* LPS in enteroendocrine cells and *Chlamydia* LPS in *lamina propria*. G-I: Immunostainings for (G) *Chlamydia* LPS (FITC, green,); (H) CD68 (Alexia 350, blue); and (I) merged showing co-localisation of CD68 and *Chlamydia* LPS in macrophages (arrows). Three enteroendocrine cells are also positive for *Chlamydia* LPS (arrowheads).

Reproduced from Dlugosz et al., *BMC Gastroenterology* 2010, Vol. 10, p. 19 doi:10.1186/1471-230X-10-19.

Thus, we found chlamydial antigens in enteroendocrine cells and macrophages of the small bowel mucosa. Chlamydial antigens were present in biopsies from 89% of patients with severe IBS but in only 14% of controls. The odds ratio for mucosal *Chlamydia* LPS being indicative for presence of IBS is much higher than any previously described pathogenetic marker in IBS (Öhman & Simrén, 2007).

In absence of DNA proof of bacterial presence several questions remain to consider. One is whether observed immunofluorescence findings represent true presence of bacterial antigens or if they are unspecific findings or artefacts. We think that unspecific or artefactual binding is unlikely in view of the difference between patients and controls. The genus-specific epitope for our anti-LPS antibody is not shared by other Gram-negative bacteria and monoclonal antibodies to this epitope do not bind to LPS from those organisms (Caldwell & Hitchcock, 1984).

Another question is if observed antigens represent an ongoing infection or remainders of a past infection. In 19 patients biopsies we had access to more than one biopsy that had been taken with a time interval of at least 1 year. *Chlamydia* LPS was present in biopsies with a median time difference of 5.2 (range 1-11) years. Such a long-term presence of chlamydial antigens is most likely attributable to replicating *Chlamydiae* residing in the diseased tissue (Beatty et al., 1994).

The finding of *C. trachomatis* antigens in EEC makes it tempting to suggest a novel pathogenetic mechanism in IBS. The enteroendocrine system is crucial in particular to the digestive functions of the gastrointestinal tract. Serotonin-producing EEC may present an ideal location for *Chlamydia* due to the abundance of tryptophan and tryptophan metabolites in these cells. Tryptophan is required for normal development in *Chlamydia* species and tryptophan metabolism has been implicated in *Chlamydia* persistence and tissue tropism (Akers & Tan, 2006). If infection of EEC leads to changes in their production or secretion of signalling substances, disturbances of gastrointestinal function are likely to occur.

4. Infection of enteroendocrine cell lines

Our findings in the small bowel mucosa of patients with IBS suggested that infection of enteroendocrine cells (EEC) with *C. trachomatis* could be involved in the pathogenesis of their disease. In order to study this mechanism in more detail we set up an *in vitro* model using enteroendocrine cell lines (Dlugosz et al., 2011). We used two different human enteroendocrine cell lines: LCC-18 (a kind gift from K. Öberg, Uppsala University Hospital, Uppsala, Sweden), derived from a neuroendocrine colonic tumour and CNDT-2 (a kind gift from L. M. Ellis, University of Texas, Houston, USA), derived from a small intestinal carcinoid. We studied the influence of acute and persistent infection with *C. trachomatis* L2 strain 434 (ATCC) on gene expression and protein distribution of enteroendocrine markers.

Growth of *C. trachomatis*, manifested through inclusions containing both elementary bodies (EB) and reticulate bodies (RB), could be observed for both cell lines. Similar growth was observed in HeLa cells, which were used as positive control. Similar to previously described infection cycles in other cell types, *C. trachomatis* successfully infected and multiplied within the confinements of the inclusion in EEC and yielded productive EBs, which can therefore be considered an active infection (Figure 2A). In order to investigate whether the persistent life-cycle could be induced in the EEC, cells were infected with *C. trachomatis* and incubated in the absence and presence of penicillin G (penG), which has been demonstrated previously to induce persistent growth of *Chlamydia* in HeLa cells. When EEC were treated with penG we observed enlarged, aberrant reticulate bodies reminiscent of persistent growth forms suggesting that persistence can be induced in both EEC tested (Figure 2B).

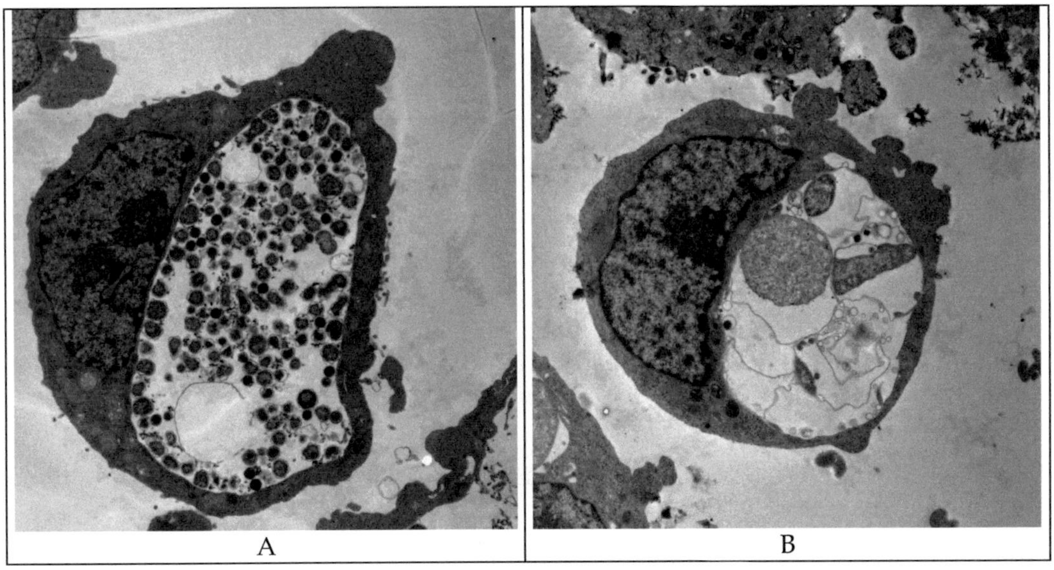

Fig. 2. Infection of enteroendocrine cells from cell line LCC-18 with *Chlamydia trachomatis*. A: Active infection. B: Persistent infection.

In order to investigate if infection with *C. trachomatis* affected the intracellular transport of signalling molecules we studied the distribution of immunoreactivity for serotonin and chromogranin-A (CgA) in infected and non-infected cells. Immunofluorescence demonstrated differences in the cellular distributions of serotonin and CgA between infected and non-infected cells (Figure 3). In infected cells serotonin and CgA were mainly localized within chlamydial inclusions, whereas in non-infected cells these markers predominantly exhibited a cytoplasmatic distribution. No serotonin or CgA was detected in infected or non-infected HeLa cells, which in this instance served as negative control.

In order to analyze the infection process at the molecular level, we investigated the expression of selected target genes using real time PCR. Genes coding for EEC protein markers (CHGA, VMAT1, mGluR4, TPH1, TRPA1), house-keeping proteins (TFCP2, GAPDH), enviromental stress marker (HSPB1) as well as TLR4, which is believed to mediate the main line of response upon *Chlamydia* infection, where subjected to PCR analysis. Transcriptomes of *C. trachomatis* infected EEC (LCC-18 and CNDT-2) were analysed after 24h. The same time-point was investigated after induction of persistence using penicillin G. We found significant down-regulation of VMAT1 expression in persistent infection compared to non-infected cells ($p<0.05$) and up-regulation of TLR4 expression in active and persistent infection ($p<0.05$). Expression of CHGA, the gene coding for CgA, as well as TPH1 and TRPA1, genes coding for proteins associated with serotonin synthesis and release, were not changed upon infection with *Chlamydia*. Gene expression changes were associated with infection and did not appear in cells exposed to heat-treated bacteria.

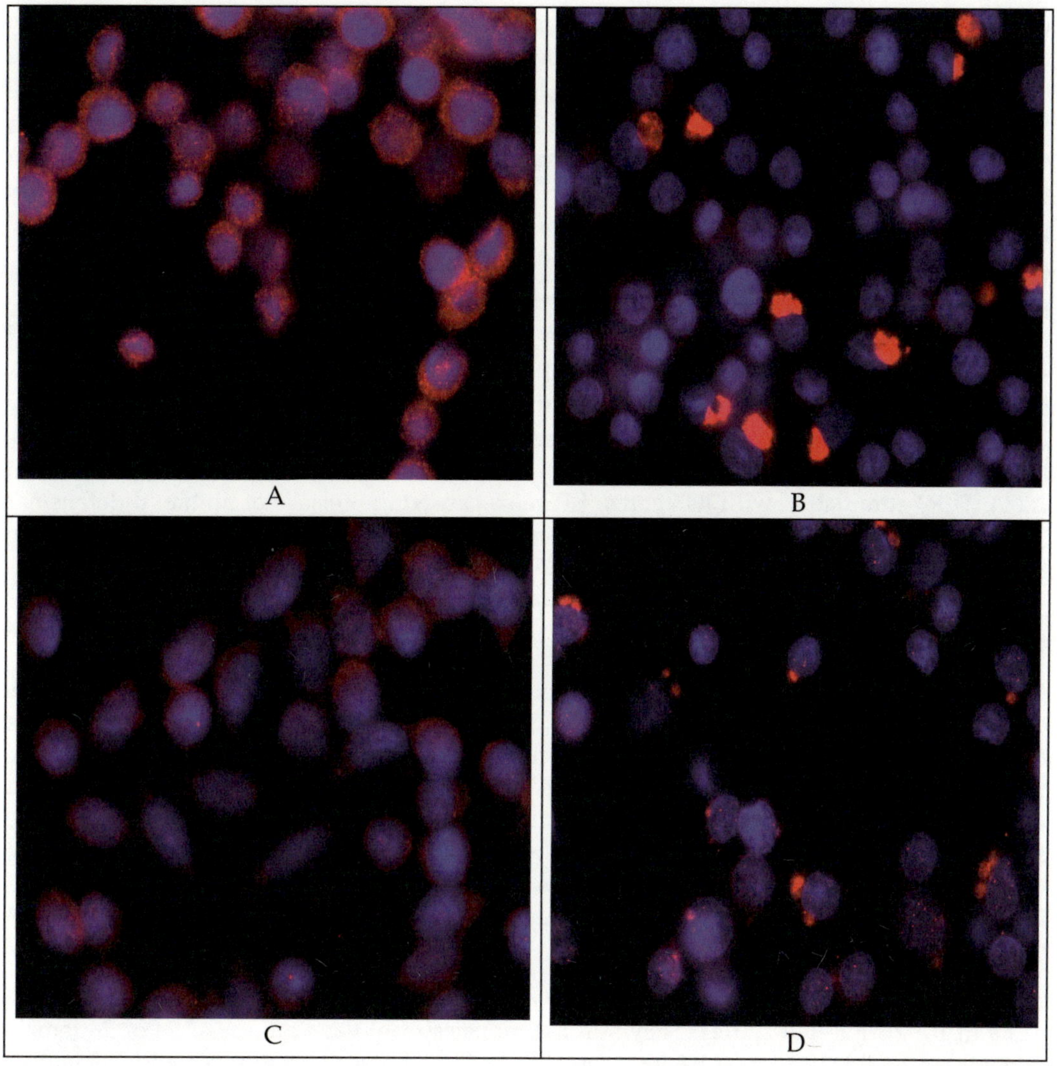

Fig. 3. Altered cellular distribution of serotonin and chromogranin A in non-infected and *Chlamydia trachomatis* L2-infected EEC. A: Cytoplasmatic distribution of chromogranin A (CgA) in non-infected LCC-18 cells (rabbit CgA antibody and Alexia 568-red and DAPI nucleus staining (blue), original magnification x63). B: Chromogranin A labeling in *Chlamydia* containing inclusions (arrows) in infected LCC-18 cells (rabbit CgA antibody and Alexia 568-red and DAPI nucleus staining (blue), original magnification x63). C: Cytoplasmatic distribution of serotonin in non-infected LCC-18 cells (rabbit serotonin antibody, Alexia 568-red and DAPI nucleus staining (blue), original magnification x63). D: Serotonin in *Chlamydia* containing inclusions (arrows) in persistently infected CNDT-2 cells (rabbit serotonin antibody and Alexia 568-red and DAPI nucleus staining (blue), original magnification x63).

Our study is the first to show that the presence of *C. trachomatis* alters the cellular distributions of serotonin and CgA in vitro. Both serotonin and CgA are important for immune activation and gut inflammation *in vivo* and several serotonergic receptors have been characterized in lymphocytes, monocytes, macrophages and dendritic cells (Cloez-Tayarani & Changeux, 2007). Serotonin has been shown to activate immune cells, which are responsible for the production of proinflammatory mediators (Khan & Ghia, 2010). Consequently, a manipulation of the serotonin system could modulate responses to gut inflammation. CgA on the other hand has antimicrobial activity (Shooshtarizadeh et al., 2010) and exhibits both proinflammatory and anti-inflammatory functions (Khan & Ghia, 2010).

We think that altered protein distribution and down-regulation of the vesicular monoamine transporter VMAT1 suggest bacterial influence on vesicular transport. The expression of genes associated with serotonin synthesis (TPH1) and release (TRPA1) was not impaired. At this stage, it is unclear if the altered distribution of serotonin and CgA in *C. trachomatis* infected EEC is induced by the bacteria themselves or is part of an innate immunity response via up-regulation of toll-like receptors. Others have reported increased LPS-induced serotonin secretion in EEC derived from patients with Crohn's disease (Kidd et al., 2009). TLR4 stimulation with its agonist LPS also caused the release of human β-defensin-2 (HBD-2) from EEC (Palazzo et al., 2007) and elevated HBD-2 levels have recently been found in patients with IBS (Langhorst et al., 2009).

5. Innate immunity in IBS

The ability of intestinal mucosa to detect bacterial cellular components requires the expression of pattern recognition receptors (PRR) that recognize repetitive patterns present on Gram-positive and Gram-negative bacteria, fungi, viruses and parasites. Toll-like receptors (TLR) belong to the family of PRRs and are present on macrophages of the lamina propria, dendritic cells, paneth cells and intestinal epithelial cells. TLR4 is regarded as the PRR for lipopolysaccharide (LPS), the toxin of Gram-negative bacteria (including *Chlamydia*). Expression of TLR4 by intestinal cells is normally down-regulated to maintain immune tolerance to the luminal microorganisms but up-regulated in gut inflammation (Gribar et al., 2008).

A a research group from Cork, Ireland recently investigated the potential involvement of TLRs in IBS (Brint et al., 2011). They studied biopsies from the sigmoid colon of 26 female patients with IBS, 19 female healthy controls and 29 disease controls (10 with ulcerative colitis and 19 with Crohn's disease) and applied quantitative real-time RT-PCR for RNA gene expression. They found that the expression of TLR4 was significantly up-regulated (5-fold) in patients with IBS compared to healthy controls. They also found a small but statistically significant up-regulation of TLR5 (1.7-fold) and down-regulation of TLR7 and TLR8 (2-fold). The increase in the expression of TLR 4 was 15-fold in patients with ulcerative colitis and 8-fold in Crohn's disease.

The authors believed that disruption of the intestinal epithelial barrier in inflammatory bowel disease, allowing translocation of commensal bacteria to the underlying submucosa, could explain the up-regulation of TLR expression observed in ulcerative colitis and Crohn's disease (Brint et al., 2011). They speculated that a similar but less pronounced disruption of the intestinal epithelial barrier could exist also in patients with IBS. The authors concluded that the differences observed in TLR expression might indicate an appropriate immune response to a pathogen or to alterations in the host microbiota.

Another recent study from the same group investigated cytokine and cortisol levels in plasma and peripheral TLR activity after stimulation of cultured whole blood with TLR agonists in 30 patients with IBS and 30 healthy controls (McKernan et al., 2011). Patients with IBS had elevated plasma levels of IL-6, IL-8 and cortisol. Release of IL-1β, IL-6, IL-8 and TNF-α was measured after stimulation with agonists for TLR1-8. Patients with IBS exhibited elevated responses to TLR2 (TNF-α), TLR3 (IL-8), TLR4 (IL-1β and TNF-α), TLR5 (IL-1β and TNF-α), TLR7 (IL-8), TLR8 (IL-1β, IL-6, IL-8 and TNF-α). No difference between patients and controls was seen in cytokine release after stimulation of TLR1, 6 and 9.

The authors concluded that patients with IBS demonstrate elevated cytokine levels, a finding that supports a previous observation from the same group (Dinan et al., 2006), and enhanced TLR activity in the periphery, which indicates that patients with IBS have some immune dysregulation (McKernan et al., 2011). They speculated that there might be a link between stress (increased plasma levels of cortisol), TLR activation and cytokine profiles in patients with IBS, similar to that observed in mice (Zhang et al., 2008).

We analysed endoscopic biopsies from the right and the left colon in 10 patients with inflammatory bowel disease (5 with Crohn's colitis and 5 with ulcerative colitis) and 10 patients with IBS (5 with diarrhoea-predominant and 5 with constipation-predominant IBS) and biopsies from the left colon in 5 healthy controls. We used rabbit polyclonal antibodies to TLR4 (Abcam, UK) and tyramide signal amplification (Invitrogen, USA) technology for immunohistochemistry and Nikon NIS-Elements (Nikon, Japan) for image analysis. TLR4 expression was calculated as a percentage of lamina propria area occupied by TLR4 positive cells.

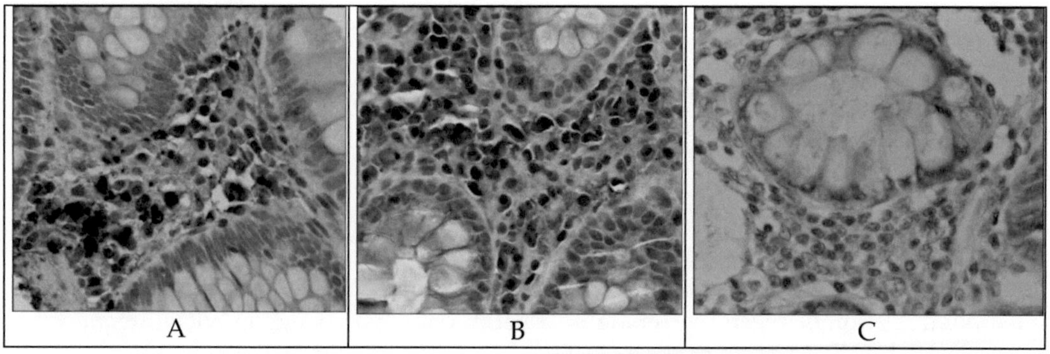

Fig. 4. Immunohistochemical expression of TLR4 in colon mucosa. A: Patient with IBS (original magnification x40). B: Patient with inflammatory bowel disease (original magnification x40). C: Healthy control (original magnification x40). Immunohistochemistry using a rabbit polyclonal antibody to TLR4 and tyramide signal amplification.

Immunohistochemical expression of TLR4 was increased in both inflammatory bowel disease and IBS (p=0.04) compared to healthy individuals. In IBS and inflammatory bowel disease the increase of TLR4 expression was mainly in cells of *l. propria* (Figure 4). Our findings support the previous observation that TLR4 gene expression is up-regulated in IBS and inflammatory bowel disesase (Brint et al., 2011). Our data again suggest the involvement of Gram-negative pathogens or dysregulation of the intestinal immune response to the commensal flora as possible pathogenetic mechanisms in IBS.

6. Discussion

Chlamydial antigens were found in enteroendocrine cells and macrophages of the small bowel mucosa in 89% of patients with IBS but in only 14% of controls. Even though we were unable to prove the presence of viable *Chlamydia,* lack of positive PCR being the major obstacle, the evidence for an intracellular organism or at least a protein structure with an antigen in common with *Chlamydia* in patients with IBS is strong. Given the crucial role of enteroendocrine cells in digestive function, our results suggest that the presence of chlamydial antigens in these cells may be involved in the pathogenesis in IBS. Chlamydial antigens have not been described in human enteroendocrine cells before. If this finding can be corroborated by DNA evidence of bacterial presence, it represents a previously unknown cell tropism of *Chlamydia.*

In an *in vitro* model we found that enteroendocrine cells from both the small bowel and the large bowel could be infected with *C. trachomatis* yielding productive infections and that persistence could be induced using penicillin G. Immunofluorescence showed different cellular distributions of serotonin and chromogranin A in non-infected (cytoplasmatic distribution) compared with infected cells (serotonin and chromogranin A mostly in chlamydial inclusions). In line with the microscopical findings, we found a significant down-regulation of the gene coding for the vesicular monoamine transporter (VMAT1) in infected compared with non-infected EEC ($P < 0.05$). Altered protein distributions together with down-regulation of VMAT1 suggest that chlamydial infection may influence vesicular transport. It is therefore possible that such an infection *in vivo* could lead to disturbances in the regulation of gut functions.

Up-regulation of TLR4 suggests the involvement of Gram-negative pathogens or dysregulation of the intestinal immune response to the commensal flora as possible pathogenetic mechanisms in IBS. This finding also lends support to the idea that a persistent infection of the gastrointestinal tract with *C. trachomatis* is part of the pathogenesis in IBS.

7. Speculations

The symptom profile of patients with IBS has long been a challenge to the medical community. The main symptoms are abdominal pain, diarrhoea or constipation or both, and a temporal relation between worsening or onset of pain and change in bowel frequency or stool consistency (Longstreth et al., 2006). However, patients with IBS may have a number of other symptoms from the gastrointestinal tract including dysphagia, dyspepsia, nausea, vomiting, anorexia, post-prandial distension, flatulence, borborygmia (noisy bowel sounds), mucus in stools, and feeling of incomplete evacuation. There is considerable overlap between IBS and other prevalent functional gastrointestinal disorders such as functional dyspepsia and patients often change their symptom profile from one to the other with time (Agréus et al., 2001). If a persistent infection of enteroendocrine cells is important in the pathogenesis of IBS, then it is reasonable to assume that this infection can affect different populations of enteroendocrine cells and lead to correspondingly different symptom profiles. Such a mechanism could explain the variability of presenting symptoms among patients with functional gastrointestinal disorders and perhaps there is no meaningful difference between IBS, functional constipation, functional diarrhoea, functional bloating, functional abdominal pain and the majority of other functional gastrointestinal syndromes (Longstreth et al., 2006).

One of the most common measurable abnormalities in patients with IBS is visceral hypersensitivity (Akbar et al., 2009). The mechanisms behind visceral hypersensitivity have remained unproven but glial cells and TLR4-activation seem important both in the CNS (Tanga et al., 2005) and in the spinal cord (Saito et al., 2010). In light of our findings of chlamydial antigens and TLR4 up-regulation in IBS it is reasonable to hypothesize that visceral hypersensitivity can arise from TLR4 activation either of enteroglial cells or of glial cells in the spinal cord or CNS.

The most commonly noted overlap syndrome with IBS is fibromyalgia (Sivri et al., 1996; Sperber et al., 1999; Triadafilopoulos et al., 1991). It has therefore been suggested that IBS and fibromyalgia may have a common pathogenesis (Veale et al., 1991). Fibromyalgia is a chronic form of diffuse muculoskeletal pain with tenderness at specific locations, often associated with persistent fatigue, cognitive and mood disorders, joint stiffness, and insomnia that occurs mainly in females (Solitar, 2010). It has long been speculated that the driving force for fibromyalgia might be an infection and similar to IBS many patients associate the onset of their condition with an acute illness or have noticed that infections may worsen their symptoms (Bennett et al., 2007). An interesting similarity between IBS and fibromyalgia is that both groups seem to have increased peripheral levels of the cytokine IL-8 (McKernan et al., 2011; Wang et al., 2009). We therefore hypothesize that the driving force for fibromyalgia and possibly also other chronic inflammatory conditions is a persistent infection in the gastrointestinal tract. In the case of fibromyalgia the overlap with IBS supports the view of a common aetiology. The gastrointestinal tract is our largest interface to the world of microbes and the most likely location of a driving force for other chronic inflammatory disorders would therefore also be the gastrointestinal tract (Scheinecker & Smolen, 2011).

8. Conclusions

The above series of studies collectively indicate a role for *C. trachomatis* in the pathogenesis of IBS. Our data suggests that patients with IBS may have a persistent infection with *C. trachomatis* of enteroendocrine cells and macrophages. So far only the small bowel has been studied and it remains to find out if also the mucosa of the large bowel exhibits the same findings. Cell line experiments indicate that enteroendocrine cells can indeed be infected by *C. trachomatis* and that persistent infection of such cells leads to profound changes of the intracellular distribution of serotonin and chromogranin A.

Patients with IBS exhibit a pronounced up-regulation of TLR4. The level of up-regulation is similar to that found in inflammatory bowel disease. It is possible that observed changes in the innate immune system reflect stimulation from chlamydial LPS. It is yet unclear if the mechanisms behind up-regulation of TLR4 are the same in IBS and inflammatory bowel disease.

Further studies are needed to confirm or refute the hypothesis that live bacteria are present in the mucosa of the small bowel in patients with IBS. It is tempting to suggest a therapeutic trial aimed at eradicating a persistent infection with *C. trachomatis*. However, it is uncertain if eradication of a persistent chlamydial infection is at all possible (Gieffers et al., 2001).

9. Acknowledgments

The studies from our group were supported by grants from Ruth and Richard Juhlin's Foundation and Foundation Olle Engkvist Byggmästare. Dr. Dlugosz is a recipient of the Rome Foundation Fellowship in Functional Gastrointestinal and Motility Disorders 2009-2010 and 2010-2011. None of the funding sources had any involvement with the study.

10. References

Agréus, L.; Svärdsudd, K.; Talley, N. J.; Jones, M. P. & Tibblin, G. (2001). Natural history of gastroesophageal reflux disease and functional abdominal disorders: a population-based study. *The American Journal of Gastroenterology*, Vol. 96, No. 10, (October 2001), pp. 2905-2914, ISSN 0002-9270

Akbar, A.; Walters, J. R. & Ghosh, S. (2009). Review article: visceral hypersensitivity in irritable bowel syndrome: molecular mechanisms and therapeutic agents. *Alimentary Pharmacology & Therapeutics*, Vol. 30, No. 5, (September 2009), pp. 423-435, ISSN 0269-2813

Akers, J. C. & Tan, M. (2006). Molecular mechanism of tryptophan-dependent transcriptional regulation in *Chlamydia trachomatis*. *Journal of Bacteriology*, Vol. 188, No. 12, (June 2006), pp. 4236-4243, ISSN 0021-9193

Akiho, H.; Ihara, E. & Nakamura, K. (2011). Low-grade inflammation plays a pivotal role in gastrointestinal dysfunction in irritable bowel syndrome. *World Journal of Gastrointestinal Pathophysiology*, Vol. 1, No. 3, (August 2011), pp. 97-105, ISSN 2150-5330

Amouretti, M.; Le Pen, C.; Gaudin, A. F.; Bommelaer, G.; Frexinos, J.; Ruszniewski, P.; Poynard, T.; Maurel, F.; Priol, G. & El Hasnaoui, A. (2006). Impact of irritable bowel syndrome (IBS) on health-related quality of life (HRQOL). *Gastroentérolgie Clinique et Biologique*, Vol. 30, No. 2, (February 2006), pp. 241-246, ISSN 0399-8320

Beatty, W. L.; Morrison, R. P. & Byrne, G. I. (1994). Persistent *Chlamydiae*: from cell culture to a paradigm for chlamydial pathogenesis. *Microbiological Reviews*, Vol. 58, No. 4, (December 1994), pp. 686-699, ISSN 0146-0749

Bennett, R. M.; Jones, J.; Turk, D. C.; Russell, I. J. & Matallana, L. (2007). An internet survey of 2,596 people with fibromyalgia. *BMC Musculoskeletal Disorders*, Vol. 8, No., (March 2007), pp. 27, ISSN 1471-2474

Brint, E. K.; MacSharry, J.; Fanning, A.; Shanahan, F. & Quigley, E. M. (2011). Differential expression of toll-like receptors in patients with irritable bowel syndrome. *The American Journal of Gastroenterology*, Vol. 106, No. 2, (February 2011), pp. 329-336, ISSN 0002-9270

Caldwell, H. D. & Hitchcock, P. J. (1984). Monoclonal antibody against a genus-specific antigen of *Chlamydia* species: location of the epitope on chlamydial lipopolysaccharide. *Infection and Immunity*, Vol. 44, No. 2, (May 1984), pp. 306-314, ISSN 0019-9567

Cloez-Tayarani, I. & Changeux, J. P. (2007). Nicotine and serotonin in immune regulation and inflammatory processes: a perspective. *Journal of Leukocyte Biology*, Vol. 81, No. 3, (March 2007), pp. 599-606, ISSN 0741-5400

Courtright, P. & West, S. K. (2004). Contribution of sex-linked biology and gender roles to disparities with trachoma. *Emerging Infectious Diseases*, Vol. 10, No. 11, (Nov 2004), pp. 2012-2016, ISSN 1080-6040

Dinan, T. G.; Quigley, E. M.; Ahmed, S. M.; Scully, P.; O'Brien, S.; O'Mahony, L.; O'Mahony, S.; Shanahan, F. & Keeling, P. W. (2006). Hypothalamic-pituitary-gut axis dysregulation in irritable bowel syndrome: plasma cytokines as a potential biomarker? *Gastroenterology*, Vol. 130, No. 2, (February 2006), pp. 304-311, ISSN 0016-5085

Dlugosz, A.; Törnblom, H.; Mohammadian, G.; Morgan, G.; Veress, B.; Edvinsson, B.; Sandström, G. & Lindberg, G. (2010). *Chlamydia trachomatis* antigens in enteroendocrine cells and macrophages of the small bowel in patients with severe irritable bowel syndrome. *BMC Gastroenterology*, Vol. 10, (February 2010), pp. 19, ISSN 1471-230X

Dlugosz, A.; Zakikhany, K.; Muschiol, S.; Hultenby, K. & Lindberg, G. (2011). Infection of human enteroendocrine cells with *Chlamydia trachomatis*: a possible model for pathogenesis in itrritable bowel syndrome. *Neurogastroenterology & Motility*, Vol. 23, No. 10, (October 2011), pp. 928-934, ISSN 1350-1925

Drossman, D. A.; Morris, C. B.; Schneck, S.; Hu, Y. J.; Norton, N. J.; Norton, W. F.; Weinland, S. R.; Dalton, C.; Leserman, J. & Bangdiwala, S. I. (2009). International survey of patients with IBS: symptom features and their severity, health status, treatments, and risk taking to achieve clinical benefit. *Journal of Clinical Gastroenterology*, Vol. 43, No. 6, (July 2009), pp. 541-550, ISSN 0192-0790

Everett, K. D.; Hornung, L. J. & Andersen, A. A. (1999). Rapid detection of the *Chlamydiaceae* and other families in the order *Chlamydiales*: three PCR tests. *Journal of Clinical Microbiology*, Vol. 37, No. 3, (March 1999), pp. 575-580, ISSN 0095-1137

Francis, C.; Prior, A.; Whorwell, P. J. & Morris, J. (1998). *Chlamydia trachomatis* infection: Is it relevant in irritable bowel syndrome? *Digestion*, Vol. 59, No. 2, (May 1998), pp. 157-159, ISSN 0012-2823

Gieffers, J.; Fullgraf, H.; Jahn, J.; Klinger, M.; Dalhoff, K.; Katus, H. A.; Solbach, W. & Maass, M. (2001). *Chlamydia pneumoniae* infection in circulating human monocytes is refractory to antibiotic treatment. *Circulation*, Vol. 103, No. 3, (January 2001), pp. 351-356, ISSN 0009-7322

Gribar, S. C.; Anand, R. J.; Sodhi, C. P. & Hackam, D. J. (2008). The role of epithelial Toll-like receptor signaling in the pathogenesis of intestinal inflammation. *Journal of Leukocyte Biology*, Vol. 83, No. 3, (March 2008), pp. 493-498, ISSN 0741-5400

Hungin, A. P.; Whorwell, P. J.; Tack, J. & Mearin, F. (2003). The prevalence, patterns and impact of irritable bowel syndrome: an international survey of 40,000 subjects. *Alimentary Pharmacology & Therapeutics*, Vol. 17, No. 5, (March 2003), pp. 643-650, ISSN 0269-2813

Jakobsen, A. M.; Andersson, P.; Saglik, G.; Andersson, E.; Kölby, L.; Erickson, J. D.; Forssell-Aronsson, E.; Wängberg, B.; Ahlman, H. & Nilsson, O. (2001). Differential expression of vesicular monoamine transporter (VMAT) 1 and 2 in gastrointestinal endocrine tumours. *The Journal of Pathology*, Vol. 195, No. 4, (November 2001), pp. 463-472, ISSN 0022-3417

Khan, W. I. & Ghia, J. E. (2010). Gut hormones: emerging role in immune activation and inflammation. *Clinical & Experimental Immunology*, Vol. 161, No. 1, (July 2010), pp. 19-27, ISSN 1365-2249

Kidd, M.; Gustafsson, B. I.; Drozdov, I. & Modlin, I. M. (2009). IL1beta- and LPS-induced serotonin secretion is increased in EC cells derived from Crohn's disease. *Neurogastroenterology & Motility*, Vol. 21, No. 4, (April 2009), pp. 439-450, ISSN 1365-2982

Kim, D. Y. & Camilleri, M. (2000). Serotonin: a mediator of the brain-gut connection. *The American Journal of Gastroenterology*, Vol. 95, No. 10, (October 2000), pp. 2698-2709, ISSN 0002-9270

Langhorst, J.; Junge, A.; Rueffer, A.; Wehkamp, J.; Foell, D.; Michalsen, A.; Musial, F. & Dobos, G. J. (2009). Elevated human beta-defensin-2 levels indicate an activation of the innate immune system in patients with irritable bowel syndrome. *The American Journal of Gastroenterology*, Vol. 104, No. 2, (Feb 2009), pp. 404-410, ISSN 0002-9270

Lindberg, G.; Törnblom, H.; Iwarzon, M.; Nyberg, B.; Martin, J. E. & Veress, B. (2009). Full-thickness biopsy findings in chronic intestinal pseudo-obstruction and enteric dysmotility. *Gut*, Vol. 58, No. 8, (August 2009), pp. 1084-1090, ISSN 0017-5749

Longstreth, G. F.; Thompson, W. G.; Chey, W. D.; Houghton, L. A.; Mearin, F. & Spiller, R. C. (2006). Functional bowel disorders. *Gastroenterology*, Vol. 130, No. 5, (April 2006), pp. 1480-1491, ISSN 0016-5085

Makharia, G. K.; Verma, A. K.; Amarchand, R.; Goswami, A.; Singh, P.; Agnihotri, A.; Suhail, F. & Krishnan, A. (2011). Prevalence of irritable bowel syndrome: a community based study from northern India. *Journal of Neurogastroenterology and Motility*, Vol. 17, No. 1, (January 2011), pp. 82-87, ISSN 2093-0879

McKernan, D. P.; Gaszner, G.; Quigley, E. M.; Cryan, J. F. & Dinan, T. G. (2011). Altered peripheral toll-like receptor responses in the irritable bowel syndrome. *Alimentary Pharmacology & Therapeutics*, Vol. 33, No. 9, (May 2011), pp. 1045-1052, ISSN 0269-2813

Monack, D. M.; Mueller, A. & Falkow, S. (2004). Persistent bacterial infections: the interface of the pathogen and the host immune system. *Nature Reviews Microbiology*, Vol. 2, No. 9, (September 2004), pp. 747-765, ISSN 1740-1526

Öhman, L. & Simrén, M. (2007). New insights into the pathogenesis and pathophysiology of irritable bowel syndrome. *Digestive and Liver Disease*, Vol. 39, No. 3, (March 2007), pp. 201-215, ISSN 1590-8658

Öhman, L. & Simrén, M. (2010). Pathogenesis of IBS: role of inflammation, immunity and neuroimmune interactions. *Nature Reviews Gastroenterology & Hepatology*, Vol. 7, No. 3, (March 2010), pp. 163-173, ISSN 1759-5045

Palazzo, M.; Balsari, A.; Rossini, A.; Selleri, S.; Calcaterra, C.; Gariboldi, S.; Zanobbio, L.; Arnaboldi, F.; Shirai, Y. F.; Serrao, G. & Rumio, C. (2007). Activation of enteroendocrine cells via TLRs induces hormone, chemokine, and defensin secretion. *The Journal of Immunology*, Vol. 178, No. 7, (April 2007), pp. 4296-4303, ISSN 0022-1767

Saito, O.; Svensson, C. I.; Buczynski, M. W.; Wegner, K.; Hua, X. Y.; Codeluppi, S.; Schaloske, R. H.; Deems, R. A.; Dennis, E. A. & Yaksh, T. L. (2010). Spinal glial TLR4-mediated nociception and production of prostaglandin E(2) and TNF. *British Journal of Pharmacology*, Vol. 160, No. 7, (August 2010), pp. 1754-1764, ISSN 0007-1188

Scheinecker, C. & Smolen, J. S. (2011). Rheumatoid arthritis in 2010: from the gut to the joint. *Nature Reviews Rheumatology*, Vol. 7, No. 2, (February 2011), pp. 73-75, ISSN 1759-4790

Shooshtarizadeh, P.; Zhang, D.; Chich, J. F.; Gasnier, C.; Schneider, F.; Haikel, Y.; Aunis, D. & Metz-Boutigue, M. H. (2010). The antimicrobial peptides derived from chromogranin/secretogranin family, new actors of innate immunity. *Regulatory Peptides*, Vol. 165, No. 1, (November 2010), pp. 102-110, ISSN 0167-0115

Sikander, A.; Rana, S. V. & Prasad, K. K. (2009). Role of serotonin in gastrointestinal motility and irritable bowel syndrome. *Clinica Chimica Acta*, Vol. 403, No. 1-2, (May 2009), pp. 47-55, ISSN 0009-8981

Sivri, A.; Cindas, A.; Dincer, F. & Sivri, B. (1996). Bowel dysfunction and irritable bowel syndrome in fibromyalgia patients. *Clinical Rheumatology*, Vol. 15, No. 3, (May 1996), pp. 283-286, ISSN 0770-3198

Solitar, B. M. (2010). Fibromyalgia: knowns, unknowns, and current treatment. *Bulletin of the NYU Hospital for Joint Diseases*, Vol. 68, No. 3, (October 2010), pp. 157-161, ISSN 1936-9719

Sperber, A. D.; Atzmon, Y.; Neumann, L.; Weisberg, I.; Shalit, Y.; Abu-Shakrah, M.; Fich, A. & Buskila, D. (1999). Fibromyalgia in the irritable bowel syndrome: studies of prevalence and clinical implications. *The American Journal of Gastroenterology*, Vol. 94, No. 12, (December 1999), pp. 3541-3546, ISSN 0002-9270

Spiller, R. C. (2007). Role of infection in irritable bowel syndrome. *Journal of Gastroenterology*, Vol. 42, No. Suppl 17, (January 2007), pp. 41-47, ISSN 0944-1174

Storz, J. & Spears, P. (1979). Pathogenesis of chlamydial polyarthritis in domestic animals: characteristics of causative agent. *Annals of the Rheumatic Diseases*, Vol. 38, No. Suppl 1, (January 1979), pp. 111-115, ISSN 0003-4967

Tanga, F. Y.; Nutile-McMenemy, N. & DeLeo, J. A. (2005). The CNS role of Toll-like receptor 4 in innate neuroimmunity and painful neuropathy. *Proceedings of the National Acadademy of Sciences of the United States of America*, Vol. 102, No. 16, (April 2005), pp. 5856-5861, ISSN 0027-8424

Thompson, W. G.; Irvine, E. J.; Pare, P.; Ferrazzi, S. & Rance, L. (2002). Functional gastrointestinal disorders in Canada: first population-based survey using Rome II criteria with suggestions for improving the questionnaire. *Digestive Diseases and Sciences*, Vol. 47, No. 1, (January 2002), pp. 225-235, ISSN 0163-2116

Thompson, W. G.; Longstreth, G. F.; Drossman, D. A.; Heaton, K. W.; Irvine, E. J. & Muller-Lissner, S. A. (1999). Functional bowel disorders and functional abdominal pain. *Gut*, Vol. 45, No. Suppl 2, (September 1999), pp. II43-47, ISSN 0017-5749

Törnblom, H.; Holmvall, P.; Svenungsson, B. & Lindberg, G. (2007). Gastrointestinal symptoms after infectious diarrhea: a five-year follow-up in a Swedish cohort of adults. *Clinical Gastroenterology and Hepatology*, Vol. 5, No. 4, (April 2007), pp. 461-464, ISSN 1542-3565

Törnblom, H.; Lindberg, G.; Nyberg, B. & Veress, B. (2002). Full-thickness biopsy of the jejunum reveals inflammation and enteric neuropathy in irritable bowel syndrome. *Gastroenterology*, Vol. 123, No. 6, (December 2002), pp. 1972-1979, ISSN 0016-5085

Triadafilopoulos, G.; Simms, R. W. & Goldenberg, D. L. (1991). Bowel dysfunction in fibromyalgia syndrome. *Digestive Diseases and Sciences*, Vol. 36, No. 1, (January 1991), pp. 59-64, ISSN 0163-2116

Veale, D.; Kavanagh, G.; Fielding, J. F. & Fitzgerald, O. (1991). Primary fibromyalgia and the irritable bowel syndrome: different expressions of a common pathogenetic process. *British Journal of Rheumatology*, Vol. 30, No. 3, (June 1991), pp. 220-222, ISSN 0263-7103

Wang, H.; Buchner, M.; Moser, M. T.; Daniel, V. & Schiltenwolf, M. (2009). The role of IL-8 in patients with fibromyalgia: a prospective longitudinal study of 6 months. *The Clinical Journal of Pain*, Vol. 25, No. 1, (January 2009), pp. 1-4, ISSN 0749-8047

Williams, R. E.; Hartmann, K. E.; Sandler, R. S.; Miller, W. C. & Steege, J. F. (2004). Prevalence and characteristics of irritable bowel syndrome among women with chronic pelvic pain. *Obstetrics & Gynecology*, Vol. 104, No. 3, (September 2004), pp. 452-458, ISSN 0029-7844

Witkin, S. S. (2002). Immunological aspects of genital chlamydia infections. *Best Practice & Research Clinical Obstetrics & Gynaecology*, Vol. 16, No. 6, (December 2002), pp. 865-874, ISSN 1521-6934

Zhang, Y.; Zhang, Y.; Miao, J.; Hanley, G.; Stuart, C.; Sun, X.; Chen, T. & Yin, D. (2008). Chronic restraint stress promotes immune suppression through toll-like receptor 4-mediated phosphoinositide 3-kinase signaling. *Journal of Neuroimmunology*, Vol. 204, No. 1-2, (November 2008), pp. 13-19, ISSN 0165-5728

Zondervan, K. T.; Yudkin, P. L.; Vessey, M. P.; Jenkinson, C. P.; Dawes, M. G.; Barlow, D. H. & Kennedy, S. H. (2001). Chronic pelvic pain in the community--symptoms, investigations, and diagnoses. *American Journal of Obstetrics & Gynecology*, Vol. 184, No. 6, (May 2001), pp. 1149-1155, ISSN 0002-9378

10

Chlamydia, Hepatocytes and Liver

Yuriy K. Bashmakov and Ivan M. Petyaev
Lycotec Ltd, Cambridge,
United Kingdom

1. Introduction

The genus *Chlamydia* includes a unique group of aerobic Gram-negative obligate intracellular parasitic bacteria of eubacterial origin which cause numerous infectious diseases in humans and animals. Despite some inherited genomic and phenotypic variations there is one distinctive feature of all chlamydial pathogens, most cases of chlamydial infection are initiated, developed and resolved within the epithelium of the bronchoalveolar system, urogenital system or conjunctivae. Generally, mucosal epithelial tissue and its residing/migrating cellular constituents serve as the primary focus of microbial insult as well as a preferential cell population supporting chlamydial growth. Despite strict tissue tropism and the unique capability of chlamydial pathogens to infect, propagate and finalize their life cycle in mucosal epithelial cells, there is a growing body of evidence that chlamydial species can grow in other cell types thereby invading multiple tissues and organs far beyond the primary locus of infection. The purpose of this chapter is to analyze some novel observations revealing the ability of chlamydial species to grow in hepatic cells along with reports on liver involvement in the pathogenesis of chlamydial infection. This has been done within the modern framework of understanding the molecular biology of chlamydial species and their growth requirements in host cells .

All chlamydial strains have a similar genetic background and share major cutoff points in their developmental cycle, phenotypic characteristics and mechanisms of infectivity . The separation of genus *Chlamydia* into two genera - *Chlamydia* and *Chlamydophila* introduced in 1999 (Everett et al 1999) reflects some variations in the clustering of the 16S rRNA gene and was disputed soon after proposal/introduction (Schachter et al., 2001) . It has been opposed recently by new data on complete chlamydial genome sequencing (Stephens et al., 2001; Myers et al., 2009). Although there are several exceptions, all chlamydial species are >97% similar by 16S rRNA gene sequence comparison which undermines taxonomic separation of the genus (Stephens et al., 2001) . With this proviso a reunited genus *Chlamydia* includes 3 clinically relevant obligate pathogens: *C. trachomatis*, *C. pneumoniae* and *C. psittaci.*

2. Chlamydia as a pathogen

The first member of genus *Chlamydia* was identified and reported by Ludwig Halberstaedter and Stanislaus von Prowazec (Halberstaedter & von Prowazec, 1907) during an expedition to the island of Java when they reproduced conjunctival lesions in orangutans by inoculation of eye scrapings from patients with trachoma . Although they did not propose a name for the new pathogen, they pointed out that the etiologic agent identified microscopically in the conjunctiva of the trachoma patients had nothing to do with the kingdom of bacteria and had to be distinguished equally from the protozoan organisms . Instead, vonProwazec introduced a new taxon "*Chlamydozoa*" to include the newly discovered pathogen under investigation (von Prowazec, 1907).

Another pathogen belonging to the genus *Chlamydia* – *Chlamydia psittaci* had been initially shown to infect birds and can be transmitted to humans via direct contact causing psittacosis or parrot fever (Verminnen et al., 2008). The first cases of the human disease were reported in 1893 in Paris, France (Morange, 1895). However, detailed insight into the microbiology of *Chlamydia psittaci* was gained only after the introduction of cell culture technique and a large epidemic of psittacosis in the USA and Europe in 1930 (Vanrompay et al., 1995).

Extensive trachoma research paved the way for the discovery of another member of genus *Chlamydia*. An atypical strain designated as TW-183 was isolated in 1965 from the eye of a child participating in a vaccine study led by Prof J. T. Grayston in Taiwan . However, it was not until 1985 that Grayston and collaborators accumulated multiple pieces of evidence to show that the Taiwanese isolate is linked to respiratory infections in adults and represents a new member of genus *Chlamydia* named *Chlamydia pneumoniae* (Saikku et al., 1985).

From 1935 all chlamydial species were categorized as viruses since they could not synthesize ATP, did not grow in media and required a eukaryotic cell for propagation (Fields & Barnes, 1992). However, in 1963 the presence of the cell wall and its major chemical component - muramic acid was confirmed in several chlamydial strains (Perkinsh & Allsona, 1963; Garrett et al., 1974). This fact along with identification of ribosomes, DNA and RNA structures revealed that all chlamydial species belong to the kingdom of bacteria (Moulder, 1982) .

Although the infections caused by chlamydial pathogens are mostly asymptomatic, exposure to chlamydial pathogens worldwide is remarkably high. About 50-80% of the human population has detectable antibodies to *C. pneumoniae*, while 10-20% of adults show seropositivity to *C. trachomatis* (den Hartog et al., 2005; Asquith et al., 2011). Antibody specific to *C. psittaci* is found in a much smaller human population (0.1-3.0 %). However, the real infection rate might be seriously underestimated (Fenga et al., 2007).

The incubation period for Chlamydia-induced infections is generally believed to vary, depending on the strain, from several days (*C. trachomatis*) to month and years (*C. pneumoniae)*. Despite of extreme fluctuations in the time span of chlamydial disease, chronic course of infection and persistency in chlamydial biovar colonization is an ultimate feature of chlamydiosis (den Hartog et al., 2005; Asquith et al., 2011; Fenga et al., 2007).

There is a remarkable variety of human disease attributable to the chlamydial pathogens. The spectrum of human disease is closely related to the subdivision of chlamydial pathogens into biological variants (biovars) and serological subtypes (serovars).

C. trachomatis is represented by two biovars relevant to human pathology: the trachoma and lymphogranuloma venereum (LGV). Serovariants belonging to both *C. trachomatis* biovars differ in major outer membrane protein (MOMP) antigenicity and are known to cause various diseases: trachoma, sexually transmitted urogenital disease, some forms of arthritis, and neonatal inclusion conjunctivitis and pneumonia (Carlson et al., 2004). The existence of different chlamydial "pathotypes" is attributed to small genomic differences (Miyairi et al., 2006). Although the original classification includes 15 MOMP serovars of *C. trachomatis,* there are currently > 20 genovars and serovariants of the pathogen (Byrne, 2010). Their propagation is limited primarily to epithelial cells of mucous membranes . In contrast, it is believed that LGV serovars are more invasive due to their ability to invade the lymphatic system (Martin-Iquacel et al., 2010) .

There are three distinct *C. pneumoniae* biovars: human biovar TWAR, equine biovar and koala biovar. All human isolates representing the TWAR group are almost indistinguishable from each other with 0.1% variation in 16S rRNA and 0.4% difference in the *ompA* gene (Kutlin et al., 2007). *C. pneumoniae* is a proven causative agent of acute and chronic respiratory infections (bronchitis, sinusitis, pneumonia *etc*) and possibly some other diseases. However, unequivocal proof of direct causal relationship between persistent *C. pneumoniae* infection and these internal diseases (atherosclerosis, multiple sclerosis, bronchial asthma and stroke) has not yet been presented (Burillo et al., 2010; Cochrane et al., 2005).

Despite the obvious possibility of zoonotic transmission and identification of animal strains in humans (Dickx et al., 2010), the clinical manifestations of *C. psittaci* infection do not seem to reflect serovar specificity. All eight serovars of *C. psittaci* have similar virulence, tissue tropism and highly conserved 16S rRNA (Grinblat-Huse et al., 2011; Fraeyman et al., 2010). Infection in birds and animals is often manifested by conjunctivitis and respiratory disease followed by septicemia and multi-organ failure in the most severe cases (Harkinezhad et al., 2009). In humans, zoonotic psittacosis is most commonly represented by flu-like symptoms, fever and pneumonia (Beeckman & Vanrompay, 2009).

3. Life cycle

Chlamydiae are aerobic non-motile pear-shaped bacteria with a circularly arranged genome typically containing one plasmid. *Chlamydia* has a unique and dual faceted life cycle involving a switch between two naturally occurring biological forms: a large (~1.0 μM) intracellular, metabolically active and self-reproducing reticulate body (RB) and an extracellular, metabolically dormant, infectious elementary body (EB) of smaller (~0.3 μM) size (Kariagina et al., 2009) .

Internalization of the chlamydial EB into eukaryotic cells is the first step of the chlamydial infectious cycle. Several mechanisms are implemented for chlamydial attachment/entry into phagocytic and non-phagocytic cells . Generally, receptor-mediated endocytosis in clathrin-coated pits, pinocytosis in non-clathrin-coated pits and phagocytosis are among them (Puolakkainen et al., 2005). However, RNA interference experiments (Hybiske & Stephens, 2007) have emphasized the predominant role of the clathrin-mediated pathway whereas caveolae, phagocytosis and macropinocytosis are less relevant, at least for *C. trachomatis* entry into non-phagocytic cells. Ligand-receptor interactions seem to be essential for chlamydial internalization, since attachment dynamics often display a saturation pattern (Hackstadt et al., 1985) . There are a number of chemical ligands on the chlamydial surface promoting attachment to eukaryotic cell membranes. Among them are heparan sulfate, major outer membrane protein, glycosaminoglycans, heat shock protein 70, and OmcB (Puolakkainen et al., 2005; Abromatis & Stephens, 2009).

Although identification of a single eukaryotic receptor responsible for chlamydial attachment and subsequent entry into host cells remains elusive, a number of membrane receptors are implemented in the internalization of chlamydial species. These include insulin-like growth factor 2, epithelial membrane protein 2, polymorphic membrane proteins (PMP), mannose 6-phosphate receptor, estrogen receptor complex, platelet-derived growth factor receptor and possibly LDL-receptor (Dautry-Varsat et al., 2004; Puolakkainen et al.,2005; Abromatis & Stephens, 2009; Bashmakov et al., 2010) . It is obvious that the variety of receptors and other polyvalent interactions between chlamydial pathogens and host cell membrane implemented for chlamydial entry reflect some differences in the mode of exposure to the pathogen, presence or absence of centrifugation force during inoculation, as well as electrolyte composition of the incubation medium. However, there is a genus-specific mechanism promoting initial interaction of *Chlamydia* with eukaryotic cell membrane. Protein disulfide isomerase (PDI) is believed to play an essential role in the internalization mechanism utilized by multiple chlamydial species and serovars (Conant & Stephens , 2007). Nevertheless, the initial attachment of chlamydial particles to the host cell membrane leads to the recruitment of actin cytoskeleton to the attachment locus, formation of actin-rich tubular structures at the base of the attachment site, membrane invagination and final internalization of the bacteria (Clifton et al., 2004). Once internalized and incorporated into a non-acidified lysosome-free vacuole, termed an inclusion body, EB within begin to transform into metabolically active RB which are capable of dividing by binary fission (Hammerschlag, 2002) . The metabolic phenotype of RB characterized by active RNA and protein synthesis becomes established within 6-8 hours of the postinfection period and continues for the next 24-48 hours until reverse transformation to EB driven by unknown developmental stimuli takes place (Scidmore et al., 2003). The classic developmental cycle of chlamydial species terminates with membrane rupture and the release of newly synthesized EB initiating a new round of infection in the host cells.

4. Dissemination

Mucosal epithelial cells are a primary target for all major chlamydial biovars. Once inoculated to susceptible mucosa, chlamydial species accomplish their infectious cycle in the epitheliocytes, rupture their apical surface and spread canalicularly to the adjacent cells (Perry & Hughes, 1999). Canalicular spread of *Chlamydia* was traditionally attributed to the cases of *C. trachomatis* infection complicated by endometritis and salpingitis (Guaschino & De Seta, 2000). However similar horizontal spread of *C. pneumoniae* and *C. psittaci* within the epithelium leading to appearance of chlamydial EB and inflammatory cells in the alveolar lumen takes place in the lungs (Gieffers et al., 2004; Theegarten et al., 2008). This initial stage of chlamydial infection provides a short window of opportunity when the mechanism of local innate immunity may terminate developing infection due to continuous exposure of the pathogen to numerous antibacterial constituents of the epithelial secretion fluid (Perry & Hughes, 1999; Jayarapu et al., 2009) . Infected epithelial cells have been shown to secrete pro-inflammatory cytokines (INF-γ, TNF-α, interleukin 1 and 6, granulocyte-macrophage colony-stimulating factor) promoting cell migration to the infection site (Roan & Starnbach, 2008). It is important that epitheliocyte-derived cytokines, rather than T-lymphocyte mediators, are believed to trigger tissue fibrosis and scarring in urogenital chlamydiosis (Derbigny et al., 2005). Regardless of the type of epithelium, granulocytes and macrophages are the first cells to migrate to the site of primary microbial insult. Both cell types can harbor viable chlamydial pathogens (Rupp et al., 2009; Chong-Cerrillo et al., 2003; Buendia et al., 1999). Although granulocytes do not re-enter the systemic circulation (Yamagata et al., 2007) they can pass on viable *Chlamydia* to the macrophages whose ability to migrate through mucosal epithelium is a well established fact (Gieffers et al., 2004; Yamagata et al., 2007). Moreover, granulocytes are responsible for initiation of long-term immune response to chlamydial pathogens. Their systemic depletion ameliorates migration of $CD4^+$ and $CD8^+$ T cells to conjunctivae infected with *C. trachomatis* (Lacy et al., 2011).

Chlamydial pathogens do not remain confined to the primary locus of infection. Identification of chlamydial pathogens in different organs and tissues reveals the obvious involvement of haemotogenic and lymphatic pathways in the generalization of chlamydial infection. The cell-mediated hypothesis for *C. pneumoniae* dissemination proposed by Gieffers and others in 2004, has remained unchallenged so far and acquired further confirmation. It has been proposed that alveolar macrophages infected by granulocytes can penetrate mucosal barriers and gain access to the systemic circulation via lymphatic efferent flow as peripheral blood mononuclear cells with further spread to the endothelium, internal organs and tissues (Gieffers et al., 2004; Blasi et al., 2004) . A crucial piece of supporting evidence comes from reports describing the detection of chlamydial biovars in the regional lymph nodes and peripheral blood (Buxton et al., 1996; Sessa et al., 2007; Castro et al., 2010).

There is ongoing discussion related to bacteremia and its role in dissemination of chlamydial infection. It is believed (Gieffers et al., 2004) that there is a low probability of free and sustained circulation of chlamydial EB in the bloodstream since chlamydial particles are likely to be the subject of rapid clearance by elements of the reticuloendothelial system. Furthermore, multiple surface-located adhesins, represented by the family of polymorphic membrane proteins (Molleken et al., 2010), are known to promote the adherence of chlamydial biovars to the endothelial cell and lymphocytes . However, according to our recently published results, EB of *C. pneumoniae* are identifiable by both electron microscopy and RT-PCR in serum specimens obtained from the patients with acute coronary syndrome (Petyaev et al., 2010). By a conservative estimate, our finding may be attributed to the partial lysis of blood cells during serum isolation. On the other hand, there is a certain possibility that free circulation of chlamydial pathogens in blood may take place *in vivo* under some pathophysiological conditions and/or stages of chlamydial disease.

Although bacteremia becomes an indisputable pathophysiological feature of chlamydial infection, determination of chlamydial pathogens in the blood of patients by nucleic acid amplification protocol and/or bacterial culture has not yet become part of the algorithm in the laboratory diagnostics of chlamydiosis. This can be explained by some clinical cases where negative blood culture and PCR readings are observed in seropositive patients with obvious clinical signs of generalized chlamydial infection (Lamas & Eykyn 2009). The unknown prognostic value of the blood tests for chlamydial pathogens creates another issue. Further investigation is required to clarify the significance of bacteremia in the clinical manifestations and outcomes of chlamydiosis.

Alternatively, the lymphatic pathway of generalization may represent a self-sufficient mechanism for sustaining dissemination of chlamydial pathogens in the human body. As an example, the nasal lymphatic system alone may provide a direct route for dissemination of bacterial pathogens colonizing the nasopharyngeal mucosa to the subarachnoid space (Filippidis & Fountas, 2009) . Similarly, liver involvement in the clinical manifestation of C.

trachomatis infection can be explained by direct connections between the pelvic lymphatic network and hepatic tissue (Park et al., 2008).

There is an unresolved controversy about the role of chlamydial pathogens in neurological disorders. Although ultimate proof of the association between chlamydial infection and neurological disease has not presented yet, there are multiple reports on the identification of chlamydial species in brain specimens (Piercy et al., 1999; Beagley et al., 2009; Hammond et al., 2010). Along with direct lymphogenic dissemination mentioned above, monocyte-mediated translocation through the blood/brain barrier is claimed to be a key mechanism for brain entry of chlamydial pathogens (Contini et al., 2010). On the other hand, cerebrospinal fluid may promote spread of chlamydial pathogens within brain structures (Contini et al., 2008). Whether chlamydial pathogens circulate in cerebrospinal fluid in free form or require macro-microphages as the vehicle for transport inside the central nervous system remains under investigation . Although axonal transport plays a definite role in the spread of some infectious agents (Kalinke et al., 2011), there is no evidence that axonal delivery is any way involved in the dissemination of chlamydial infection in the nervous system. Reports on rare cases of sepsis induced by *C. pneumoniae* (Bustamante et al., 2002), *C. psittaci* (Janssen et al., 2006) and *C. trachomatis* (Kaan et al., 2002) require thorough evaluation and further conformation.

5. Liver involvement: Clinical evidence

Fitz-Hugh-Curtis syndrome is a complication of inflammatory pelvic disease involving inflammation of the hepatic capsule (perihepatitis) in patients infected with *C. trachomatis* and/or *N. gonorrhoeae.* From a clinical point of view, Fitz-Hugh-Curtis syndrome mimics the basic clinical features of acute cholecystitis and affects almost exclusively young women. This medical condition was initially observed by Carlos Stajano in 1920 who noticed formation of adhesion between Glisson's liver capsule and the anterior abdominal wall in patients with venereal infection complaining of abdominal pain in the right upper quadrant (Stajano, 1920). Thomas Fitz-Hugh and Arthur Curtis gave a detailed description of the syndrome in the 1930s, establishing causative relation between "violin-string" adhesions on the liver capsule, inflammatory pelvic disease and gonococcal infection (Curtis, 1930; Fitz-Hugh, 1934). It was not until the late 1970s, however, that *C. trachomatis* was linked to the etiology of Fitz-Hugh-Curtis syndrome (Wang et al., 1980). Presence of *C. trachomatis* in urogenital specimens, confirmed by PCR assay, is seen in up to 87% of patients with Fitz-Hugh-Curtis syndrome (Yang et al., 2008). According to modern understanding, clinical manifestations of the syndrome arise from the direct colonization of the liver capsule by *C. trachomatis* . Canalicular spread of the pathogen in peritoneal fluid via the right paracolic gutter as well as lymphogenic and hematogenous dissemination are believed to be implicated in the pathogenesis of perihepatitis (Peter et al., 2004). Despite the long-lasting belief that Fitz-Hugh-Curtis syndrome is exclusively attributed to inflammation within the hepatic capsule, perihepatic space and diaphragm, there is some evidence that the liver parenchyma, especially subcapsular regions of the liver, are involved in the course of disease (Lee et al., 2008). Subcapsular enhancement of the liver parenchyma and mildly elevated liver function tests in Fitz-Hugh-Curtis patients have been reported by many researchers (Kim et al., 2007; Lee et al., 2008) . These abnormalities are correctable with antibiotic treatment suggesting their direct association with infection. Moreover, *C. trachomatis* is reportedly isolated not only from the liver capsule of patients (Wolner-Hansen et al., 1982), but also from hepatic parenchyma obtained by biopsy (Dan et al., 1987).

To date there is neither an independent nosologic entity nor liver disease attributable specifically to *C. pneumoniae.* However, there are some reports on *C. pneumoniae* identification in human liver. The pathogen was identified in hepatocytes and sinusoidal cells of the periportal zone in a significant number of patients with acute liver allograft rejection (Lotz et al., 2004). A high occurrence rate of *C. pneumoniae* is also reported in both the explanted livers and hepatic biopsies of patients with primary biliary cirrhosis (Abdulkarim et al., 2004) . Although causative association between *C. pneumoniae* infection and primary biliary cirrhosis has been disputed by other researchers (Taylor-Robinson et al., 2005) there have been new attempts to link some other hepatobiliary diseases (acute intrahepatic cholestasis, nonalcoholic steatohepatitis) to persistent *C. pneumoniae* infection (Bolukbas et al., 2005; Bogdanos & Vergani, 2009).

In contrast, there is a relatively extensive body of scientific literature suggesting that identification of *C. psittaci* in the internal organs is quite a common phenomenon in cases of avian chlamydiosis. Recent advances in the molecular diagnostics of infection in birds have allowed routine detection of *C. psittaci* markers in different tissues, including liver (Nordentoft et al., 2011). The pathogen was identified by using PCR and immunohistochemistry protocols in the livers of budgerigars (Perpinan et al., 2010), canaries (Ferreri et al., 2007) and Amazon parrots (Raso et al., 2004). It has also been isolated from the livers of laying hens (Jizhang et al., 2010). A crucial piece of evidence comes from the analysis of human cases of *C. psittaci* infection. It is widely reported that the clinical manifestation of psittacosis is often associated with abnormal liver function in the patients (Ciftci et al., 2008; Maegawa et al., 2001., Goupil et al., 1998).

6. Hepatotropism

The tissue distribution of chlamydial pathogens has been extensively studied by many researchers using different routes of administration, dosage, strain virulence and type of experimental animals. Irrespective of these variables, the liver was a major site for clearance of *C . trachomatis* (Tuffrey et al., 1984), *C. pneumoniae* (Saikku et al.,1998) and *C. psittaci* (Iversen et al., 1976). Cell-mediated retention of the pathogens has also been seen in the spleen, bone morrow and lungs with the appearance of infected immune cells in their structure.

The liver is one of the largest organs of the human body receiving about a quarter of cardiac output and releasing half of the lymph flow into the thoracic lymphatic duct (Bertolino et al., 2002) . This unique positioning results in the constant exposure of liver cells to different foreign agents such as bacteria, viruses and parasites as well as immune cells infected with them. Very little is known about how and why chlamydial pathogens enter the liver tissue.

In order to enter hepatocytes, chlamydial particles have first to depart from the site of primary colonization and navigate through the systemic circulation in cell-associated (neutrophils, monocytes and lymphocytes) or free form. It is believed that "sense of direction" in the migrating cells is driven by coordinated expression of cytokines and cell adhesion molecules on the surface of endothelium in the tissues and organs. Indeed, it has been recently shown (Jupelli et al., 2010) that the involvement of internal organs in chlamydial infection is somehow controlled by Th1-type immune mediators, interleukin 12 (IL-12) and interferon–γ (IFN-γ). In particular, mice genetically deficient in IL-12, IFN-γ or IFN-γ receptor-1 showed 100% mortality and markedly enhanced liver dissemination of *C. muridarum* after intranasal challenge with the pathogen. This observation is well supported by previously published results. A similar finding has been reported with anti-IFN-γ monoclonal antibody treatment in mice infected with *C. psittaci* (McCafferty et al., 1994) . Moreover, liver has been recently shown to express in a constitutive manner Intercellular Adhesion Molecule-1 (ICAM-1), a protein facilitating leukocyte endothelial transmigration, whose participation in dissemination of chlamydial pathogens has been recently discussed (Ochietti et al., 2002).

Once chemotactic stimuli are recognized, bacterial pathogens in cell-associated form, enter the liver via highly fenestrated sinusoid capillaries, which are composed of sinusoidal lining cells - endothelial cells, macrophages and Kupffer cells (Celton-Morizur & Desdouets, 2010). In their concert action these cells implement clearance of bacteria, endotoxins and microbial debris from the bloodstream and regulate intra-sinusoidal cell migration (Gregory et al., 2002). Kupffer cells are known to ingest and destroy adherent granulocytes containing infectious pathogens (Holub et al., 2009). In this regard, it becomes extremely important that Kupffer cells are shown to support chlamydial growth resulting in productive *C. pneumoniae* infection under "*in vitro*" and "*in vivo*" conditions (Marangoni et al., 2006). Kupffer cells can migrate to Disse's space and establish direct contact with hepatocytes through their cytoplasmic extensions delivering some internal constituents (pro-inflammatory cytokines, mediators *etc*) to the liver trabeculae (Perrault & Pecheur, 2009). In this setting, initial attachment of Chlamydia-infected granulocytes to Kupffer cells with further propagation of chlamydial pathogens in Kupffer cells and their final transmission to the hepatic microenvironment becomes a conceivable chain of events explaining the appearance of chlamydial pathogens in the liver.

It is worth noting that some other infectious pathogens use a similar strategy to invade hepatocytes. As an example, hepatitis B virus is revealed to invade liver tissue by scavenging liver sinusoidal endothelial cells, rather than hepatocytes themselves (Breiner et al., 2001). Therefore, initial invasion of non-hepatic cells might be a general mechanism in the development of hepatocyte infection.

Hepatocytes are polarized epithelial cells with basolateral and apical poles facing blood or bile respectively. The integrity of hepatic trabeculae and separation of blood and bile flows are maintained by tight junctions among adjacent hepatocytes. The basolateral surface of hepatocytes is considered to be a major gate for infectious pathogens delivered to the liver with the blood flow (Perrault & Pecheur, 2009). General mechanisms underlying chlamydial entry in hepatocytes are very likely to resemble those seen in other epithelial cells. Hepatocytes express most of the receptors required for chlamydial attachment and entry into the eukaryotic host cell. Liver has a remarkably high expression level for insulin-like growth factor 2, estrogen receptor complex and platelet-derived growth factor receptor required for chlamydial entry (Leung et al., 2004) . Moreover, liver is known to express abundantly LDL-receptor (Dietschy & Turley, 2002), which can be implemented in our view in the pathogenesis of chlamydiosis. Using an immunoprecipitation approach we have found (Petyaev et al., 2010) that two chlamydial biovars – *C. trachomatis* and *C. pneumoniae* can bind ApoB-containing lipoproteins under "*in vitro*" conditions. This was strikingly distinct from no interaction with the HDL fraction. Furthermore, preincubation of the chlamydial pathogens with LDL particles enhanced in our experiments their ability to infect an immortalized hepatic HepG2 cell line, known to express abundantly LDL receptor. Association of bacterial particles with plasma lipoproteins and subsequent receptor-facilitated uptake does not seem to be an absolute requirement for chlamydial entry since it is possible to establish productive chlamydial infection under serum-free conditions . However, LDL- receptor appears to play an as yet poorly understood role in the initial stages of chlamydial infection. The likelihood of the *Chlamydia*-lipoprotein interactions under *in vivo* conditions becomes even more clear due to our recent identification of cross-reactive antibodies against chlamydial lipopolysaccharide and human ApoB (Petyaev et al., 2011). Besides adding a new variant to the physico-chemical aspect of interaction between *Chlamydia* and lipoproteins, the cross-protective immunological response and subsequent emergence of lipoprotein–specific antibodies may have a detrimental impact on the vascular endothelium. LDL-containing immune complexes are known to be taken up by lipid-laden macrophages and extensively deposited in atherosclerotic plaque (Miller et al., 2010). Therefore association of immune complexes with *Chlamydia* encouraged with cross-reactive antibody will endorse the pathogen delivery into atherosclerotic plaque.

It is worth mentioning that other infectious pathogens utilize lipoproteins and lipoprotein receptors in mechanisms of infectivity. It is well known that hepatitis C virus particles in human plasma are bound to very low density lipoproteins (VLDL) and low density lipoproteins (LDL) forming "viral lipoparticles" (Andre et al., 2005) . Their attachment and entry into hepatocytes requires LDL-receptor and surface receptor CD81 providing a dual receptor mechanism for viral attachment and entry into the target cells (Bartosch et al., 2003). Therefore, the ability of some infectious agents to invade hepatocytes seems to exploit the mechanism of molecular mimicry when an infectious particle "hijacks" a eukaryotic ligand and utilizes the corresponding eukaryotic membrane receptor as well as cross-reactive immunity for invasion of the host cell.

7. Hepatocytes

Extensive *in vitro* studies using cultured hepatocytes are required to understand the molecular mechanisms of liver involvement in chlamydial disease and its outcomes. A major methodological problem emerges from the fact that hepatocytes lose their tissue-specific phenotype and expression of liver-specific genes within 24-48 hours of isolation. For this reason immortalized hepatic cell lines have only a remote resemblance to the metabolic phenotype of whole liver (Guillouzo & Guguen-Guillouzo, 2008). This difficulty can be partially overcome by the use of freshly isolated hepatocytes plated onto collagen-coated dishes in the presence of certain hormones (Shimomura et al., 1999). It has been shown during the last few years that major chlamydial species can efficiently propagate in cultured hepatoma cells (Wang et al., 2007; Bashmakov et al., 2010) and accomplish their entire developmental cycle with the final release of infective progeny from ruptured hepatocytes. A similar observation has been made in experiments with freshly isolated hepatocytes from rat liver (I.M. Petyaev *et al*, 2011, unpublished results). Nevertheless, the nature of the multifaceted relationship emerging between *Chlamydia* and hepatocytes during infection can be understood only in the context of the unique properties of chlamydial pathogens as obligate intracellular parasites.

The chlamydial genome is relatively conserved. Among 1009 genes of *C. caviae* (formerly *C. psittaci*), 798 have orthologs present in *C. pneumoniae* and *C. trachomatis* (Read et al., 2003). These genes supposedly embody a nominal set of genetic material required for the survival of chlamydial species in host cells. The chlamydial genome contains genes encoding complete glycogen turnover, aerobic respiration and various transporter systems. However, genes responsible for biosynthesis of purine/pyrimidine bases, lipids and amino acids are absent or poorly represented (Vandahl et al., 2004). Moreover, the *C. trachomatis* genome encodes some genes for *de novo* synthesis of fatty acids, phosphatidylethanolamine and phosphatidylglycerol, although genes involved in polyunsaturated fatty acid pathways, biosynthesis of cholesterol, sphingolipids and glycerophospholipids have not been identified (Stephens et al., 1998) . Therefore chlamydial inclusions have to acquire major lipids such as cholesterol, sphingomyelin, and neutral lipids from the host cells by intercepting Golgi-derived lipid-containing vesicles (Moore et al., 2008) . Chlamydial pathogens are obligate parasites completely relying on the host cell metabolism. Nutrient deficiency in the host cells is not a matter of "discomfort" for replicating chlamydial pathogens it is rather a matter of ultimate survival and their ability to propagate. As an example, *C. trachomatis* is unable to replicate in the Chinese hamster ovary-derived cell line SPB-1, a mutant cell line deficient in sphingolipid biosynthesis (van Ooij et al., 2000). Similarly, severe tryptophan deficiency in the host cells leads to early developmental arrest of *C. trachomatis* and other chlamydial pathogens (Leonhardt et al., 2007). The metabolic profile of host cells predetermines the efficiency of chlamydial growth. It is believed, that endothelial cells provide a better metabolic environment for *C. pneumoniae* than monocytes due to distinct differences in iron homeostasis (Bellmann-Weiler et al., 2010).

If availability of substrates were the single requirement for sustaining chlamydial infection in eukaryotic cells, hepatocytes would certainly be a most advantageous type of host cell for chlamydial pathogens. Hepatocytes contain an enormous variety of compounds essential for *Chlamydia* . Liver is the organ with the highest rate of 3-hydroxy-3-methyl-glutaryl-CoA (HMG-CoA) reductase expression, a rate limiting enzyme of cholesterol biosynthesis (Dietschy & Turley, 2002). Hepatic cells also synthesize and store various fatty acids, triglycerides and phospholipids. They also operate a highly sophisticated system for endoplasmic vesicular transport of lipids (Jump, 2011). In addition, liver is the central organ of tryptophan turnover (Brandacher et al., 2007) with a remarkable ability to synthesize and catabolize different amino acids .

Recent studies demonstrate that chlamydial pathogens affect hepatocyte-specific functions. *C. trachomatis* infection in hepatocytes has been shown to be accompanied by enhanced transcription of fatty acid binding protein (FABP) leading to increased fatty acid uptake, while overexpression of FABP promotes chlamydial growth in transfected hepatocytes (Wang et al., 2007) . *C. trachomatis* infection also impairs endogenous transcription of another crucial gene of lipid homeostasis - LDL-receptor (LDL-R). We found that the decline in LDL-R mRNA in HepG2 hepatoma cells reflects multiplicity of infection and can be reversed by treatment with mevastatin, an inhibitor of HMG-CoA reductase. A similar tendency has been observed in HepG2 cells infected with *C. pneumoniae* (Y.Bashmakov *et al*, 2010 unpublished results). In both cases mevastatin treatment also reduced infection rate in cultured cells . First of all these results are in good agreement with the anti-chlamydial effects of statins reported in animal studies (Erkkaila et al., 2005; Tiirola et al., 2007). Secondly, the anti-chlamydial effects of statins observed under *in vivo* and *in vitro* conditions open a new perspective in treatment of chlamydiosis whose "signature feature" is drug-resistance of the intracellular bacterial pathogen. Unlike other anti-microbial agents, statins have recently been shown to mediate their effects on infection by inhibiting post-translational protein prenylation in both host cell and infectious agent in a manner independent of cholesterol depletion (Khan et al., 2009; Amet et al., 2008). At the same time, protein prenylation is vital for *Chlamydia* and the functioning of the chlamydial Rab protein family represented by almost 70 members . Silencing of Rab 6 and Rab 11 by siRNA inhibits replication of *C. trachomatis* and impairs lipid acquisition from the host cells (Capmany et al., 2010). Extensive studies are required to show if targeting the geranylgeranylation system does indeed hold promise in the treatment of persistent chlamydial infection.

8. Conclusions

To the best of our knowledge, this chapter represents the very first attempt to discuss the small but growing body of evidence suggesting liver involvement in chlamydiosis. The variety of extragenital and extraocular manifestations of *C. trachomatis* infection as well as the frequent appearance of *C. pneumoniae* and *C. psittaci* in extra-respiratory tissues suggest the systemic character of chlamydial disease and validate a systemic therapeutic approach to the treatment of chlamydiosis. However, conventional diagnostic interventions in modern hepatology impose a substantial limit on direct assessment of chlamydial pathogens in the liver. Nevertheless, presence of chlamydial pathogens in the liver tissue can be verified in a considerable number of patients in particular those with inflammatory hepatobiliary disease. According to our recent results, genomic and immunohistochemical markers of *C. pneumoniae* are identifiable in the liver biopsies of 10.2% of patients with calculous cholecystitis, whereas *C. trachomatis* markers were found in 20.5% of patients from the same category (I.M. Petyaev *et al*, 2011, unpublished results). It has yet to be addressed whether the identification of chlamydial markers in the liver has any pathophysiological significance and possible relation to the course of disease or viability of the bacteria. Thorough bacteriological analysis of liver isolates, their susceptibility to antibiotics and their ability to cause aberrant and persistent variants of infection need to be studied .

To date, liver involvement in chlamydiosis constitutes a subject of rare and often casuistic communications overshadowed by reports on association of chlamydial infection with atherosclerosis and other inflammatory diseases . However, the apparent hepatotropism of chlamydial pathogens creates in our opinion a missing link between chlamydial infection and vascular disease since the liver plays an indispensable role in both lipid homeostasis and systemic inflammatory response. LDL receptor-mediated hepatic clearance of pro-atherogenic lipoproteins is a main route for cholesterol disposal in the human body. Therefore, the negative effect of chlamydial pathogens on LDL receptor expression in cultured hepatocytes may constitute an extremely important mechanism in explaining abnormalities of plasma lipid profile in the patient with chlamydiosis . It remains to be answered in future if the presence of chlamydial pathogens in liver or hepatocytes has any impact respectively on hepatic clearance or uptake of plasma lipoproteins via the LDL receptor-mediated mechanism.

Special consideration should be given to the evaluation of the possible clinical significance of interaction between chlamydial biovars with ApoB-containing lipoproteins. It is conceivable that persistent increase in plasma LDL and VLDL can promote dissemination of chlamydial pathogens, in particular *C. pneumoniae,* to host cell with high or moderate expression of LDL-receptor. Finally, a question as to what extent chlamydial pathogen propagation in liver may affect systemic inflammatory response and hepatic insulin sensitivity has to be explored in the future.

9. References

[1] Abdulkarim AS, Petrovic LM, Kim WR, Angulo P, Lloyd RV, Lindor KD, Tuffrey M, Falder P, Thomas B, Taylor-Robinson D. (2004). Primary biliary cirrhosis: an infectious disease caused by Chlamydia pneumoniae? *Journal of Hepatology,* Vol. 40, No.3, (March 2004), pp. 380-384, ISSN 0168-8278

[2] Abromaitis S, Stephens RS. (2009). Attachment and entry of Chlamydia have distinct requirements for host protein disulfide isomerase. *PLoS Pathogens,* Vol.5, No.4, (April 2009), e1000357. ISSN 1553-7366

[3] Amet T, Nonaka M, Dewan MZ, Saitoh Y, Qi X, Ichinose S, Yamamoto N, Yamaoka S. (2008). Statin-induced inhibition of HIV-1 release from latently infected U1 cells reveals a critical role for protein prenylation in HIV-1replication. *Microbes and Infection,.* Vol.10, No.5, (April 2008), pp.471-480. ISSN 1286-4579

[4] André P, Perlemuter G, Budkowska A, Bréchot C, Lotteau V. (2005). Hepatitis C virus particles and lipoprotein metabolism. *Seminars of Liver Disease,* Vol. 25, No.4, pp. 93-104, ISSN 0272-8087

[5] Asquith KL, Horvat JC, Kaiko GE, Carey AJ, Beagley KW (2011) . Interleukin-13 Promotes Susceptibility to Chlamydial Infection of the Respiratory and Genital Tracts. *PLoS Pathogens,* Vol.7, No.5, e1001339. ISSN 1553-7366

[6] Bartosch B, Vitelli A, Granier C, Goujon C, Dubuisson J, Pascale S, Scarselli E, Cortese R, Nicosia A, Cosset FL. (2003). Cell entry of hepatitis C virus requires a set of co-receptors that include the CD81 tetraspanin and the SR-B1 scavenger receptor. *Journal of Biological Chemistry* . Vol.278, No.43, (October 2003), pp. 41624-30, ISSN 0021-9258

[7] Bashmakov YK, Zigangirova NA, Gintzburg LA, Bortsov PA, Petyaev IM . (2010). ApoB-containing lipoproteins promote infectivity of chlamydial species in human hepatoma cell line. *World Journal of Hepatology.* Vol.2, No.2, (February 2010), pp. 74-80, ISSN 1948-5182

[8] Bashmakov YK, Zigangirova NA, Pashko YP, Kapotina LN, Petyaev IM. (2010). Chlamydia trachomatis growth inhibition and restoration of LDL-receptor level in HepG2 cells treated with mevastatin. *Comparative Hepatology.* (January 2010), pp. 9:3, ISSN 14765926

[9] Beagley KW, Huston WM, Hansbro PM, Timms P. (2009). Chlamydial infection of immune cells: altered function and implications for disease. *Critical Reviews in Immunology* . Vol.29, No.4, (April 2009), pp. 275-305, ISSN 1040-8401

[10] Beeckman, DS, Vanrompay, DC (2009). Zoonotic Chlamydophila psittaci infections from a clinical perspective. *Clinical Microbiology and Infection,* Vol.15, No.1, (January 2009), pp. 11–17, ISSN 1198-743X

[11] Bellmann-Weiler R, Martinz V, Kurz K, Engl S, Feistritzer C, Fuchs D, Rupp J, Paldanius M, Weiss G. (2010). Divergent modulation of Chlamydia pneumoniae infection cycle in human monocytic and endothelial cells by iron, tryptophan availability

and interferon gamma. *Immunobiology,* Vol.215, No.9-10 (September 2010), pp.842-848, ISSN 0171-2985
[12] Bertolino P, McCaughan GW, Bowen DG. (2009). Role of primary intrahepatic T-cell activation in the 'liver tolerance effect'. *Biochemical Journal.* Vol. 423, No.3, (October 2009), pp. 303-14, ISSN 0264-6021
[13] Blasi F, Centanni S, Allegra L. (2004). Chlamydia pneumoniae: crossing the barriers? *European Respiratory Journal.* Vol.23, No.4, (April 2004), pp. 499-500, ISSN 0903-1936
[14] Bogdanos DP, Vergani D. (2009). Bacteria and primary biliary cirrhosis. *Clinical Reviews in Allergy and Immunolology.* Vol.36, No.1, (February 2009), pp.30-39, ISSN 1080-0549
[15] Bolukbas FF, Bolukbas C, Zeyrek F, Aslan M, Bahcecioglu HI, Ozardali I. (2005). High rate of seropositivity of Chlamydia pneumoniae IgA in male patients with nonalcoholicsteatohepatitis. *Digestive Disease Sciences.* Vol. 50, No.6, (June 2005), pp.; 1141-1145, ISSN 0163-2116
[16] Brandacher G, Margreiter R, Fuchs D. (2007) . Implications of IFN-gamma-mediated tryptophan catabolism on solid organ transplantation. *Current Drug Metabolism.* Vol.8, No.3, (April 2007), pp 273-282, ISSN 1389-2002
[17] Breiner KM, Schaller H, Knolle PA . (2001). Endothelial cell-mediated uptake of a hepatitis B virus: a new concept of liver targeting of hepatotropic microorganisms. *Hepatology.* Vol.34, No.4, (October 2001), pp. 803-808, ISSN 1527-1746
[18] Buendía AJ, De Oca RM, Navarro JA, Sánchez J, Cuello F, Salinas J. (1999). Role of polymorphonuclear neutrophils in a murine model of Chlamydia psittaci-induced abortion. *Infection and Immunity.* Vol.67, No.5, (May 1999), pp.2110-2116, ISSN 1098-5522
[19] Burillo A, Bouza E (2010). Chlamydophila pneumoniae. *Infectious Diseases Clinics North America.* Vol.24, No.1, (March 2010); pp. 61-71, ISSN 0891-5520
[20] Bustamante RR, Zalba EB, Boldova AR, Suárez MA. (2002). Community-acquired pneumonia, acute respiratory distress syndrome, and severe sepsis due to Chlamydia pneumoniae. *Revista Clinica Espanola.* Vol. 202, No.11, (November 2002), pp.623-627, ISSN 0014-2565
[21] Buxton D, Rae AG, Maley SW, Thomson KM, Livingstone M, Jones GE, Herring AJ. (1996). Pathogenesis of Chlamydia psittaci infection in sheep: detection of the organism in a serial study of the lymph node. *Journal of Comparative Pathology.* Vol. 114, No.3, (April 1996), pp. 221-230, ISSN 0021-9975
[22] Byrne GI. (2010). Chlamydia trachomatis strains and virulence: rethinking links to infection prevalence and disease severity. *Journal of Infectious Diseases* . Vol.201, No.2, (June 2010), pp.126-133, ISSN 0022-1899
[23] Capmany A, Damiani MT. (2010).Chlamydia trachomatis intercepts Golgi-derived sphingolipids through a Rab14-mediated transport required for bacterial development and replication. *PLoS One.* Vol.5, No.11, (November 2010), e14084, ISSN 1932-6203
[24] Carlson JH, Hughes S, Hogan D. (2004). Polymorphisms in the Chlamydia trachomatis cytotoxin locus associated with ocular and genital isolates. *Infection and Immunity* Vol.72, No.12, (December 2004), pp. 7063-7072, ISSN 1098-5522
[25] Castro R, Baptista T, Vale A, Nunes H, Prieto E, Araújo C, Mansinho K, da Luz Martins Pereira F. (2010). Lymphogranuloma venereum serovar L2b in Portugal.

International Journal of STD and AIDS. Vol.21, No.4, (April 2010), pp. 265-269, ISSN 0956-4624

[26] Celton-Morizur S, Desdouets C. (2010). Polyploidization of liver cells . *Advances in Experimental Medicine and Biology*. Vol.676, (April 2010), pp.123-135. ISSN 0065-2598

[27] Chong-Cerrillo C, Selsted ME, Peterson EM, de la Maza LM. (2003). Susceptibility of human and murine Chlamydia trachomatis serovars to granulocyte- and epithelium-derived antimicrobial peptides. *Journal of Peptide Research*. Vol.61, No.5, (May2003), pp.237-242, ISSN 1399-3011

[28] Ciftçi B, Güler ZM, Aydoğdu M, Konur O, Erdoğan Y. (2008). Familial outbreak of psittacosis as the first Chlamydia psittaci infection reported from Turkey. *Tuberkuloz Toraks*. ; Vol.56, No.2, (February 2008), pp.215-220, ISSN 0494-1373

[29] Clifton DR, Fields KA, Grieshaber SS, Dooley CA, Fischer ER, Mead DJ, Carabeo RA, Hackstadt T . (2004). A chlamydial type III translocated protein is tyrosine-phosphorylated at the site of entry and associated with recruitment of actin. *Proceedings of National Academy of Sciences USA*. ul 6; Vol.101, No.27, (July 2004), pp. 10166-10171, ISSN 1091-6490

[30] Cochrane, M., Walker, P., Gibbs, H. & Timms, P. (2005). Multiple genotypes of Chlamydia pneumoniae identified in human carotid plaque. *Microbiology*, Vol.151, No.7, (July 2005), pp. 2285–2290, ISSN 1350-0872

[31] Conant CG, Stephens RS (2007). Chlamydia attachment to mammalian cells requires protein disulfide isomerase. *Cellular Microbiology*, Vol.9, No.1, (January 2007), pp.222-232, ISSN 1462-5822

[32] Contini C, Seraceni S, Cultrera R, Castellazzi M, Granieri E, Fainardi E. (2010). Chlamydophila pneumoniae Infection and Its Role in Neurological Disorders. *Interdisciplinary Perspective on Infectious Diseases.*, 2010:273573, ISSN 1687-708X

[33] Contini C, Seraceni S, Cultrera R, Castellazzi M, Granieri E, Fainardi E. (2008). Molecular detection of Parachlamydia-like organisms in cerebrospinal fluid of patients with multiple sclerosis. *Multiple Sclerosis Journal* . Vol.14, No.4, (May 2008), pp.564-566, ISSN 1352-4585

[34] Curtis A. (1930). A cause of adhesions in the right upper quadrant. *JAMA*, vol.94, pp.1221–1222, ISSN 0098-7484

[35] Dan M, Tyrrell LD, Goldsand G. (1987). Isolation of Chlamydia trachomatis from the liver of a patient with prolonged fever. *Gut.*, Vol. 28, No.11, (November 1987), pp.1514-1516, ISSN 0017-5749

[36] Dautry-Varsat, A., Balañá, M. E. and Wyplosz, B. (2004). Chlamydia– Host Cell Interactions: Recent Advances on Bacterial Entry and Intracellular Development. Traffic, Vol. 5, No.8, (August 2004), pp. 561–570, ISSN 1600-0854

[37] den Hartog JE, Land JA, Stassen FR, Slobbe-van Drunen ME, Kessels AG, Bruggeman CA. (2004). The role of chlamydia genus-specific and species-specific IgG antibody testing in predicting tubal disease in subfertile women. *Human Reproduction.*, Vol. 19, No.6, (June 2004), pp.1380-1384, ISSN 0268-116

[38] Derbigny WA, Kerr MS, Johnson RM. (2005). Pattern recognition molecules activated by Chlamydia muridarum infection of cloned murine oviduct epithelial cell lines. *Journal of Immunology*. Vol.175, No.9, (November 2005), pp 6065-6075, ISSN 0022-1767

[39] Dickx V, Beeckman DS, Dossche L, Tavernier P, Vanrompay D. (2010). Chlamydophila psittaci in homing and feral pigeons and zoonotic transmission. *Journal of Medical Microbiology*. Vol.59, No.11, (November2010), pp.1348-1353, ISSN 1473-5644

[40] Dietschy JM, Turley SD. (2002). Control of cholesterol turnover in the mouse. *Journal of Biological Chemistry*. Vol.277, No.6, (February 2002), pp.3801-4, ISSN 0021-8258

[41] Erkkilä L, Jauhiainen M, Laitinen K, Haasio K, Tiirola T, Saikku P, Leinonen M. (2005). Effect of simvastatin, an established lipid-lowering drug, on pulmonary Chlamydia pneumoniae infection in mice. *Antimicrobial Agents and Chemotherapy*., Vol. 49, No.9, (September 2005), pp. 3959-3962, ISSN 1098-6596

[42] Everett KD, Bush RM, Andersen AA. (1999). Emended description of the order Chlamydiales, proposal of Parachlamydiaceae fam. nov. and Simkaniaceae fam. nov., each containing one monotypic genus, revised taxonomy of the family Chlamydiaceae, including a new genus and five new species, and standards for the identification of organisms. *International Journal of Systemic Bacteriology*, Vol.49, No.2, (February 1999), pp.415–440, ISSN 0020-7713

[43] Fenga C, Cacciola A, Di Nola C, Calimeri S, Lo Giudice D, Pugliese M, Niutta PP, Martino LB (2007). Serologic investigation of the prevalence of Chlamydophila psittaci in occupationally-exposed subjects in eastern Sicily. *Annals of Agricultural and Environmental Medicine* . Vol. 14, No.1, (January 2007), pp.93-96, ISSN 1232-1966

[44] Ferreri AJ, Dolcetti R, Magnino S, Doglioni C, Cangi MG, Pecciarini L, Ghia P, Dagklis A, Pasini E, Vicari N, Dognini GP, Resti AG, Ponzoni M. (2007). A woman and her canary: a tale of chlamydiae and lymphomas. *Journal of National Cancer Institute*. Vol.99, No.18, (September 2007), 19; pp.1418-1419, ISSN 0027-8874

[45] Fields, P. I. & Barnes, R. C. (1992). The genus Chlamydia, In: The Prokaryotes, A. Balows (Ed.), 3691–3709, ISBN 10: 0387254994, New York: Springer, USA

[46] Filippidis A, Fountas KN (2009). Nasal lymphatics as a novel invasion and dissemination route of bacterial meningitis. *Medical Hypotheses*,. Vol.72, No.6, (June 2009), pp.694-697, ISSN 0306-9877

[47] Fitz-Hugh T Jr. (1934). Acute gonococcic peritonitis of the right upper quadrant in women. *JAMA*, Vol.102, pp.2094–2096. ISSN 0098-7484.

[48] Fraeyman A, Boel A, Van Vaerenbergh K, De Beenhouwer H. (2010). Atypical pneumonia due to Chlamydophila psittaci: 3 case reports and review of literature. *Acta Clinica Belgica*, Vol.65, No.3, (May-June 2010), pp.192-196, ISSN 0001-5512

[49] Garrett AJ, Harrison MJ, Manire GP (1974).A search for the bacterial mucopeptide component, muramic acid, in Chlamydia. *Journal General Microbiology*., Vol.80, No.1, (January 1974), pp.315-318, ISSN 0022-1287

[50] Gieffers J, van Zandbergen G, Rupp J, Sayk F, Krüger S, Ehlers S, Solbach W, Maass M. (2004). Phagocytes transmit Chlamydia pneumoniae from the lungs to the vasculature. *European Respiratory Journal*. Vol.23, No.4, (April 2004), pp.506-510, ISSN 1399-3003

[51] Goupil F, Pellé-Duporté D, Kouyoumdjian S, Carbonnelle B, Tuchais E . (1998). Severe pneumonia with a pneumococcal aspect during an ornithosis outbreak. *Presse Medicale*. Vol.27, No.22, (June 1998), 20; pp.1084-1088, ISSN 0755-4982

[52] Gregory SH, Cousens LP, van Rooijen N, Döpp EA, Carlos TM, Wing EJ. (2002). Complementary adhesion molecules promote neutrophil-Kupffer cell interaction

and the elimination of bacteria taken up by the liver. *Journal of Immunology*. Vol.168, No.1, (January 2002), pp.308-315, ISSN 0022-1767

[53] Grinblat-Huse V, Drabek EF, Huot Creasy H, Daugherty SC, Jones KM, Santana-Cruz I, Tallon LJ, Read TD, Hatch TP, Bavoil P, Myers GS. (2011). Genome sequences of the zoonotic pathogens Chlamydia psittaci 6BC and Cal10. *Journal of Bacteriology* . Vol.193, No15, (August 2011), pp.4039-4040, ISSN 1098-5530

[54] Guaschino S, De Seta F. (2000). Update on Chlamydia trachomatis. *Annals of the New York Academy of Sciences*, Vol.900, pp. 293–300. ISSN 0077-8923.

[55] Guillouzo A, Guguen-Guillouzo C. (2008). Evolving concepts in liver tissue modeling and implications for in vitro toxicology. *Expert Opinion on Drug Metabolism and Toxicology* . Vol.4, No.10, (October 2008), pp.1279-1294, ISSN 1744-7607

[56] Hackstadt, T., Todd, W.J., and Caldwell, H.D. (1985). Disulfide-mediated interactions of the chlamydial major outer membrane protein: role in the differentiation of chlamydiae? *Journal of Bacteriology*. Vol.161, No.1, (January 1985), pp.25–31, ISSN 1098-5530

[57] Halberstaedter L, von Prowazek S . (1907). Ueber Zelleinschlusse parasitirer Natur Beim Trachom . *Gesundheitsamt*, No.3, pp. 44– 47, ISSN 1865-0686

[58] Hammerschlag MR. (2002). The intracellular life of chlamydiae. *Seminars Pediatric Infectious Diseases*. Vol.13, No.4, (October 2002), pp.239-248, ISSN 1045-1870

[59] Hammond CJ, Hallock LR, Howanski RJ, Appelt DM, Little CS, Balin BJ. (2010). Immunohistological detection of Chlamydia pneumoniae in the Alzheimer's disease brain. *BMC Neuroscience*. Vol.23, No.11, (September 2010), pp.1-8, ISSN 1471-2202

[60] Harkinezhad T, Geens T, Vanrompay D. (2009). Chlamydophila psittaci infections in birds: a review with emphasis on zoonotic consequences. *Veterinary Microbiology*. Vol.135, No.1-2, (March 2009), pp.68-77, ISSN 0378-1135

[61] Holub M, Cheng CW, Mott S, Wintermeyer P, van Rooijen N, Gregory SH. (2009). Neutrophils sequestered in the liver suppress the proinflammatory response of Kupffer cells to systemic bacterial infection. *Journal of Immunology, Vol.183, No.5,* (September 2009), pp. 3309-3316, ISSN 1550-6606

[62] Hybiske K, Stephens RS. (2007). Mechanisms of Chlamydia trachomatis entry into nonphagocytic cells. *Infection and Immunity*. Vol.75, No.8, (August 2007), pp.3925-3934, ISSN 1098-5522

[63] Iversen JO, Hanson RP, Spalatin J. (1976). Experimental chlamydiosis in wild and domestic lagomorphs. *Journal Wildlife Diseases,* Vol.12, No.2, (April 1976), pp.215-220, ISSN 0090-3558

[64] Janssen MJ, van de Wetering K, Arabin B. (2006). Sepsis due to gestational psittacosis: A multidisciplinary approach within a perinatological center--review of reported cases . *International Journal of Fertility and Women's Medicine*. Vol.51, No.1, (January 2006), pp.17-20, ISSN 1534-892X

[65] Jayarapu K, Kerr MS, Katschke A, Johnson RM. (2009). Chlamydia muridarum-specific CD4 T-cell clones recognize infected reproductive tract epithelial cells in an interferon-dependent fashion. *Infection and Immunity*. Vol.77, No.10, (October 2009), pp.4469-79, ISSN 1098-5522

[66] Jizhang Zhou, Changqing Qiu, Guozhen Lin, Xiaoan Cao, Fuying Zheng, Xiaowei Gong, Guanghua Wang. (2010). Isolation of Chlamydophila psittaci from Laying

Hens in China. Veterinary Research, Vol.21, No.3, (March 2010), pp.43-45, ISSN 1297-9716

[67] Jump DB. (2011). Fatty acid regulation of hepatic lipid metabolism. *Current Opinion in Clinical Nutrition and Metabolic Care.* Vol.14, No.2, (March 2011), pp.115-120, ISSN 1363-1950

[68] Jupelli M, Selby DM, Guentzel MN, Chambers JP, Forsthuber TG, Zhong G, Murthy AK, Arulanandam BP. (2010). The contribution of interleukin-12/interferon-gamma axis in protection against neonatal pulmonary Chlamydia muridarum challenge. *Journal of Interferon and Cytokine Research* . Vol.30, No.6, (June 2010), ISSN 1079-9907

[69] Kaan JA, Branger J, van Ampting JM, Speelman P (2002). Fitz-Hugh-Curtis syndrome: 2 patients with perihepatitis and sepsis. *Nederlands Tijdschrift voor Geneeskunde* . Vol.146, No.20, (May 2002), pp.954-957, ISSN 0028-2162

[70] Kalinke U, Bechmann I, Detje CN. (2011). Host strategies against virus entry via the olfactory system. *Virulence.* Vol.2, No.4, (July 2011), pp. 37-41, ISSN 2150-5608

[71] Kariagina AS, Alekseevskiĭ AV, Spirin SA, Zigangirova NA, Gintsburg AL. (2009). Effector proteins of Clamidia. *Molecular Biology (Moskow).* Vol.43, No.6, (November 2009), pp.963-983, ISSN 0006-2979

[72] Khan MA, Gallo RM, Renukaradhya GJ, Du W, Gervay-Hague J, Brutkiewicz RR. (2009). Statins impair CD1d-mediated antigen presentation through the inhibition of prenylation. *Journal of Immunology.* Vol.182, No.8, (April 2009), pp.4744-50, ISSN 0022-1767

[73] Kim S, Kim TU, Lee JW, Lee TH, Lee SH, Jeon TY, Kim KH. (2007). The perihepatic space: comprehensive anatomy and CT features of pathologic conditions. *Radiographics* . Vol.27, No.1, (January 2007), pp.129-43, ISSN 0271-5333

[74] Kutlin A, Roblin PM, Kumar S, Kohlhoff S, Bodetti T, Timms P, Hammerschlag MR. (2007). Molecular characterization of Chlamydophila pneumoniae isolates from Western barred bandicoots. *Journal of Medical Microbiology.* Vol.56, No.3, (March 2007), pp.407-417, ISSN 0022-2615

[75] Lacy HM, Bowlin AK, Hennings L, Scurlock AM, Nagarajan UM, Rank RG. (2011). Essential role for neutrophils in pathogenesis and adaptive immunity in Chlamydia caviae ocular infections. *Infection and Immunity.* Vol.79, No.5, (May 2011), pp.1889-1897, ISSN 1098-5522

[76] Lamas CC, Eykyn SJ. (2003). Blood culture negative endocarditis: analysis of 63 cases presenting over 25 years. *Heart.* Vol. 89, No.3, (March 2003), pp.258-262, ISSN 1355-6037

[77] Lee JW, Kim S, Kwack SW, Kim CW, Moon TY, Lee SH, Cho M, Kang DH, Kim GH. (2008). Hepatic capsular and subcapsular pathologic conditions: demonstration with CT and MR imaging. *Radiographics.* Vol.28, No.5, (September 2008), pp. 1307-1323, ISSN 0271-5333

[78] Leonhardt RM, Lee SJ, Kavathas PB, Cresswell P (2007). Severe tryptophan starvation blocks onset of conventional persistence and reduces reactivation of Chlamydia trachomatis. *Infection and Immunity.* Vol. 75, No.11, (November 2007), pp.5105-5117, ISSN 1098-5522

[79] Leung KC, Johannsson G, Leong GM, Ho KK. (2004). Estrogen regulation of growth hormone action. *Endocrine Reviews*. Vol.25, No.5, (October 2004), pp.693-721, ISSN 0013-7227
[80] Lotz G, Simon S, Patonai A, Sótonyi P, Nemes B, Sergi C, Glasz T, Füle T, Nashan B, Schaff Z. (2004). Detection of Chlamydia pneumoniae in liver transplant patients with chronic allograft rejection. *Transplantation*. Vol.77, No.10, (May 2004), pp.1522-1528. ISSN 0041-1337
[81] Maegawa N, Emoto T, Mori H, Yamaguchi D, Fujinaga T, Tezuka N, Sakai N, Ohtsuka N, Fukuse T. (2001). 2 cases of Chlamydia psittaci infection occurring in employees of the same pet shop. *Nihon Kokyuki Gakkai Zasshi* . Vol.39, No.10, (October 2001), pp.753-757, ISSN 1343-3490
[82] Marangoni A, Donati M, Cavrini F, Aldini R, Accardo S, Sambri V, Montagnani M, Cevenini R. (2006). Chlamydia pneumoniae replicates in Kupffer cells in mouse model of liver infection. *World Journal of Gastroenterology* . Vol.12, No.40, (October 2006), pp. 6453-6457, ISSN 1007-9327
[83] Martin-Iguacel R, Llibre JM, Nielsen H, Heras E, Matas L, Lugo R, Clotet B, Sirera G. (2010). Lymphogranuloma venereum proctocolitis: a silent endemic disease in men who have sex with men in industrialized countries. *European Journal of Clinical Microbiology & Infectious Diseases* . Vol.29, No.8, (August 2010), pp.917-925, ISSN 0934-9723
[84] McCafferty MC, Maley SW, Entrican G, Buxton D. (1994). The importance of interferon-gamma in an early infection of Chlamydia psittaci in mice. *Immunology*. Vol.81, No.4, (April 1994), pp.631-636, ISSN 0022-1767
[85] Miller YI, Choi SH, Fang L, Tsimikas S. (2010). Lipoprotein modification and macrophage uptake: role of pathologic cholesterol transport in atherogenesis. *Subcellular Biochemistry*, Vol.51, No.2, (April 2010), pp.229-251, ISSN 0306-0225
[86] Miyairi I, Mahdi OS, Ouellette SP, Belland RJ, Byrne GI. (2006). Different growth rates of Chlamydia trachomatis biovars reflect pathotype. *Journal of Infectious Diseases*, Vol. 194, No.3, (August 2006), pp.350-357, ISSN 0022-1899
[87] Mölleken K, Schmidt E, Hegemann JH (2010). Members of the Pmp protein family of Chlamydia pneumoniae mediate adhesion to human cells via short repetitive peptide motifs. *Molecular Microbiology*. Vol.78, No.4, (November 2010), pp.1004-1017, ISSN 1365-2958
[88] Moore ER, Fischer ER, Mead DJ, Hackstadt T . (2008). The chlamydial inclusion preferentially intercepts basolaterally directed sphingomyelin-containing exocytic vacuoles. *Traffic*. Vol.9, No.12, (December 2008), pp.2130-2140, ISSN 1600-0854
[89] Morange, A. 1895. De la psittacose, ou infection speciale determinee par des perruches. Academie de Paris, 1895, Paris, France.
[90] Moulder JW. (1982). The relation of basic biology to pathogenic potential in the genus Chlamydia. *Infection* . Vol.10, Suppl 1, (November 1982), pp.10-18, ISSN 0300-8126
[91] Myers GS, Mathews SA, Eppinger M, Mitchell C, O'Brien KK, White OR, Benahmed F, Brunham RC, Read TD, Ravel J, Bavoil PM, Timms P. (2009). Evidence that human Chlamydia pneumoniae was zoonotically acquired. *Journal of Bacteriology*. Vol.191, No.23, (December 2009), pp. 727225-33, ISSN 1098-5530
[92] Nordentoft S, Kabell S, Pedersen K. (2011). Real-Time detection and identification of Chlamydophila species in veterinary specimens using SYBR Green based PCR

Assays. *Applied and Environmental Microbiology*. Vol.77, No.14, (July 2011), pp.4705-4711, ISSN 0099-2240

[93] Ochietti B, Lemieux P, Kabanov AV, Vinogradov S, St-Pierre Y, Alakhov V. (2002). Inducing neutrophil recruitment in the liver of ICAM-1deficient mice using polyethyleneimine grafted with Pluronic P123 as an organ-specific carrier for transgenicICAM-1. *Gene Therapy* . Vol.9, No.14, (July 2002), pp. 939-945, ISSN 0969-7128

[94] Park JY, Lim MC, Lim SY, Bae JM, Yoo CW, Seo SS, Kang S, Park SY. (2008). Port-site and liver metastases after laparoscopic pelvic and para-aortic lymph node dissection for surgical staging of locally advanced cervical cancer. *International Journal of Gynecological Cancer* . Vol.18, No.1, (January 2008), pp.176-180, ISSN 1048-891X

[95] Perkinsh R, Allisona C . (1963). Cell-wall constituents of rickettsiae and psittacosis-lymphogranuloma organisms. *Journal of General Microbiology;* Vol.30, (March 1963), pp. 469-480, ISSN 0022-1287

[96] Perpiñán D, Garner MM, Wellehan JF, Armstrong DL. (2010) Mixed infection with reovirus and Chlamydophila in a flock of budgerigars (Melopsittacus undulatus). *Journal Avian Medicine and Surgery*. Vol.24, No.4, (December 2010), pp.316-321. ISSN 1082-6742

[97] Perrault M, Pécheur EI. (2009). The hepatitis C virus and its hepatic environment: a toxic but finely tuned partnership. *Biochemical Journal*. Vol.12, No.3, (October 2009), pp. 303-314, ISSN 0264-6021

[98] Perry LL, Hughes SA. (1999). Chlamydial colonization of multiple mucosae following infection by any mucosal route. *Infection and Immunity*. Vol.67, No.7, (July 1999), pp.3686-3689, ISSN 1098-5522

[99] Peter NG, Clark LR, Jaeger JR. (2004). Fitz-Hugh-Curtis syndrome: a diagnosis to consider in women with right upper quadrant pain. *Cleveland Clinic Journal of Medicine*. Vol.71, No.3, (March 2004), pp. 233-239, ISSN 0891-1150

[100] Petyaev IM, Zigangirova NA, Petyaev AM, Pashko UP, Didenko LV, Morgunova EU, Bashmakov YK. (2010). Isolation of Chlamydia pneumoniae from serum samples of the patients with acute coronary syndrome. *International Journal of Medical Science*. Vol.10, No.4, (June 2010), pp. 181-190, ISSN 0974-5343.

[101] Petyaev IM, Zigangirova NA, Tsibezov VV, Ross A, Bashmakov YK. (2011). Monoclonal antibodies against lipopolysaccharide of Chlamydia trachomatis with crossreactivity to human ApoB. *Hybridoma (Larchmt)* . Vol. 30, No.2, (April 2011), pp.131-136, ISSN 1554-0014

[102] Piercy DW, Griffiths PC, Teale CJ. (1999). Encephalitis related to Chlamydia psittaci infection in a 14-week-old calf. *Veterinary Record* . Vol.144, No.5, (January 1999), pp.126-128, ISSN 0042-4900

[103] Puolakkainen M, Kuo CC, Campbell LA (2005). Chlamydia pneumoniae uses the mannose 6-phosphate/insulin-like growth factor 2 receptor for infection of endothelial cells. *Infection and Immunity* . Vol.73, No.8, (August 2005), pp.4620-4625, ISSN 1098-5522

[104] Raso Tde F, Godoy SN, Milanelo L, de Souza CA, Matuschima ER, Araújo Júnior JP, Pinto AA. (2004). An outbreak of chlamydiosis in captive blue-fronted Amazon

parrots (Amazona aestiva) in Brazil. *Journal of Zoo and Wildlife Medicine*. Vol.35, No.1, (March 2004), pp.94-96, ISSN 1042-7260

[105] Read TD, Myers GS, Brunham RC, Nelson WC, Paulsen IT, Heidelberg J, Holtzapple E, Khouri H, Federova NB, Carty HA, Umayam LA, Haft DH, Peterson J, Beanan MJ,White O, Salzberg SL, Hsia RC, McClarty G, Rank RG, Bavoil PM, Fraser CM . (2003). Genome sequence of Chlamydophila caviae (Chlamydia psittaci GPIC): examining the role of niche-specific genes in the evolution of the Chlamydiaceae. *Nucleic Acids Research* . Vol.31, No.8, (April 2003), pp.2134-2147, ISSN 1362-4962

[106] Roan NR, Starnbach MN. (2008). Immune-mediated control of Chlamydia infection. *Cellular Microbiology* . Vol.10, No.1, (January 2008), pp.9-19, ISSN 1462-5288

[107] Rupp J, Pfleiderer L, Jugert C, Moeller S, Klinger M. (2009). Chlamydia pneumoniae Hides inside Apoptotic Neutrophils to Silently Infect and Propagate in Macrophages. *PLoS ONE* Vol.4, No.6, e6020, ISSN 1932-6203

[108] Saikku P, Laitinen K, Leinonen M. (1998).Animal models for Chlamydia pneumoniae infection. *Atherosclerosis* . Vol. 140, Suppl.1, (October 1998), pp.; 140, 17-19, ISSN 0021-9150

[109] Saikku P, Wang SP, Kleemola M, Brander E, Rusanen E, Grayston JT. (1985). An epidemic of mild pneumonia due to an unusual strain of Chlamydia psittaci. *Journal of Infectious Diseases*, Vol. 151, No.5, (May 1985), pp.832-839, ISSN 0022-1899

[110] Schachter J, Stephens RS, Timms P. (2001). Radical changes to chlamydial taxonomy are not necessary just yet. *International Journal of Systematic and Evolutionary Microbiology*, Vol.51, No.1, (January 2001), pp.251-253, ISSN 0020-7713

[111] Scidmore MA, Fischer ER, Hackstadt T. (2003). Restricted fusion of Chlamydia trachomatis vesicles with endocytic compartments during the initial stages of infection. *Infection and Immunity* . Vol.71, No.2, (February 2003), pp.973-984, ISSN 1098-5522

[112] Sessa R, Di Pietro M, Schiavoni G, Petrucca A, Cipriani P, Zagaglia C, Nicoletti M, Santino I, del Piano M. (2007). Measurement of Chlamydia pneumoniae bacterial load in peripheral blood mononuclear cells may be helpful to assess the state of chlamydial infection in patients with carotid atherosclerotic disease. *Atherosclerosis* . Vol.195, No.1, (November 2007), pp.224-230, ISSN 0021-9150

[113] Shimomura I, Bashmakov Y, Ikemoto S, Horton JD, Brown MS, Goldstein JL. (1999). Insulin selectively increases SREBP-1c mRNA in the livers of rats with streptozotocin-induced diabetes. *Proceedings of National Academy of Sciences USA*. Vol.96, No.24, (November 1999), pp.13656-13661, ISSN 1091-6490

[114] Stajano C. (1920). La reaccion frenica en ginecologica. *Semana Medica Beunoa Airea*, Vol.27, (May 1920), pp.243–248.

[115] Stephens RS, Myers G, Eppinger M, Bavoil PM (2009). Divergence without difference: phylogenetics and taxonomy of Chlamydia resolved. *FEMS Immunology and Medical Microbiology*. Vol.55, No.2, (March 2009), pp.115-119, ISSN 1574-695X

[116] Stephens RS, Kalman S, Lammel C, Fan J, Marathe R, Aravind L, Mitchell W, Olinger L, Tatusov RL, Zhao Q, Koonin EV, Davis RW (1998). Genome sequence of an obligate intracellular pathogen of humans: Chlamydia trachomatis. *Science*. Vol.282, No.5389, (October 1998), pp. 754-759, ISSN 1095-9203

[117] Taylor-Robinson D, Sharif AW, Dhanjal NS, Taylor-Robinson SD. (2005). Chlamydia pneumoniae infection is an unlikely cause of primary biliary cirrhosis. *Journal of Hepatology,* Vol.42, No.5, (May 2005), pp.779-780, ISSN 0168-8278
[118] Theegarten D, Sachse K, Mentrup B, Fey K, Hotzel H, Anhenn O. (2008). Chlamydophila spp. infection in horses with recurrent airway obstruction: similarities to human chronic obstructive disease. *Respiratory Research.* Vol.29, No.9, (July 2008), pp.9-14, ISSN 1465-9921
[119] Tiirola T, Jauhiainen M, Erkkilä L, Bloigu A, Leinonen M, Haasio K, Laitinen K, Saikku P. (2007). Effect of pravastatin treatment on Chlamydia pneumoniae infection, inflammation and serum lipids in NIH/S mice. *International Journal of Antimicrobial Agents.* Vol.29, No.4, (June 2007), pp.741-746, ISSN 0924-8579
[120] Tuffrey M, Falder P, Thomas B, Taylor-Robinson D. (1984). The distribution and effect of Chlamydia trachomatis in CBA mice inoculated genitally, intra-articularly or intravenously. *Medical Microbiology and Immunology.* Vol.173, No.1, (January 1984), pp.29-35, ISSN 1574-695X
[121] van Ooij C, Kalman L, van Ijzendoorn, Nishijima M, Hanada K, Mostov K, Engel JN. (2000). Host cell-derived sphingolipids are required for the intracellular growth of Chlamydia trachomatis. *Cellular Microbiology.* Vol.2, No.6, (December 2000), pp.627-637, ISSN 1462-5822
[122] Vandahl BB, Birkelund S, Christiansen G. (2004). Genome and proteome analysis of Chlamydia. Proteomics . Vol.4, No.10, (October 2004), pp.2831-2842, ISSN 1615-9853
[123] Vanrompay D, Ducatelle R, Haesebrouck F. (1995). Chlamydia psittaci infections: a review with emphasis on avian chlamydiosis. *Veterinary Microbiology.* Vol.45, No.2-3, (July 1995), pp.93-119, ISSN 0378-1135
[124] Verminnen K, Duquenne B, De Keukeleire D, Duim B, Pannekoek Y, Braeckman L, Vanrompay D. (2008). Evaluation of a Chlamydophila psittaci infection diagnostic platform for zoonotic risk assessment. *Journal of Clinical Microbiology.* Vol.46, No.1, (January 2008), pp.281-285, ISSN 1098-660X.
[125] von Prowazek S. (1907). Chlamydoeoa Zuzammenfassende Uebersicht. *Arch Protistenkunde,* Vol.10, pp.336-358.
[126] Wang G, Burczynski F, Anderson J, Zhong G. (2007) . Effect of host fatty acid-binding protein and fatty acid uptake on growth of Chlamydia trachomatis L2 . *Microbiology,* Vol.153, No.6, (June 2007), pp.1935–1939, ISSN 1350-0872
[127] Wang SP, Eschenbach DA, Holmes KK, Wager G, Grayston JT. (1980). Chlamydia trachomatis infection in Fitz-Hugh-Curtis syndrome. *American Journal Obstetrics and Gynecology.* Vol.138, No.2, (December1980), pp.1034-1038, ISSN 0002-9378
[128] Wølner-Hanssen P, Svensson L, Weström L, Mårdh PA. (1982). Isolation of Chlamydia trachomatis from the liver capsule in Fitz-Hugh-Curtis syndrome. *New England Journal of Medicine,* Vol.306, No.2, (January 1982), pp.113-117, ISSN 0028-4798
[129] Yamagata T, Sugiura H, Yokoyama T, Yanagisawa S, Ichikawa T, Ueshima K, Akamatsu K, Hirano T, Nakanishi M, Yamagata Y, Matsunaga K, Minakata Y. (2007). Overexpression of CD-11b and CXCR1 on circulating neutrophils: its possible role in COPD . *Chest* . Vol. 132, No.3, (September 2007), pp.890-899, ISSN 0012-3692

[130] Yang HW, Jung SH, Han HY, Kim A, Lee YJ, Cha SW, Go H, Choi GY, Cho SH, Lim SH. (2008). Clinical feature of Fitz-Hugh-Curtis syndrome: analysis of 25 cases]. *Korean Journal of Hepatology*. Vol.14, No.2, (June 2008), pp.178-184, ISSN 1738-222X

11

Chlamydia trachomatis Infection and Reproductive Health Outcomes in Women

Luis Piñeiro and Gustavo Cilla
Microbiology Service, Hospital Donostia and Biodonostia Research Institute
Spain

1. Introduction

Chlamydia trachomatis infection is a major and increasing public health problem worldwide and is currently the main cause of sexually-transmitted infections (STI). The incidence of this infection is highest in young women and is especially important in this population group due to the potential consequences in the female reproductive tract, such as pelvic inflammatory disease, tubal damage, and infertility. During pregnancy, *C. trachomatis* infection has been associated with adverse outcomes, including spontaneous abortion, ectopic pregnancy, premature rupture of membranes, preterm birth. Moreover, the infection can be transmitted perinatally to women's offspring causing neonatal conjunctivitis, nasopharyngitis and pneumonia.

Because of the particular characteristics of this intracellular microorganism (unique biphasic division cycle, slow metabolism) and its interaction with the host's immune response, *C. trachomatis* infection may often pass unnoticed and be under-diagnosed, facilitating its spread, which is mainly associated with sexual risk behaviour. *C. trachomatis* is currently classified in 18 genotypes, or serovars, based on the genetic variation of the major outer membrane protein (MOMP). The genotypes most frequently producing genitourinary tract infection are genotypes D, E, F, G, H, I, J and K. In the last decade, the microbiological diagnosis of *C. trachomatis* infection has improved due to the development of nucleic acid amplification techniques (NAATs) and their progressive introduction in laboratories. Contact tracing is essential in the management of this infection to avoid reinfections. Due to the high and growing impact of *C. trachomatis* infection in public health, the main international agencies involved in STI surveillance (Centers for Disease Control and Prevention [CDC], European Centre for Disease Prevention and Control [ECDC]...) have proposed various prevention measures and levels of intervention to improve its control.

This chapter discusses the transmission and epidemiological data of *C. trachomatis* infection in women of reproductive age, especially pregnant women, and the etiopathogenic mechanisms causing its symptoms and sequelae on fertility and pregnancy. The management of this infection in pregnancy will be analysed in detail, focusing on diagnosis and appropriate treatment, information on the possible effects of this infection, and partner management, which may raise particularly delicate issues. Finally, the screening strategies established in several countries for the population groups with the highest prevalence of this infection will be described and their effectiveness in controlling its spread and in preventing its adverse effects on fertility, pregnancy and vertical transmission, will be analysed.

2. Epidemiology

2.1 Transmission

Transmission of *C. trachomatis* infection is through direct contact between the mucous membranes of two individuals during sexual activity or through an infected birth canal. Because of the anatomical characteristics of the female genital tract, the risk of contracting an STI is higher in women than in men.

As with other STI, the risk of *C. trachomatis* transmission is directly related to certain sexual activities, such as starting sexual relations at an early age, their frequency, and a recent change of partner, and especially to risk behaviours, such as sexual activity without protection or incorrect condom use, multiple sexual partners and promiscuity. Other risk factors are a history of contact with *C. trachomatis* or other STI, a previous STI, etc. Pregnant women are not free of these risks.

In the last few years, the incidence of this infection has increased, partly due to a false sense of security created by antiviral HIV therapy in some sectors of the population, leading to carelessness in the use of preventive methods during sexual relations, thus facilitating STI. A higher risk of infection has been described in persons with a low socioeconomic position and in substance abusers, due to lower awareness of and compliance with preventive measures in these population groups. Adolescents are the group most likely to engage in high-risk behaviours, such us unprotected sex, especially when they are under the influence of drugs or alcohol.

A major feature of the epidemiology of *C. trachomatis* infection is the high percentage of the infected population that may be asymptomatic, often for several months. While the percentage of asymptomatic infected men is estimated to be up to 50%, in women this percentage may be as high as 70-75% (18). Asymptomatic infected individuals may spread undiagnosed infection among the sexually active population. Consequently, to improve *C. trachomatis* infection control, in many countries screening strategies have been recommended in the population with the highest prevalence, in addition to treatment of cases and partner management to prevent reinfections.

Transmission of *C. trachomatis* infection among the population can also be facilitated by the emergence of mutated strains, as occurred in Sweden in 2006 with the new variant of *C. trachomatis* (nvCT), which was not detected with the molecular techniques used in some regions due to a 377 bp deletion in the cryptic plasmid (74). The nvCT caused many false-negative diagnoses, allowing this variant to spread to other northern European countries (91). Fortunately, spread beyond these countries has been limited (70).

Another important issue is that other microorganisms causing an STI, including HIV, hepatitis B virus, herpes simplex viruses, *Neisseria gonorrhoeae, Treponema pallidum,* can be transmitted in the same episode as that leading to *C. trachomatis* infection. Moreover, in *C. trachomatis*-infected individuals, there is a greater risk of acquiring and, in the case of coinfection, of transmitting other STI due to the inflammatory alterations produced in affected genital mucous membranes (28).

2.2 Incidence rate

C. trachomatis affects over 600 million people worldwide with more than 90 million new cases occurring globally each year (98). In the USA, more than 1.2 million new cases were reported in 2009, a rate of 409/100,000 people, the most frequently affected being young black women aged 15-24 years (22). In Europe, an incidence rate of 150/100,000 inhabitants has been reported, with an incidence of 1,200/100,000 among women aged between 15 and 24 years (35). The real figures are probably higher since cases are under-reported due to the marked differences in national surveillance and reporting systems. Indeed, some European countries do not provide data, others report very low incidence rates (<1/100,000 inhabitants), and some regions, such as Nordic countries or the UK, report incidence rates of >250/100,000 inhabitants. Consequently, the reported data should be interpreted with caution: a low rate could under estimate the real incidence if the diagnostic measures and reporting systems are inadequate; however an increasing rate may not reflect greater transmission of the infection in countries implementing screening programs that allow detection of asymptomatic cases. Nevertheless, the tendencies in data from several countries show that the reported incidence of *C. trachomatis* infection has increased considerably in the last few years (Figure 1). This increase may be due to the sum of multiple factors: the rise in sexual risk behaviours, decreased compliance with preventive measures, greater knowledge and awareness of *C. trachomatis* infection - leading to more frequent diagnosis -, increased sensitivity of diagnostic methods, and improvement in reporting systems, among other factors.

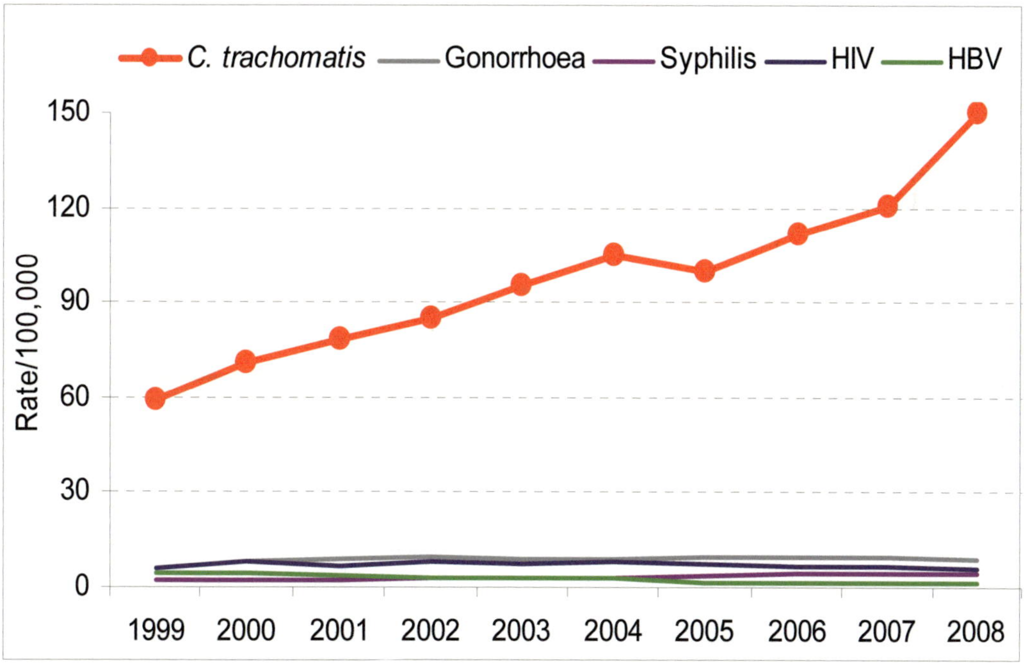

Fig. 1. Incidence rate of *C. trachomatis* and other sexually transmitted infections in the EU per 100,000 inhabitants (ECDC data). (HBV: hepatitis B virus).

Author, country, study period, (reference)	Samples	Population	Women analysed (prevalence)	Factors associated with higher prevalence
X.S. Chen et al, China (Fuzhou, Fujian), Jul-Sep/02 (25)	Cervix	Antenatal care attendees (first prenatal visit)	504 (10.1%)	Younger (18% in ≤25 years), higher monthly income
Pinto et al, Brazil (national study), Mar-Nov/09 (67)	Urine	Parturient women 15-24 years	2071 (9.8%)	Younger (13% in <20 years), first sexual intercourse <15 years, >1 partners/yr.
Romoren et al, Bostwana (Gaberone), Oct/00-Feb/01 (76)	Cervix	Antenatal care attendees	703 (8%)	Younger (<20 years), unmarried, <1 year in relationship
Kilmarx et al, Thailand (Bangkok and Chiang Rai), Jun-Dec/96 (51)	Urine	Antenatal care attendees (first prenatal visit)	1021 (5.7%)	Younger (13% in <20 years), higher gestational age
Silveira et al, USA (Baltimore, Maryland), Jul/05-Feb/08 (RS) (85)	Not provided	Parturient women with antenatal care information available	2127 (4.7%)	Younger (12% in <20 years), ethnicity (black), single, smoking, NG during pregnancy
Roberts et al, USA (Dallas, Texas), May-Sep/09 (75)	Cervix and urine	Pregnant women at 35-37 weeks' gestation	2018 (cervix: 4.3%) (urine: 4.1%)	Not provided
Rours et al, The Netherlands (Rotterdam), Feb/03-Jan/05 (77)	Urine	Pregnant women attending midwifery practice or antenatal clinic	4055 (3.9%)	Younger (13% in <21 years), ethnicity (16% in Antillean), single (12%)
McMillan et al, Ireland (Dublin), Jun/03-May/04 (60)	Urine	Asymptomatic pregnant women	783 (3.8%)	Younger and single
M.Y. Chen et al., Australia (Melbourne), Oct/06-Jul/07 (24)	Urine	Pregnant women 16-25 years	987 (3.2%)	>1 sexual partner in the past year (12%)
Böhm et al., Germany (national study), Apr-Dec/08 (RS) (14)	Cervix (group1), urine (group 2)	Asymptomatic (g1 and 2) or symptomatic (g 3) pregnant women	51164 (3.1%) g1: 31856 (3.3%) g2: 18169 (2.9%) g3: 1139 (2.0%)	Younger (10% in ≤20 years)

Author, country, study period, (reference)	Samples	Population	Women analysed (prevalence)	Factors associated with higher prevalence
Oakeshott et al, United Kingdom (south London), Jun/98-Jul/00 (63)	Vaginal (self taken), urine	Pregnant women <10 weeks' gestation (general practice and family planning clinic)	1216 (2.4%)	Younger (9% in <25 years, 14% in teenagers), ethnicity (9% in blacks)
Hospital Donostia, Spain (Data not yet published, Oct/10-May/11)	Urine	Pregnant women with complications and unselected parturient women	551 (1.5%)	Younger (5.2% in <30 years)

Abbreviations: NG: *Neisseria gonorrhoeae*; RS: retrospective study

Table 1. Prevalence of *C. trachomatis* infection determined by nucleic acid amplification techniques in studies performed in pregnant women (attending antenatal services) or parturient women throughout the world (if not otherwise specified, prospective, cross-sectional, observational studies).

In the last few years, numerous epidemiological studies have aimed to determine the prevalence of *C. trachomatis* infection in pregnant women, an essential step for the design of appropriate infection control programs in distinct geographical regions (Table 1). The results of these studies are influenced by the sociodemographic characteristics of the population studied, such as age, setting of the population tested, and risk factors, etc., as well as by the type of sample and the diagnostic method used. Currently, the methods of choice in these studies are based on NAATs, generally indicating a prevalence of between 1 and 10%, the highest prevalence being found among young pregnant women and single pregnant women. Specifically, the prevalence in women aged less than 20-22 years was >10% in studies performed in countries as far apart as Botswana, Brasil, Germany, the USA and Ireland.

3. Symptoms, etiopathogenesis, and sequelae

The main target of *C. trachomatis* are columnar epithelial cells, particularly in the cervix and urethra, as well as in the rectum, throat, and conjunctiva; in adult women, the squamous epithelium of the vagina is unreceptive to infection. Most infections in women start in the endocervix and the main clinical manifestation in symptomatic infections is cervicitis, sometimes with intermenstrual or postcoital bleeding or dyspareunia. Symptoms usually begin 2 to 6 weeks after infection. Vaginal discharge is present in 50% and is usually mucous and less abundant and purulent than in *Neisseria gonorrhoeae* infections. Dysuria and pollakiuria are infrequent, but urethritis can be associated with cervicitis. In women with hypogastric pain, pelvic inflammatory disease (PID) should be suspected. Depending on sexual practices, other local symptoms (pharyngeal, rectal) may be present. Without an accurate and rapid diagnosis, untreated infections (symptomatic or asymptomatic), may spread among the sexually active population and give rise to complications and sequelae.

The consequences of *C. trachomatis* infection for women's reproductive health can be severe. This pathogen may spread upward from the endocervix, possibly due to binding to spermatozoids or the passive transport mechanisms of the genital tract, causing endometritis, salpingitis or PID, which can lead to sequelae in 10-20% of patients, mainly infertility and ectopic pregnancy (19). The risk of PID is increased in women with *C. trachomatis* infection who undergo uterine instrumentation, which can reactivate the bacteria or provoke upward spread (4). In addition, *C. trachomatis* can occasionally cause HLA-B27-associated reactive arthritis, Reiter's syndrome, perihepatitis, and Fitz-Hugh-Curtis syndrome. Another complication of *C. trachomatis* infection is its possible role as a carcinogenic co-factor in the development of cervical neoplasms caused by high-risk human papillomavirus (HPV) types (66).

During pregnancy, these infections have been associated with premature rupture of membranes, premature delivery, low birth weight neonates, and miscarriage. Women can infect their neonates through the birth canal, causing conjunctivitis, nasopharyngitis and pneumonia. The risk of perinatal transmission has been estimated to be 20-50% for conjunctivitis (manifesting at 5-12 days after birth), frequently associated with nasopharyngeal infection, and 10-20% for pneumonia (at 1-3 months) (16). Postpartum endometritis can also be associated with *C. trachomatis* infection.

3.1 Factors involved in etiopathogenesis

Knowledge of the etiopathogenesis and mechanisms of interaction among microorganisms and their hosts is important to adopt the most appropriate prevention and control strategies, such as screening of high-risk populations, optimal screening intervals, etc., and will help in the development of future vaccines. Paradoxically, in some patients, the defense mechanisms against *C. trachomatis* infection - mainly the inflammatory and adaptive immune responses - could be harmful to tissues. Tissue lesions giving rise to sequelae could be of immunopathological origin rather than due to the direct action of chlamydia.

Epithelial cells are the first defense against *C. trachomatis* infection. On becoming infected, these cells secrete chemokines and cytokines, which stimulate the cellular inflammatory response (leucocytes, natural killer cells, dendritic cells...). The continuous release of some of these cytokines (interleukin [IL]-1, IL-8...), especially during chronic or repeated infections, can cause direct tissue damage and scarring (17,87).

In addition, shortly after *C. trachomatis* infection, an innate cellular immune response is produced, mediated mainly by $CD4^+$ T cells, with production of Th1-type cytokines, such as tumor necrosis factor (TNF)-α and interferon (INF)-γ, which inhibit intracellular chlamydial replication (39). If the infection is not eradicated and persists, or in repeat infections, adaptive T cell immune responses against *C. trachomatis* antigens can be produced, which could collaterally contribute to the development of inflammatory sequelae through autoimmune or delayed hypersensitivity mechanisms, which are still not well understood (17). In experimental animal models, in repeat infections, the enhanced inflammatory response may be mediated by cytotoxic $CD8^+$ T cells primed against chlamydial heat shock protein 60 (cHSP60), producing greater tissue destruction and fibrosis than in the initial infection, this risk increasing with each additional reinfection (56,71). Serum and genital mucosal IgA and IgG antibodies to specific *C. trachomatis* proteins such as cHSP and to chlamydial elementary bodies (EBs) are usually detected during active infection in women (37), but their precise role in the resolution of infection remains unclear.

In vitro studies have revealed that the peculiar metabolic cycle of *C. trachomatis* can be altered by INF-γ and other inducers. In a normal cycle, the infectious but metabolically inactive extracellular EBs infect cells, and once inside, they differentiate to non-infectious but metabolically active intracellular reticulate bodies (RBs) that multiply by binary fission within vacuoles. In turn, these RBs reorganize back to EBs that are released to the extracellular medium. In the altered cycle, morphologically enlarged, aberrant, and nondividing RBs are found in a viable but noncultivable state (100). This mechanism may contribute to persistent *C. trachomatis* infection in humans, avoiding the immune system and inducing an immunopathogenic response. However, the question of whether these altered RBs appear *in vivo* and are involved in the development of sequelae remains to be elucidated.

Other determining factors in the development of PID and sequelae may be the natural duration of untreated *C. trachomatis* infection in the host and the number of infections acquired. Approximately half of infections resolve spontaneously in the first year after initial chlamydia testing, but in some women infections may persist for several years. The duration of infection and the chlamydial load in repeat infections seem to be lower than in the first infection, suggesting the existence of some degree of partial immunity (37). However, repeat infections are common and are associated with a higher risk of PID and sequels (41). The sooner an infection is detected, the lower the microorganism's opportunity to ascend the upper genital tract and the lesser the time of action of the immunopathological mechanisms involved in the development of sequelae.

Only a minority of infected women develop reproductive disorders, due to differences in numerous factors including the type of dendritic cell, co-stimulatory molecule expression, the cytokine secretion pattern and hormone levels (1). Therefore, there may be a greater genetic predisposition linked to expression of specific *C. trachomatis* cell receptors, as well as differentiated mechanisms in the immunological response (HLA class I and II variants and functional polymorphisms in cytokine) that determines the result of infection in the host and its potential consequences (3,88).

Although the *ompA* gene of *C. trachomatis* evolves more rapidly than the remaining genome, and its product (MOMP) is exposed on the surface of EBs, there is no evidence that any genotypic *C. trachomatis* variant (MOMP serovars) has a greater capacity than other variants to spread or avoid the immune response and produce greater clinical severity (30,92). The possible roles of other *C. trachomatis* biomarkers, such as the polymorphic outer membrane autotransporter family of proteins (89), type III secretion system effectors (29), and the putative large cytotoxin (9) are currently being studied. These biomarkers could help to identify strain-specific variants with distinct pathogenic characteristics. Further studies that analyse the phenotypic behaviour of this microorganism together with the clinical and epidemiological features of the population studied are required. Furthermore, new studies should attempt to gain greater insight into the molecular epidemiology of the strains involved through techniques allowing high genotypic discrimination, such as multilocus sequence typing (MLST), variable number tandem repeat (VNTR)...

3.2 Main reproductive health sequelae in women

3.2.1 PID

PID includes several genital tract disorders among women, such as endometritis, salpingitis, tubo-ovarian abscess and pelvic peritonitis. For PID to occur, *C. trachomatis, N. gonorrhoeae,* or other microorganisms must spread upward from the lower genital tract, infecting and causing inflammation of the uterus, fallopian tubes, and ovaries. The most frequent cause of PID is *C. trachomatis* genital infection, and studies in women with laparoscopically proven PID have described a prevalence of 10-60% (86). However, the risk of developing PID among *C. trachomatis*-infected women is not well known since few prospective studies have been performed and the number of cases included has generally been small. Despite these limitations, the risk seems to be high: the results of a recent randomised controlled trial performed in the UK that included 75 women with untreated, asymptomatic *C. trachomatis* infection found that 9.5% (95% CI 4.7%-18.3%) developed PID over 1 year (63). Although current data are limited, the risk of developing PID seems to be higher in the first few weeks of infection (41).

The main clinical manifestation of PID is abdominal pain. However, particularly in the initial stages, the symptoms may be non-specific, consisting of abnormal discharge, intermenstrual or postcoital bleeding, fever, urinary frequency, low back pain, nausea/vomiting, etc., and several consultations are required to reach a diagnosis. After a PID - which can be symptomatic or subclinical - gynecological and reproductive sequelae may appear, such as infertility (15-20%), ectopic pregnancy (an increased risk of 6-10-fold) and chronic pelvic pain, as a result of alterations in the cilia lining the fallopian tubes, destruction of ciliated cells, tubal occlusion, scarring, or adhesion formation among pelvic organs. However, the risk of developing sequelae after PID caused by *C. trachomatis* and that caused by other etiologies seems to be similar (41). Genetic studies of individual immunopathogenetic factors have suggested that a single nucleotide polymorphism in inflammasome-associated NLRP3 is related to the severity of *C. trachomatis* infection (95). Screening for chlamydia infection and treatment can prevent PID, although, as mentioned in the section on prevention, some authors have questioned the cost-effectiveness of screening in the prevention of sequelae.

3.2.2 Tubal factor infertility

An estimated 5-15% of women of reproductive age are infertile, representing a major problem for more than 70 million women worldwide (15). According to the WHO, *C. trachomatis* postinfection damage of the fallopian tubes may cause 30–40% of cases of female infertility (99), the most common cause being PID.

Multiple mechanisms can contribute to the development of this severe repercussion of *C. trachomatis* infection. Studies in the murine model have demonstrated that interstitial cells of Cajal (ICC), which form a dense network associated with the smooth muscle cells of the oviduct, are the source of the electrical pacemaker activity responsible for oviduct motility and egg transport, and that these cells are damaged by the inflammatory responses released by chlamydia infection. The destruction of the oviduct ICC networks might contribute to oviduct stasis and pseudo-obstruction, functional block of oocyte transport and retention of secretions, which could progress to fibrosis, tubal occlusion and finally infertility (32). Hydrosalpinx, a result of tubal obstruction, is present in about 30% of women with tubal factor infertility (TFI), and the fluid can reflux into the uterine cavity, inhibiting implantation of embryos in the endometrium. In addition, cystic fibrosis transmembrane conductance regulator (CFTR), an AMP-activated chloride channel that regulates epithelial electrolyte and fluid secretion and whose expression is elevated in the reproductive tract of

C. trachomatis-infected women, has been implicated in the pathogenesis of hydrosalpinx formation (2). Moreover, CFTR expression has another effect on fertility in the uterus, given that this substance plays a role in the regulation of the balance between the fluid volume in the endometrial mucous membrane during the estrous cycle, which is involved in blastocyst implantation. In the murine model, CFTR overexpression induced by cytokine release during *C. trachomatis* infection leads to abnormal fluid accumulation in uterus at diestrus and to a reduced implantation rate (43).

In addition, individual genetic variations may play a major role in the immune response to *C. trachomatis* and in the pathogenesis of complications and sequelae. More specifically, functional polymorphisms in specific cytokine genes and other components of the host's immune and proinflammatory response (IL-10, IL-12, TNF-α, NRLP3...) are involved in the regulation of the immune response and contribute to the distinct manifestations of the disease and its outcomes (66). Lastly, the sequence identity shared between cHSP60 and human HSP60 (48.5%) has traditionally been considered to cause cross-reactivity and consequently autoimmunity, which could play a role in the pathogenesis of TFI. However, TFI has recently been associated with antibodies against cHSP60, but not against human HSP60, pointing to an infectious rather than an autoimmune inflammation and suggesting antibody testing as a supplement in TFI diagnosis (44).

3.2.3 Ectopic pregnancy

Approximately 1-2% of pregnancies are ectopic, and 97-98% occur in the Fallopian tubes, representing the main cause of maternal death in the first trimester of pregnancy (94). The risk of ectopic pregnancy is higher in women with Fallopian tube damage due to pelvic infections mainly by *C. trachomatis* or pelvic surgery, previous ectopic pregnancy, smoking and *in vitro* fertilization. Therefore, most of the above-mentioned etiopathogenic mechanisms of TFI can also cause an ectopic pregnancy.

Tubal ectopic pregnancy is caused by a combination of factors that allow embryo retention in the Fallopian tube due to limitations in tubal transport and/or alterations in the tubal environment that favour early egg implantation. The Fallopian tubes in women with ectopic pregnancies show altered expression of prokineticin receptors (PROKRs), a molecule involved in the control of smooth muscle contractility. Through ligation of tubal Toll-like receptor 2 and activation of NFκB (nuclear factor kappa-light-chain enhancer of activated B cells), *C. trachomatis* infection leads to increased tubal PROKR2, probably predisposing the tubal microenvironment to ectopic implantation (84). In addition, an increase in the expression of activins and inducible nitric oxide synthasa (iNOS) within the human Fallopian tube of patients with an ectopic pregnancy and antibodies against *C. trachomatis* has been observed, suggesting that these proteins may be involved in the microbial-mediated immune response that contributes to tubal damage and ectopic pregnancy (72). Nitric oxide production is considered to be part of the innate immune response (being bactericidal for intracellular pathogens, including *C. trachomatis*), but chronic chlamydia infections can lead to an excess of iNOS-derived nitric oxide, damaging tubal epithelial cells and possibly leading to an ectopic pregnancy (83). Lastly, the elafin molecule has anti-protease, anti-microbial, innate immune defence and anti-inflammatory properties and is found in various human mucosal membranes such as those of the female genital tract, and whose expression is increased in the Fallopian tubes of women with ectopic pregnancy. Elafin is also up-regulated in an *in-vitro* model in response to *C. trachomatis* infection (52).

3.2.4 Pregnancy outcomes

C. trachomatis infection during pregnancy has been associated with adverse outcomes such as premature rupture of membranes (PRM), premature delivery, low birth-weight and miscarriage. However, the results of studies on this topic have often been distinct and even contradictory. Many of these publications included a small number of women and used inappropriate serological methods to distinguish between current and past infection.

Recently, two large population-based studies (each with about 4000 women) have shed new light on the potential role of *C. trachomatis* in this context. A population-based retrospective cohort study carried out in Washington State (USA) using birth certificate data found that chlamydia-infected women had a higher risk of preterm delivery and PRM than a non-infected control group (13). Premature delivery (<37 weeks) occurs in 9.6% of all births worldwide and can be due to multiple factors, with 30% being related to PRM (8). The mechanism through which chlamydia causes PRM is not well known, but could be produced through choriodecidual inflammation and chorioamnionitis generated through some of the above-mentioned etiopathogenetic mechanisms. Interestingly, this risk has been reported to decrease in successfully treated patients, given that the frequency of PRM was lower than in patients who were treated but who had either persistent or recurrent chlamydia infection at the end of pregnancy; furthermore, the risk was not significantly different to the risk in those without *C. trachomatis* detection in pregnancy (27). In the second population-based cohort study, a prospective and non-interventional analysis during pregnancy performed in Holland, *C. trachomatis* infection detected with NAATs was significantly associated with prematurity before 35 weeks of pregnancy, this risk being higher before 32 weeks (78). Of deliveries before 32 and 35 weeks of pregnancy, 14.9% and 7.4%, respectively, were associated with *C. trachomatis* infection, suggesting that chlamydia contributes more to early than to late prematurity. In this study, pregnancy was shorter in chlamydia-positive women. Neither of these two population-based studies found that low birth weight (<2,500 g) or small-for-gestational-age neonates, or miscarriage were associated with maternal *C. trachomatis* infection.

A recent Polish study found that the prevalence of *C. trachomatis* detected by NAATs and serology was higher in women who miscarried than in other pregnant women, suggesting that chlamydial infection can cause spontaneous pregnancy loss (97). However, studies designed to analyse the possible role of *C. trachomatis* in miscarriage are lacking and this issue continues to be controversial. Finally, postpartum endometritis is a common complication in *C. trachomatis*-infected women.

3.2.5 Cervical neoplasia

Cervical neoplasia is the second most common cancer in women worldwide, the main cause being persistent infection with high-risk HPV. However, only a small proportion of HPV infections are persistent and progress to cervical cancer, suggesting that co-factors may also be involved in its carcinogenesis. Some seroepidemiological studies have associated *C. trachomatis* with the development of cervical squamous cell carcinoma, and it has even been suggested that this association could be greater with specific serotypes (G, I, D and B) (6,65). The results of two large (8441 women), multinational, clinical trials that evaluated the safety and efficacy of an HPV vaccine suggested that *C. trachomatis* is an independent, but moderate, co-factor for the development of cervical neoplasia. In addition, *C. trachomatis* seems to be involved only in the early stages of cervical carcinogenesis, as no increased risk associated with *C. trachomatis* was found for CIN-3 (55).

The mechanisms causing this association are unknown. *C. trachomatis* modulates the host immune response and inhibits apoptosis, which could encourage the persistence of infected HPV cells. Moreover, *C. trachomatis* induces inflammation and cervical metaplasia, favouring the access and propagation of HPV, given that metaplastic cells are potential targets for HPV. Chlamydia infection may increase the access of HPV to the basal epithelium and increases HPV viral load (66). Therefore, some authors argue that associations between *C. trachomatis* and cervical premalignancy could be caused, in part, by an increased susceptibility to HPV infection (79). In contrast, new molecular evidence now suggests that chlamydial protease-like activity factor induces centrosome amplification, which may help to explain the role of chlamydia in cervical carcinogenesis (49).

4. Microbiological diagnosis

This section aims to outline the microbiological diagnostic methods most commonly used in *C. trachomatis* infection and to define the most appropriate samples for diagnosis in women. Diagnostic techniques, which are discussed in another chapter, will not be described in detail. A general consideration when approaching the diagnosis of an STI in the clinical setting is that other microorganisms that could cause coinfection should always be investigated. Consequently, other bacterial causes, such as *N. gonorrhoeae* and *Trichomonas vaginalis*, among others, must be excluded and a serum sample must be requested to investigate HIV, hepatitis B and C viruses and syphilis infection. Obviously, this practice is not applied in most screening programmes.

Appropriate samples for *C. trachomatis* detection are cervical exudates, vaginal swabs and urine samples. Depending on the symptoms, conjunctival, pharyngeal and rectal exudates can also be obtained, as well as other samples in specific cases. Cervical exudates should be obtained by a gynecologist. Vaginal swabs can be self-collected or collected by a physician, with no differences in sensitivity or specificity (81). With urine sampling, it is essential to collect first-void urine, defined as the first 10-30mL of the urine, and for the patient not to have urinated for at least 2 hours previously. Self-collected vaginal swabs and first-void urine are samples that are widely accepted by women (12), and can be collected in-house and mailed to laboratories, thus facilitating epidemiological studies and screening programmes in asymptomatic women. In addition, urine allows samples to be grouped into pools and increases the cost-effectiveness of studies, with little reduction in sensitivity (77). A large German study, using 5 urine pools, obtained a negative predictive value of 98.1% for the pooling system (14).

A wide variety of techniques are available for *C. trachomatis* detection. Cell culture, antigen-based detection methods, such as direct fluorescent assay, immunochromatography and enzyme immunoassay, and nucleic acid hybridization tests have been widely used in clinical laboratories. Due to their lower sensitivity, all these techniques are being substituted by NAATs, which increase detection by 20-40% and are the currently recommended techniques. However, NAATs are expensive and their introduction for *C. trachomatis* detection may be difficult in some laboratories. The chlamydial load is lower in urine than in vaginal swabs and is lower in the latter than in endocervical swabs (61). Therefore, vaginal swabs and urine should only be analysed through molecular amplification methods. These distinct chlamydial loads probably explain the lower sensitivity found by some authors when using first-void urine rather than vaginal or endocervical swabs (14), although this difference has not been found in all studies (75). The most recent NAATs use specific primers and probes that target two cryptic plasmid fragments or a fragment of the cryptic plasmid and another fragment of the *ompA* gene. These new NAATs are able to detect variants with deletions in the cryptic plasmid such as the new Swedish *C. trachomatis* variant (nvCT), first detected in 2006. The nvCT variant contains a 377-bp deletion in the cryptic plasmid that covers the single targets originally utilized in some commercial NAATs (74). The use of modern automatic nucleic acid extraction devices also helps to improve the sensitivity of techniques that perform manual extraction through lysis (69).

Numerous point-of-care tests, based on immunological methods and providing rapid diagnosis have been designed for *C. trachomatis* detection. The sensitivity of these tests is currently considered to be inadequate, at around <50%, as is their specificity, given that most are based on lipopolysaccharide detection, which often presents cross-reaction with the lipopolysaccharide of Gram-negative bacteria, leading to the possibility of false-positive results. Given this possibility, the development of a point-of-care tests that detects *C. trachomatis* with sufficient sensitivity (>90%) is currently a pressing need (48). Recently, new tests based on signal amplification systems have shown a higher sensitivity of around 80% (59).

Serological methods are not useful in the diagnosis of uncomplicated *C. trachomatis* infection. The antibody profile generated in acute and chronic infection is not well known. Moreover, the serological response can been inconsistent or weak, since the infection is usually limited to the mucosal surface. Nevertheless, antibody detection is considered important in women with TFI, as serological evidence of past infection is associated with a significantly increased risk of women suffering TFI (4). Likewise, serological methods are useful in epidemiological studies (53).

C. trachomatis typing can be performed through serotyping with monoclonal antibodies against the MOMP protein or genotyping of the *ompA* gene, whether through restriction fragment length polymorphism analysis or sequencing. Genotyping through sequencing is easier to implement in clinical laboratories and can be performed directly in the clinical sample, which explains its increasing use. This technique is allowing the worldwide distribution of distinct genotypes of *C. trachomatis* to be determined and its possible geographical features and temporal evolution to be compared (68). Other techniques allowing greater discrimination and differentiation among strains, such as MLST and VNTR, have been developed; these techniques will help to generate further insight into the natural history of the infection, thus enabling detailed clinical-epidemiological studies and aiding vaccine design.

5. Treatment

In addition to accurate diagnosis and appropriate antibiotic therapy, the management of uncomplicated *C. trachomatis* infection also requires counseling and treatment of the sexual partner(s), which reduces the possibility of reinfection of the original partner and infection of possible other partners, thus decreasing transmission within the community.

C. trachomatis is usually susceptible to tetracyclines, macrolides, fluoroquinolones, amoxicillin, rifampin and sulfonamides, among other antibiotics. With rare exceptions, such as rifampin, chlamydiae do not easily develop resistances to antibiotics and, because these microorganisms are obligate intracellular bacteria they are unlikely to acquire resistance genes from other bacteria through horizontal transmission (45). Although there are few studies of antimicrobial susceptibility in *C. trachomatis*, reports of isolates in patients with resistance strains are scarce, and in most of these reports, the isolates screened displayed characteristics of heterotypic resistance, affecting only a small part of the bacterial population. This type of resistance often disappears with the spread of the bacteria (80). However, heterotypic resistance could cause treatment failure in patients with high chlamydial load (46). A recent European study that included *C. trachomatis* isolates from all the urogenital serovars (D through K, n=45) found that all the isolates were susceptible to the antimicrobials tested: levofloxacin, erythromycin, doxycycline, clarithromycin, and azithromycin (33). Nevertheless, in India, decreased antibiotic susceptibility to azithromycin and doxycycline has been reported in 38% - a significant proportion - of the strains isolated in patients with recurrent infections (10). The advisability of monitoring the development of *C. trachomatis* resistance is hampered by the lack of standardized antimicrobial susceptibility tests, which currently require cell cultures.

The standard treatment regimens for uncomplicated lower genital tract infections are one dose of azithromycin or two doses/day of doxycycline for 7 days (Table 2). Both regimens have shown an efficacy of >95% in the microbial cure of *C. trachomatis* (54), although compliance is lower with doxycycline. A single dose of azithromycin should be the treatment of choice in persons who may not be able to comply with longer treatment regimens. Other alternatives are erythromycin, which is associated with a higher rate of adverse effects, and ofloxacin and levofloxacin, which are more expensive. The treatment of HIV-infected women is similar. Treatment should be started as soon as possible, especially in women with urethritis/cervicitis with clear secretion and/or more then 5 leukocytes per field in the Gram stain, even when an etiologic diagnosis is unavailable. In these patients, the recommended empirical treatment includes an oral dose of azithromycin and an intramuscular dose of ceftriaxone to cover possible infection by - or coinfection with -*N. gonorrhoeae*. After starting treatment, patients should abstain from sexual contact for 7 days.

Infection	Antibiotic treatment
Urethritis/cervicitis	Azithromycin 1 g po 1 dose Doxycycline 100 mg/12h po 7 days
Lymphogranuloma venereum	Doxycycline 100 mg/12h po 21 days
PID	Cefoxitin 2 g/6h IV + doxycycline 100 mg/12h po Clindamycin 900 mg/8h IV + gentamicin 1.5 mg/kg/8h IM/IV
Pregnancy	Azithromycin 1 g po 1 dose Amoxicillin 500 mg/8h po 7 days
Ophthalmia neonatorum	Erythromycin base or ethylsuccinate 50 mg/kg/day (4 doses) po 14 days
Infant pneumonia	Erythromycin base or ethylsuccinate 50 mg/kg/day (4 doses) po 14 days

Table 2. Recommended regimens of antibiotic treatment in *C. trachomatis* infections

An indispensable component of treatment is partner management. This strategy is often difficult but it is essential to strongly advise patients to inform their sexual partners of their infection and for their partners to be examined. All sexual partners in the 60 days prior to symptom onset in the index case - or the last contact, if more than 60 days previously - must be diagnosed and treated. When attendance by sexual partners is highly unlikely, the index patient may be given the partner's treatment and instructed in its use, a practice known as expedited partner therapy, which is easier if azithromycin is used. Lack of partner management is usually the most frequent cause of reinfection, and expedited partner therapy has been shown to be useful in ensuring partner treatment among men and in reducing repeat infections among women (20).

A cure test is not routinely recommended if treatment of the index case has been adequate. This test is recommended in pregnancy (see below) and when there is doubt about treatment compliance, suspected reinfection or persistent symptoms. When a cure test is performed, NAATs should be used 3-5 weeks after the end of treatment. *C. trachomatis* nucleic acids can persist in cells for up to 3 weeks (23). Nevertheless, since reinfection is frequent in persons with previous *C. trachomatis* infection (47), a new test of *C. trachomatis* detection is recommended approximately 3 months after the end of treatment (23).

In pregnancy, tetracyclines and fluoroquinolones are contraindicated. The recommended antibiotics are azithromycin, amoxicillin and erythromycin and the current first-line choice is a single oral dose of 1 g of azithromycin. Erythromycin produces a higher frequency of gastrointestinal adverse effects, requiring treatment withdrawal; moreover, in pregnant women, liver clearance of this drug is increased, which could reduce its plasma concentration, thus increasing the risk of treatment failure (66). Due to the lower effectiveness of antimicrobials in pregnancy, as well as the possible adverse effects on pregnancy course and the possibility of neonatal transmission, a cure test is recommended 3-5 weeks after the end of treatment, as well as a further test at 3 months to exclude reinfection. In pregnant women with risk factors, such as those aged ≤25 years or with several sexual partners or a new sexual partner, an additional test should be performed in the third trimester of pregnancy (23).

The treatments recommended in other situations are shown in table 2. Treatment of PID falls beyond the scope of this chapter. However, since *C. trachomatis* is one of the most common causes of PID, the etiology of PID is often polymicrobial and *C. trachomatis* detection in cases of PID is far from easy - especially without samples from the upper-genital tract - treatment of *C. trachomatis* should be covered in all patients with PID.

Lastly, prophylaxis or specific treatment in the neonates of mothers with genital C. trachomatis infection is not recommended. These neonates should be monitored clinically to allow microbiological diagnosis and treatment if symptoms develop: up to one month should be allowed for the development of conjunctivitis, and up to 3 months for pneumonia.

6. Prevention

In addition to being easily treated with antibiotics, *C. trachomatis* infection is preventable. Because of the increasing incidence rates of this infection, the high percentage of the population that may have asymptomatic infection, and the severity of its potential sequelae, various control programs have been developed. The CDC in the USA recommend annual chlamydia screening in all sexually active women aged ≤25 years and in older women with risk factors. Screening of all pregnant women is also recommended (23). In Europe, the ECDC have described four levels of intervention in *C. trachomatis* infection control (34): A) primary prevention: sexual health promotion and information; B) case management: guidelines for clinical and microbiological diagnosis, as well as for patient treatment, which includes contact tracing, and a system for case reporting; C) "opportunistic" testing: screening in asymptomatic persons from specified groups considered at risk to detect new cases, mainly in young persons and/or those with several sexual partners when attending health services for other reasons; and D) proactive systematic population-based screening, aimed at covering a substantial portion of a defined population to reduce the prevalence of infection. Although most European countries carry out the first two levels, fewer have experience and knowledge of the third and fourth levels. In this context, no consistent association between the economic resources of a country and the intensity of chlamydia control activities has been found (57). In their guidelines, the ECDC recognizes that there is insufficient epidemiological information for decision making and aims to obtain sufficient data between 2010-11.

The increase in the last few years in the incidence rates of several STI such as *C. trachomatis* infection highlights the need to maintain and, if possible, intensify primary prevention through health education and safe sex campaigns, such as correct and consistent condom use. Information campaigns are essential to raise awareness of STI not only among young people but also among their parents and even the physicians involved in the management of these infections (96), since the stigma commonly associated with STI is usually a handicap to their management and to adherence to prevention programmes. Primary prevention of *C. trachomatis* infection through vaccination is not yet feasible. The complex antigen structure of this pathogen and still insufficient knowledge of the protective *C. trachomatis* antigens involved in the immune response have proven to be a barrier to the development of effective vaccines.

Secondary prevention through opportunistic or systematic screening is still the most important intervention to limit the adverse effects of *C. trachomatis* infection on reproductive health (66). Screening for chlamydia in females aged <25 years has been described as one of the most beneficial and cost-effective preventive services that can be offered in medical practice (58), and has been considered as an A-rated recommended preventive service (strongest recommendation) (93). Screening of men has not been shown to be cost-efficient and, although this practice could prevent many infections in women, its impact on the burden of disease in women by testing young men or specific risk groups is controversial (38,50).

Preventive strategies should focus especially on the young, because the incidence rates of infection are much higher in this population group and the increase observed in the last decade has affected mainly this age group, with little variation in other age groups (73). To comply with the objectives of public health programmes and reduce transmission among the population as far as possible, both wide acceptance among the target population and high coverage and regular uptake are essential (53). Unfortunately, screening coverage rates do not usually exceed 60%, partly due to lack of knowledge among some young women about the need for screening and the social stigma attached to STI (21,58). Publicity campaigns and strategies such as "Get Yourself Tested" (available at http://www.gytnow.org) aim to improve these results and avoid the formation of core groups with high reinfection rates, such as sexually active adolescent girls or young men with a previous history of STI (7,36,66). The various screening modalities have contributed to the increase in the number of detected cases, without this increase representing a real rise in incidence, given that it essentially reveals previously undetected asymptomatic infections. Moreover, recent studies using mathematical models suggest that screening reduces the prevalence of infection (50,90).

Opportunistic screenings aim to halt spread of infection and avoid its sequelae through detection of new cases in asymptomatically infected risk groups. The most common target groups are usually sexually active young persons, especially those with frequent changes of partner, pregnant women, women seeking pregnancy termination, and those undergoing instrumentation of the uterus. Partly due to differences in the local epidemiology and burden of disease, various policies and practices are underway in several countries such as the USA, England, Denmark, Estonia, Iceland, Latvia, Norway, and Sweden, although not all of these policies are nationwide and some are implemented in specific regions only (19,34,50,57). Women are usually more willing than men to undergo diagnostic tests for STI. For example, in Sweden, less than 30% of all persons tested for chlamydia are men (42). Since 2003 in Stockholm and currently in other Swedish counties, there is an opportunistic screening called "Chlamydia Monday", because the campaign takes place annually one Monday in September. Every year, the number of chlamydia cases reported in Sweden is higher in September and October, since the opportunities of finding a new sexual partner and becoming infected increase in summer. During the campaign, massive media activity provides information and promotes condom use to prevent STI, and encourages people to get tested for chlamydia with the aim of recruiting young men in particular, who request testing less than women. "Chlamydia Monday" helps to raise awareness of the importance of STI among the public and is a cost-effective intervention to decrease the prevalence of chlamydia and its complications in Sweden, encouraging both men and women to seek testing (31).

Systematic screening for chlamydia using the internet and self-sampling kits has been implemented in certain regions of The Netherlands among 16 to 29 year-olds and its results in terms of the impact on population prevalence and cost-effectiveness evaluation will allow the advisability of implementing a nationwide chlamydia screening programme to be assessed and the optimal strategy to be designed. The acceptability of this home-based screening was high, the response rate being 63% (40); however, increasing this response remains difficult. Innovative strategies such as those used in this programme that combine confidentiality, simplicity and perception of the benefit of screening could increase the participation achieved in opportunistic screenings.

Knowledge of the impact of chlamydia screening on individuals and public health is limited (39,53). The health gains and cost-savings obtained by *C. trachomatis* screening programmes may have been overestimated, especially in epidemiological studies using serological techniques. The effect of screenings on reducing the risk of developing complications and sequelae has been analysed in some studies that have reached distinct conclusions; furthermore, comparison of these studies is difficult due to their various limitations, such as the study type and duration, the age groups analysed, and the multifactorial causes of the sequelae, among other factors. A large nonrandomized cohort study in female US Army recruits found no differences in hospitalizations for PID among women who were screened compared with those who were not (26). Equally, a randomised study with 9-year follow-up in women aged 21-23 years performed in Denmark found no differences between screened and non-screened women in the rates of PID and long-term risk of reproductive complications as the outcome (5). In contrast, two randomized trials comparing chlamydia screening in young women with a control group not invited for testing found a 50% reduction in PID over the subsequent year (64,82). Finally, in another randomised trial, limited evidence was observed suggesting that screening for chlamydia reduces PID rates: 10% of asymptomatic infected women not treated developed PID within a year, versus 2% of screened and treated women (63). Further studies evaluating the effectiveness of chlamydia screening are clearly needed.

The risk of longer-term reproductive health consequences, such as infertility and ectopic pregnancy, is low after treatment of a single episode (62,66); however, as previously mentioned, the development of sequelae is influenced by the immunopathological changes produced after successive reinfections and by the length of the infection (39). Therefore, the optimal frequency for testing is currently estimated to be once a year or with each change of partner. In this context, tertiary prevention - i.e. accurate diagnosis and appropriate treatment - shortens the duration of infection, and, if partner management is included, prevents transmission chains and reinfections.

In countries with a high prevalence of *C. trachomatis* infection, screening in pregnant or puerperal women increases infection control by including a substantial proportion of the target population. There is evidence of improved pregnancy and birth outcomes for pregnant women aged <25 years treated for chlamydia, and screening has been recommended (93). No studies have evaluated the effectiveness of screening in pregnant women aged >25 years old, but this practice could prevent adverse pregnancy outcomes and vertical infection. For these reasons, universal screening in pregnancy should be considered unless selective criteria can be validated (85). If the screening is performed at the beginning of pregnancy, there is a risk of not preventing possible reinfections, and if performed at the end, some of the complications of infection during pregnancy cannot be avoided. The CDC has recommended screening in all women at the first antenatal visit with rescreening in the third trimester in women aged ≤25 years and those who have a new or more than one sexual partner, as these are the women at highest risk. Women usually have little awareness of the transmission and effects of chlamydia before being tested, and the high acceptance of screening demonstrated in young women who have previously been informed of the sequels of this infection and its possible consequences on the health of their neonates will be essential to the uptake of chlamydia screening in future antenatal screening strategies (11).

In summary, most chlamydia infections are undetected and therefore the potential complications and sequels that can arise are not prevented. In the next few years, improvement in screening programs due to the knowledge currently being gained will probably enhance not only individual benefit, but also the impact on public health.

7. Conclusion

C. trachomatis genital infection is an increasing public health problem worldwide and has major adverse effects on women's reproductive health and in pregnancy. This infection may go unnoticed in up to 75% of infected women. The development of molecular amplification techniques in the last few years has increased the sensitivity and specificity of the detection of this intracellular bacterium. Infection is easily treated with antibiotics, while single-dose therapy improves adherence. An essential part of treatment is contact management. However, the most effective weapon is prevention. The adoption of the optimal preventive measures for each country is helped by better knowledge of the incidence, prevalence and impact of this infection. National health systems should make every effort to improve surveillance and to provide information on this infection, its potential consequences and the possibilities of prevention to the public. Special emphasis should be placed on young persons and on the core groups that are least likely to follow these preventive measures. Prevention can be enhanced through screening, which is especially important in pregnant women to reduce complications in both the pregnancy and the neonate. Despite the progress made in the last few years in the knowledge of etiopathogenesis, diagnosis, treatment and prevention of *C. trachomatis*, further research is required to reduce the burden of this infection.

8. Acknowledgment

This study was partially funded by a grant from the *Fondo de Investigación Sanitaria* (FIS PI10/02191).

9. References

[1] Agraval, T., Vats, V., Wallace, P.K., Salhan, S. & Mittal, A. (2008). Role of cervical dendritic cell subsets, co-stimulatory molecules, cytokine secretion profile and beta-estradiol in development of sequalae to Chlamydia trachomatis infection. *Reproductive Biology and Endocrinology*, Vol. 1. No. 6, (October 2008), pp. 46, ISSN 1477-7827

[2] Ajonuma, L.C., Chan, P.K., Ng, E.H., Fok, K.L., Wong, C.H., Tsang, L.L., Tang, X.X., Ho, L.S., Lau, M.C., Chung, C.M., He, Q., Huang, H.Y., Yang, D.Z., Rowlands, D.K., Chung, Y.W. & Chan, H.C. (2008). Involvement of cystic fibrosis transmembrane conductance regulator (CFTR) in the pathogenesis of hydrosalpinx induced by Chlamydia trachomatis infection. *The Journal of Obstetrics and Gynaecology Research*, Vol. 34, No. 6, (December 2008), pp. 923-930, ISSN 1341-8076

[3] Ajonuma, L.C., Fok, K.L., Ho, L.S., Chan, P.K., Chow, P.H., Tsang, L.L., Wong, C.H., Chen, J., Li, S., Rowlands, D.K., Chung, Y.W. & Chan, H.C. (2010). CFTR is required for cellular entry and internalization of Chlamydia trachomatis. *Cell Biology International*, Vol. 34, No. 6, (April 2010), pp. 593-600, ISSN 1065-6995

[4] Akande, V., Turner, C., Horner, P., Horne, A. & Pacey, A; British Fertility Society. (2010). Impact of Chlamydia trachomatis in the reproductive setting: British Fertility Society Guidelines for practice. *Human Fertility (Cambridge, England)*, Vol. 13, No.3, (September 2010), pp. 115-125, ISSN 1464-7273

[5] Andersen, B., van Valkengoed, I., Sokolowski, I., Møller, J.K., Østergaard, L. & Olesen, F. (2011). Impact of intensified testing for urogenital Chlamydia trachomatis infections: a randomised study with 9-year follow-up. *Sexually Transmitted Infections*, Vol. 87, No. 2, (March 2011), pp. 156-161, ISSN 1368-4973

[6] Anttila, T., Saikku, P., Koskela, P., Bloigu, A., Dillner, J., Ikäheimo, I., Jellum, E., Lehtinen, M., Lenner, P., Hakulinen, T., Närvänen, A., Pukkala, E., Thoresen, S.,

Youngman, L. & Paavonen, J. (2001). Serotypes of Chlamydia trachomatis and risk for cervical squamous cell carcinoma. *The Journal of American Medical Association*, Vol. 285, No. 1 (January 2001), pp. 47–51, ISSN 0098-7484

[7] Batteiger, B.E., Tu, W., Ofner, S., Van Der Pol, B., Stothard, D.R., Orr, D.P., Katz, B.P. & Fortenberry, J.D. (2010). Repeated Chlamydia trachomatis genital infections in adolescent women. *The Journal of Infectious Diseases*, Vol. 201, No. 1, (January 2010), pp. 42-51, ISSN 0022-1899

[8] Beck, S., Wojdyla, D., Say, L., Betran, A.P., Merialdi, M., Requejo, J.H., Rubens, C., Menon, R. & Van Look, P.F. (2010). The worldwide incidence of preterm birth: a systematic review of maternal mortality and morbidity. *Bulletin of the World Health Organization*, Vol. 88 No. 1, (January 2010), pp. 31-38, ISSN 0042-9686

[9] Belland, R.J., Scidmore, M.A., Crane, D.D., Hogan, D.M., Whitmire, W., McClarty, G. & Caldwell, H.D. (2001). *Chlamydia trachomatis* cytotoxicity associated with complete and partial cytotoxin genes. *Proceedings of the National Academy of Sciences of the United States of America*, Vol. 98, No. 24, (November 2001), pp. 13984–13989, ISSN 0027-8424

[10] Bhengraj, A.R., Vardhan, H., Srivastava, P., Salhan, S. & Mittal, A. (2010). Decreased susceptibility to azithromycin and doxycycline in clinical isolates of Chlamydia trachomatis obtained from recurrently infected female patients in India. *Chemotherapy*, Vol. 56, No. 5, (October 2010), pp. 371-377, ISSN 0009-3157

[11] Bilardi, J.E., De Guingand, D.L., Temple-Smith, M.J., Garland, S., Fairley, C.K., Grover, S., Wallace, E., Hocking, J.S., Tabrizi, S., Pirotta, M. & Chen, M.Y. (2010). Young pregnant women's views on the acceptability of screening for chlamydia as part of routine antenatal care. *BioMed Central Public Health*, Vol. 19, No. 10, (August 2010), pp. 505, ISSN 1471-2458

[12] Blake, D.R., Maldeis, N., Barnes, M.R., Hardick, A., Quinn, T.C. & Gaydos, C.A. (2008). Cost-effectiveness of screening strategies for Chlamydia trachomatis using cervical swabs, urine, and self-obtained vaginal swabs in a sexually transmitted disease clinic setting. *Sexually Transmitted Diseases*, Vol 35, No. 7, (July 2008), pp. 649-655, ISSN 0148-5717

[13] Blas, M.M., Canchihuaman, F.A., Alva, I.E. & Hawes, S.E. (2007). Pregnancy outcomes in women infected with Chlamydia trachomatis: a population-based cohort study in Washington State. *Sexually Transmitted Infections*, Vol 83, No. 4, (July 2007), pp. 314-318, ISSN 1368-4973

[14] Böhm, I., Gröning, A., Sommer, B., Müller, H.W., Krawczak, M. & Glaubitz, R. (2009). A German Chlamydia trachomatis screening program employing semi-automated real-time PCR: results and perspectives. *Journal of Clinical Virology*, Vol. 46, Suppl. 3, (November 2009), pp. 27-32, ISSN 1386-6532

[15] Boivin, J., Bunting, L., Collins, J.A. & Negron KG. (2007). International estimates of infertility prevalence and treatment-seeking: potential need and demand for infertility medical care. *Human Reproduction (Oxford, England)*, Vol. 22, No. 6, (June 2007), pp. 1506-1512, ISSN 0268-1161

[16] Brocklehurst. P. & Rooney G. Interventions for treating genital Chlamydia trachomatis infection in pregnancy. (2009). *Cochrane Database of Systematic Reviews* 1998, Issue 4, Art. No. CD000054, (June 1998, updated 2009), DOI: 10.1002/14651858.CD000054, ISSN 1361-6137

[17] Carey, A.J. & Beagley, K.W. (2010). Chlamydia trachomatis, a hidden epidemic: effects on female reproduction and options of treatment. American *Journal of Reproductive Immunology*, Vol. 63, No. 6, (June 2010), pp. 576-586, ISSN 0165-0378

[18] Cates, W. & Wasserheit, J.N. (1991). Genital chlamydial infections: epidemiology and reproductive sequelae. *American Journal of Obstetetrics and Gynecology*, Vol. 164, No. 6 Pt 2, (June 1991), pp. 1771-81, ISSN 0002-9378

[19] Centers for Disease Control and Prevention. (2002). Screening tests to detect Chlamydia trachomatis and Neisseria gonorrhoeae infections - 2002. *Morbidity and Mortality Weekly Report*, Vol. 51, No. RR15, (October 2002), pp. 1-39, ISSN 0149-2195

[20] Centers for Disease Control and Prevention. (2006). Expedited partner therapy in the management of sexually transmitted diseases. Atlanta, GA: US Department of Health and Human Services, CDC; 2006. In: *CDC*, 03.08.2011, Available from: http://www.cdc.gov/std/treatment/eptfinalreport2006.pdf.

[21] Centers for Disease Control and Prevention. (2009). Chlamydia screening among sexually active young female enrollees of health plans–United States, 2000–2007. *Morbidity and Mortality Weekly Report*, Vol. 58, No. 14, (April 2009), pp. 362–365, ISSN 0149-2195

[22] Centers for Disease Control and Prevention. (2010). Trends in Sexually Transmitted Diseases in the United States: 2009 National Data for Gonorrhea, Chlamydia and Syphilis, In: *CDC*, 30/05/2011, Available from : http://www.cdc.gov/std/stats09/trends2009.pdf

[23] Centers for Disease Control and Prevention, Workowski, K.A., Berman, S.M. (2010). Sexually transmitted diseases treatment guidelines, 2010. *Morbidity and Mortality Weekly Report*, Vol. 59, No. RR-12, (December 2010), pp. 1-110, ISSN 0149-2195

[24] Chen, M.Y., Fairley, C.K., De Guingand, D., Hocking, J., Tabrizi, S., Wallace, E.M., Grover, S., Gurrin, L., Carter, R., Pirotta, M. & Garland, S. (2009). Screening pregnant women for chlamydia: what are the predictors of infection? *Sexually Transmitted Infections*, Vol. 85, No. 1, (February 2009), pp. 31-5, ISSN 1368-4973

[25] Chen, X.S., Yin, Y.P., Chen L.P., Yu, Y.H., Wei, W.H., Thuy N.T., et al. (2006). Sexually transmitted infections among pregnant women attending an antenatal clinic in Fuzhou, China. *Sexually Transmited Diseases*, Vol. 33, No. 5, (May 2006), pp. 296 - 301, ISSN 0148-5717

[26] Clark, K.L., Howell, M.R., Li, Y., Powers, T., McKee, K.T. Jr., Quinn, T.C., Gaydos, J.C. & Gaydos, C.A. (2002). Hospitalization rates in female US Army recruits associated with a screening program for Chlamydia trachomatis. *Sexually Transmitted Diseases*, Vol. 29, No. 1, (January 2002), pp.1–5, ISSN 0148-5717

[27] Cohen, I., Veille, J.C. & Calkins, B.M. (1990). Improved pregnancy outcome following successful treatment of chlamydial infection. *The Journal of American Medical Association*, Vol. 263, No. 23 (June 1990), pp. 3160-3163, ISSN 0098-7484

[28] Cohen, M.S. (1998). Sexually transmitted diseases enhance HIV transmission: no longer a hypothesis. *The Lancet*, Vol. 351, Suppl 3, (June 1998), pp. 5-7, ISSN 0140-6736

[29] Cornelis, G.R. & Van, G.F. (2000). Assembly and function of type III secretory systems. *Annual Review of Microbiology*, Vol. 54, (October 2000), pp. 735–774, ISSN 0066-4227

[30] Dean, D., Bruno, W.J., Wan, R., Gomes, J.P., Devignot, S., Mehari, T., de Vries, H.J., Morré, S.A., Myers, G., Read, T.D. & Spratt BG. (2009). Predicting phenotype and emerging strains among Chlamydia trachomatis infections. *Emerging Infectious Diseases*, Vol. 15, No. 9, (September 2009), 1385-94, ISSN 1080-6059

[31] Deogan, C.L., Bocangel, M.K., Wamala, S.P. & Månsdotter, A.M. (2010). A cost-effectiveness analysis of the Chlamydia Monday--a community-based intervention to decrease the prevalence of chlamydia in Sweden. *Scandinavian Journal of Public Health,* Vol. 38, No. 2 (March 2010), pp. 141-150, ISSN 1403-4948

[32] Dixon, R.E., Hwang, S.J., Hennig, G.W., Ramsey, K.H., Schripsema, J.H., Sanders, K.M. & Ward, S.M. (2009). Chlamydia infection causes loss of pacemaker cells and inhibits oocyte transport in the mouse oviduct. *Biology of Reproduction,* Vol. 80, No. 4, (April 2009), pp. 665-673, ISSN 0006-3363

[33] Donati, M., Di Francesco, A., D'Antuono, A., Delucca, F., Shurdhi, A., Moroni, A., Baldelli, R. & Cevenini, R. (2010). In vitro activities of several antimicrobial agents against recently isolated and genotyped Chlamydia trachomatis urogenital serovars D through K. *Antimicrobial Agents and Chemotherapy,* Vol. 54, No. 12, (December 2010), pp. 5379-5380, ISSN 0066-4804

[34] European Centre for Disease Prevention and Control. (June 2009). Chlamydia control in Europe, In: *ECDC,* 12.05.2011, Available from: http://www.ecdc.europa.eu/en/files/pdf/Health_topics/0906_GUI_Chlamydia_Control_in_Europe.pdf

[35] European Centre for Disease Prevention and Control. (2010). Annual epidemiological report on communicable diseases in Europe 2010, In: *ECDC,* 03.08.2011, Available from:
http://www.ecdc.europa.eu/en/publications/Publications/1011_SUR_Annual_Epidemiological_Report_on_Communicable_Diseases_in_Europe.pdf

[36] Fung, M., Scott, K.C., Kent, C.K. & Klausner, J.D. (2007). Chlamydial and gonococcal reinfection among men: a systematic review of data to evaluate the need for retesting. *Sexually Transmitted Infections,* Vol 83, No. 4, (July 2007), pp. 304-309, ISSN 1368-4973

[37] Geisler, W.M. (2010). Duration of untreated, uncomplicated Chlamydia trachomatis genital infection and factors associated with chlamydia resolution: a review of human studies. *The Journal of Infectious Diseases,* Vol. 201, Suppl 2 (June 2010), pp. S104-113, ISSN 0022-1899

[38] Gift, T.L., Blake, D.R., Gaydos, C.A. & Marrazzo, J.M. (2008). The cost-effectiveness of screening men for Chlamydia trachomatis: a review of the literature. *Sexually Transmitted Diseases,* Vol. 35, Suppl. 11, (November 2008), pp. S51-60, ISSN 0148-5717

[39] Gottlieb, S.L., Martin, D.H., Xu, F., Byrne, G.I. & Brunham RC. (2010). Summary: The natural history and immunobiology of Chlamydia trachomatis genital infection and implications for Chlamydia control. *The Journal of Infectious Diseases,* Vol. 201, Suppl 2 (June 2010), pp. S190-204, ISSN 0022-1899

[40] Greenland, K.E., Op de Coul, E.L., van Bergen, J.E., Brouwers, E.E., Fennema, H.J., Götz, H.M., Hoebe, C.J., Koekenbier, R.H., Pars, L.L., van Ravesteijn, S.M. & van den Broek, I.V. (2011). Acceptability of the Internet-Based Chlamydia Screening Implementation in the Netherlands and Insights Into Nonresponse. *Sexually Transmitted Diseases,* Epub ahead of print, (January 2011), ISSN 0148-5717

[41] Hagerty, C.L., Gottlieb, S.L., Taylor, B.D., Low, N., Xu, F. & Ness R.B. (2010). Risk of sequelae after Chlamydia trachomatis genital infection in women. *The Journal of Infectious Diseases,* Vol. 201, Suppl 2 (June 2010), pp. S134-55, ISSN 0022-1899

[42] Hansdotter, F. & Blaxhult, A. (2008). 'Chlamydia Monday' in Sweden. *Euro Surveillance,* Vol. 13, No. 38 (September 2008), pp. 18984, ISSN 1560-7917

[43] He, Q., Tsang, L.L., Ajonuma, L.C. & Chan HC. (2010). Abnormally up-regulated cystic fibrosis transmembrane conductance regulator expression and uterine fluid accumulation contribute to Chlamydia trachomatis-induced female infertility. *Fertility and Sterility*, Vol. 93, No. 8, (May 2010), pp. 2608-2614, ISSN 0015-0282

[44] Hjelholt, A., Christiansen, G., Johannesson, T.G., Ingerslev, H.J. & Birkelund, S. (2011). Tubal factor infertility is associated with antibodies against Chlamydia trachomatis heat shock protein 60 (HSP60) but not human HSP60. *Human Reproduction (Oxford, England)*, Vol. 26, No. 8, (August 2011), pp. 2069-2076, ISSN 0268-1161

[45] Hong, K.C., Schachter, J., Moncada, J., Zhou, Z., House, J. & Lietman, T.M. (2009). Lack of macrolide resistance in *Chlamydia trachomatis* after mass azithromycin distributions for trachoma. *Emerging Infectious Diseases*, Vol. 15, No. 7, (July 2009), pp. 1088-1090, ISSN 1080-6040

[46] Horner, P. (2006). The case for further treatment studies of uncomplicated genital Chlamydia trachomatis infection. *Sexually Transmitted Infections*, Vol. 82, No. 4, (August 2006), pp. 340-343, ISSN 1368-4973

[47] Hosenfeld, C.B., Workowski, K.A., Berman, S., Zaidi, A., Dyson, J., Mosure, D., Bolan, G. & Bauer, H.M. (2009). Repeat infection with Chlamydia and gonorrhea among females: a systematic review of the literature. *Sexually Transmitted Diseases*, Vol. 36, No. 8, (August 2009), pp. 478-489, ISSN 0148-5717

[48] Hsieh, Y.H., Gaydos, C.A., Hogan, M.T., Uy, O.M., Jackman, J., Jett-Goheen, M., Albertie, A., Dangerfield, D.T. 2nd., Neustadt, C.R., Wiener, Z.S. & Rompalo, A.M. (2011). What qualities are most important to making a point of care test desirable for clinicians and others offering sexually transmitted infection testing? *PLoS One*, Vol.6, No. 4, (April 2011), pp. e19263, ISSN 1932-6203

[49] Johnson, K.A., Chen, A.L., Tan, M. & Sütterlin, C. (2010). The role of the protease CPAF in chlamydia-induced centrosome amplification, *Proceedings of the Twelfth International Symposium on Human Chlamydial Infections*, Salzburg, Austria, (June 2010), oral presentation

[50] Kalwij, S., Macintosh, M. & Baraitser, P. (2010). Screening and treatment of Chlamydia trachomatis infections. *British Medical Journal*, Vol. 340, c1915, (April 2010), doi: 10.1136/bmj.c1915, ISSN 0959-8138

[51] Kilmarx, P.H., Black, C.M., Limpakarnjanarat, K., Shaffer, N., Yanpaisarn, S., Chaisilwattana, P., Siriwasin, W., Young, N.L., Farshy, C.E., Mastro, T.D. & St Louis, M.E. (1998). Rapid assessment of sexually transmitted diseases in a sentinel population in Thailand: prevalence of chlamydial infection, gonorrhoea, and syphilis among pregnant women--1996. *Sexually Transmitted Infections*, Vol. 74, No. 3, (June 1998), pp. 189-93, ISSN 1368-4973

[52] King, A.E., Wheelhouse, N., Cameron, S., McDonald, S.E., Lee, K.F., Entrican, G., Critchley, H.O. & Horne, A.W. (2009). Expression of secretory leukocyte protease inhibitor and elafin in human fallopian tube and in an in-vitro model of Chlamydia trachomatis infection. *Human Reproduction (Oxford, England)*, Vol 24, No. 3, (March 2009), pp. 679-686, ISSN 0268-1161

[53] Land, J.A., Van Bergen, J.E., Morré, S.A. & Postma, M.J. (2010). Epidemiology of Chlamydia trachomatis infection in women and the cost-effectiveness of screening. *Human Reproduction Update*, Vol. 16, No. 2, (March-April 2010), pp. 189-204, ISSN 1355-4786

[54] Lau, C.Y. & Qureshi, AK. (2002). Azithromycin versus doxycycline for genital chlamydial infections: a meta-analysis of randomized clinical trials. *Sexually Transmitted Diseases*, Vol. 29, No. 9, (September 2002), pp. 497-502, ISSN 0148-5717

[55] Lehtinen, M., Ault, K.A., Lyytikainen, E., Dillner, J., Garland, S.M., Ferris, D.G., Koutsky, L.A., Sings, H.L., Lu, S., Haupt, R.M. & Paavonen, J.; for the FUTURE I and II Study Group. (2011). Chlamydia trachomatis infection and risk of cervical intraepithelial neoplasia. *Sexually Transmitted Infections*, Vol. 87, No. 5, (August 2011), pp. 372-376, ISSN 1368-4973

[56] Lichtenwalner, A.B., Patton, D.L., Van Voorhis, W.C., Sweeney, Y.T. & Kuo, C.C. (2004). Heat shock protein 60 is the major antigen which stimulates delayed-type hypersensitivity reaction in the macaque model of Chlamydia trachomatis salpingitis. *Infection and Immunity*, Vol. 72, No. 2, (February 2004), pp. 1159-1161, ISSN 0019-9567

[57] Low, N., Cassell, J.A., Spencer, B., Bender, N., Martin Hilber, A., van Bergen, J., Andersen, B., Herrmann, B., Dubois-Arber, F., Hamers, F.F., van de Laar, M. & Stephenson, J.M. (2011). Chlamydia control activities in Europe: cross-sectional survey. *European Journal of Public Health*, Epub ahead of print, (April 2011), ISSN 1101-1262

[58] Maciosek, M., Coffield, A., Edwards, N., Flottemesch, T.J., Goodman, M.J. & Solberg, L.I. (2006). Priorities among effective clinical preventive services: results of a systematic review and analysis. *American Journal of Preventive Medicine*, Vol. 31, No. 1, (July 2006), pp. 52–61, ISSN 0749-3797

[59] Mahilum-Tapay, L., Laitila, V., Wawrzyniak, J.J., Lee, H.H., Alexander, S., Ison, C., Swain, A., Barber, P., Ushiro-Lumb, I. & Goh, B.T. (2007). New point of care Chlamydia Rapid Test--bridging the gap between diagnosis and treatment: performance evaluation study. *British Medical Journal*, Vol. 335, No. 7631, (December 2007), pp. 1190-1194, ISSN 0959-8138

[60] McMillan, H.M., O'Carroll, H., Lambert, J.S., Grundy, K.B., O'Reilly, M., Lennon, B., et al. (2006). Screening for Chlamydia trachomatis in asymptomatic women attending outpatient clinics in a large maternity hospital in Dublin, Ireland. *Sexually Transmitted Infections*, Vol. 82, No. 6, (December 2006), pp. 503-5, ISSN 1368-4973

[61] Michel, C.E., Sonnex, C., Carne, C.A., White, J.A., Magbanua, J.P., Nadala, E.C. Jr. & Lee, H.H. (2007). Chlamydia trachomatis load at matched anatomic sites: implications for screening strategies. *Journal of Clinical Microbiology*, Vol. 45, No. 5, (May 2007), pp. 1395-1402, ISSN 0095-1137

[62] Moss, N.J., Ahrens, K., Kent, C.K. & Klausner, J.D. (2006). The decline in clinical sequelae of genital Chlamydia trachomatis infection supports current control strategies. *The Journal of Infectious Diseases*, Vol. 193, No. 9, (May 2006), pp. 1336–1338, ISSN 0022-1899

[63] Oakeshott, P., Kerry, S., Aghaizu, A., Atherton, H., Hay, S., Taylor-Robinson, D., Simms, I. & Hay P. (2010). Randomised controlled trial of screening for Chlamydia trachomatis to prevent pelvic inflammatory disease: the POPI (prevention of pelvic infection) trial. *British Medical Journal*, Vol. 340, No. c1642, (April 2010), doi: 10.1136/bmj. c1642, ISSN 0959-8138

[64] Ostergaard, L., Andersen, B., Moller, J.K. & Olesen, F. (2000). Home sampling versus conventional swab sampling for screening of Chlamydia trachomatis in women: a cluster-randomized 1-year follow-up study. Clinical of Infectious Diseases, Vol. 31, No. 4, (October 2000), pp. 951–957, ISSN 1058-4838

[65] Paavonen, J., Karunakaran, K.P., Noguchi, Y., Anttila, T., Bloigu, A., Dillner, J., Hallmans, G., Hakulinen, T., Jellum, E., Koskela, P., Lehtinen, M., Thoresen, S., Lam, H., Shen, C. & Brunham, R.C. (2003). Serum antibody response to the heat shock protein 60 of Chlamydia trachomatis in women with developing cervical cancer. *American Journal of Obstetrics and Gynecology*, Vol. 189, No. 5, (November 2003), pp. 1287–1292, ISSN 0002-9378

[66] Paavonen, J. (2011). Chlamydia trachomatis infections of the female genital tract: State of the art. *Annals of Medicine*, Epub ahead of print, (February 2011), ISSN 0785-3890

[67] Pinto, V.M., Szwarcwald, C.L., Baroni, C., Stringari, L.L., Inocêncio, L.A. & Miranda, A.E. (2011). Chlamydia trachomatis prevalence and risk behaviors in parturient women aged 15 to 24 in Brazil. *Sexually Transmitted Diseases*, Vol. 38, No. 12, (December 2011), pp. 1-5, ISSN 0148-5717

[68] Piñeiro, L., Montes, M., Gil-Setas, A., Camino, X., Echeverria, M.J. & Cilla, G. (2009). Genotyping of Chlamydia trachomatis in an area of northern Spain. Enfermedades Infecciosas y Microbiología Clínica, Vol 27, No. 8, (October 2009), pp. 462-464, ISSN 0213-005X

[69] Piñeiro, L., Vicente, D., Echeverría, M.J. & Cilla, G. (2009). Application of an automatic nucleic acid extraction method to improve the detection of Chlamydia trachomatis. *Enfermedades Infecciosas y Microbiología Clínica*, Vol. 27, No. 9, (November 2009), pp. 549-550, ISSN 0213-005X

[70] Piñeiro, L., Unemo, M. & Cilla, G. (2011). Absence of the Swedish new variant of Chlamydia trachomatis (nvCT) and C. trachomatis genotype distribution in Gipuzkoa, Spain, 2009-2010. *Acta Dermato-Venereologica*, Epub ahead of print, (November 2011), doi 10.2340/00015555-1234, ISSN 0001-5555

[71] Rank, R.G., Bowlin, A.K. & Kelly, K.A. (2000). Characterization of lymphocyte response in the female genital tract during ascending Chlamydial genital infection in the guinea pig model. *Infection and Immunity*, Vol. 68, No. 9, (September 2000), pp. 5293–5298, ISSN 0019-9567

[72] Refaat, B., Al-Azemi, M., Geary, I., Eley, A., Ledger & W. (2009). Role of activins and inducible nitric oxide in the pathogenesis of ectopic pregnancy in patients with or without Chlamydia trachomatis infection. *Clinical and Vaccine Immunology*, Vol. 16, No. 10, (October 2009), pp. 1493-1503, ISSN 1556-6811

[73] Riera-Montes, M. & Velicko, I. (2011). The Chlamydia surveillance system in Sweden delivers relevant and accurate data: results from the system evaluation, 1997-2008. *Eurosurveillance*, Vol. 16, No. 27, (July 2011), ISSN 1560-7917

[74] Ripa, T. & Nilsson, P. (2006). A variant of Chlamydia trachomatis with deletion in cryptic plasmid: implications for use of PCR diagnostic tests. *Euro Surveillance*, Vol. 11, No. 11, (November 2006), E061109.2, ISSN 1560-7917

[75] Roberts, S.W., Sheffield, J.S., McIntire, D.D. & Alexander, J.M. (2011). Urine screening for Chlamydia trachomatis during pregnancy. *Obstetrics & Gynecology*, Vol. 117, No. 4, (April 2011), pp. 883-85, ISSN 0029-7844

[76] Romoren, M., Sundby, J., Velauthapillai, M., Rahman, M., Klouman, E. & Hjortdahl, P. (2007). Chlamydia and gonorrhoea in pregnant Batswana women: time to discard the syndromic approach? *BMC Infectious Diseases*, Vol. 16, No. 7, (April 2007), pp. 27, ISSN 1471-2334

[77] Rours, G.I., Verkooyen, R.P., Willemse, H.F., van der Zwaan, E.A., van Belkum, A., de Groot, R., Verbrugh, H.A. & Ossewaarde, J.M. (2005). Use of pooled urine samples and automated DNA isolation to achieve improved sensitivity and cost-

effectiveness of large-scale testing for Chlamydia trachomatis in pregnant women. *Journal of Clinical Microbiology*, Vol. 43, No. 9, (September 2005), pp. 4684-4690, ISSN 0095-1137

[78] Rours, G.I., Duijts, L., Moll, H.A., Arends, L.R., de Groot, R., Jaddoe, V.W., et al. (2011). Chlamydia trachomatis infection during pregnancy associated with preterm delivery: a population-based prospective cohort study. *European Journal of Epidemiology*, Vol. 26, No. 6, (June 2011), pp. 493-502, ISSN 0393-2990

[79] Safaeian, M., Quint, K., Schiffman, M., Rodriguez, A.C., Wacholder, S., Herrero, R., Hildesheim, A., Viscidi, R.P., Quint, W. & Burk, R.D. (2010). Chlamydia trachomatis and risk of prevalent and incident cervical premalignancy in a population-based cohort. *Journal of the National Cancer Institute*, Vol. 102, No. 23, (December 2010), pp. 1794-1804, ISSN 0027-8874

[80] Sandoz, K.M. & Rockey, D.D. (2010). Antibiotic resistance in Chlamydiae. *Future Microbiology*, Vol. 5, No. 9, (September 2010), pp. 1427-1442, ISSN 1746-0913

[81] Schachter, J., Chernesky, M.A., Willis, D.E., Fine, P.M., Martin, D.H., Fuller, D., Jordan, J.A., Janda, W. & Hook, E.W. 3rd. (2005). Vaginal swabs are the specimens of choice when screening for *Chlamydia trachomatis* and *Neisseria gonorrhoeae*: results from a multicenter evaluation of the APTIMA assays for both infections. *Sexually Transmitted Diseases*, Vol. 32, No. 2, (December 2005), pp. 725-728, ISSN 0148-5717

[82] Scholes, D., Stergachis, A., Heidrich, F.E., Andrilla, H., Holmes, K.K. & Stamm, W.E. (1996). Prevention of pelvic inflammatory disease by screening for cervical chlamydial infection. *The New England Journal of Medicine*, Vol. 334, No. 21, (May 1996), pp. 1362–1366, ISSN 0028-4793

[83] Shao, R., Zhang, S.X., Weijdegård, B., Zou, S., Egecioglu, E., Norström, A., Brännström, M. & Billig, H. (2010). Nitric oxide synthases and tubal ectopic pregnancies induced by Chlamydia infection: basic and clinical insights. *Molecular Human Reproduction*, Vol. 16, No. 12, (December 2010), pp. 907-915, ISSN 1360-9947

[84] Shaw, J.L., Wills, G.S., Lee, K.F., Horner, P.J., McClure, M.O., Abrahams, V.M., Wheelhouse, N., Jabbour, H.N., Critchley, H.O., Entrican, G. & Horne, A.W. (2011). Chlamydia trachomatis infection increases fallopian tube PROKR2 via TLR2 and NFκB activation resulting in a microenvironment predisposed to ectopic pregnancy. *The American Journal of Pathology*, Vol. 178, No. 1, (January 2011), pp. 253-260, ISSN 0002-9440

[85] Silveira, M.F., Erbelding, E.J., Ghanem, K.G., Johnson, H.L., Burke, A.E. & Zenilman, J.M. (2010). Risk of Chlamydia trachomatis infection during pregnancy: effectiveness of guidelines-based screening in identifying cases. *International Journal of STD & AIDS*, Vol. 21, No. 5, (May 2010), pp. 367-70, ISSN 0956-4624

[86] Simms, I. & Stephenson, J.M. (2000). Pelvic inflammatory disease epidemiology: what do we know and what do we need to know? *Sexually Transmitted Infections*, Vol. 76, No. 2, (April 2000), pp. 80-87, ISSN 1368-4973

[87] Stephens, R.S. (2003). The cellular paradigm of chlamydial pathogenesis. *Trends in Microbiology*, Vol. 11, No. 3, (January 2003), pp. 44–51, ISSN 0966-842X

[88] Srivastava, P., Jha, R., Bas, S., Salhan, S. & Mittal, A. (2008). In infertile women, cells from Chlamydia trachomatis infected sites release higher levels of interferon-gamma, interleukin-10 and tumor necrosis factor-alpha upon heat-shock-protein stimulation than fertile women. *Reproductive Bioloy and Endocrinology*, Vol. 6, No. 20, (May 2008), pp. 1-10, ISSN 1477-7827

[89] Tan, C., Spitznagel, J.K., Shou, H.-Z., Hsia, R.C. & Bavoil, P.M. (2006). The polymorphic membrane protein gene family of the chlamydiaceae. In: *Chlamydia genomics and pathogenesis,* Bavoil, P.M. & Wyrick, P.B., pp. 195-218, Horizon Bioscience, ISBN 1904933211, Norfolk, United Kingdom

[90] Turner, K.M., Adams, E.J., Lamontagne, D.S., Emmett, L., Baster, K. & Edmunds, W.J. (2006). Modelling the effectiveness of chlamydia screening in England. *Sexually Transmitted Infections,* Vol. 82, No. 6, (December 2006), pp. 496-502, ISSN 1368-4973

[91] Unemo, M. & Clarke, I.N. (2011). The Swedish new variant of Chlamydia trachomatis. *Current Opinion in Infectious Diseases,* Vol. 24, No. 1, (February 2011), pp. 62-9, ISSN 0951-7375

[92] Unemo, M., Seth-Smith, H.M., Cutcliffe, L.T., Skilton, R.J., Barlow, D., Goulding, D., Persson, K., Harris, S.R., Kelly, A., Bjartling, C., Fredlund, H., Olcén, P., Thomson, N.R. & Clarke, I.N. (2010). The Swedish new variant of Chlamydia trachomatis: genome sequence, morphology, cell tropism and phenotypic characterization. *Microbiology,* Vol. 156, Pt. 5, (May 2010), pp. 1394-404, ISSN 1350-0872

[93] U.S. Preventive Services Task Force. (2007). Screening for chlamydial infection: U.S. Preventive Services Task Force recommendation statement. *Annals of Internal Medicine,* Vol. 147, No. 2, (July 2007), pp. 128-134, ISSN 0003-4819

[94] Varma, R. & Gupta, J. (2009). Tubal ectopic pregnancy. *Clinical Evidence (Online),* Vol. 4, (April 2009), pp. 1406, ISSN 1462-3846

[95] Wang, W., Stassen, F.R., Surcel, H.-M., Öhman, H., Tiitinen, A., Paavonen, J., de Vries, H.J., Heijmans, R., Pleijster, J., Morré, S.A. & Ouburg S. (2009). Analyses of polymorphism in inflammasome-associated NLRP3 and miRNA-146A genes in the susceptibility to and tubal pathology of Chlamydia trachomatis infection. *Drugs of Today (Barcelona, Spain: 1998),* Vol. 45, Suppl B, (November 2009), pp. 95–103, ISSN 1699-3993

[96] Wiesenfeld, H.C., Dennard-Hall, K., Cook, R.L., Ashton, M., Zamborsky, T. & Krohn, M.A. (2005). Knowledge about sexually transmitted diseases in women among primary care physicians. *Sexually Transmitted Diseases,* Vol. 32, No. 11, (November 2005), pp. 649-653, ISSN 0148-5717

[97] Wilkowska-Trojniel, M., Zdrodowska-Stefanow, B., Ostaszewska-Puchalska, I., Redźko, S., Przepieść, J. & Zdrodowski, M. (2009). The influence of Chlamydia trachomatis infection on spontaneous abortions. *Advances in Medical Sciences,* Vol. 54, No. 1, (June 2009), pp. 86-90, ISSN 1896-1126

[98] World Health Organization. (2001). Global prevalence and incidence of selected curable sexually transmitted infections: overview and estimates, In: *WHO,* 03.08.2011, Available from: http://www.who.int/hiv/pub/sti/who_hiv_aids_2001.02.pdf

[99] World Health Organization. (2007). Global strategy for the prevention and control of sexually transmitted infections: 2006–2015: breaking the chain of transmission. In: *WHO,* 19.06.2011, Available from: www.who.int/entity/reproductivehealth/publications/rtis/9789241563475/en/

[100] Wyrick, P.B. (2010). Chlamydia trachomatis persistence in vitro: an overview. The Journal of Infectious Diseases, Vol. 201, Suppl 2, (June 2010), pp. S88-95, ISSN 0022-1899

12

Correlation Between *Chlamydia trachomatis* IgG and Pelvic Adherence Syndrome

Demetra Socolov et al.*
Grigore T. Popa University of Medicine and Pharmacy, Iassy
Romania

1. Introduction

Chlamydia trachomatis genital tract infections are prevalent worldwide (Stamm 2008), with 92 million new *chlamydia* cases occured every year: 3–4 million new cases occur every year in the US, 5 million in Western Europe, and 16 million in Sub-Saharan Africa (World Health Organization 2001; Weinstock et al., 2004). *Chlamydia* prevalence has been reported to range from 3%-7% among asymptomatic populations in men, and in women range from 3.0% in the general population to 9.5% among university students (World Health Organization 2001; Stamm 2008; Patel et al.,. 2008; Forhan et al., 2009; Imai et al., 2010; Satterwhite et al., 2010).

Chlamydia is a pathogenic obligate intracellular bacterium with a biphasic developmental cycle that takes place inside a *parasitophorous vacuole* termed an inclusion. This implies cell types adapted for extracellular survival (elementary bodies, EBs) and intracellular multiplication (reticulate bodies, RBs). Within 2 hours after entry into host cells, *Chlamydia trachomatis* EBs are trafficked to the perinuclear region of the host cell and remain in close proximity to the Golgi apparatus, where they begin to fuse with a subset of host vesicles containing sphingomyelin, demonstrating that *chlamydial* migration from the cell periphery to the peri-Golgi region resembles host cell vesicular trafficking (Grieshaber et al., 2003).

Due to their obligate intracellular nature, the detection and manipulation of *Chlamydia* have proved challenging. Novel techniques such as real-time PCR facilitate the diagnosis of infections due to these pathogens, but in the absence of organized screening programs, asymptomatic infections are not treated, leading to several serious diseases. The development of tests based on nucleic acid amplification technology represented an important advance in the field of STD (sexually transmitted disease) diagnosis. Nucleic acid amplification detection technique is more sensitive and specific and offers the

* Coralia Bleotu[2], Nora Miron[1], Razvan Socolov[1], Lucian Boiculese[1], Mihai Mares[3], Sorici Natalia[4], Moshin Veaceslav[4], Anca Botezatu[2] and Gabriela Anton[2]
[1]*Grigore T. Popa University of Medicine and Pharmacy, Iassy, Romania*
[2]*Stefan S. Nicolau Institute of Virology, Bucharest, Romania*
[3]*Ion Ionescu de la Brad, University, Iassy, Romania*
[4]*National Center of Reproductive Health and Medical Genetics, Chisinau, Republic of Moldavia*

opportunity to screen for infections in asymptomatic individuals, using noninvasive sampling.

Generaly, in female genital tract *Chlamydia trachomatis* produce asymptomatic infections in approximately 80% of women (Zimmerman et al., 1990), but is associated with serious reproductive morbidity causing cervicitis (Marazzo & Martin, 2007; Stamm et al., 2008; Falk 2010) and is also associated with urethritis.(Dieterle, 2008), PID (Howie et al., 2011), infertility (Forti G. & Krausz C.,1998).

The pathogenic processes causing the sequelae are thought to be partly immunological (Beatty et al., 1994) When initiation and propagation of infection occurs, both humoral and cellular immune response are triggered. In damaged area an influx of immune cells (lymphocytes, macrophages, dendritic cells) occurs. At the site of infection there is a strong inflammatory reaction characterized by a mucopurulent vaginal discharge and formation of immune complexes, a process that may contribute to the immunopathology of the disease. However, the absence of tools for genomic manipulation has limited the understanding of factors involved in host cell interactions.

However, all factors that induce inflammatory reaction (intrauterine devices for contraception, sexually transmitted diseases, etc) increase the risk of pelvic inflammatory disease (PID). Generally, the *Chlamydia trachomatis* infection resolves without sequelae, but occasionally it spreads from the lower to the upper genital tract and pelvic inflammatory disease may develop (Paavonen et al., 1985; Morre et al., 2002), leading to scarring of the fallopian tube, causing occlusion, resulting in ectopic pregnancy or tubal factor infertility. The diagnosis of the adherential syndrome is performed tardily using laparoscopy, an invasive method. In order to find markers that would impose the needing to perform laparoscopy from the beginning our aim was to evaluate possible correlations between various microbiological agents involved in infertility caused by pelvic adherence syndrome. We also evaluate a possible correlation between the presence of Ig G for *Chlamydia Trachomatis* and the adhesion syndrome.

2. Methods and materials

2.1 Patients

174 infertile women (with a mean age of 31.38± 4.3) were enrolled in the study between 2008- 2010. The study received the approval of ethical committee of Grigore T. Popa University of Medicine and Pharmacy.

2.2 Methods

Anamnestic data included: history of surgery in pelvic-abdominal area, obstetric history (pregnancies, births, abortions, SEU). All women performed an analysis set: assessment of ovarian reserve by second day hormonal dosage, ultrasonographic monitoring ovulation, spermogram and sperm culture of the male partner, uterotubal assessment component of infertility using the HYCOSY, HSG and hysteroscopy coupled with laparoscopy with Dye Test, considered to be the gold standard technique.

Hysteroscopies coupled with laparoscopies with blue methylene test, were carried out under general endotracheal anesthesia, in the operating room, using Karl Storz®

Tuttingen Germany equipment. We always started by a diagnostic hysteroscopy with the intention to visualise the entire cavity, the mucosal aspect and the tubal proximal ostia. After the cannulation of the uterus, we continued with the laparoscopic time, consisting in a peritoneal CO2 insuflation and a transabdominal insertion of a 10mm laparoscope. We performed the visual inspection of the pelvic area, recording the aspect of the uterus and both adnexes (ovaries and tubes), the presence of the intraperitoneal adhesions and the foci of endometriosis. Adherence syndrome was framed according to the AFS classification (1998) in the following categories: minimal 1-5 points, mild 6-10 points, medium 11-20 points, severe 21-32 points. After completion of the pelvic inspection, the right upper quadrant was evaluated for the presence of perihepatic adhesions (Fitz Hugh Curtis Syndrome).

During pelvic surgery, attention was given to minimise the tissue handling, excision of all adhesions when possible and constant irrigation of tissue with warm saline solution during adhesiolysis. We used the electro surgery in bipolar or monopolar mode for dissection and only bipolar mode for coagulation. Adnexa adherent to the uterus were separated and tubes were detached from the ovaries and other pelvic organs. The ovary was separated from the underlying peritoneum of the ovarian fossa or uterosacral ligament. Omental adhesions to the anterior parietal peritoneum or bowel adhesions to pelvic structures were detached. In some patients, both adnexa were completely frozen with dense adhesions to bowel and vital organs. In these cases, operative surgery was not performed and patients were referred to AMP (Assisted Medical Procreation) techniques. Endometriosis foci of the peritoneum were inspected and if superficial, coagulated. Ovarian cysts (serous or endometriotic) were operated by cystectomy. At the end, patency of fallopian tubes was assessed by injecting dilute solution of methylene blue into the uterine cavity through the uterine canula. The passage was considered to be present if the methylene blue was visualised through the external tubal orifice and negative if no methylene blue passage was seen. The tubal obstruction was considered proximal if the tube did not change in volume or colour during the injection of the dye solution and distal, if the external end of the tube dilated and became blue. We performed for these last cases a neosalpingostomy (a new orifice into the external extremity of the tube) if the obstruction was ampullar, or a fimbrioplasty (the dilatation of the fimbrial end of the tube when fimbrial plis were conserved but agglutinated).

2.3 Sample collection and storage

Endocervical samples have been collected in duplicate from all patients using *Chlamydia* Swab/Brush Collection Kit (Bio-Rad Laboratories, France). The process of the samples was performed immediately after collection or samples were stored at 2–8 °C for 24 hours, or freeze at -20/80°C. Serum samples were obtained from each patient. Sera were aliquoted, stored at −80°C and thawed only once.

2.4 DNA isolation

For DNA isolation was used the recommended DNA-Sorb-A (Sacace, REF K-1-1/A) kit. DNA was extracted according to the manufacturer's instructions. 10 µl of Internal Control was added in each isolation mixture. Internal Control was the same for all urogenital infectious kits.

2.5 Real Time PCR for bacteria detection in cervical smear

Bacteria detection was performed using STD Real-TM (Saccace) Kit that detects the most important bacterial infections with *Chlamydia trachomatis, Ureaplasma urealyticum, Mycoplasma genitalium/hominis, Neisseria gonorrhoeae.*

2.6 Serological assay

Serological assay was done using NovaLisaTM Chlamydia trachomatis IgA/IgG/IgM ELISA kits (NovaTec Immundiagnostica GmbH, Dietzenbach - Germany).

2.7 Statistical calculations

Statistical calculations were performed using SPSS software (version 16), and P values of 0.05 or less being considered significant.

3. Results

Patients: From 174 women enrolled in our study, 97 cases were primary infertility and 77 cases presented secondary infertility.

In assessing the laparoscopic diagnostic with Dye test 71 adherence syndrome patients were classified according to American Fertility Society, within the following categories: minimal-39 cases, mild-28cases, medium-4 cases, severe-0 cases 7 patients had absent tubes (salpingectomy for ectopic pregnancy in history), (4 right, 3 left).

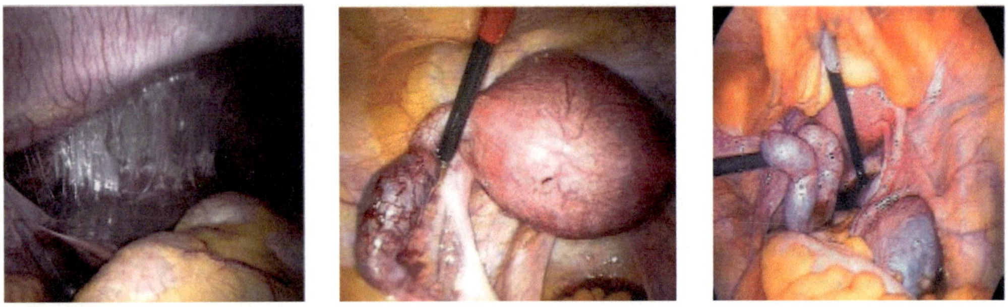

Fig. 1. Laparoscopic aspect: a) Fitz Hugh Curtis Syndrome; b) Left distal tube obstruction-hydrosalpinx; c) Dye test negative-hydrosalpinx

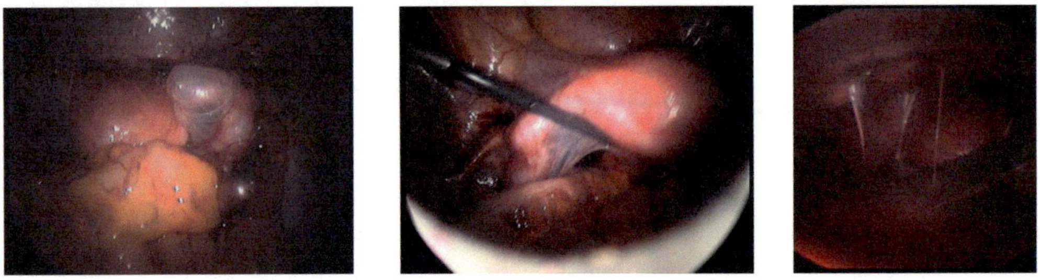

Fig. 2. Another laparoscopic aspect of diffuse adhesions,involving: a) right adnexa; b) left adenxa; c) perihepatic adhesions (Fitz Hugh Curtis)

Impairment was bilateral in 12 cases and unilateral in 27. Proximal localization of obstruction was observed in 37 patients, and distal in 12. In 2 cases, Fitz Hugh Curtis syndrome was present, one case in correlation with pelvic adhesions and the other with apparently intact internal genitalia, negative PCR results for all the germs tested and Ig G *Chlamydia trachomatis* (IgGCT) negative. Figure 1 show some laparoscopic aspect.

3.1 Bacterial diagnostic

In order to prove bacterial presence, real time PCR was performed. *Chlamydia trachomatis* DNA was detected in two smears, *Mycoplasma hominis* in 7, *Ureaplasma urealyticum* in 54 and only one was positive for *Neisseria gonorrhoeae* according to table 2.

	Positive
Chlamydia trachomatis	2/174 (1.15%)
Mycoplasma hominis	7/174 (4.02%)
Ureaplasma urealyticum	54/174 (31.03%)
Neisseria gonorrhoeae	1/174 (0.57%)

Table 1. Detection of bacterial DNA.

Serological detection of IgG specific for *Chlamydia trachomatis* was associated with presence of adherences in 40 cases from 52 positive cases (76.9%). However, 38 cases that test negative for IgG (31.1%) presented adherence, but only 12 cases that didn't show adherence have IgG positive test (table 3).

		adherence	
		present	absent
IgG CT	present	40/52 (76.9%)	12/52 (23.07%)
	absent	38/122 (31.1%)	84/122 (68.9%)
	total	78/174 (44.8%)	96/174 (55.2%)

Table 2. Association of *Chlamydia trachomatis* IgG with presence of adherence,

Evaluating CT IgG positivity as possible marker for tubal obstructions (distal and proximal summed), we found:

- For tubal passage: sensitivity 36.5%, specificity 73.8%, PPV (positive predictive value) 44.2%, NPV (negative predictive value) 67.2%;
- For pathological tubal aspect: sensitivity 37.1%, specificity 79.2%, PPV 69.2%, NPV 50%.

		left and/or right tubal passage		tubal aspect	
		present	absent	present	absent
IgG CT	present	23/52 (44.2%)	29/52 (55.8%)	36/52 (69.2%)	16/52 (30.8%)
	absent	40/122 (32.79%)	82/122 (67.21%)	61/122 (50%)	61/122 (50%)
	total	63/174 (36.2%)	111/174 (63.8%)	97/174 (55.75%)	77/174 (44.25%)

Table. 3. Association of *Chlamydia trachomatis* IgG with tubal disorders

Evaluation of outbreaks of endometriosis as a marker of adherent pelvic syndrome gave the following results:

		endometriosis	
		present	absent
adherences	present	4/78 (5.22%)	74/78 (94.87%)
	absent	2/96 (2.08%)	94/96 (97.92%)
	Total	6/174 (3.45%)	168/174 (96.55%)

Table 4. Association of endometriosis with presence of adherence

Regarding the classification performance of endometriosis with adhesions, we found the following values: sensitivity 66%, specificity 56%, PPV 5.2%, NPV 97.9%

adherences	Previous surgical interventions	
	present	absent
present	25/78 (30.05%)	53/78 (67.95%)
absent	18/96 (18.75%)	78/96 (81.25%)
Total	43/174 (24.71%)	131/174 (75.29%)

Table. 5. Association of previous surgical pelvic interventions with presence of adhesions

The statistical measures of classification performance are: sensititvity 58%, specificity 59%, PPV 32%, NPV 81%.

We also used logistic regression with adherence the dichotomous dependant variable and the predictors defined by endometriosis, previous pelvic surgery and IgG CT. Hosmer and Lemeshow test concludes if the model adequately describes the data. We had obtained a "p" value greater than 0.9 which confirms the applicability.

Not all the variables have a consistent contribution to the model. Thus the procedure is selecting at each step the predictor with the highest score that has statistical significance (stepwise regression).

			Score	df	Sig.
Step 0	Variables	endometriosis	1.198	1	.274
		IgCT	30.890	1	.000
		Previous surgery	4.092	1	.043
	Overall Statistics		34.937	3	.000

Table 6. Statistical significance of endometriosis, IgG CT, and previous surgery in relation with pelvic adhesions

Next table shows that only two of the predictors appear to be important in prediction:

- For endometriosis, we got a significance of p=0.274, so no statistical relevance
- For IgG CT and previous surgery, p<0.001 and p=0.043, therefore statistically significant means to be added to the model in adhesions prediction.

We have calculated the usefulness of the predictors by means of the B coefficients with the Wald statistic for the two predictors selected in the model.

		B	**S.E.**	**Wald**	**df**	**Sig.**	**Exp(B)**	**95% C.I.for EXP(B)**	
								Lower	**Upper**
Step 1	Surgical intervention	.786	.391	4.036	1	.045	2.196	1.019	4.729
	Ig G CT	2.024	.388	27.151	1	.000	7.567	3.535	16.202
	Constant	-.999	.227	19.402	1	.000	.368		

Table 7. Wald evaluation for IgG CT, and previous surgery.

The B coefficients meanings have not straightforward interpretation of the logistic regression. Therefore an exponentiation operation of the coefficients is applicable for a better and easier interpretation. The Exp(B) represents the ratio of the odds (odd=risk/(1-risk)) of the dependent variable for an unit increase of the predictor that is in charge. For example the odds of having adherence are 2.196 times bigger for a person with pelvic surgery compared with one that has no pelvic surgery. Similarly the odds ratio of having adherence by Ig G CT may be interpreted.

Both variables have statistical significance, but the largest Exp (B) value expresses that the odds ratio increases 7.56 times for a person with Ig G CT in order to get adherence, compared with no Ig CT presence.

4. Discussions

The attempt of using Ig G to *Chlamydia trachomatisas a marker for* pelvic adherence syndrome, in order to establish the need of performing laparoscopy from the beginning, we obtained a low sensitivity (36%), but a good specificity (76%). That means that there is not a good correlation established between *Chlamydia trachomatis* IgG positivity and tubal obstructions, and some women with disease may be lost in this screening. However, in our study, it seems that most adherences were given by *Chlamydia*, while in the majority of studies coming from countries with screening programmes for *Chlamydia trachomatis* and for the prevention of STD (sexual transmitted diseases),endometriosis is far on the first place.

Several methods currently used for diagnosis of *chlamydia* infection have its own advantages and limitations. Cytological method (Romanovski-Giemsa staining of smear) is almost not used any more due to its low sensitivity and specificity. Culturing remain the golden tool of diagnosing as it has the highest specificity, and good sensitivity (aprox. 80%), but this method is very labor intensive as *chlamydiae* do not grow on artificial nutrient and isolation of *chlamydiae* need a monolayer of McCoy, L-929 or HeLa cells. Serological detection remain a usefull tool in detecting chronic and acute infections with *Chlamydia trachomatis*. Generaly, there is an immunoassay test used to detect different classes of circulating antibodies IgG, IgA, IgM. However, their clinical utility is burdened by heterogeneity of humoral immune response, individual factor being especially important for proportion of false negative results. In superficial genital infections (cervicitis, urethritis), serological test did not have diagnosis relevance because of the superficial location of infection and low circulating antibodies titer subsequent infection. However, IgM is detected early after infection and persists aproximatively one month, so it is transient and rises in Ig M titres are infrequently found and IgG have low titer. In contrast, in severe infection, like pelvic inflammatory syndrome, detection of a high titre of IgG indicates an older or evolving infection. However, in order to capture the antibodies dynamics, it is recommend a new sampling and retest. Therefore, according to our results IgG serological detection can be used for evaluate older infections that can cause infertility.

In our study sensitivity for IgG *Chlamydia trachomatis* in adhesion and tubal obstruction was lower than in other studies. Land et al.,(2003) reports a Ig G antibodies for *Chlamydia trachomatis* sensitivity of about 60% for tubal pathology with a 85-90%specificity.

Veenemans et al.,(2002) evaluated HSG and IgG for *Chlamydia Trachomatis* testing in predicting tubal factor infertility and found for HSG a sensitivity of 57% with a specificity of 66% and for IgG CT, a sensitivity of 80% with a specificity of 55%. The authors concluded that both tests have poor predictive value, but because both tests cause minimal inconvenience to the patient, both should be maintained in the infertility primary examination.

There is evident difference in results between published studies and the clinical significance of the the igG CT however has its limitations due to false positive and false negative test results (Land 2003).Patients with false negative CT antibody test results may have not *chlamydia* related causes of adhesions or tubal oclusions or no antibodies may be found after a previous CT infection.

Between other causes of adhesions or tubal occlusions, the most frequent are: pelvic endometriosis, previous pelvic surgery (for infertility, apendicitis, peritonitis,)(Smart et al., 1995, Moll et al., 1997), previous pelvic minimal invasive investigations (HSG, Histeroscopy, dilatation and curretage, IUD applications, past history of abortion) and genital infections with other microorganisms than *Chlamydia trachomatis : Neisseria gonorrhoeae, Ureaplasma urealyticum, Mycoplasma genitalium/hominis* and other germs associated with *bacterial vaginosis.*

To analyze the effects of infection with *Mycoplasma genitalium and hominis* on human faloppian tubes (HFT) and to compare them with the effects of infection with the classical genital pathogens: *Chlamydia trachomatis* and *Neisseria gonorrhoeae,* Baczynsta (2007) used in vitro models in which, pieces of normalHFT were infected with different bacteria and analysed by scanning electron microscopy and confocal microscopy.The conclusion was that tubal infection with *Mycoplasma genitalium and hominis* affected the tubal epithelium resulting in cilia damage but effect was very moderate when compared with the extensive damage of the epithelium caused by *Chlamydia trachomatis* and *Neisseria gonorrhoeae.*

As a cause of false negative result for CT antibodies tests, it has been postulated that IgG CT antibodies may decline over time after CT infection, between the primary infection in adolescence and the in fertility investigations in adulthood. But Gijsen (2002) demonstrated that, despite the decrease in the antibody titers over time, they do not completely disappear.

Between the false positive values, it was postulated that there are many cross reactions with other Chlamydia species and that the current ELISA method of determining IgG CT antibodies may not be very specific.

According to Ossewaarde (1998)cited by Veenemans (2002), the border values and interpretation " clear indication for an infection in the past", depend mostly on the type of the test used, antibody, conjugation, fluorescence lamp and population. Therefore, comparison of titers from different laboratories and different tests is not possible.

Another question raised was, if testing Ig G antibodies for both *Chlamydia trachomatis* and *Chlamydia pneumoniae* will not enhance the detection rate of adhesions and tubal occlusions in subfertile population.

Gijsen (2001) demonstrated that tubal factor subfertility seem to be more common in subfertile women with IgG antibodies to both CT and CP (49%) versus CT antibodies only (30%), but the difference was not statistically significant.

Another reason for differences in sensitivity and specificity of IgG CT dosages is the threshold point chose by the laboratory for a positive result. If the threshold point is high, sensitivity decrease and specificity increase.

Veenemans(2002) reported a sensitivity of 80% with a specificity of 55% for a threshold of 1/32 and a sensibility of 66% for a specificity of 68% when the threshold was 1/32.In our study, the threshold value was 1/32.

Some research groups were able to correlate prevalence and high serum-titre of immunoglobulin IgG antibodies against *Chlamydia trachomatis* with tubal factor infertility

(Machado et al., 2007; Malik et al., 2009). Hjelholt et al., (2011) confirm an association between tubal factor infertility and antibodies to major outer membrane protein and heat shock protein 60 from *Chlamydia trachomatis*, suggesting antibody testing as a supplement in tubal factor infertility diagnosis. No connection was observed between tubal factor infertility and antibodies to human HSP60, pointing to an infectious rather than an autoimmune inflammation as the cause of tubal factor infertility.

The probability that *Chlamydia trachomatis* produces pelvic and tubal lesions is correlated with the persistence of the untreated uncomplicated genital *chlamydial* infections and with the presence of recurent infections. In a review study (Geisler, 2010), *chlamydia* resolution occured in 54% of participants at one year follow up, 83% at two years, 91% at three years and 95% at four years. Clinical and biological factors found to be involved in the resolution of untreated uncomplicated *Chlamydia trachomatis*, were: older age, caucasian race to which the clearence is higher.

Cohen et al., (2005) found that select peripherical blood mononuclear cell lymphoproliferative responses to *Chlamydia* EBS and heat shock protein 60 (cHSP60) correlated with protection against incident *Chlamydia* but not with a reduction in incident *chlamydial* infection. Cervical lymphoproliferative response to cHSP10 were higher in reccurent infection, while lymphoproliferative response to OmpA was higher in primary infection (Agrawal et al., 2007). The presence of OmpA A type E protein favour the persistence of infection at 1 year follow up (Morre et al., 2002), as well as infection load (a quantitative measure of persistence organism burden and pressumably a surogate for *Chlamydia trachomatis* replication. Some other factors were associated with reccurent infections (interferon gamma levels were found higher in cervical wash samples from women with reccurent infections), or protective effects against recurrent *chlamydia* (IL10 gene promoter variant, promoter positions -1082, -819, -592) (Wang et al., 2005).

In our study, it is interesting that the values of sensitivity and specificity are somewhat similar for the presence of adhesions and tubal obstruction. That means that when injuries occur appear equally both tubal adhesions and tubal touching.

Perihepatic adhesions are generally considered pathognomonic for pelvic inflammatory disease. This syndrome, named after the individuals who first described it: Fitz-Hugh (1934) and Curtis (1930) is composed of two phases: acute and chronic.

The acute phase presents as a sharp, pleuritic type pain in the right upper quadrant, worsened with coughing, deep inspiration and movement. A laparoscopy performed in this precise moment could surprise inflammation of the peritoneum, overlying the liver and the anterior abdominal wall.

Usually, in laparoscopy, we can see the chronic phase characterised by typical violin string adhesions between the anterior abdominal wall, inferior surface of the diaphragm and the upper/anterior surface of the liver. It is classically correlated with pelvic inflammatory disease, but Hanjani et al., (1992) and Chatwani et al., (1995) described a subgroup of female patients with perihepatic adhesions and no evidence of acute or chronic PID at the time of laparoscopy. One of our cases can be included in this category too, the infertility seeming to be related to the male factor. The patient denied previous liver disease, right upper quadrant pain or surgery involving the liver, gallbladder or billiary tree.

Potential causes proposed by the previous authors (Hanjani et al., 1992; Chatwani et al., 1995) include:

- subclinical infections or immunologic process of the liver that would not have been recognised;
- a possible prior episode of perihepatitis, secondary to Neisseria Gonorrhoeae, as there is no reliable test to detect prior episodes of gonococcal infection, but there is no clinical evidence of the tubal lesion in this patient;
- another possibility was a mild subclinical non *chlamydial* pelvic infection with no histological or biological evidence of past infection.

5. Conclusion

In countries with low resources without prevention programmes for STD (sexual transmitted diseases), *chlamydial* infection remains on the first place as an etiological factor for pelvic adhesions and tubal obstruction in infertility. In our study Ig G for *Chlamydia trachomatis* didn't correlate well with pelvic adhesions, to be able to indicate a laparoscopy only on its presence. We recommend therefore the HYCOSY or HSG to screen patients who need laparoscopy, but because testing for IgG CT causes minimal inconvenience to patient in contrast with HSG and HYCOSY, it still can be maintained in the infertility work up. We are still looking for other infection or immunological markers to indicate the presence of adhesions and therefore, the laparoscopy from the beginning.

6. Acknowledgment

Acknowledgement: to the ANCS bilateral project Romania –Republic of Moldavia, no 423/04.06.2010

7. References

Agrawal, T.; Vats, V.; Salhan, S. & Mittal, A. (2007). Mucosal and peripheral immune responses to *chlamydial* heat shock proteins in women infected with *Chlamydia trachomatis. Clin Exp Immunol.* Vol. 148, pp. 461-468.

Baczynska, A.; Funch, P.; Fedde,r J.; Knudsen, H.J.; Birkelund, S.; Christiansen, G.; (2007) Morphology of human Fallopian tubes after infection with Mycoplasma genitalium and Mycoplasma hominis--in vitro organ culture study.*Hum Reprod.* Vol.22,No.4,pp968-79.

Beatty, W.L.; Byrne, G.I. & Morrison, R.P. (1994). Repeated and persistent infection with *Chlamydia* and the development of chronic inflammation and disease.Trends Microbiol, vol 2, pp. 94–98.

Chatwani, A.; Mohamed, N.; Amin-Hanjani, S.; Nyirjesy, P. (1995). Perihepatic adhesions: another look. *Infectious diseases in Obstetrics and Gynecology*.Vol. 2, pp.263-266

Curtis, A.H. (1930). Causes of adhesion in the right up quadrant. *JAMA*.Vol. 94, pp.1221-1223.

Cohen, C.R.; Koochesfahani, K.M.; Meier, A.S.; Shen, C.; Karunakaran, K.; Ondondo, B.; Kinyari, T.; Mugo, N.R.; Nguti, R. & Brunham, R.C. (2005). Immunoepidemiologic profile of *Chlamydia trachomatis* infection: importance of heat shock protein 60 and interferon -gamma.*J Infect Dis*. Vol. 192, pp. 591-599.

Dieterle, S. (2008). Urogenital infections in reproductive medicine. *Andrologia*. Vol. 40, No. 2, 117-119.

Falk, L. (2010). The overall agreement of proposed definitions of mucopurulent cervicitis in women at high risk of *Chlamydia* infection., *Acta Derm Venereol*. Vol. 90, No. 5, pp. 506-511.

Fitz-Hugh, T.J. (1934). Acute gonococcal peritonitis of right upper quadrant in women. *JAMA*. Vol. 102, pp. 2094.

Forhan, S.E.; Gottlieb, S.L.; Sternberg, M.R.; Xu, F.; Datta, S.D.; McQuillan, G.M.; Berman, S.M. & Markowitz, L.E. (2009). Prevalence of sexually transmitted infections among female adolescents aged 14 to 19 in the United States. *Pediatrics*. Vol. 124, No. 6, pp. 1505–1512.

Forti, G. & Krausz, C. (1998). Evaluation and Treatment of the Infertile Couple, *J Clin Endocrinol. Metabolism*, Vol. 83, No. 12, pp. 4177-4188.

Geisler, W.M. (2010). Duration of untreated, uncomplicated *Chlamydia trachomatis* Genital Infection and Factors Associated with *Chlamydia* Resolution: a review of Human studies. *Journal of Infection Disease*. Vol. 201, suppl 2, pp. S104-112.

Gijsen, A.P.; Land, J.A.; Goossens, V.J.; Slobbe, M.E.; Bruggeman, C.A.(2002).Chlamydia antibody testing in screening for tubal factor subfertility: the significance of IgG antibody decline over time.*Hum Reprod*. Vol.17, no3,pp699-703.

Grieshaber, S.S.; Grieshaber, N.A. & Hackstadt T. (2003). *Chlamydia trachomatis* uses host cell dynein to traffic to the microtubule-organizing center in a p50 dynamitin-independent process. *J Cell Sci*., Vol. 116, No. Pt 18, pp. 3793-3802.

Hanjani, S.; Neely, T. & Chatwani, A. (1992). Perihepatic adhesions; not neccessarly pathognomonic of pelvic infection. *Am J Obstet Gynecol*. Vol. 167, pp. 115-117

Hjelholt, A.; Christiansen, G.; Johannesson, T.G.; Ingerslev H.J. & Birkelund S. (2011). Tubal factor infertility is associated with antibodies against *Chlamydia trachomatis* heat shock protein 60 (HSP60) but not human HSP60, Human Reproduction, Vol.26, No.8 pp. 2069–2076.

Howie, S.E.; Horner, P.J. & Horne, A.W. (2011). *Chlamydia trachomatis* infection during pregnancy - known unknowns. *Discov Med*. Vol. 12, No. 62, pp.57-64.

Imai, H.; Nakao, H.; Shinohara, H.; Fujii, Y.; Tsukino, H.; Hamasuna, R.; Osada, Y.; Fukushima, K.; Inamori, M.; Ikenoue, T. & Katoh, T. (2010). Population-based study of asymptomatic infection with *Chlamydia trachomatis* among female and male students. *Int J STD AIDS*. Vol. 21, No. 5, pp. 362–366.

Land,J.A.;Gijsen,A.P.; Kessels,A.G.H.;Slobbe,M.E.P.;Bruggeman,C.A.(2003).Performance of five serological *Chlamydia* antibody tests in subfertile women. *Hum Reprod.*vol 18:2621-2627

Machado, A.C.; Guimaraes, E.M.; Sakurai, E.; Fioravante, F.C.; Amaral, W.N. & Alves, M.F. (2007). High titers of *Chlamydia trachomatis* antibodies in Brazilian women with tubal occlusion or previous ectopic pregnancy. *Infect Dis Obstet Gynecol*, Vol. 2007, Article ID 24816, 6 pages, doi:10.1155/2007/24816

Madeleine, M.M.; Anttila, T.; Schwartz, S.M.; Saikku, P.; Leinonen, M.; Carter, J.J.; Wurscher, M.; Johnson, L.G.; Galloway, D.A. & Daling, J.R. (2007). Risk of cervical cancer associated with *Chlamydia trachomatis* antibodies by histology, HPV type and HPV cofactors. *Int J Cancer. Vol.* 120, No. 3, pp. 650-655.

Malik, A.; Jain, S.; Rizvi, M.; Shukla, I. & Hakim, S. (2009). *Chlamydia trachomatis* infection in women with secondary infertility. *Fertil Steril.* Vol. 91, pp. 91–95.

Marazzo, J. & Martin, D. (2007). Management of women with cervicitis. *Clin Infect Dis.* Vol. 44, Suppl 3, pp. S102–S110.

Mol, B.W.; Dijkman, B.; Wertheim, P.; Lijmer, J.; van der Veen, F.; Bossuyt, P.M.(1997). The accuracy of serum chlamydial antibodies in the diagnosis of tubal pathology: a meta-analysis. *Fertil Steril.* ,Vol. 67,No.6,pp1031-7

Morre, S.A.; van den Brule, A.J.; Rozendaal, L.; Boeke, A.J.; Voorhorst, F.J.; de Blok, S. & Meijer, C.J. (2002). The natural course of asymptomatic *Chlamydia trachomatis* infections: 45% clearance and no development of clinical PID after one-year follow-up. *Int J STD AIDS*, Vol. 13, Suppl. 2, pp. 12–18.

Paavonen, J.; Kiviat, N.; Brunham, R.C.; Stevens, C.E.; Kuo, C.C.; Stamm, W.E.; Miettinen, A.; Soules, M.; Eschenbach, D.A. & Holmes, K.K. (1985). Prevalence and manifestations of endometritis among women with cervicitis. *Am JObstet Gynecol*, Vol. 152, pp. 280–286.

Patel, A.; Rashid, S.; Godfrey, E. & Panchal, H. (2008). Prevalence of *Chlamydia trachomatis* and *Neisseria gonorrhoeae* genital infections in a publicly funded pregnancy termination clinic: Empiric vs. indicated treatment? *Contraception.* Vol. 78, No. 4, pp.328–331.

Satterwhite, C.; Tian, L.; Braxton, J. & Weinstock, H. (2010). *Chlamydia* prevalence among women and men entering the National Job Training Program: United States, 2003–2007. *Sex Transm Dis.*, Vol. 37, No. 2, pp. 63–74.

Swart, P,; Mol, B.W.; van der Veen, F.; van Beurden, M.; Redekop, W.K.; Bossuyt, P.M. (1995).The accuracy of hysterosalpingography in the diagnosis of tubal pathology: a meta-analysis.*Fertil Steril.* Vol.64,No 3,pp486-91.

Stamm, W. (2008). *Chlamydia trachomatis* infections of the adult. In: Homes K, Sparling P, Mardh P-A, et al, editors. *Sexually Transmitted Diseases.* New York, NY: McGraw Hill; 2008.

Veenemans,L.M.W.; van der Linden P.J.(2002).The value of Chlamydia trachomatis antibody testing in predicting tubal factor infertility..*Hum Reprod.* 2002 Mar;17(3):695-8.

Wang, C.; Tahg, J.; Geisler, W.M.; Crowley-Nowick, P.A., Wilson, C.M.; Kaslow, R.A. (2005). Human leucocyte antigen and cytokine gene variants as predictors of recurrent

Chlamydia trachomatis infection in high risk adolescents. *J Infect Dis.* Vol 191, No. 7, pp.1084-1092.

Weinstock, H.; Berman, S. & Cates, W.Jr. (2004). Sexually transmitted diseases among American youth: Incidence and prevalence estimates, 2000. *Perspect Sex Reprod Health.* Vol. 36, No. 1, pp. 6–10.

World Health Organization. Global prevalence and incidence of selected curable sexually transmitted infections: Overview and estimates. Available from: http://whqlibdoc.who.int/hq/2001/WHO_HIV_AIDS_2001.02.pdf.

Zimmerman, H.L.; Potterat, J.J.; Dukes, R.L.; Muth, J.B.; Zimmerman, H.P.; Fogle, J.S. & Pratts, C.I. (1990). Epidemiologic differences between *chlamydia* and gonorrhea. *Am J Public Health.* Vol. 80, No. 11, pp. 1338–1342.

13

The Role of *Chlamydia trachomatis* in Male Infertility

Gilberto Jaramillo-Rangel et al.*
Department of Pathology, School of Medicine, Autonomous University of Nuevo Leon, Monterrey, Nuevo Leon, Mexico

1. Introduction

1.1 Cell biology of *Chlamydia trachomatis* (*C. trachomatis*)

Chlamydia spp. are associated with a broad clinical spectrum of human diseases, including cardiovascular disease, and pulmonary, ocular and urogenital tract infections [1]. *C. trachomatis* is an obligate intracellular pathogen. The infection cycle starts with the entry of an infectious particle (elementary body or EB) into an epithelial cell. The EB-laden cytoplasmic vacuole (inclusion) migrates to the peri-Golgi region as the EB differentiates into a noninfectious but metabolically active reticulate body (RB). After replication, progeny RBs differentiate back to EBs for exiting the infected cells to disseminate to adjacent cells [2].

Over 18 serological variants (serovars) of *C. trachomatis* have been identified based on monoclonal antibody typing of the major outer membrane protein (MOMP). Serovars A, B, Ba and C cause trachoma, the leading cause of infectious blindness worldwide. Serovars Ba and C are also rarely associated with urogenital infections. Serovars D to K, Da, Ia and Ja are responsible for sexual transmitted diseases (STD) worldwide. The lymphogranuloma venereum (LGV) serovars L1-L3 and L2a, along with serovars D and G, are prevalent in anorectal infections unlike other genital serovars [3].

The clinical course of *C. trachomatis* infection shows remarkable interindividual differences in transmission, symptomatic course, persistence or clearance of infection, and development of late complications. In general, the described differences in clinical course could be explained by interaction between the host (host factors), pathogen (virulence factors), and environmental factors (such as coinfections) [4].

---

* Guadalupe Gallegos-Avila[1], Benito Ramos-González[1], Salomón Alvarez-Cuevas[1], Andrés M. Morales-García[1], José Javier Sánchez[2], Ivett C. Miranda-Maldonado[1], Alberto Niderhauser-García[1], Jesús Ancer-Rodríguez[1] and Marta Ortega-Martínez[1]
[1]*Department of Pathology, School of Medicine, Autonomous University of Nuevo Leon, Monterrey, Nuevo Leon, Mexico*
[2]*Department of Preventive Medicine, Public Health and Microbiology, School of Medicine, Autonomous University of Madrid, Madrid, Spain*

1.2 Urogenital infections with *C. trachomatis* in women and men

C. trachomatis is the most prevalent bacterial cause of sexually transmitted infections in the world and can result in severe genital disease. Over 90 million chlamydial infections are detected annually worldwide and various studies have estimated that there are four to five million new cases of chlamydial infection each year in the USA alone [5, 6]. However, the reported incidence rates of genital chlamydial infections in the population likely are an underestimate because of the highly asymptomatic nature of the pathogen. Approximately 75% of infected women and 50% of infected men have asymptomatic urogenital infections, which represents a huge population of untreated individuals who can transmit the organism [5].

In women, genital tract infections caused by *C. trachomatis* cause major complications as pelvic inflammatory disease (PID), ectopic pregnancy, infertility and infant pneumonia. The risks factors vary in different population groups. However, in most cases, higher prevalence rates in sexually active individuals have been associated with younger age, unmarried status, low socioeconomic conditions and the use of oral contraceptives. *C. trachomatis* is recovered more often from women who acquire gonorrhea than from similarly exposed women who do not acquire gonorrhea [7, 8].

Non-gonococcal urethritis (NGU) is the most common clinical genital syndrome seen in the male, and *C. trachomatis* is the most important etiological agent for NGU. According to the Centers for Disease Control and Prevention (CDC), reported cases of men infected with *C. trachomatis* in the USA raised from 210,955 in 2004 to 315,065 in 2008, and infection rate per 100,000 population in the same period raised from 144.0 to 209.1 [9].

Infection is primarily through penetrative sexual intercourse. In view of the increased practice of oral sex this has become a more important potential route of transmission for genital pathogens, including *C. trachomatis*, not only in homo/bisexual men, but also in heterosexual men [10, 11]. Cell-to-cell transmission, systemic dissemination, and autoinoculation of infectious fluids may contribute to chlamydial spread in the organism [12].

NGU may be complicated by epididymitis and orchitis. Thus, a role of *C. trachomatis* infection in the development of urethritis, epididymitis and orchitis is now well accepted, but a role for this pathogen in the development of prostatitis remains controversial [13, 14]. These disorders caused by *C. trachomatis* in men will be discussed in the next section.

2. Clinical manifestations of male urogenital infection with *C. trachomatis*

2.1 Urethritis

The symptoms of urethritis are variable. In acute urethritis, the patient notices a urethral discharge and dysuria. Others have no symptoms or are symptom-free throughout the day and only notice a drop of pus in the morning prior to the first voiding of urine. Sometimes the glans or meatus urethrae may present with some redness as a sign of inflammation [15].

Urethritis can be caused by several microorganisms. The most relevant are *Neisseria (N.) gonorrhoeae, C. trachomatis, Ureaplasma (U.) urealyticum, Mycoplasma (M.) genitalium* and *Trichomonas (T.) vaginalis* [15, 16]. *C. trachomatis* is the most common pathogen identified in NGU; up to 42% of NGU cases may be caused by this bacterium [17]. Furthermore, there are three cases of chlamydia per case of gonorrhea each year in the USA [18]. Overall, the reported frequency of *C. trachomatis* in male urethritis ranges from 15 to 56% [15, 19].

C. trachomatis infection appears to be equally prevalent in symptomatic and asymptomatic urethral disease, again reiterating the highly asymptomatic nature of this pathogen [13, 20, 21]. When the infection is asymptomatic and undiagnosed, may have potentially serious consequences, like upper genital tract complications.

2.2 Epididymitis

The role of *C. trachomatis* as an etiological agent for the development of epididymitis also is widely accepted [13]. Untreated chlamydial infection of the urethra can spread to the epididymis. Patients usually have unilateral testicular pain with scrotal erythema, tenderness, or swelling over the epididymis [22]. The occurrence of chlamydial epididymitis is not always preceded by symptoms of urethritis and only in some cases they are accompanied by the increase of polymorphonuclear (PMN) leukocytes in urethral discharge. Chlamydial epididymitis is of milder course when compared to epididymitis of another etiology [23].

C. trachomatis is the causative agent in most cases of acute epididymitis in men younger than 35 years, whereas common urinary tract pathogens account for the etiology of the majority of acute and chronic epididymal inflammations in men above this age [24-26]. For example, Zdrodowska-Stefanow et al. found *C. trachomatis* infection in 45.8% of patients of epididymitis below 35 years, whereas in older men the presence of the bacterium was detected in 6.7% [26].

2.3 Epididymo-orchitis

Left untreated, the infection will progress from epididymitis to epididymo-orchitis. In the young patient it must be differentiated from torsion. In the older patient, subacute scrotal pain is most likely epididymo-orchitis. As in torsion, the testicle and/or epididymis is painful and tender; however, in this case, scrotal pain is more gradual in onset, there is no nausea or vomiting, the testicle is not high riding, and there is associated erythema and edema [27].

The causes of epididymo-orchitis reflect common causes of genitourinary infection in men based on particular age groups. In children and older men (>35 years), the most common cause of epididymitis is coliform organisms that result in bacteriuria. In contrast, the organisms that cause urethritis or STD are the common etiologies of epididymitis and orchitis in young adult men (<35 years) [28]. Chlamydial antigen has been detected in urethral or urine samples from 11 to 35% of men presenting with epididymo-orchitis [13].

2.4 Prostatitis

Prostatitis is one of the most common urological disorders and can affect men of any age. Approximately one-third of all men during their lifetime will experience symptoms consistent with prostatitis [29]. The early classification of prostatitis described four syndromes for which pelvic pain in the male was the common factor [30]. In 1995 and 1998, two consensus meetings of the National Institutes of Health (NIH) attempted to refine the four traditional classes of prostatitis. The NIH classification system designates categories I and II for cases in which bacteria clearly cause acute or chronic prostatitis, respectively. NIH category III incorporates the third (nonbacterial) and fourth (prostadynia) traditional classes and designates the entire cohort as Chronic Prostatitis/Chronic Pelvic Pain Syndrome (CP/CPPS), for which current clinical evidence does not indicate a clear bacterial cause. The fourth NIH category includes patients with prostatic inflammation in expressed prostatic secretions or on biopsy specimens performed for other clinical indications [31, 32].

In acute bacterial prostatitis, patients can present with voiding complaints, such as dysuria, frequency, urgency, or hesitancy. Other symptoms can include suprapubic pain, hematuria, or systemic symptoms such as fever, chills, nausea, vomiting, or malaise. Physical examination often reveals a warm, swollen, painful prostate. In chronic bacterial prostatitis a hallmark of a small minority of men is recurrent episodes of urinary tract infection. There may be irritative or lees often obstructive lower urinary tract symptoms and patients often complain of pain in perineum, lower abdomen, genitalia, back and lower rectum. These men also present with exacerbations of acute urinary infection with worsening of symptoms of bladder irritation, occasionally pyrexia, abdominal and loin pain. Pain is the most severe and commonly reported symptom in patients with CP/CPPS. The "classic" presentation is that of a patient who presents with pelvic, perineal, or genital pain associated with voiding and/or sexual dysfunction, characterized by a relapsing, remitting course. Finally, patients included in the fourth NIH category of prostatitis are asymptomatic, but there is evidence of inflammation, infection or both in prostate-specific specimens after massage and/or in cytological or histological investigations of prostatic biopsy specimens which have been obtained on account of elevation of the serum prostate-specific antigen (PSA). [29, 33- 35].

The most important agents of acute and chronic bacterial prostatitis are *Escherichia coli* (accounting for up to 87% of cases), *Pseudomonas* spp., *Enterobacter* spp., *Proteus* spp., *Klebsiella* spp. and *Enterococcus* spp. [35-37]. It is still under debate if and to what extent *C. trachomatis* can cause prostatitis. The definitive association between isolation of the bacterium and a prostatic origin is limited by the fact that diagnostic material from the prostate may reflect only urethral contamination. The prevalence of *C. trachomatis* infection in patients with prostatitis has ranged from 3 to 40% approximately [for reviews see 13, 23].

3. Which is the role of *C. trachomatis* in male infertility?

3.1 Role of the inflammation of the urogenital tract

Both acute and chronic infection and/or inflammation can cause partial or complete obstruction of sperm transport with, respectively, oligozoospermia or azoospermia. Bilateral obstruction of the epididymis is common after recurrent infection with *C. trachomatis* [38, 39]. On the other hand, chronic inflammatory changes in the seminiferous tubules observed in orchitis, would be expected to disrupt the normal process of spermatogenesis and cause alterations both in sperm number and quality [40].

Besides of the anatomical consequences of obstruction, inflammation may act as a co-factor in the etiopathogenesis of infertility. Pressure-induced rupture of the epididymal duct or ductuli efferentes will disrupt the blood-testis barrier, activating an immunological defense reaction and inducing the production of anti-sperm antibodies (ASA) [38]. The presence of ASA can lead to the immobilization and/or agglutination of spermatozoa, which may significantly impair sperm motility affecting acrosome reaction, cervical mucus penetration, zona pellucida binding, and sperm-oocyte function. Also, ASA can prevent implantation and/or arrest embryo development. ASAs were observed in the serum and/or in the seminal plasma or on the sperm surface in approximately 10% of infertile male partners [41, 42].

An increased prevalence of an autoimmune response to sperm in men with *C. trachomatis* in semen suggests that a subclinical chlamydial infection may activate an immune response to sperm [8]. Witkin et al. demonstrated that the presence of a humoral immune response to *C. trachomatis* is correlated with the development of an autoimmune response to spermatozoa [43]. Also, other authors found that chronic male genital infection with *C. trachomatis* could be associated with the development of ASA [44]. However, other groups found no association between chlamydial antibodies in semen and the presence of ASA [45], or between chronic inflammatory or infectious disease of the male reproductive tract with *C. trachomatis* and presence of ASA in semen [46].

On the other hand, heat shock proteins (HSP) are essential mammalian and bacterial stress proteins. At the cellular level, they act as chaperones, have important regulatory functions, and are considered to be an essential factor for reproduction. Members of the 60 kDa HSP family (HSP-60) in particular have been recognized as immunodominant antigens of many microbial pathogens, including *C. trachomatis*. Since the amino acid homology between many microbial HSP (e.g. chlamydial HSP-60) and the human 60 kDa HSP is high, the development of an autoimmune response to the human HSP-60 in susceptible individuals with chronic infections has been suggested [47-49]. According to one study, HSP-60 was present in a soluble form in semen primarily in men with evidence of immune system activation within their genital tract, and this presence correlated with the occurrence of antichlamydial immunoglobulin-A (IgA) [50]. However, Karinen et al. found that in male partners of subfertile couples serum antibody levels to HSP chlamydial antigens were lower than in controls [51]. Future research is necessary to assess the possible role of immunoresponse to bacterial HSP in reproductive function.

Cytokines are regulatory proteins produced by leukocytes and other cells that control inflammation. Controversy exists as to whether elevated cytokine levels are related to semen quality. Kokab et al. found that men infected with *C. trachomatis* had lower percent progressive sperm motility, a higher leukocyte count, and a raised concentration of IL-8 in semen compared with men without infection. However, when median IL-6 concentrations in *C. trachomatis*-infected and -noninfected groups were compared, there was no statistical significance between them [52]. Eggert-Kruse et al. found only one subfertile male patient (1/137) who was positive for *C. trachomatis* and had high IL-8 concentration in seminal plasma [53]. Thus, more studies are necessary in this area.

3.2 Direct interaction of *C. trachomatis* with sperm function and its impact on semen parameters

Attachment of *C. trachomatis* to human spermatozoa was first observed in *in vitro* experiments using immunofluorescence tests with monoclonal antibodies to the bacterium, and transmission electron microscopy. Furthermore, sperm penetration tests revealed that spermatozoa, when progressing forward, can carry chlamydiae attached to them [54]. Also, electron microscope observations on male ejaculates revealed the presence of EBs and RBs of *C. trachomatis* in spermatozoa. After the passage of the infectious EB into the nucleus, all stages of RB formation in the head of the spermatozoon were detected. Thus, was postulated that *C. trachomatis* can infect and be transmitted by spermatozoa to the female partner and cause infertility [55].

Friberg et al. observed that *C. trachomatis* was attached to spermatozoa recovered from the peritoneal cavity of patients with salpingitis, and suggested that spermatozoa may serve as vectors for *C. trachomatis* and spread this pathogen to the peritoneal surfaces of the uterus and fallopian tubes [56]. Also, Vigil et al. suggested that the possible effect of *C. trachomatis* on male fertility is not due to alterations in sperm quality or function, but rather to the transmission of the disease to female partners, causing inflammatory processes and promoting the generation of ASA [57].

However, other studies suggested that *C. trachomatis* may cause a direct damage to spermatozoon. Diquelou et al. observed abnormal sperm movements in men with positive culture for *C. trachomatis* [58]. Hosseinzadeh et al. showed that following incubation with EBs of *C. trachomatis* serovar E, the tyrosine phosphorylation of two major sperm epitopes of 80 and 95 kDa is significantly increased. As a result, these authors hypothesized that *C. trachomatis* serovar E may compromise sperm function by accelerating sperm capacitation, since tyrosine phosphorylation of sperm proteins is closely associated with capacitation *in vitro* [59]. However, a further series of experiments demonstrated that serovar E was causing sperm death, suggesting that the chlamydial-induced increase in tyrosine phosphorylation was associated more with cell death than with capacitation [60]. Finally, in another work Hosseinzadeh et al. demonstrated that *C. trachomatis*-induced death of human spermatozoa is caused primarily by lipopolysaccharide (LPS) [61].

On the other hand, the impact of *C. trachomatis* on semen quality is controversial. *In vitro* studies (see above) show that co-incubation of spermatozoa with chlamydia causes a significant decline in numbers of motile sperm and results in premature sperm death. By, contrast, *in vivo* studies of *C. trachomatis* in men have provided conflicting evidence as to whether it is associated with reduced fertility [62]. Idahl et al. demonstrated that the presence of IgA and IgG antibodies to *C. trachomatis* in serum of male partners of infertile couples was significantly correlated with reduced motility of the spermatozoa, increased number of dead spermatozoa, higher prevalence of leukocytes in semen, decrease in sperm concentration, decrease in the number of progressive spermatozoa and a rise in the teratozoospermia index [63]. Veznik et al. examined 627 sperm samples. Sperm analysis showed significant differences between Chlamydia-positive and –negative samples. The Chlamydia-contaminated group showed lower values of normal sperm morphology, volume, concentration, motility and velocity, than the Chlamydia-negative samples [64]. However, Vigil et al. did not found significant differences between *C. trachomatis*-infected and –noninfected male partners of infertile couples in any of the sperm parameters assessed (sperm concentration, motility and morphology) [57]. Gdoura et al. reported that the mean values of seminal volume, sperm concentration, sperm viability, sperm motility, sperm morphology, and leukocyte count were not significantly related to the detection of *C. trachomatis* DNA in semen specimens of male partners of infertile couples [65]. Finally, another example of the controversial role of *C. trachomatis* in semen parameters is observed in prostatitis patients. Whereas Mazzoli et al. found that *C. trachomatis* affects sperm concentration, percentage of motile sperm and normal morphological forms in prostatitis patients [66], Motrich et al. found that chlamydial infection has no detrimental effects on sperm quality [67]. Thus, for a number of reasons, mostly based on methodological aspects, the impact of *C. trachomatis* on semen parameters is controversial and further investigations should be performed to understand the disparities seen among the available studies.

3.3 The controversial role of leukocytospermia on fertility

Leukocytes are present throughout the male reproductive tract, are found in most ejaculates, and are thought to play an important role in immunosurveillance and phagocytic clearance of abnormal sperm [68]. PMN leukocytes are the most prevalent type of leukocyte in semen (50 to 60%), followed by macrophages/monocytes (20 to 30%), and T-lymphocytes (2 to 5%) [69]. Leukocytospermia is defined by the World Health Organization (WHO) as the presence of peroxidase-positive leukocytes in concentrations greater than $1x10^6$/mL of semen [70].

Leukocytospermia may be due to either a genital tract infection or an inflammatory immunologic response. Other possible etiologies of leukocytospermia besides infection need to be considered. Environmental factors, such as smoking, alcohol consumption, and marijuana use, increase leukocytes in semen. Prolonged abstinence and certain sexual practices (use of vaginal products or anal intercourse) can produce leukocytospermia. Increased leukocytes in semen may be seen in men with abnormal spermatogenesis as a mechanism for the removal of defective sperm from the ejaculate. Finally, varicocele or vasovasostomy can result in a high number of leukocytes in semen [71, 72].

Neofytou et al. found a statistical significance between leukocytospermia and the presence of DNA of the Epstein-Barr virus (EBV) but not with the detection of other members of the Herpesviridae family [73]. Most studies show no correlation between the presence of leukocytes and bacteria in semen [74-76]. However, Punab et al. observed a positive correlation between the leukocyte count and the number of different bacteria detected in semen, and also between the leukocyte count and the total count of microorganisms in semen samples [77]. In fact, these authors along with Gdoura et al. [78] demonstrated that the WHO-defined cut-off point ($1x10^6$ leukocytes per mL) has very low sensitivity for discriminating between patients with and without significant bacteriospermia, as a more optimal sensitivity/specificity ratio appears at $0.2x10^6$ leukocytes per mL of semen.

EBs of *C. trachomatis* incubated in the presence of complement or specific antibody or both caused chemotaxis of human PMN leukocytes *in vitro* [79]. Four types of *C. trachomatis*-leukocyte interaction were observed *in vitro*: (i) minimal to no bacterial binding, (ii) bacterial binding, followed by ingestion and high-level multiplication, (iii) bacterial binding, followed by ingestion but minimal multiplication, and (iv) bacterial binding, but minimal entrance or replication [80]. *In vivo*, was observed that men whose ejaculates were positive for chlamydial DNA had a significantly higher mean concentration of leukocytes than in those whose ejaculates were negative for the presence of DNA of the pathogen. Leukocytospermia was twice as common in men that were positive for chlamydial DNA, but it was not always associated with the presence of chlamydial DNA in semen [81]. Also, Idahl et al. showed that *C. trachomatis* serum IgA was significantly correlated with a higher prevalence of leukocytes in semen [63]. However, Bezold et al. found no difference in prevalence of *C. trachomatis* and other pathogens between asymptomatic male infertile patients with and without leukocytospermia [82]. Also, other authors found no relation between infection with *C. trachomatis* and leukocyte count in semen [65, 83, 84].

The effect of leukocytospermia on male fertility is controversial: whereas some studies found an adverse effect of leukocytospermia on semen quality, others found no effect on semen parameters or even an improvement. This is probably due to different detection methods, different populations studied and to the fact that leukocyte subtypes in semen may have different functions [69, 85-88].

Thus, according to the reviewed literature, the impact of *C. trachomatis* on leukocyte count and male fertility is controversial. In previous works, we presented ultrastructural findings encountered in semen samples of infertile men infected with *C. trachomatis* and/or mycoplasmas: a) structural damage of spermatozoa, b) phagocytosis of damaged spermatozoa by leukocytes, c) destruction of bacteria by leukocytes, d) persistence of bacteria in leukocytes, and e) phagocytosis of damaged spermatozoa and leukocytes by epithelial cells of the genital tract. However, less than 1% of the samples analyzed presented leukocytospermia. Taken together, these data suggest that leukocytes might have a biological impact in fertility in some patients regardless of their count in semen [89-91].

Henkel et al. found that leukocyte counts $<1x10^6$/mL caused a significant decrease of motility and DNA integrity of spermatozoa [92]. Sharma et al. were unable to identify a safe lower limit for leukocyte count in semen because the presence of any leukocytes, no matter how few, was associated with elevated oxidative stress [93]. Aitken et al. concluded that low concentrations of leukocytes in the human ejaculate caused reactive oxygen species (ROS) generation and sperm damage [94]. Thus, the WHO threshold value for leukocytospermia has seriously been questioned by our data and those of others and should be re-evaluated.

3.4 Sperm DNA damage

3.4.1 Oxidative stress

ROS are short-lived chemical intermediates which contain one or more electrons with unpaired spin. In order to overcome this state of unpaired electrons, they are highly and unspecifically reactive molecules able to oxidize proteins, lipids and nucleic acids. In many cases this oxidation causes irreversible damage to biological systems [95].

ROS leads to oxidative damage of the sperm membrane, which reduces fluidity of the membrane and disrupts the fusion events of the acrosome reaction. Sperm damaged by ROS lose motility, especially progressive motility, and have decreased viability and diminished fertilizing ability in the hamster egg sperm penetration assay and in *in vitro* fertilization [71]. Strong evidence suggests that high levels of ROS mediate the occurrence of high frequencies of single- and double-strand DNA breaks commonly observed in the spermatozoa of infertile men. Furthermore, studies in which the sperm was exposed to artificially produced ROS resulted in a significant increase in DNA damage in the form of modification of all bases, production of base-free sites, deletions, frame shifts, DNA cross-links and chromosomal rearrangements [96].

ROS are associated with both increased apoptosis leading to spermatozoa DNA damage and decreased sperm variables (motility, concentration, and morphology) in semen of infertile men [97]. Also, several studies demonstrated an increased ROS generation in the ejaculates of infertile men [98, 99].

In the context of infections, either the pathogen itself may induce an increased generation of ROS or the invading inflammatory cells could generate ROS during the respiratory burst, consuming the antioxidants present. In the male genital tract, ROS are generated by the pathogen, leukocytes (PMNs and macrophages) and defective spermatozoa [100, 101].

Studies with cell cultures infected with *C. trachomatis* demonstrated the production of ROS, which was associated with formation of lipid peroxides in host cell membranes [102]. More recently, other authors also have demonstrated that infection with *C. trachomatis* elicits the production of ROS [103, 104]. These data and the fact that *C. trachomatis* infection has been associated with a raised leukocyte count and the presence of damaged spermatozoa in semen (see precedent sections), indicate that *C. trachomatis* might have a role in male infertility trough the production of ROS.

3.4.2 Apoptosis

The apoptotic mode of cell death is an active and defined process which plays an important role in the development of multicellular organisms and in the regulation and maintenance of the cell populations in tissues upon physiological and pathological conditions [105]. Apoptosis controls the overproduction of male gametes and restricts the normal proliferation levels during conditions unsuitable for sperm development [106]. Also, apoptosis has been involved in the removal of abnormal cells from the testicles of patients with spermatogenetic failures [107].

Oosterhuis et al. found that about 20% of ejaculated spermatozoa are apoptotic, and that the concentration of spermatozoa is lower in men with more apoptotic spermatozoa [108]. Apoptosis has been observed in ejaculated spermatozoa from infertile men. Baccetti et al. observed that apoptosis is abnormally frequent in the sperm cells of the ejaculate of sterile men, and that it shows the classical biochemical and ultrastructural pattern in spermatozoa, spermatids, and apoptotic bodies [109]. Barroso et al. found that spermatozoa from infertile men display hallmarks of apoptosis, such as translocation of membrane phosphatidylserine (PS) and DNA strand breaks [110]. McVicar et al. found that the apoptotic marker Fas was expressed in sperm of infertile men, although DNA fragmentation was observed in all sperm of fertile and infertile men [111].

On the other hand, Shen et al. found that the detection of apoptotic cells in sperm of subfertile patients was inversely correlated to sperm motility and vitality, and positively correlated to total sperm counts, sperm concentration and abnormal sperm morphology [112]. These results support the abortive apoptosis theory, which establishes that apoptosis in mature sperm is initiated during spermatogenesis, after which some cells earmarked for elimination via apoptosis may escape the removal mechanism and contribute to poor sperm quality [113, 114].

Several studies show that *C. trachomatis* causes apoptosis of spermatozoon. Eley et al. observed that co-incubation of sperm with *C. trachomatis* LPS results in cellular death which is in part due to apoptosis [115]. Satta et al. observed that the experimental *C. trachomatis* infection causes sperm PS externalization and DNA fragmentation [116]. Gallegos et al. determined that patients with genitourinary infection by *C. trachomatis* and mycoplasmas have increased sperm DNA fragmentation in comparison with fertile controls [117]. We identified spermatozoa showing ultrastructural features resembling apoptosis in semen samples of infertile men infected with *C. trachomatis* and mycoplasmas. These features included: loose fibrillar-microgranular chromatin network, presence of vacuoles in the chromatin, partially disrupted nuclear membranes and membranous bodies within the vacuoles of the chromatin [90, 91]. Lastly, Sellami et al. showed that inoculation of fertile male Swiss mice in the meatus urethra with *C. trachomatis* could lead to alteration of semen parameters, induction of apoptosis in spermatozoa, and decrease of the reproductive performance of male mice [118]. Taken together, these data support a role of *C. trachomatis* on sperm apoptosis. However, more research is needed to assess the real effect of this process in male fertility.

3.4.3 Other phenomena associated with sperm DNA damage

Besides of oxidative stress and apoptosis, defective sperm chromatin packaging may be another mechanism by which DNA damage arise in human spermatozoa. A variety of causes have been correlated with increased levels of sperm DNA damage, such as cigarette smoking, iatrogenic processes, malignancies (mainly testicular cancer, Hodgkin's disease and leukemia), environmental toxicants, physical agents as radiation and heat, drugs, increasing male age, elevated body mass index and medical conditions as insulin dependent diabetes (for reviews see 96, 119, 120].

4. *C. trachomatis* coinfections and male infertility

Urethritis has traditionally been classified as gonoccocal or NGU. However, the replacement of Gram stain testing of urethral discharge with combined laboratory testing for both gonococcal and chlamydial infections makes this distinction less important [16]. In addition, many studies have shown that some men with gonococcal urethritis are coinfected with *C. trachomatis*.

The frequency of *C. trachomatis* and *N. gonorrhoeae* coinfection in men can vary dramatically depending on several factors, as the individual incidence and prevalence of each of these microorganisms in the studied population, the type of sample analyzed, the method used to detect the bacteria, etcetera. For example, whereas Barbosa et al. reported a coinfection prevalence of 4.4% in Brazil [121], Papadogeorgakis et al. found gonococcal coinfection in 30% of the *C. trachomatis*-infected patients in Greece [122]. Kahn et al. found that 51% of males with gonorrhea were coinfected with chlamydia in US juvenile detention centers [123]. Thus, most of the studies are geographically limited and targeted to a certain portion of the population. However, the fact that some men with gonococcal urethritis are coinfected with *C. trachomatis* has led to the recommendation that men treated for gonoccocal urethritis should be treated routinely with a regimen that is effective against chlamydial infection [124].

Besides of *C. trachomatis* and *N. gonorrhoeae*, obligate pathogenic microorganisms in the male urogenital tract are *Mycobacterium tuberculosis, Treponema pallidum, Haemophilus ducreyi, Klebsiella (Calymmatobacterium) granulomatis*, herpes simplex virus (HSV) 2, human papilloma viruses (HPVs), and *T. vaginalis*. In systemic disease human immunodeficiency viruses, hepatitis B virus (HBV), hepatitis C virus, hepatitis D virus, and cytomegalovirus (CMV) may be excreted with semen, often in high concentrations [37]. Mixed infections are common and failure to diagnose and treat may lead to serious complications and continued transmission.

About 200 established species have already been described within the class Mollicutes, and this number continues to rise [125]. Several Mollicutes species have been isolated from humans. For six of them: *U. urealyticum, M. hominis, M. genitalium, M. primatum, M. spermatophilum* and *M. penetrans*, the genital tract is the main site of colonization [126]. These microorganisms can be found commensal in lower genitourinary tracts of sexually active men and women. Moreover, they cause many disorders such as nonchlamydial NGU [127, 128]. The role of mycoplasmas and ureaplasmas in male infertility has been discussed controversially. Dieterle found no evidence that *U. urealyticum* has a significant impact on male infertility [129]. However, Zeighami et al. found that *U. urealyticum* was more common in semen of infertile men that in semen of healthy controls. Also, in infertile patients infected with ureaplasmas, the volume, count and morphology of semen samples were lower than in infertile patients negatives for the detection of the microorganisms [130]. Gdoura et al. reported that the comparison of the semen parameters of infertile men with and without genital mycoplasmas and ureaplasmas showed no significant differences, apart from the sperm concentration in the infection of *M. hominis* and *M. genitalium* and sperm morphology in the infection of *M. hominis*. Mixed species of mycoplasmas and ureaplasmas were detected in 6.7% of semen samples [131].

The identification of *C. trachomatis* in men infected with other sexually transmitted pathogens and their impact on male fertility have been reported in the literature. Gunyeli et al. determined the prevalence of *C. trachomatis, M. hominis* and *U. urealyticum* infections among infertile couples and effects of these infections on infertility. No difference was found between fertile and infertile couples in terms of the effects of these infections on sperm parameters and infertility. Moreover, the prevalence of these infections was found to be the same in fertile and infertile groups [132]. Gdoura et al. found that the mean values of seminal volume, sperm concentration, sperm viability, sperm motility, sperm morphology, and leukocyte count were not significantly related either to the detection of *C. trachomatis* DNA or to that of genital ureaplasma or mycoplasma DNA in semen specimens of asymptomatic male partners of infertile couples [65]. Bezold et al. detected the presence of DNA of CMV, HPV, human herpesvirus type 6, HSV, HBV, EBV, and *C. trachomatis* in semen from asymptomatic infertile men. The presence of DNA of the pathogens was associated with a decrease in sperm concentration, motile sperm concentration, total sperm count, and neutral alpha-glucosidase concentration [82]. Lastly, we found *C. trachomatis* and mycoplasmas coinfection in semen samples of 25% of the infertile men analyzed. Ultrastructural data suggested that leukocytes might have a role in fertility of some individuals infected with these bacteria [90, 91].

5. Diagnosis and treatment of *C. trachomatis* infections

Laboratory testing of *C. trachomatis* has traditionally consisted of cell culture of inocula prepared from urogenital specimens and later, the antigen and nucleic acid detection technologies were developed [23]. Antibodies to *Chlamydia* spp. are best detected with a microimmunofluorescent (MIF) assay, but these assays are not widely available [133]. The MIF test is valuable in the diagnosis of urogenital infections but is expensive and labor-intensive while the complement fixation (CF) test yields reliable results only for LGV. The value of *Chlamydia*-specific antibodies (IgM, IgG, IgA) in the diagnosis of urogenital infections using indirect immunofluorescence (IF) and immunoperoxidase (IPO) methods is limited since these antibodies are genus-specific and thus will also be elevated in infections with *Chlamydophila pneumoniae* [37].

With regard to its high specificity, the bacteriological culture has been the method of choice for diagnosis. Another advantage is that these cultures maintain the viability of the microorganisms for additional studies such as genotyping or antimicrobial susceptibility tests. One disadvantage of the culture is the low sensitivity of 70-85%. Furthermore, the costs, the high level of technical expertise necessary and the time required to obtain results, are significant disadvantages of this method [8, 134]. Cycloheximide-treated McCoy or HeLa cell lines are used most frequently to isolate *C. trachomatis*. Centrifugation techniques appear to enhance absorption of chlamydiae to cells. Intracytoplasmic inclusions can be detected at 48 to 72 hours with species-specific immunofluorescent monoclonal antibodies for *C. trachomatis* and Giemsa or iodine stains [133].

Rapid methods for diagnosis of a *C. trachomatis* infection include a direct fluorescent-antibody stain (DFA) and enzyme immunoassays (EIA) to detect antigens of the bacterium. Both types of assay have low sensitivities compared to culture and DNA amplification methods. Compared to culture, the sensitivity of these assays, depending on many variables including the population examined and the culture technique used for comparison has been reported to vary from 50 to 90% [135]. However, the use of the DFA technique enables to detect *C. trachomatis in situ* in tissue biopsies, which is not possible with serological or DNA amplification methods (Gallegos et al., personal communication), and its specificity ranges from 98 to 99% [136].

Because of their high sensitivity and specificity, and their possible use for a large range of sample types, nucleic acid amplification tests (NAATs) are the tests of choice for the diagnosis of *C. trachomatis* genital infections. Several commercial NAATs are available and make use of different technologies: polymerase chain reaction (PCR) and real-time PCR, strand displacement amplification, transcription-mediated amplification, and nucleic acid sequence-based amplification. The major targets for amplification-based tests are generally multiple-copy genes, e.g. those carried by the cryptic plasmid of *C. trachomatis*, or gene products such as rRNAs [137].

A new genetic variant of *C. trachomatis* was discovered in Sweden in 2006. The variant has a 377 base pair deletion in the plasmid which was the target for the commonly used NAATs. Therefore this new variant was initially not detected by the NAATs. So far the variant has been only occasionally detected outside Sweden or other Scandinavian countries. Many recent studies have focused on the new variant and disease syndromes associated with this variant. The clinical manifestations seem not to differ from the clinical manifestations caused by the wild types. Subsequently, NAATs have been modified so that this variant can now be detected by all NAATs commonly used in microbiology laboratories [138].

New guidelines for the treatment of patients with sexually transmitted chlamydial infection have been recently published. Recommended regimens are azithromycin 1 g orally in a single dose or doxycycline 100 mg orally twice a day for 7 days. Alternative regimens include erythromycin base 500 mg orally four times a day for 7 days, or erythromycin ethylsuccinate 800 mg orally four times a day for 7 days, or levofloxacin 500 mg orally once daily for 7 days, or ofloxacin 300 mg orally twice a day for 7 days [139].

Clinical trials demonstrate equivalent efficacy and tolerability of azithromycin versus doxycycline regimens for chlamydial infections. Each antibiotic regimen has advantages or disadvantages in terms of cost, convenience, and compliance, yet both regimens will remain recommended as first-line therapy for uncomplicated chlamydial infection in nonpregnant individuals [140]. However, in patients who have erratic health-care-seeking behavior, poor treatment compliance, or unpredictable follow-up, azithromycin might be more cost-effective in treating chlamydia because it enables the provision of a single-dose of directly observed therapy [139, 141].

6. Conclusions

Infection with *C. trachomatis* accounts for the most common bacterial sexually transmitted infection in the world. In men, *C. trachomatis* can cause urethritis, epididymitis, epididymo-orchitis and prostatitis, although asymptomatic infections are quite common. Both acute and chronic infection and/or inflammation can cause partial or complete obstruction of sperm transport with, respectively, oligozoospermia or azoospermia. A subclinical chlamydial infection may activate an immune response to sperm. Infection of the testis and prostate is implicated in a deterioration of sperm, possibly affecting fertility. Also, there is increasing evidence that the function of human spermatozoa can be significantly affected by direct exposure to the bacterium or by the host immune response induced by it. The role of leukocytospermia in the pathogenesis of male infertility remains controversial. The mechanisms by which leukocytes and *C. trachomatis* may lead to sperm damage include ROS generation and the induction of sperm apoptosis. On the other hand, the co-infection with *C. trachomatis* and other microorganisms may be a cause of the impairment of sperm quality, motility and function. Because of their high sensitivity, NAATs are the more reliable methods for the diagnosis of *C. trachomatis* infection. However, in tissue biopsies a DFA assay may be more useful to detect the bacterium. Treatments options for uncomplicated urogenital infections include therapy with azithromycin or doxycycline.

7. References

[1] Ojcius, D.M., Darville, T. & Bavoil, P.M. (2005). Can chlamydia be stopped? *Scientific American*, Vol. 292, No. 5, (May 2005), pp. 72-79, ISSN 0036-8733.

[2] Zhong, G., Lei, L., Gong, S., Qi, M. & Fan, H. (2010). Molecular basis of chlamydial interactions with host cells, *Proceedings of the Twelfth International Symposium on Human Chlamydial Infections*, pp. 69-78, ISBN 0-9664383-3-7, Lake Fuschl, Hof bei Salzburg, Austria, June 20-25, 2010.

[3] Dean, D., Myers, G.S. & Read, T.D. (2006). Lessons and challenges arising from the "first wave" of Chlamydia genome sequencing, In: *Chlamydia: Genomics and Pathogenesis*, P.M. Bavoil & P.B. Wyrick (Eds.), pp. 11-12, Horizon Bioscience, ISBN 978-1-904933-21-2, Norfolk, UK.

[4] Karimi, O., Ouburg, S., de Vries, H.J., Peña, A.S., Pleijster, J., Land, J.A. & Morré, S.A. (2009). TLR2 haplotypes in the susceptibility to and severity of Chlamydia trachomatis infections in Dutch women. *Drugs Today*, Vol. 45 (Suppl. B), (November 2009), pp. 67-74, ISSN 1699-3993.

[5] Dean, D. (2009). Chlamydia trachomatis today: treatment, detection, immunogenetics and the need for a greater global understanding of chlamydial disease pathogenesis. *Drugs Today*, Vol. 45 (Suppl. B), (November 2009), pp. 25-31, ISSN 1699-3993.

[6] World Health Organization. (2011). Chlamydia trachomatis, In: *Initiative for Vaccine Research (IVR): Sexually Transmitted Diseases*, 07.06.2011, Available from http://www.who.int/vaccine_research/diseases/soa_std/en/index1.html

[7] Creighton, S., Tenant-Flowers, M., Taylor, C.B., Miller, R. & Low, N. (2003). Co-infection with gonorrhoea and chlamydia: how much is there and what does it mean? *International Journal of STD & AIDS*, Vol. 14, No. 2, (February 2003), pp. 109-113, ISSN 0956-4624.

[8] Gonzales, G.F., Muñoz, G., Sánchez, R., Henkel, R., Gallegos-Avila, G., Díaz-Gutierrez, O., Vigil, P., Vásquez, F., Kortebani, G., Mazzolli, A. & Bustos-Obregón, E. (2004). Update on the impact of Chlamydia trachomatis infection on male fertility. *Andrologia*, Vol. 36, No. 1, (February 2004), pp. 1-23, ISSN 0303-4569.

[9] Centers for Disease Control and Prevention. (November 2009a). Table 5. Chlamydia-men-reported cases and rates by state/area and region listed in alphabetical order: United States and outlying areas, 2004-2008, In: *2008 Sexually Transmitted Diseases Surveillance*, 18.08.2011, Available from http://www.cdc.gov/std/stats08/tables/5.htm

[10] Edwards, S. & Carne, C. (1998). Oral sex and transmission of non-viral STIs. *Sexually Transmitted Infections*, Vol. 74, No. 2, (April 1998), pp. 95-100, ISSN 1368-4973.

[11] Karlsson, A., Osterlund, A. & Forssen, A. (2011). Pharyngeal Chlamydia trachomatis is not uncommon any more. *Scandinavian Journal of Infectious Diseases*, Vol. 43, No. 5, (May 2011), pp. 344-348, ISSN 0036-5548.

[12] Perry, L.L. & Hughes, S. (1999). Chlamydial colonization of multiple mucosae following infection by any mucosal route. *Infection and Immunity*, Vol. 67, No. 7, (July 1999), pp. 3686-3689, ISSN 0019-9567.

[13] Cunningham, K.A. & Beagley, K.W. (2008). Male genital tract chlamydial infection: implications for pathology and infertility. *Biology of Reproduction*, Vol. 79, No. 2, (August 2008), pp. 180-189, ISSN 0006-3363.

[14] Paavonen, J. & Eggert-Kruse, W. (1999). Chlamydia trachomatis: impact on human reproduction. *Human Reproduction Update*, Vol. 5, No. 5, (September-October 1999), pp. 433-447, ISSN 1355-4786.

[15] Ochsendorf, F.R. (2006). Urethritis, Sexually Transmitted Diseases (STD), Aquired Immunodeficiency Syndrome (AIDS), In: *Andrology for the Clinician*, W.B. Schill, F. Comhaire & T.B. Hargreave (Eds.), pp. 327-338, SpringerLink, ISBN 978-3-540-23171-4, Heidelberg, Germany.

[16] Brill, J.R. (2010). Sexually transmitted infections in men. *Primary Care: Clinics in Office Practice*, Vol. 37, No. 3, (September 2010), pp. 509-525, ISSN 0095-4543.

[17] Stamm, W.E., Batteiger, B.E., McCormack, W.M., Totten, P.A., Sternlicht, A., Kivel, N.M. & Rifalazil Study Group. (2007). A randomized, double-blind study comparing single-dose rifalazil with single-dose azithromycin for the empirical treatment of nongonococcal urethritis in men. *Sexually Transmitted Diseases*, Vol. 34, No. 8, (August 2007), pp. 545-552, ISSN 0148-5717.

[18] Centers for Disease Control and Prevention. (November 2009b). National surveillance data for Chlamydia, Gonorrhea, and Syphilis, In: *Sexually Transmitted Diseases in the United States, 2008*, 10.06.2011, Available from http://www.cdc.gov/std/stats08/trends.htm

[19] Bakare, R.A., Oni, A.A., Umar, U.S., Okesola, A.O., Kehinde, A.O., Fayemiwo, S.A. & Fasina, N.A. (2002). Non-gonoccocal urethritis due to Chlamydia trachomatis: the Ibadan experience. *African Journal of Medicine and Medical Sciences*, Vol. 31, No. 1, (March 2002), pp. 17-20, ISSN 0309-3913.
[20] Tait, I.A. & Hart, C.A. (2002). Chlamydia trachomatis in non-gonococcal urethritis patients and their heterosexual partners: routine testing by polymerase chain reaction. *Sexually Transmitted Infections*, Vol. 78, No. 4, (August 2002), pp. 286-288, ISSN 1368-4973.
[21] Takahashi, S., Takeyama, K., Kunishima, Y., Takeda, K., Suzuki, N., Nishimura, M., Furuya, R. & Tsukamoto, T. (2006). Analysis of clinical manifestations of male patients with urethritis. *Journal of Infection and Chemotherapy*, Vol. 12, No. 5, (October 2006), pp. 283-286, ISSN 1341-321X.
[22] Miller, K.E. (2006). Diagnosis and treatment of Chlamydia trachomatis infection. *American Family Physician*, Vol. 73, No. 8, (April 2006), pp. 1411-1416, ISSN 0002-838X.
[23] Wagenlehner, F.M., Weidner, W. & Naber, K.G. (2006). Chlamydial infections in urology. *World Journal of Urology*, Vol. 24, No. 1, (February 2006), pp. 4-12, ISSN 0724-4983.
[24] Melekos, M.D & Asbach, H.W. (1988). The role of chlamydiae in epididymitis. *International Urology and Nephrology*, Vol. 20, No. 3, (May 1988), pp. 293-297, ISSN 0301-1623.
[25] Terho, P. (1982). Chlamydia trachomatis and clinical genital infections: a general review. *Infection*, Vol. 10 (Suppl. 1), (January 1982), pp. 5-9, ISSN 0300-8126.
[26] Zdrodowska-Stefanow, B., Ostaszewska, I., Darewicz, B., Darewicz, J., Badyda, J., Pucilo, K., Bulhak, V. & Szczurzewski, M. (2000). Role of Chlamydia trachomatis in epididymitis. Part I: Direct and serologic diagnosis. *Medical Science Monitor*, Vol. 6, No. 6, (November-December 2000), pp. 1113-1118, ISSN 1234-1010.
[27] Alsikafi, N.F, Elliott, S.P, Garcia, M.M. & McAninch, J.W. (2007). Urogenital tract, In: *Acute Care Surgery. Principles and Practice*, L.D. Britt, D.D. Trunkey & D.V. Feliciano (Eds.), pp. 561-588, Springer, ISBN 978-0-387-34470-6, New York, USA.
[28] Tran, K.B. & Wessells, H. (2005). Genital and infectious emergencies. Prostatitis, urethritis, and epididymo-orchitis, In: *Urological Emergencies. A Practical Guide*, H. Wessells & J.W McAninch (Eds.), pp. 135-146, Humana Press, ISBN 978-1-58829-256-8, New York, USA.
[29] Nguyen, C.T. & Shoskes, D.A. (2008). Evaluation of the prostatitis patient, In: *Chronic Prostatitis/Chronic Pelvic Pain Syndrome*, D.A. Shoskes (Ed.), pp. 1-16, Humana Press, ISBN 978-1-934115-27-5, New York, USA.
[30] Drach, G.W., Fair, W.R., Meares, E.M. & Stamey, T.A. (1978). Classification of benign diseases associated with prostatic pain: prostatitis or prostatodynia? *The Journal of Urology*, Vol. 120, No. 2, (August 1978), pp. 226, ISSN 0022-5347.
[31] Hua, V.N., Williams, D.H. & Schaeffer, A.J. (2005). Role of bacteria in chronic prostatitis/chronic pelvic pain syndrome. *Current Urology Reports*, Vol. 6, No. 4, (July 2005), pp. 300-306, ISSN 1527-2737.
[32] Krieger, J.N., Nyberg, L. Jr. & Nickel, J.C. (1999). NIH consensus definition and classification of prostatitis. *The Journal of the American Medical Association*, Vol. 282, No. 3, (July 1999), pp. 236-237, ISSN 0098-7484.

[33] Bishop, M.C. (2006). Prostatitis, In: *Andrology for the Clinician*, W.B. Schill, F. Comhaire & T.B. Hargreave (Eds.), pp. 217-224, SpringerLink, ISBN 978-3-540-23171-4, Heidelberg, Germany.

[34] Potts, J.M. (2000). Prospective identification of National Institutes of Health category IV prostatitis in men with elevated prostate specific antigen. *The Journal of Urology*, Vol. 164, No. 5, (November 2000), pp. 1550-1553, ISSN 0022-5347.

[35] Rothman, J.R. & Jaffe W.I. (2007). Prostatitis: updates on diagnostic evaluation. *Current Urology Reports*, Vol. 8, No. 4, (July 2007), pp. 301-306, ISSN 1527-2737.

[36] Millán-Rodríguez, F., Palou, J., Bujons-Tur, A., Musquera-Felip, M., Sevilla-Cecilia, C., Serrallach-Orejas, M., Baez-Angles, C. & Villavicencio-Mavrich, H. (2006). Acute bacterial prostatitis: two different sub-categories according to a previous manipulation of the lower urinary tract. *World Journal of Urology*, Vol. 24, No. 1, (February 2006), pp. 45-50, ISSN 0724-4983.

[37] Schiefer, H.G. & von Graevenitz, A. (2006). Clinical Microbiology, In: *Andrology for the Clinician*, W.B. Schill, F. Comhaire & T.B. Hargreave (Eds.), pp. 401-407, SpringerLink, ISBN 978-3-540-23171-4, Heidelberg, Germany.

[38] Depuydt, C., Mahmoud, A. & Everaert, K. (2006). Infection/inflammation of the male genital tract as cause of abnormal spermatozoa. In: *Andrology for the Clinician*, W.B. Schill, F. Comhaire & T.B. Hargreave (Eds.), pp. 322-327, SpringerLink, ISBN 978-3-540-23171-4, Heidelberg, Germany.

[39] Dohle, G.R., van Roijen, J.H., Pierik, F.H., Vreeburg, J.T & Weber, R.F. (2003). Subtotal obstruction of the male reproductive tract. *Urological Research*, Vol. 31, No. 1, (March 2003), pp. 22-24, ISSN 0300-5623.

[40] Weidner, W., Krause, W. & Ludwig, M. (1999). Relevance of male accessory gland infection for subsequent fertility with special focus on prostatitis. *Human Reproduction Update*, Vol. 5, No. 5, (September-October 1999), pp. 421-432, ISSN 1355-4786.

[41] Lenzi, A., Gandini, L., Lombardo, F., Rago, R., Paoli, D. & Dondero, F. (1997). Antisperm antibody detection: 2. Clinical, biological, and statistical correlation between methods. *American Journal of Reproductive Immunology*, Vol. 38, No. 3, (September 1997), pp. 224-230, ISSN 1600-0897.

[42] Silva, C.A.A., Ferreira Borba, A., Cocuzza, M., Freire de Carvalho, J. & Bonfá, E. (2008). Autoimmune orchitis, In: *Diagnostic Criteria in Autoimmune Diseases*, Y. Shoenfeld, R. Cervera & M.E. Gershwin (Eds.), pp. 281-284, Humana Press, ISBN 978-1-60327-472-2, Totowa, NJ, USA.

[43] Witkin, S.S., Kligman, I. & Bongiovanni, A.M. (1995). Relationship between an asymptomatic male genital tract exposure to Chlamydia trachomatis and an autoimmune response to spermatozoa. *Human Reproduction*, Vol. 10, No. 11, (November 1995), pp. 2952-2955, ISSN 0268-1161.

[44] Martínez-Prado, E. & Camejo-Bermúdez, M.I. (2010). Expression of IL-6, IL-8, TNF-alpha, IL-10, HSP-60, anti-HSP-60 antibodies, and anti-sperm antibodies, in semen of men with leukocytes and/or bacteria. *American Journal of Reproductive Immunology*, Vol. 63, No. 3, (March 2010), pp. 233-243, ISSN 1600-0897.

[45] Eggert-Kruse, W., Buhlinger-Gopfarth, N., Rohr, G., Probst, S., Aufenanger, J., Naher, H. & Runnebaum, B. (1996). Antibodies to Chlamydia trachomatis in semen and

relationship with parameters of male fertility. *Human Reproduction*, Vol. 11, No. 7, (July 1996), pp. 1408-1417, ISSN 0268-1161.

[46] Marconi, M., Pilatz, A., Wagenlehner, F., Diemer, T. & Weidner, W. (2009). Are antisperm antibodies really associated with proven chronic inflammatory and infectious diseases of the male reproductive tract? *European Urology*, Vol. 56, No. 4, (October 2009), pp. 708-715, ISSN 0302-2838.

[47] Domeika, M., Domeika, K., Paavonen, J., Mardh, P.A. & Witkin, S.S. (1998). Humoral immune response to conserved epitopes of Chlamydia trachomatis and human 60-kDa heat-shock protein in women with pelvic inflammatory disease. *The Journal of Infectious Diseases*, Vol. 177, No. 3, (March 1998), pp. 714-719, ISSN 0022-1899.

[48] Neuer, A., Spandorfer, S.D., Giraldo, P., Dieterle, S., Rosenwaks, Z. & Witkin, S.S. (2000). The role of heat shock proteins in reproduction. *Human Reproduction Update*, Vol. 6, No. 2, (March-April 2000), pp. 149-159, ISSN 1355-4786.

[49] Eggert-Kruse, W., Neuer, A., Clussmann, C., Boit, R., Geissler, W., Rohr, G. & Strowitzki, T. (2002). Seminal antibodies to human 60kd heat shock protein (HSP 60) in male partners of subfertile couples. *Human Reproduction*, Vol. 17, No. 3, (March 2002), pp. 726-735, ISSN 0268-1161.

[50] Munoz, M.G., Jeremias, J. & Witkin, S.S. (1996). The 60 kDa heat shock protein in human semen: relationship with antibodies to spermatozoa and Chlamydia trachomatis. *Human Reproduction*, Vol. 11, No. 12, (December 1996), pp. 2600-2603, ISSN 0268-1161.

[51] Karinen, L., Pouta, A., Hartikainen, A.L., Bloigu, A., Paldanius, M., Leinonen, M., Saikku, P. & Jarvelin, M.R. (2004). Antibodies to Chlamydia trachomatis heat shock proteins Hsp60 and Hsp10 and subfertility in general population at age 31. *American Journal of Reproductive Immunology*, Vol. 52, No. 5, (November 2004), pp. 291-297, ISSN 1600-0897.

[52] Kokab, A., Akhondi, M.M., Sadeghi, M.R., Modarresi, M.H., Aarabi, M., Jennings, R., Pacey, A.A. & Eley, A. (2010). Raised inflammatory markers in semen from men with asymptomatic chlamydial infection. *Journal of Andrology*, Vol. 31, No. 2, (March-April 2010), pp. 114-120, ISSN 0196-3635.

[53] Eggert-Kruse, W., Boit, R., Rohr, G., Aufenanger, J., Hund, M. & Strowitzki, T. (2001). Relationship of seminal plasma interleukin (IL)-8 and IL-6 with semen quality. *Human Reproduction*, Vol. 16, No. 3, (March 2001), pp. 517-528, ISSN 0268-1161.

[54] Wolner-Hanssen, P. & Mardh, P.A. (1984). In vitro tests of the adherence of Chlamydia trachomatis to human spermatozoa. *Fertility and Sterility*, Vol. 42, No. 1, (July 1984), pp. 102-107, ISSN 0015-0282.

[55] Erbengi, T. (1993). Ultrastructural observations on the entry of Chlamydia trachomatis into human spermatozoa. *Human Reproduction*, Vol. 8, No. 3, (March 1993), pp. 416-421, ISSN 0268-1161.

[56] Friberg, J., Confino, E., Suarez, M. & Gleicher, N. (1987). Chlamydia trachomatis attached to spermatozoa recovered from the peritoneal cavity of patients with salpingitis. *The Journal of Reproductive Medicine*, Vol. 32, No. 2, (February 1987), pp. 120-122, ISSN 0024-7758.

[57] Vigil, P., Morales, P., Tapia, A., Riquelme, R. & Salgado, A.M. (2002). Chlamydia trachomatis infection in male partners of infertile couples: incidence and sperm function. *Andrologia*, Vol. 34, No. 3, (June 2002), pp. 155-161, ISSN 0303-4569.

[58] Diquelou, J.Y, Pastorini, E., Feneux, D. & Gicquel, J.M. (1989). The role of Chlamydia trachomatis in producing abnormal movements by spermatozoa. *Journal de gynécologie, obstétrique et biologie de la reproduction*, Vol. 18, No. 5, pp. 615-625, ISSN 0368-2315.

[59] Hosseinzadeh, S., Brewis, I.A., Pacey, A.A, Moore, H.D. & Eley, A. (2000). Coincubation of human spermatozoa with Chlamydia trachomatis in vitro causes increased tyrosine phosphorylation of sperm proteins. *Infection and Immunity*, Vol. 68, No. 9, (September 2000), pp. 4872-4876, ISSN 0019-9657.

[60] Hosseinzadeh, S., Brewis, I.A., Eley, A. & Pacey, A.A. (2001). Co-incubation of human spermatozoa with Chlamydia trachomatis serovar E causes premature sperm death. *Human Reproduction*, Vol. 16, No. 2, (February 2001), pp. 293-299, ISSN 0268-1161.

[61] Hosseinzadeh, S., Pacey, A.A. & Eley, A. (2003). Chlamydia trachomatis-induced death of human spermatozoa is caused primarily by lipopolysaccharide. *Journal of Medical Microbiology*, Vol. 52, No. 3, (March 2003), pp. 193-200, ISSN 0022-2615.

[62] Eley, A., Pacey, A.A., Galdiero, M., Galdiero, M. & Galdiero, F. (2005a). Can Chlamydia trachomatis directly damage your sperm? *The Lancet Infectious Diseases*, Vol. 5, No. 1, (January 2005), pp. 53-57, ISSN 1473-3099.

[63] Idahl, A., Abramsson, L., Kumlin, U., Liljeqvist, J.A. & Olofsson, J.I. (2007). Male serum Chlamydia trachomatis IgA and IgG, but not heat shock protein 60 IgG, correlates with negatively affected semen characteristics and lower pregnancy rates in the infertile couple. *International Journal of Andrology*, Vol. 30, No.2, (April 2007), pp. 99-107, ISSN 0105-6263.

[64] Veznik, Z., Pospisil, L., Svecova, D., Zajicova, A. & Unzeitig, V. (2004). Chlamydiae in the ejaculate: their influence on the quality and morphology of sperm. *Acta Obstetricia et Gynecologica Scandinavica*, Vol. 83, No. 7, (July 2004), pp. 656-660, ISSN 0001-6349.

[65] Gdoura, R., Kchaou, W., Ammar-Keskes, L., Chakroun, N., Sellemi, A., Znazen, A., Rebai, T. & Hammami, A. (2008a). Assessment of Chlamydia trachomatis, Ureaplasma urealyticum, Ureaplasma parvum, Mycoplasma hominis, and Mycoplasma genitalium in semen and first void urine specimens of asymptomatic male partners of infertile couples. *Journal of Andrology*, Vol. 29, No. 2, (March-April 2008), pp. 198-206, ISSN 0196-3635.

[66] Mazzoli, S., Cai, T., Addonisio, P., Bechi, A., Mondaini, N. & Bartoletti, R. (2010). Chlamydia trachomatis infection is related to poor semen quality in young prostatitis patients. *European Urology*, Vol. 57, No. 4, (April 2010), pp. 708-714, ISSN 0302-2838.

[67] Motrich, R.D., Cuffini, C., Oberti, J.P., Maccioni, M. & Rivero, V.E. (2006). Chlamydia trachomatis occurrence and its impact on sperm quality in chronic prostatitis patients. *Journal of Infection*, Vol. 53, No. 3, (September 2006), pp. 175-183, ISSN 0163-4453.

[68] Tomlinson, M.J., White, A., Barratt, C.L., Bolton, A.E. & Cooke, I.D. (1992). The removal of morphologically abnormal sperm forms by phagocytes: a positive role for seminal leukocytes? *Human Reproduction*, Vol. 7, No. 4, (April 1992), pp. 517-522, ISSN 0268-1161.

[69] Wolff, H. (1995). The biologic significance of white blood cells in semen. *Fertility and Sterility*, Vol. 63, No. 6, (June 1995), pp. 1143-1157, ISSN 0015-0282.

[70] World Health Organization. (2010). *WHO Laboratory Manual for the Examination and Processing of Human Semen* (5th edition), World Health Organization, ISBN 978-92-4-154778-9, New York, USA.

[71] Branigan, E.F. (2005). Infection and male infertility, In: *Office Andrology*, P.E. Patton & D.E. Battaglia (Eds.), pp. 189-200, Humana Press, ISBN 978-1-58829-318-3, Totowa, NJ, USA.

[72] Close, C.E., Roberts, P.L. & Berger, R.E. (1990). Cigarettes, alcohol and marijuana are related to pyospermia in infertile men. *The Journal of Urology*, Vol. 144, No. 4, (October 1990), pp. 900-903, ISSN 0022-5347.

[73] Neofytou, E., Sourvinos, G., Asmarianaki, M., Spandidos, D.A. & Makrigiannakis, A. (2009). Prevalence of human herpes virus types 1-7 in the semen of men attending an infertility clinic and correlation with semen parameters. *Fertility and Sterility*, Vol. 91, No. 6, (June 2009), pp. 2487-2494, ISSN 0015-0282.

[74] Eggert-Kruse, W., Pohl, S., Naher, H., Tilgen, W. & Runnebaum, B. (1992). Microbial colonization and sperm-mucus interaction: results in 1000 infertile couples. *Human Reproduction*, Vol. 7, No. 5, (May 1992), pp. 612-620, ISSN 0268-1161.

[75] Lackner, J., Schatzl, G., Horvath, S., Kratzik, C. & Marberger, M. (2006). Value of counting white blood cells (WBC) in semen samples to predict the presence of bacteria. *European Urology*, Vol. 49, No. 1, (January 2006), pp. 148-153, ISSN 0302-2838.

[76] Rodin, D.M, Larone, D. & Goldstein, M. (2003). Relationship between semen cultures, leukospermia, and semen analysis in men undergoing fertility evaluation. *Fertility and Sterility*, Vol. 79 (Suppl 3), (June 2003), pp. 1555-1558, ISSN 0015-0282.

[77] Punab, M., Loivukene, K., Kermes, K. & Mandar, R. (2003). The limit of leucocytospermia from the microbiological viewpoint. *Andrologia*, Vol. 35, No. 5, (October 2003), pp. 271-278, ISSN 0303-4569.

[78] Gdoura, R., Kchaou, W., Znazen, A., Chakroun, N., Fourati, M., Ammar-Keskes, L. & Hammami, A. (2008b). Screening for bacterial pathogens in semen samples from infertile men with and without leukocytospermia. *Andrologia*, Vol. 40, No. 4, (August 2008), pp. 209-218, ISSN 0303-4569.

[79] Register, K.B., Morgan, P.A. & Wyrick, P.B. (1986). Interaction between Chlamydia spp. and human polymorphonuclear leukocytes in vitro. *Infection and Immunity*, Vol. 52, No. 3, (June 1986), pp. 664-670, ISSN 0019-9567.

[80] Bard, J.A. & Levitt, D. (1985). Binding, ingestion, and multiplication of Chlamydia trachomatis (L2 serovar) in human leukocyte cell lines. *Infection and Immunity*, Vol. 50, No. 3, (December 1985), pp. 935-937, ISSN 0019-9567.

[81] Hosseinzadeh, S., Eley, A. & Pacey, A.A. (2004). Semen quality of men with asymptomatic chlamydial infection. *Journal of Andrology*, Vol. 25, No. 1, (January-February 2004), pp. 104-109, ISSN 0196-3635.

[82] Bezold, G., Politch, J.A., Kiviat, N.B., Kuypers, J.M, Wolff, H. & Anderson, D.J. (2007). Prevalence of sexually transmissible pathogens in semen from asymptomatic male infertility patients with and without leukocytospermia. *Fertility and Sterility*, Vol. 87, No. 5, (May 2007), pp. 1087-1097, ISSN 0015-0282.

[83] El Feky, M.A., Hassan, E.A., El Din, A.M., Hofny, E.R., Afifi, N.A., Eldin, S.S. & Baker, M.O. (2009). Chlamydia trachomatis: methods for identification and impact on semen quality. *Egyptian Journal of Immunology*, Vol. 16, No. 1, pp. 49-59, ISSN 1110-4902.

[84] Munuce, M.J., Bregni, C., Carizza, C. & Mendeluk, G. (1999). Semen culture, leukocytospermia, and the presence of sperm antibodies in seminal hyperviscosity. *Archives of Andrology*, Vol. 42, No.1, (January-February 1999), pp. 21-28, ISSN 0148-5016.

[85] Aziz, N., Agarwal, A., Lewis-Jones, I., Sharma, R.K. & Thomas, A.J. Jr. (2004). Novel associations between specific sperm morphological defects and leukocytospermia. *Fertility and Sterility*, Vol. 82, No. 3, (September 2004), pp. 621-627, ISSN 0015-0282.

[86] Keck, C., Gerber-Schafer, C., Clad, A., Wilhelm, C. & Breckwoldt, M. (1998). Seminal tract infections: impact on male fertility and treatment options. *Human Reproduction Update*, Vol. 4, No. 6, (November-December 1998), pp. 891-903, ISSN 1355-4786.

[87] Kiessling, A.A., Lamparelli, N., Yin, H.Z, Seibel, M.M. & Eyre, R.C. (1995). Semen leukocytes: friends or foes? *Fertility and Sterility*, Vol. 64, No. 1, (July 1995), pp. 196-198, ISSN 0015-0282.

[88] Tomlinson, M.J., Barratt, C.L & Cooke, I.D. (1993). Prospective study of leukocytes and leukocyte subpopulations in semen suggests they are not a cause of male infertility. *Fertility and Sterility*, Vol. 60, No. 6, (December 1993), pp. 1069-1075, ISSN 0015-0282.

[89] Gallegos-Avila, G., Alvarez-Cuevas, S., Niderhauser-García, A., Ancer-Rodríguez, J., Jaramillo-Rangel, G. & Ortega-Martínez, M. (2009a). Phagocytosis of spermatozoa and leucocytes by epithelial cells of the genital tract in infertile men infected with Chlamydia trachomatis and mycoplasmas. *Histopathology*, Vol. 55, No. 2, (August 2009), pp. 232-234, ISSN 1365-2559.

[90] Gallegos-Avila, G., Ortega-Martínez, M., Ramos-González, B., Tijerina-Menchaca, R., Ancer-Rodríguez, J. & Jaramillo-Rangel, G. (2009b). Ultrastructural findings in semen samples of infertile men infected with Chlamydia trachomatis and mycoplasmas. *Fertility and Sterility*, Vol. 91, No.3, (March 2009), pp. 915-919, ISSN 0015-0282.

[91] Gallegos-Avila, G., Ancer-Rodríguez, J., Ortega-Martínez, M. & Jaramillo-Rangel, G. (2010). Infection and phagocytosis: analysis in semen with transmission electron microscopy. In: *Microscopy: Science, Technology, Applications and Education*, A. Mendez-Vilas & J. Diaz (Eds.), pp. 85-92, Formatex Research Center, ISBN 978-84-614-6189-9, Badajoz, Spain.

[92] Henkel, R., Kierspel, E., Stalf, T., Mehnert, C., Menkveld, R., Tinneberg, H.R., Schill, W.B. & Kruger, T.F. (2005). Effect of reactive oxygen species produced by spermatozoa and leukocytes on sperm functions in non-leukocytospermic patients. *Fertility and Sterility*, Vol. 83, No. 3, (March 2005), pp. 635-642, ISSN 0015-0282.

[93] Sharma, R.K., Pasqualotto, A.E, Nelson, D.R., Thomas, A.J. Jr. & Agarwal, A. (2001). Relationship between seminal white blood cell counts and oxidative stress in men treated at an infertility clinic. *Journal of Andrology*, Vol. 22, No. 4, (July-August 2001), pp. 575-583, ISSN 0196-3635.

[94] Aitken, R.J., Buckingham, D.W., Brindle, J., Gomez, E., Baker, H.W. & Irvine, D.S. (1995). Analysis of sperm movement in relation to the oxidative stress created by

leukocytes in washed sperm preparations and seminal plasma. *Human Reproduction*, Vol. 10, No. 8, (August 1995), pp. 2061-2071, ISSN 0268-1161.

[95] Sanocka, D. & Kurpisz, M. (2004). Reactive oxygen species and sperm cells. *Reproductive Biology and Endocrinology*, Vol. 23, No. 2, (March 2004), pp. 12, ISSN 1477-7827.

[96] Agarwal, A. & Said, T.M. (2003). Role of sperm chromatin abnormalities and DNA damage in male infertility. *Human Reproduction Update*, Vol. 9, No. 4, (July-August 2003), pp. 331-345, ISSN 1355-4786.

[97] Wang, X., Sharma, R.K., Sikka, S.C, Thomas, A.J. Jr., Falcone, T. & Agarwal, A. (2003). Oxidative stress is associated with increased apoptosis leading to spermatozoa DNA damage in patients with male factor infertility. *Fertility and Sterility*, Vol. 80, No. 3, (September 2003), pp. 531-535, ISSN 0015-0282.

[98] Iwasaki, A. & Gagnon, C. (1992). Formation of reactive oxygen species in spermatozoa of infertile patients. *Fertility and Sterility*, Vol. 57, No.2, (February 1992), pp. 409-416, ISSN 0015-0282.

[99] Mazzilli, F., Rossi, T., Marchesini, M., Ronconi, C. & Dondero, F. (1994). Superoxide anion in human semen related to seminal parameters and clinical aspects. *Fertility and Sterility*, Vol. 62, No. 4, (October 1994), pp. 862-868, ISSN 0015-0282.

[100] Ochsendorf, F.R. (1999). Infections in the male genital tract and reactive oxygen species. *Human Reproduction Update*, Vol. 5, No. 5, (September-October 1999), pp. 399-420, ISSN 1355-4786.

[101] Vicari, E. (2000). Effectiveness and limits of antimicrobial treatment on seminal leukocyte concentration and related reactive oxygen species production in patients with male accessory gland infection. *Human Reproduction*, Vol. 15, No. 12, (December 2000), pp. 2536-2544, ISSN 0268-1161.

[102] Azenabor, A.A. & Mahony, J.B. (2000). Generation of reactive oxygen species and formation and membrane lipids peroxides in cells infected with Chlamydia trachomatis. *International Journal of Infectious Diseases*, Vol. 4, No. 1, (March 2000), pp. 46-50, ISSN 1201-9712.

[103] Abdul-Sater, A.A., Said-Sadier, N., Lam, V.M., Singh, B., Pettengill, M.A., Soares, F., Tattoli, I., Lipinski, S., Girardin, S.E., Rosenstiel, P. & Ojcius, D.M. (2010). Enhancement of reactive oxygen species production and chlamydial infection by the mitochondrial Nod-like family member NLRX1. *The Journal of Biological Chemistry*, Vol. 285, No. 53, (December 2010), pp. 41637-41645, ISSN 0021-9258.

[104] Boncompain, G., Schneider, B., Delevoye, C., Kellermann, O., Dautry-Versat, A. & Subtil, A. (2010). Production of reactive oxygen species is turned on and rapidly shut down in epithelial cells infected with Chlamydia trachomatis. *Infection and Immunity*, Vol. 78, No. 1, (January 2010), pp. 80-87, ISSN 0019-9567.

[105] Gewies, A. (2003). Introduction to apoptosis, In: *ApoReview*, 15.07.2011, Available from www.ihcworld.com/_books/apointro.pdf

[106] Sinha Hikim, A.P. & Swerdloff, R.S. (1999). Hormonal and genetic control of germ cell apoptosis in the testis. *Reviews of Reproduction*, Vol. 4, No. 1, (January 1999), pp. 38-47, ISSN 1359-6004.

[107] Tesarik, J., Greco, E., Cohen-Bacrie, P. & Mendoza, C. (1998). Germ cell apoptosis in men with complete and incomplete spermiogenesis failure. *Molecular Human Reproduction*, Vol. 4, No. 8, (August 1998), pp. 757-762, ISSN 1360-9947.

[108] Oosterhuis, G.J., Mulder, A.B., Kalsbeek-Batenburg, E., Lambalk, C.B., Schoemaker, J. & Vermes, I. (2000). Measuring apoptosis in human spermatozoa: a biological assay for semen quality? *Fertility and Sterility*, Vol. 74, No. 2, (August 2000), pp. 245-250, ISSN 0015-0282.

[109] Baccetti, B., Collodel, G. & Piomboni, P. (1996). Apoptosis in human ejaculated sperm cells (notulae seminologicae 9). *Journal of Submicroscopic Cytology and Pathology*, Vol. 28, No. 4, (October 1996), pp. 587-596, ISSN 1122-9497.

[110] Barroso, G., Morshedi, M. & Oehninger, S. (2000). Analysis of DNA fragmentation, plasma membrane translocation of phosphatidylserine and oxidative stress in human spermatozoa. *Human Reproduction*, Vol. 15, No. 6, (June 2000), pp. 1338-1344, ISSN 0268-1161.

[111] McVicar, C.M., McClure, N., Williamson, K., Dalzell, L.H. & Lewis, S.E. (2004). Incidence of Fas positivity and deoxyribonucleic acid double-stranded breaks in human ejaculated sperm. *Fertility and Sterility*, Vol. 81 (Suppl. 1), (March 2004), pp. 767-774, ISSN 0015-0282.

[112] Shen, H.M., Dai, J., Chia, S.E., Lim, A. & Ong, C.N. (2002). Detection of apoptotic alterations in sperm in subfertile patients and their correlations with sperm quality. *Human Reproduction*, Vol. 17, No. 5, (May 2002), pp. 1266-1273, ISSN 0268-1161.

[113] Sakkas, D., Mariethoz, E., Manicardi., G., Bizzaro, D., Bianchi, P.G. & Bianchi, U. (1999a). Origin of DNA damage in ejaculated human spermatozoa. *Reviews of Reproduction*, Vol. 4, No. 1, (January 1999), pp. 31-37, ISSN 1359-6004.

[114] Sakkas, D., Mariethoz, E. & St John, J.C. (1999b). Abnormal sperm parameters in humans are indicative of an abortive apoptotic mechanism linked to the Fas-mediated pathway. *Experimental Cell Research*, Vol. 251, No. 2, (September 1999), pp. 350-355, ISSN 0014-4827.

[115] Eley, A., Hosseinzadeh, S., Hakimi, H., Geary, I. & Pacey, A.A. (2005b). Apoptosis of ejaculated human sperm is induced by co-incubation with Chlamydia trachomatis lipopolysaccharide. *Human Reproduction*, Vol. 20, No. 9, (September 2005), pp. 2601-2607, ISSN 0268-1161.

[116] Satta, A., Stivala, A., Garozzo, A., Morello, A., Perdichizzi, A., Vicari, E., Salmeri, M. & Calogero, A.E. (2006). Experimental Chlamydia trachomatis infection causes apoptosis in human sperm. *Human Reproduction*, Vol. 21, No.1, (January 2006), pp. 134-137, ISSN 0268-1161.

[117] Gallegos, G., Ramos, B., Santiso, R., Goyanes, V., Gosálvez, J. & Fernández, J.L. (2008). Sperm DNA fragmentation in infertile men with genitourinary infection by Chlamydia trachomatis and Mycoplasma. *Fertility and Sterility*, Vol. 90, No. 2, (August 2008), pp. 328-334, ISSN 0015-0282.

[118] Sellami, H., Gdoura, R., Mabrouk, I., Frikha-Gargouri, O., Keskes, L., Mallek, Z., Aouni, M. & Hammami, A. (2011). A proposed mouse model to study male infertility provoked by genital serovar E, Chlamydia trachomatis. *Journal of Andrology*, Vol. 32, No. 1, (January-February 2011), pp. 86-94, ISSN 0196-3635.

[119] Aitken, R.J. & De Iuliis, G.N. (2010). On the possible origins of DNA damage in human spermatozoa. *Molecular Human Reproduction*, Vol. 16, No. 1, (January 2010), pp. 3-13, ISSN 1360-9947.

[120] Pacey, A.A. (2010). Environmental and lifestyle factors associated with sperm DNA damage. *Human Fertility (Cambridge)*, Vol. 13, No. 4, (December 2010), pp. 189-193, ISSN 1464-7273.

[121] Barbosa, M.J., Moherdaui, F., Pinto, V.M., Ribeiro, D., Cleuton, M. & Miranda, A.E. (2010). Prevalence of Neisseria gonorrhoeae and Chlamydia trachomatis infection in men attending STD clinics in Brazil. *Revista da Sociedade Brasileira de Medicina Tropical*, Vol. 43, No. 5, (September-October 2010), pp. 500-503, ISSN 0037-8682.

[122] Papadogeorgakis, H., Pittaras, T.E., Papaparaskevas, J., Pitiriga, V., Katsambas, A. & Tsakris, A. (2010). Chlamydia trachomatis serovar distribution and Neisseria gonorrhoeae coinfection in male patients with urethritis in Greece. *Journal of Clinical Microbiology*, Vol. 48, No. 6, (June 2010), pp. 2231-2234, ISSN 0095-1137.

[123] Kahn, R.H., Mosure, D.J., Blank, S., Kent, C.K., Chow, J.M., Boudov, M.R., Brock, J., Tulloch, S. & Jail STD Prevalence Monitoring Project. (2005). Chlamydia trachomatis and Neisseria gonorrhoeae prevalence and coinfection in adolescents entering selected US juvenile detention centers, 1997-2002. *Sexually Transmitted Diseases*, Vol. 32, No. 4, (April 2005), pp. 255-259, ISSN 0148-5717.

[124] Centers for Disease Control and Prevention, Workowski, K.A. & Berman, S.M. (2006). Sexually transmitted diseases treatment guidelines, 2006. *MMWR. Recommendations and reports: Morbidity and Mortality Weekly Report. Recommendations and Reports/Centers for Disease Control*. Vol. 55 (RR-11), (August 2006), pp. 1-94, ISSN 1057-5987.

[125] Razin, S. (2006). The genus Mycoplasma and related genera (class Mollicutes), In: *The Prokaryotes. A Handbook on the Biology of Bacteria. Volume 4: Bacteria: Firmicutes, Cyanobacteria*, M. Dworkin, S. Falkow, E. Rosenberg, K.H. Schleifer & E. Stackebrandt (Eds.), pp. 836, Springer Science+Business Media LLC, ISBN 978-0387-25494-4, New York, USA.

[126] Uuskula, A. & Kohl, P.K. (2002). Genital mycoplasmas, including Mycoplasma genitalium, as sexually transmitted agents. *International Journal of STD & AIDS*, Vol. 13, No. 2, (February 2002), pp. 79-85, ISSN 0956-4624.

[127] Jensen, J.S. (2004). Mycoplasma genitalium: the aetiological agent of urethritis and other sexually transmitted diseases. *Journal of the European Academy of Dermatology and Venereology*, Vol. 18, No. 1, (January 2004), pp. 1-11, ISSN 0926-9959.

[128] Kilic, D., Basar, M.M., Kaygusuz, S., Yilmaz, E., Basar, H. & Batislam, E. (2004). Prevalence and treatment of Chlamydia trachomatis, Ureaplasma urealyticum, and Mycoplasma hominis in patients with non-gonococcal urethritis. *Japanese Journal of Infectious Diseases*, Vol. 57, No. 1, (February 2004), pp. 17-20, ISSN 1344-6304.

[129] Dieterle, S. (2008). Urogenital infections in reproductive medicine. *Andrologia*, Vol. 40, No. 2, (April 2008), pp. 117-119, ISSN 0303-4569.

[130] Zeighami, H., Peerayeh, S.N., Yazdi, R.S. & Sorouri, R. (2009). Prevalence of Ureaplasma urealyticum and Ureaplasma parvum in semen of infertile and healthy men. *International Journal of STD & AIDS*, Vol. 20, No. 6, (June 2009), pp. 387-390, ISSN 0956-4624.

[131] Gdoura, R., Kchaou, W., Chaari, C., Znazen, A., Keskes, L., Rebai, T. & Hammami, A. (2007). Ureaplasma urealyticum, Ureaplasma parvum, Mycoplasma hominis and Mycoplasma genitalium infections and semen quality of infertile men. *BMC Infectious Diseases*, Vol. 8, No. 7, (November 2007), pp. 129, ISSN 1471-2334.

[132] Gunyeli, I., Abike, F., Dunder, I., Aslan, C., Tapisiz, O.L., Temizkan, O., Payasli, A. & Erdemoglu, E. (2011). Chlamydia, Mycoplasma and Ureaplasma infections in infertile couples and effects of these infections on fertility. *Archives of Gynecology and Obstetrics*, Vol. 283, No. 2, (February 2011), pp. 379-385, ISSN 0932-0067.

[133] Darville, T. (2006). Chlamydia trachomatis genital infection in adolescents and young adults, In: *Hot Topics in Infection and Immunity in Children*, A.J. Pollard & A. Finn (Eds.), pp. 85-100, Springer, ISBN 978-0-387-31783-0, New York, USA.

[134] Black, C.M. (1997). Current methods of laboratory diagnosis of Chlamydia trachomatis infections. *Clinical Microbiology Reviews*, Vol. 10, No. 1, (January 1997), pp. 160-184, ISSN 0893-8512.

[135] De la Maza, L.M., Pezzlo, M.T., Shigei, J.T. & Peterson, E.M. (2004). *Color Atlas of Medical Bacteriology*, American Society for Microbiology Press, ISBN 1-55581-206-6, Washington, DC, USA.

[136] Quinn, T.C., Gupta, P.K., Burkman, R.T., Kappus, E.W., Barbacci, M. & Spence, M.R. (1987). Detection of Chlamydia trachomatis cervical infection: a comparison of Papanicolaou and immunofluorescent staining with cell culture. *American Journal of Obstetrics and Gynecology*, Vol. 157, No. 2, (August 1987), pp. 394-399, ISSN 0002-9378.

[137] Bebear, C. & de Barbeyrac, B. (2009). Genital Chlamydia trachomatis infections. *Clinical Microbiology and Infection*, Vol. 15, No. 1, (January 2009), pp. 4-10, ISSN 1198-743X.

[138] Paavonen, J. (2010). Chlamydia trachomatis infections of the genital tract: selected highlights, *Proceedings of the Twelfth International Symposium on Human Chlamydial Infections*, pp. 379-388, ISBN 0-9664383-3-7, Lake Fuschl, Hof bei Salzburg, Austria, June 20-25, 2010.

[139] Centers for Disease Control and Prevention. (January 2011). Sexually transmitted diseases treatment guidelines 2010. Chlamydial infections, In: *Sexually Transmitted Diseases*, 02.08.2011, Available from http://www.cdc.gov/std/treatment/2010/chlamydial-infections.htm

[140] Geisler, W.M. (2007). Management of uncomplicated Chlamydia trachomatis infections in adolescents and adults: evidence reviewed for the 2006 Centers for Disease Control and Prevention sexually transmitted diseases treatment guidelines. *Clinical Infectious Diseases*, Vol. 44 (Suppl. 3), (April 2007), pp. S77-83, ISSN 1058-4838.

[141] Lau, C.Y. & Qureshi, A.K. (2002). Azithromycin versus doxycycline for genital chlamydial infections: a meta-analysis of randomized clinical trials. *Sexually Transmitted Diseases*, Vol. 29, No. 9, (September 2002), pp. 497-502, ISSN 0148-5717.

14

Chlamydial Infection in Urologic Diseases

Young-Suk Lee[1] and Kyu-Sung Lee[2]
[1]*Sungkyunkwan University School of Medicine, Samsung Changwon Hospital,*
[2]*Sungkyunkwan University School of Medicine, Samsung Medical Center,*
Republic of Korea

1. Introduction

Chlamydiae are small gram-negative obligate intracellular microorganisms that preferentially infect squamocolumnar epithelial cells. *Chlamydia* species which can cause infections in humans are *C. pneumoniae, C. psittaci* and *C. trachomatis*. Of the three species, *C. trachomatis* is responsible for sexually transmitted diseases (STDs) in men and women. Identified in 1907, *C. trachomatis* was the first chlamydial agent discovered in humans. The life cycle of *C. trachomatis* consists of an extracellular form (the elementary body) and the intracellular form (the reticulate body). The elementary body attaches to and penetrates columnar epithelial cells, where it transforms into the reticulate body, the active reproductive form of the organism. The reticulate body forms large inclusions within cells and then begins to reorganize into small elementary bodies. *C. trachomatis* can be differentiated into 18 serovars (serologically variant strains) based on monoclonal antibody-based typing assays. Serovars A, B, Ba, and C are associated with trachoma (a serious eye disease that can lead to blindness), serovars D-K are associated with genital tract infections, and L1-L3 are associated with lymphogranuloma venereum.

The pathophysiologic mechanisms of *chlamydiae* are poorly understood. The initial response to infected epithelial cells is a neutrophilic infiltration followed by lymphocytes, macrophages, plasma cells, and eosinophilic invasion. The release of cytokines and interferons by the infected epithelial cell initializes this inflammatory cascade. Infection with chlamydial organisms invokes a humoral cell response, resulting in secretory immunoglobulin A (IgA) and circulatory immunoglobulin M (IgM) and immunoglobulin G (IgG) antibodies and a cellular immune response.

C. trachomatis infections are prevalent worldwide, but current research, screening, and treatment are focused on females, with the burden of disease and infertility sequel considered to be a predominantly female problem. *C. trachomatis* is responsible for a wide spectrum of diseases that include vaginitis, cervicitis, salpingitis, endometritis, conjunctivitis, and neonatal pneumonia. A role for this pathogen in the development of male urethritis, epididymitis, and orchitis is widely accepted. Also, *C. trachomatis* can cause chronic prostatitis and infertility.

This chapter covers *C. trachomatis* infection in urologic diseases focusing on male problems such as urethritis, epididymitis and orchitis; chronic prostatitis and infertility in terms of the epidemiology, screening, clinical manifestations, diagnosis, treatment and complication.

2. Epidemiology of *C. trachomatis*

In contrast to gonorrhea infection, most men and women who are infected are asymptomatic, and, therefore, diagnosis is delayed until a positive screening result or upon discovering a symptomatic partner. *Chlamydia* has been isolated in approximately 40-60% of males presenting with nongonococcal urethritis. Recent epidemiological studies indicate a high prevalence rate of asymptomatic men who act as a reservoir for chlamydial infections.

Chlamydia is the most common bacterial sexually transmitted infection in the world, causing an estimated 89 million new cases of infection each year (World Health Organization [WHO], 2001). Ethnic group or socioeconomic deprivation, introducing a screening program that is less available and accessible, and less acceptable to people from vulnerable and disadvantaged groups, could create or widen existing inequalities in *chlamydia* prevalence. According to the Centers for Disease Control and Prevention, the last 5 years have seen an increasing rate of infection (43.5%) and it is more common in women than in men (3:1) in USA (Centers for Disease Control and Prevention [CDC], 2010).

According to Low and colleagues (Low et al., 2007), in UK in 2004, 104,155 cases of *chlamydia* were diagnosed in genitourinary medicine clinics. The number of diagnosed infections has been increasing steadily since 1995, partly owing to increased numbers of people being tested; nearly 700,000 genital infections and sexually transmitted infections were diagnosed in genitourinary clinics in 2003 compared with 442,000 in 1995. In 2007, National Chlamydia Screening Programme was conducted with 4731 men and women aged 16–39 years participated in the cross-sectional screening survey in UK. There were 219 people with positive *chlamydia* results. Prevalence in 16–24-year-olds was 6.2% in women and 5.3% in men. The prevalence in young men was the same as in young women. The examination of risk factors for *chlamydia* in the prevalence and case-control studies did not find any factors, other than young age. The number of new partners in the past 12 months was the strongest predictor of infection.

Population based studies in Europe and the USA suggest that the prevalence of *chlamydia* in men and women aged 15-24 years is 2–6% (Andersen et al., 2002; Fenton et al., 2001; Miller et al., 2004; van Bergen et al., 2005). The peak age group for infection is 16–19 years in women and 20–24 years in men (CDC, 2010).

3. Screening

Asymptomatic chlamydial infection is common among both men and women, and detection often relies on screening. Routine laboratory screening for common STDs is indicated for sexually active adolescents. The CDC and the US Preventive Services Task Force each recommend annual chlamydial screening for all sexually active women ≤ 25 years of age and also for older women with risk factors (e.g., those who have a new sex partner or multiple sex partners). For the persons in correctional facilities, universal screening of adolescent females for *chlamydia* should be conducted at intake in juvenile detention or jail facilities. Universal screening of adult females should be conducted at intake among adult females up to 35 years of age or on the basis of local institutional prevalence data (CDC, 2010).

The benefits of screening could be demonstrated in areas where the prevalence of infection and rates of pelvic inflammatory diseases are decreasing since the screening programs began (Kamwendo et al., 1996; Scholes et al., 1996; Mertz et al., 1997; CDC, 2010). Evidence is insufficient to recommend routine screening for *C. trachomatis* in sexually active young men based on feasibility, efficacy, and cost-effectiveness. However, screening of sexually active young men should be considered in clinical settings associated with high prevalence of *chlamydia* (e.g., adolescent clinics, correctional facilities, and STD clinics) (CDC, 2010).

4. Clinical manifestation of chlamydial urethritis, epididymitis, prostatitis

C. trachomatis is a bacterium whose sexually transmitted strains D–K cause genital tract infections in women (cervicitis and urethritis) and men (urethritis, epididymitis, prostatitis). However, *chlamydia* is known as a 'silent' disease because about three-quarters of infected women and about half of infected men have no symptoms (van de Laar & Morre, 2007). Symptoms of chlamydial urethritis, if present, include discharge of mucopurulent or purulent material, dysuria, urethral pruritis, urinary frequency or urgency, and show up about 1-3 weeks after being infected. One of the most common symptoms for in cases of *chlamydia* in men is a painful urination.

In the worst cases *chlamydia* infection can, without treatment, lead on to other problems such as epididymitis or orchitis if the infection has made it to the epididymis or the testicles. This is particularly worrisome because it can occasionally cause a man to become sterile. In men younger than the age of 35 who are sexually active with women, the most common offending organisms causing epididymitis are *N. gonorrhoeae* and *C. trachomatis*. Approximately 45–85% of men with epididymitis have had prior *C. trachomatis* infections and/or gonococcal infections (Berger et al., 1978; Berger et al, 1979; Melekos & Asbach, 1988). Acute epididymitis represents sudden occurrence of pain and swelling of the epididymis associated with acute inflammation of the epididymis. Physical examination localizes the tenderness to the epididymis (although in many cases the testis is also involved in the inflammatory process and subsequent pain—referred to as epididymo-orchitis). The spermatic cord is usually tender and swollen. Early on in the process, only the tail of the epididymis is tender, but the inflammation quickly spreads to the rest of the epididymis and if it continues to the testis, the swollen epididymis becomes indistinguishable from the testis. Although the process is usually unilateral, it is sometimes bilateral. Physical examination may reveal a toxic and febrile patient. The skin of the involved hemiscrotum is erythematous and edematous, and the testis is quite tender to palpation or can be associated with a transilluminating hydrocele. If the diagnosis is not evident from the history, physical examination, and these simple tests, scrotal ultrasonography should be performed (to rule out malignancy in patients with chronic orchitis/orchialgia). The most important differential diagnosis in young men and boys is testicular torsion. Testicular torsion is often difficult to differentiate from an acute inflammatory condition. Scrotal ultrasound (with use of Doppler imaging to determine testicular blood flow) is especially helpful in differential diagnosis, but occasionally it will miss the diagnosis (particularly with intermittent or partial torsion) and the clinician should err in favor of the surgically correctable diagnosis of torsion.

Another potential problem without treatment of the *chlamydia* infection is chronic prostatitis. The evidence supporting the role of *C. trachomatis* in chronic prostatitis is conflicting. The predominant symptom of chronic prostatitis is pain, which is most commonly localized to the perineum, suprapubic area, and penis but can also occur in the testes, groin, or low back. Pain during or after ejaculation is one of the most prominent, important, and bothersome feature in many patients. Irritative and obstructive voiding symptoms including urgency, frequency, hesitancy, and poor interrupted flow are associated. Infertility and chronic prostatitis will be discussed in the '7. Complications'.

The *C. trachomatis* strains L1, L2 and L3 cause lymphogranuloma venereum. This tropical sexually transmitted infection is currently responsible for outbreaks of ulcerative proctitis mainly affecting homosexual men (many with HIV infection) in various European countries and the USA (Blank et al., 2005; Nieuwenhuis et al., 2004; Nieuwenhuis et al., 2003).

5. Diagnosis

Detection of current *chlamydia* infection is based on demonstration of the organism. Tissue culture methods, direct fluorescent antibody tests or enzyme-linked immunosorbent assays (EIA) have now been largely replaced by nucleic acid amplification tests (NAATs). Culture and hybridization tests require urethral swab specimens, whereas NAATs can be performed on urine specimens. The sensitivity and specificity of the NAATs are clearly the highest of any of the test platforms for the diagnosis of chlamydial infections. Since accurate diagnosis is the goal, there is no justification for the ongoing use of other technologies. Non-culture tests such as EIA and DNA probe assays are inferior to NAATs with respect to performance. According to the Expert Consultation Meeting Summary Report 2009, NAATs are recommended for detection of reproductive tract infections caused by *C. trachomatis* in men and women with and without symptoms.

Optimal specimen types for NAATs are first catch urine from men and vaginal swabs from women. There is little need for urethral swab specimens and in some studies these samples are less sensitive than urine; urethral swab specimens and male urine were equivalent in specificity. For female screening, vaginal swab specimens are the preferred specimen type. Vaginal swab specimens are as sensitive as cervical swab specimens and there is no difference in specificity. Cervical samples are acceptable when pelvic examinations are done, but vaginal swab specimens are an appropriate sample type even when a full pelvic exam is being performed. Cervical sample specimens are certainly acceptable for NAAT testing in those settings that combine Pap and sexually transmitted infection testing from the same sample, such as liquid cytology. There was some concern about some liquid cytology samples being more likely to result in inhibition of amplification or contamination in some assays, as well as, a concern that liquid cytology samples lead to testing of populations at low risk for infection. Female urine, while acceptable, may have reduced performance when compared to genital swab samples. NAATs are also recommended for the detection of rectal and oropharyngeal infections caused by *C. trachomatis*. However, these specimen types have not been cleared by the FDA for use with NAATs and laboratories must establish performance specifications to satisfy CMS regulations for CLIA compliance prior to reporting results for patient management. Ninety five percent of testing for *chlamydia* performed using a test of choice or acceptable test (Table 1).

Test	Sites FCU	Cervix	Urethra	Pharynx	Rectum	Vulvo-vaginal
NAAT	1	1	1	3	3	3
EIA	4	2	2	5	5	5
DFA	2	2	2	2	2	5
TC	5	2	2	1	1	5

FCU, First catch urine; NAAT, nucleic acid amplification test; EIA, enzyme immunoassay; DFA, direct fluorescent antibody; TC, tissue culture.
1, test of choice; 2, acceptable, but not first choice; 3, not licensed, although encouraging work being performed; 4, only for use in asymptomatic males; 5, not recommended.
All recommendations are at grade B unless stated otherwise.

Table 1. Summary of recommended tests for use with different sites of samples (Carder et al., 2006)

These tests are very accurate, but are laboratory dependent, creating a delay between testing and receipt of diagnosis, caused by the time it takes to transport the test sample to the laboratory and process the result. This delay is problematic, as a number of infected patients will not return for treatment, following their positive diagnosis. Point-of-care testing methods can provide results within hours after the tests are carried out, which could allow infected patients to be treated immediately, as well as allowing the immediate identification of recent sexual partners who should also be tested. The Chlamydia Rapid Test is a point-of-care test that has reported improved accuracy. However, according to the recent systematic review of the clinical effectiveness and cost-effectiveness of rapid point-of-care tests for the detection of genital *chlamydia* infection, NAATs was found to be less costly and more effective, although there were circumstances under which point-of-care testing could become a viable alternative (i.e. if uptake rates for testing were increased using this point-of-care method) (Hislop et al., 2010). There are currently no point-of-care assays on the market that are suitable for routine use, although some may be of use in high risk populations where immediate treatment is the overriding concern due to poor follow up. The group felt that development of improved point-of-care tests desirable.

Laboratory tests should include Gram stains of a urethral smear and a midstream urine specimen. A urethral swab and midstream urine specimen should be sent for culture and sensitivity testing. When a boy or young man is diagnosed with epididymitis or orchitis, and the diagnosis is uncertain, he should be further evaluated with duplex Doppler scrotal ultrasonography to rule out torsion.

To detect recent or past exposure to *C. trachomatis*, both systemic and local antibodies in secretions can be used. In order to be considered as a diagnostic test the specificity must be high. The microimmunofluorescence test is considered the gold standard but is difficult to perform and the specificity of the test has been questioned. Antibodies to the chlamydial lipopolysaccharide could cause cross-reactivity but specific antibodies to *C. pneumoniae* and *C. trachomatis* can usually be distinguished by the test. ELISA tests based on peptides from the major outer-membrane protein polyantigen of *C. trachomatis* have so far showed high specificities. Although IgG antibodies can be detected in serum in 40-100% of infected women, demonstrated by cell culture or NAAT, 16-87% of *C. trachomatis*-negative women also have such antibodies. The situation is similar for serum IgA antibodies but at a lower level. The predictive values therefore become unacceptably low to use IgG or IgA antibodies in serum to diagnose current lower genital tract infection. The shorter half-life of IgA antibodies compared to IgG has suggested that IgA antibodies could reflect persistent infection. There is no solid ground as yet for the use of IgA antibodies as a marker of persistent or unresolved infection by *C. trachomatis.* IgM antibodies may have a better positive predictive value but the sensitivity is too low, which precludes their use for the diagnosis of genital chlamydial infection (Persson, 2002).

6. Treatment

Uncomplicated lower genital tract *chlamydia* infections can be cured by a single dose or short course of antibiotics. The guidelines for the treatment of persons who have or are at risk for STDs were updated by CDC after consultation with a group of professionals knowledgeable in the field of STDs who met in Atlanta on April 18–30, 2009. The approach to the management of uncomplicated genital chlamydial infection in adults includes (1) treatment of patients (to reduce complications and prevent transmission to sex partners), (2) treatment of sex partners (to prevent reinfection of the index patient and infection of other partners), (3) risk-reduction counseling, and (4) repeat chlamydial testing in women a few months after treatment (to identify recurrent/persistent infections). In the guidelines, the CDC convened an advisory group to examine recent abstracts and published literature addressing management of *C. trachomatis* infections in adolescents and adults. Key questions were posed and answered on the basis of quality of evidence and expert opinion. Clinical trials continue to demonstrate equivalent efficacy and tolerability of azithromycin and doxycycline regimens, and both remain recommended as first-line therapy in nonpregnant individuals. Azithromycin 1g and doxycycline 100mgs bd for 7 days have been shown to be >95% effective in the treatment of uncomplicated lower genital tract *C. trachomatis* infection (Horner, 2008; Horner & Boag, 2006). For those with upper genital tract disease i.e., pelvic inflammatory disease, a prolonged course of treatment for up to 14 days is recommended (Royal College of Obstetricians and Gynaecologists [RCOG], 2008). More data and clinical experience are available to support the efficacy, safety, and tolerability of azithromycin in pregnant women. Evidence is building that expedited partner therapy, with provision of treatment or a prescription, may be just as effective as or more effective than standard partner referral in ensuring partner treatment and preventing *chlamydia* recurrence in women. Although there are more studies needed and barriers to be addressed before its widespread use, expedited partner therapy will be recommended as an option for partner management.

Test of cure is not routinely recommended if standard treatment has been given, there is confirmation that the patient has adhered to therapy, and there is no risk of re-infection. However, if these criteria cannot be met or if the patient is pregnant a test of cure is advised. This should be taken using the same technique as was used for the initial testing. Ideally, a minimum of 3–5 weeks post-treatment is required as NAATs will demonstrate residual DNA/RNA even after successful treatment of the organism (recommendation grade A).

7. Complications

C. trachomatis can cause damage to both women and men's reproductive organs. If *chlamydia* is left untreated, men may develop chronic complications or irreversible damage which may cause male infertility. There is not thought to be any lasting immunity following a *chlamydia* infection that has resolved spontaneously or been treated with antibiotics, so repeated infections can occur (Holmes et al., 1999).

7.1 Chronic prostatitis

Prostatitis is the most common urologic diagnosis in men younger than 50 years and represents 8% of urology office visits (Collins et al., 1998). Chronic pelvic pain syndrome (CPPS) which is divided into two categories, inflammatory CPPS (Category ⅢA which corresponds to the former chronic nonbacterial prostatitis), and non-inflammatory CPPS (Category ⅢB which corresponds to the former prostatodynia), is the most common type of prostatitis. It is condition that many clinicians find difficult to treat effectively. The problem is that although in semen and expressed prostatic secretions there is evidence of inflammation, no pathogens are usually found in samples analyzed when routine culture methods are used. The clinical symptoms of patients with CPPS IIIA and IIIB are similar, perineal pain, often radiating to the genital area, urinary symptoms, ejaculatory disturbance, and are of chronic nature. The cause of CPPS has not yet been established and there is a lot of controversy regarding its etiology (Motrich et al., 2005). However, there is some substantial empirical support for a potential role of genitourinary tract infections in chronic prostatitis/CPPS as the etiology of this disease. Many patients relate the onset to sexual activity, often to an episode of urethritis (Krieger et al., 1999). Antimicrobials often provide transient or partial relief of symptoms and standard practice is to provide multiple courses of antimicrobials (Nickel et al., 1994; Nickel & Costerton, 1992). For many years attempts have been made to prove the role of certain microorganisms in the pathogenesis of CPPS. Attention has focused on *C. trachomatis,* the most frequent cause of non-gonococcal urethritis in sexually active men. It is believed that these bacteria can spread via intracanalicular ascension from the urethra. However, the evidence supporting the role of *C. trachomatis* as an etiologic agent in chronic prostatitis is conflicting. Mardh and Colleen (Mardh et al., 1972) found that one third of men with chronic prostatitis had antibodies to *C. trachomatis* compared with 3% of controls. Shortliffe and coworkers (Shortliffe et al., 1992) found that 20% of patients with nonbacterial prostatitis had antichlamydial antibody titers in the prostatic fluid. Bruce and colleagues (Bruce et al., 1981) found that 56% of patients with "subacute or chronic prostatitis" were infected with *C. trachomatis* (examining early morning urine, prostatic fluid, or semen). In a follow-up study, Bruce and Reid (Bruce & Reid, 1989) found that 6 of 55 men with abacterial prostatitis, including 31 believed to have chlamydial prostatitis, met strict criteria for positive diagnosis for chlamydial prostatitis based on identification of the organisms by culturing or immunofluorescence. *Chlamydia* has also been isolated in prostate tissue specimens. Poletti and coworkers (Poletti et al., 1985) isolated *C. trachomatis* from prostate samples obtained by transrectal aspiration biopsy of men with "nonacute abacterial prostatitis." Abdelatif and colleagues (Abdelatif et al., 1991) identified intracellular *chlamydia* employing "in-situ hybridization techniques" in transurethral prostate chips from 30% of men with histologic evidence of "chronic abacterial prostatitis." Shurbaji and associates (Shurbaji et al., 1988) identified *C. trachomatis* in paraffin-embedded secretions in 31% of men with histologic evidence of prostatitis compared with none in patients with BPH without inflammation.

Although Mardh and Colleen (Mardh et al., 1972) suggested that *C. trachomatis* may be implicated in as many as one third of men with CP, their follow-up studies employing culturing and serologic tests could not confirm *C. trachomatis* as an etiologic agent in idiopathic prostatitis (Mardh & Colleen, 1975; Mardh et al., 1978). Shortliffe and Wehner (Shortliffe & Wehner, 1986) came to a similar conclusion when they evaluated antichlamydial antibody titers in prostatic fluid. Twelve percent of controls compared with 20% of patients with nonbacterial prostatitis had detectable antibodies. Berger and coworkers (Berger et al., 1989) could not culture *C. trachomatis* from the urethras in men with CP nor did they find a serologic or local immune response to *C. trachomatis* in such patients. Doble and associates (Doble et al., 1989) were not able to culture or detect by immunofluorescence *chlamydia* in transperineal biopsies of abnormal areas of the prostate in men with chronic abacterial prostatitis. Krieger and colleagues (Krieger et al., 1996) were only able to find *chlamydia* in 1% of prostate tissue biopsies in men with CP. A further localization and culture series by Krieger and associates (Krieger et al., 2000) also failed to culture *chlamydia* from either urethral or prostate specimens. Further elucidation of the role of chlamydial etiology of prostate infection is required to make any definitive statement on the association between isolation of this organism and its prostatic origin and effect (Weidner et al., 2002). In the follow-up of standardized prostatitis patients, a combination of urological tests in EPS and seminal plasma combined with genital chlamydial DNA material, may further elucidate the chlamydial aetiology of prostate infection.

7.2 Infertility

There are some studies of *C. trachomatis* in men and women undergoing investigations for infertility using modern screening methods. The major sequelae of *C. trachomatis* infection in women are tubal factor infertility and tubal ectopic pregnancy. Sequelae of *C. trachomatis* infection in men may include male factor infertility but why this occurs remains uncertain . There have been a number of studies on the relationship between *C. trachomatis* infection and sperm quality, with conflicting results. However, there have been major differences in study design with: significant variation in the methodology used to measuring the history of chlamydial infection (i.e. serology versus molecular methods); as well as variable and sometimes inadequate methods to assess semen quality. More recent studies (Hosseinzadeh et al., 2004; Bezold et al., 2007; Al-Mously et al., 2009), using molecular methods to detect infection, and robust methods of laboratory andrology to examine semen, have generally found that men with a current infection of *C. trachomatis* have poorer quality ejaculates compared than men who do not. It is unclear whether this is because of reduced levels of spermatogenesis in the presence of the bacterium, or whether infection causes an altered ejaculatory response. However, it has been observed that persistent infection can result in the scarring of ejaculatory ducts or loss of stereocilia (Gonzalez-Jimenez & Villanueva-Diaz, 2006). In addition to any changes in semen quality, there is growing evidence to suggest that exposure to *C. trachomatis* can affect sperm function (Pacey & Eley, 2004; Eley et al., 2005a). In vitro experiments have shown that *C. trachomatis* triggers tyrosine phosphorylation of sperm proteins (Hosseinzadeh et al., 2000), induces premature sperm death (Hosseinzadeh et al., 2001) and stimulates an apoptosis-like response in sperm (Eley et al., 2005b; Satta et al., 2006), leading to increased levels of sperm DNA fragmentation (Gallegos et al., 2008; Satta et al., 2006). At least some of these effects are caused by lipopolysaccharides (Hosseinzadeh et al., 2003).

With regard to infertility patients receiving treatments such as IVF, the Royal College of Obstetricians and Gynaecologists recommended that women should be screened for *C. trachomatis*, or given appropriate antibiotic prophylaxis, before any uterine instrumentation takes place (RCOG, 2008). This was reiterated in the later NICE guidelines (UK Collaborative Group for HIV and STI Surveillance, 2005). However, Sowerby and Parsons (Sowerby & Parsons, 2004) noted that 53% of UK clinics either screen the female partner or give appropriate antibiotic prophylaxis. In the recruitment of sperm, egg and embryo donors the most recent UK guidelines produced by the Association of Biomedical Andrologists, Association of Clinical Embryologists, British Andrology Society, British Fertility Society and Royal College of Obstetricians and Gynaecologists (RCOG, 2008) recommend that all donors be screened for *C. trachomatis* prior to donation, and this is reiterated in the 8th Edition of the Human Fertilisation and Embryology Authority (HFEA) Code of Practice (HFEA Code of Practice, 2009).

Since it is known *C. trachomatis* can survive in liquid nitrogen (Sherman & Jordan, 1985) and that infection following insemination with cryopreserved donor semen is possible (Broder et al., 2007), the freezing and storage of gametes and embryos from patients with an active *C. trachomatis* infection is of obvious concern. This is not only to prevent women who receive treatment with thawed gametes and embryos from becoming infected with *C. trachomatis*, but because of the theoretical concern that the bacteria may cross-contaminate other (*C. trachomatis* negative) samples being stored in the same cryostorage vessel. To date, such cross contamination has only been shown with regard to Hepatitis B during storage of peripheral blood stem cells. (Tedder et al., 1995) and has never been demonstrated during reproductive tissue storage. However, the HFEA now require that all patients placing material in storage be screened for bloodborn viruses prior to placing material in storage (HFEA Code of Practice, 2009). For patients undergoing planned IVF treatment, a similar level of risk reduction will be achieved if both partners are screened and treated for *C. trachomatis*.

8. Conclusion

Population based studies in Europe and the USA suggest that the prevalence of *C. trachomatis* in men and women aged 15–24 years is 2–6%. The prevalence in young men was the same as in young women.The peak age group for infection is 16–19 years in women and 20–24 years in men. A role for *C. trachomatis* in the development of male urologic diseases such as urethritis, epididymitis, and orchitis is widely accepted. Also, *C. trachomatis* can cause chronic prostatitis and infertility. NAATs are recommended for detection of reproductive tract infections caused by *C. trachomatis* in men and women. Optimal specimen types for NAATs are first catch urine from men and vaginal swabs from women. Clinical trials continue to demonstrate equivalent efficacy and tolerability of azithromycin and doxycycline regimens, and both remain recommended as first-line therapy. Ascending chlamydial infections have been thought to be an infective cause of prostatitis. Unfortunately, the definitive association between *C. trachomatis* and prostatitis is limited by various factors. Sequelae of *C. trachomatis* infection in men may include male factor infertility but why this remains uncertain.

9. References

Abdelatif OM, Chandler FW, McGuire BS, Jr. (1991). Chlamydia trachomatis in chronic abacterial prostatitis: demonstration by colorimetric in situ hybridization. *Hum Pathol* 22(1):41-44.

Al-Mously N, Cross NA, Eley A, Pacey AA. (2009). Real-time polymerase chain reaction shows that density centrifugation does not always remove Chlamydia trachomatis from human semen. *Fertil Steril* 92(5):1606-1615.

Andersen B, Olesen F, Moller JK, Ostergaard L. (2002). Population-based strategies for outreach screening of urogenital Chlamydia trachomatis infections: a randomized, controlled trial. *J Infect Dis* 185(2):252-258.

Berger R, Alexander E, Monda G, Ansell J, McCormick G, Holmes K. (1978) Chlamydia trachomatis as a cause of acute "idiopathic" epididymitis. *N Engl J Med.* 298(6):301–304.

Berger R, Alexander E, Harnisch J, et al. (1979) Etiology, manifestations and therapy of acute epididymitis: Prospective study of 50 cases. *J Urol.* 121(6):750–754.

Berger RE, Krieger JN, Kessler D, Ireton RC, Close C, Holmes KK, Roberts PL. (1989). Case-control study of men with suspected chronic idiopathic prostatitis. *J Urol* 141(2):328-331.

Bezold G, Politch JA, Kiviat NB, Kuypers JM, Wolff H, Anderson DJ. (2007). Prevalence of sexually transmissible pathogens in semen from asymptomatic male infertility patients with and without leukocytospermia. *Fertil Steril* 87(5):1087-1097.

Blank S, Schillinger JA, Harbatkin D. (2005). Lymphogranuloma venereum in the industrialised world. *Lancet* 365(9471):1607-1608.

Broder S, Sims C, Rothman C. (2007). Frequency of postinsemination infections as reported by donor semen recipients. *Fertil Steril* 88(3):711-713.

Bruce AW, Chadwick P, Willett WS, O'Shaughnessy M. (1981). The role of chlamydiae in genitourinary disease. *J Urol* 126(5):625-629.

Bruce AW, Reid G. (1989). Prostatitis associated with Chlamydia trachomatis in 6 patients. *J Urol* 142(4):1006-1007.

Carder C, Mercey D, Benn P. (2006). Chlamydia trachomatis. *Sex Transm Infect* 82 Suppl 4:iv10-12.

Centers for Disease Control and Prevention. (2010). Sexually Transmitted Disease Surveillance 2009. Department of Health and Human Services. Atlanta: U.S.

Collins MM, Stafford RS, O'Leary MP, Barry MJ. (1998). How common is prostatitis? A national survey of physician visits. *J Urol* 159(4):1224-1228.

Doble A, Thomas BJ, Walker MM, Harris JR, Witherow RO, Taylor-Robinson D. (1989). The role of Chlamydia trachomatis in chronic abacterial prostatitis: a study using ultrasound guided biopsy. *J Urol* 141(2):332-333.

Eley A, Pacey AA, Galdiero M, Galdiero F. (2005a). Can Chlamydia trachomatis directly damage your sperm? *Lancet Infect Dis* 5(1):53-57.

Eley A, Hosseinzadeh S, Hakimi H, Geary I, Pacey AA. (2005b). Apoptosis of ejaculated human sperm is induced by co-incubation with Chlamydia trachomatis lipopolysaccharide. *Hum Reprod* 20(9):2601-2607.

Fenton KA, Korovessis C, Johnson AM, McCadden A, McManus S, Wellings K, Mercer CH, Carder C, Copas AJ, Nanchahal K, Macdowall W, Ridgway G, Field J, Erens B. (2001). Sexual behaviour in Britain: reported sexually transmitted infections and prevalent genital Chlamydia trachomatis infection. *Lancet* 358(9296):1851-1854.

Gallegos G, Ramos B, Santiso R, Goyanes V, Gosalvez J, Fernandez JL. (2008). Sperm DNA fragmentation in infertile men with genitourinary infection by Chlamydia trachomatis and Mycoplasma. *Fertil Steril* 90(2):328-334.

Gonzalez-Jimenez MA, Villanueva-Diaz CA. (2006). Epididymal stereocilia in semen of infertile men: evidence of chronic epididymitis? *Andrologia* 38(1):26-30.

Hislop J, Quayyum Z, Flett G, Boachie C, Fraser C, Mowatt G. Epub ahead of print. (2010). Systematic review of the clinical effectiveness and cost-effectiveness of rapid point-of-care tests for the detection of genital chlamydia infection in women and men. *Health Technol Assess* 14(29):1-97, iii-iv.

Holmes KK, Sparling PF, Mardh P-A, Lemon SM, Piot P, Wasserheit JN. (1999). Sexually transmitted diseases. McGraw-Hill. New York.

Horner P. (2008). Chlamydia (uncomplicated, genital). *Clin Evid (Online)* 2008.

Horner P, Boag F. (2006). 2006 UK National Guideline for the Management of Genital Tract Infection with C. trachomatis.

Hosseinzadeh S, Brewis IA, Eley A, Pacey AA. (2001). Co-incubation of human spermatozoa with Chlamydia trachomatis serovar E causes premature sperm death. *Hum Reprod* 16(2):293-299.

Hosseinzadeh S, Brewis IA, Pacey AA, Moore HD, Eley A. (2000). Coincubation of human spermatozoa with Chlamydia trachomatis in vitro causes increased tyrosine phosphorylation of sperm proteins. *Infect Immun* 68(9):4872-4876.

Hosseinzadeh S, Eley A, Pacey AA. (2004). Semen quality of men with asymptomatic chlamydial infection. *J Androl* 25(1):104-109.

Hosseinzadeh S, Pacey AA, Eley A. (2003). Chlamydia trachomatis-induced death of human spermatozoa is caused primarily by lipopolysaccharide. *J Med Microbiol* 52(Pt 3):193-200.

Kamwendo F, Forslin L, Bodin L, Danielsson D. (1996). Decreasing incidences of gonorrhea- and chlamydia-associated acute pelvic inflammatory disease. A 25-year study from an urban area of central Sweden. *Sex Transm Dis* 23(5):384-391.

Krieger JN, Jacobs R, Ross SO. (2000). Detecting urethral and prostatic inflammation in patients with chronic prostatitis. *Urology* 55(2):186-191; discussion 191-182.

Krieger JN, Riley DE, Roberts MC, Berger RE. (1996). Prokaryotic DNA sequences in patients with chronic idiopathic prostatitis. *J Clin Microbiol 34*(12):3120-3128.

Krieger JN, Ross SO, Berger RE, Riley DE. (1999). Textbook of prostatitis. Oxford: Isis Medical Media.

Low N, McCarthy A, Macleod J, Salisbury C, Campbell R, Roberts TE, Horner P, Skidmore S, Sterne JA, Sanford E, Ibrahim F, Holloway A, Patel R, Barton PM, Robinson SM, Mills N, Graham A, Herring A, Caul EO, Davey Smith G, Hobbs FD, Ross JD, Egger M. (2007). Epidemiological, social, diagnostic and economic evaluation of population screening for genital chlamydial infection. *Health Technol Assess* 11(8):iii-iv, ix-xii, 1-165.

Mardh P, Colleen S, Holmquist B. (1972). Chlamydia in chronic prostatitis. *Br Med J* 4(5836):361.

Mardh PA, Colleen S. (1975). Search for uro-genital tract infections in patients with symptoms of prostatitis. Studies on aerobic and strictly anaerobic bacteria, mycoplasmas, fungi, trichomonads and viruses. *Scand J Urol Nephrol* 9(1): 8-16.

Mardh PA, Ripa KT, Colleen S, Treharne JD, Darougar S. (1978). Role of Chlamydia trachomatis in non-acute prostatitis. *Br J Vener Dis* 54(5):330-334.

Melekos M, Asbach H. (1988) The role of chlamydiae in epididymitis. *Int Urol Nephrol.* 20(3):293–297.

Mertz KJ, Levine WC, Mosure DJ, Berman SM, Dorian KJ. (1997). Trends in the prevalence of chlamydial infections. The impact of community-wide testing. *Sex Transm Dis* 24(3):169-175.

Miller WC, Ford CA, Morris M, Handcock MS, Schmitz JL, Hobbs MM, Cohen MS, Harris KM, Udry JR. (2004). Prevalence of chlamydial and gonococcal infections among young adults in the United States. *JAMA* 291(18):2229-2236.

Motrich RD, Maccioni M, Molina R, Tissera A, Olmedo J, Riera CM, Rivero VE. (2005). Presence of INFgamma-secreting lymphocytes specific to prostate antigens in a group of chronic prostatitis patients. *Clin Immunol* 116(2):149-157.

Nickel JC, Bruce AW, Reid G. (1994). Clinical urology Krane RJ, Siroky MB, Fitzpatrick JM, editors. J.B. Lippincott. Philadelphia.

Nickel JC, Costerton JW. (1992). Coagulase-negative staphylococcus in chronic prostatitis. *J Urol* 147(2):398-400

Nieuwenhuis RF, Ossewaarde JM, Gotz HM, Dees J, Thio HB, Thomeer MG, den Hollander JC, Neumann MH, van der Meijden WI. (2004). Resurgence of lymphogranuloma venereum in Western Europe: an outbreak of Chlamydia trachomatis serovar l2 proctitis in The Netherlands among men who have sex with men. *Clin Infect Dis* 39(7):996-1003.

Nieuwenhuis RF, Ossewaarde JM, van der Meijden WI, Neumann HA. (2003). Unusual presentation of early lymphogranuloma venereum in an HIV-1 infected patient: effective treatment with 1 g azithromycin. *Sex Transm Infect* 79(6):453-455.

Pacey AA, Eley A. (2004). Chlamydia trachomatis and male fertility. *Hum Fertil* 7(4):271-276.

Persson K. (2002) The role of serology, antibiotic susceptibility testing and serovar determination in genital chlamydial infections. *Best Pract Res Clin Obstet Gynaecol.* 16(6):801-814.

Poletti F, Medici MC, Alinovi A, Menozzi MG, Sacchini P, Stagni G, Toni M, Benoldi D. (1985). Isolation of Chlamydia trachomatis from the prostatic cells in patients affected by nonacute abacterial prostatitis. *J Urol* 134(4):691-693.

HFEA Code of Practice (2009) 8th Edition. Human Fertilisation and Embryology Authority. London Royal College of Obstetricians and Gynaecologists. (1998). The initial investigation and management of the infertile couple. Royal College of Obstetricians and Gynaecologists. London

Royal College of Obstetricians and Gynaecologists. (2008). Management of acute pelvic inflammatory disease. Green top guideline No 32.

Satta A, Stivala A, Garozzo A, Morello A, Perdichizzi A, Vicari E, Salmeri M, Calogero AE. (2006). Experimental Chlamydia trachomatis infection causes apoptosis in human sperm. *Hum Reprod* 21(1):134-137.

Scholes D, Stergachis A, Heidrich FE, Andrilla H, Holmes KK, Stamm WE. (1996). Prevention of pelvic inflammatory disease by screening for cervical chlamydial infection. *N Engl J Med* 334(21):1362-1366.

Sherman JK, Jordan GW. (1985). Cryosurvival of Chlamydia trachomatis during cryopreservation of human spermatozoa. *Fertil Steril* 43(4):664-666.

Shortliffe LM, Sellers RG, Schachter J. (1992). The characterization of nonbacterial prostatitis: search for an etiology. *J Urol* 148(5):1461-1466.

Shortliffe LM, Wehner N. (1986). The characterization of bacterial and nonbacterial prostatitis by prostatic immunoglobulins. *Medicine* 65(6):399-414.

Shurbaji MS, Gupta PK, Myers J. (1988). Immunohistochemical demonstration of Chlamydial antigens in association with prostatitis. *Mod Pathol* 1(5):348-351.

Sowerby E, Parsons J. 2004. Prevention of iatrogenic pelvic infection during in vitro fertilization--current practice in the UK. *Hum Fertil* 7(2):135-140.

UK Collaborative Group for HIV and STI Surveillance. *(2005)*. Mapping the issues. Focus on prevention. HIV and other sexually transmitted infections in the UK. Health Protection Agency Centre for Infections. London.

Tedder RS, Zuckerman MA, Goldstone AH, Hawkins AE, Fielding A, Briggs EM, Irwin D, Blair S, Gorman AM, Patterson KG, et al. (1995). Hepatitis B transmission from contaminated cryopreservation tank. *Lancet* 346(8968):137-140.

van Bergen J, Gotz HM, Richardus JH, Hoebe CJ, Broer J, Coenen AJ. (2005). Prevalence of urogenital Chlamydia trachomatis increases significantly with level of urbanisation and suggests targeted screening approaches: results from the first national population based study in the Netherlands. *Sex Transm Infect* 81(1): 17-23.

van de Laar MJ, Morre SA. (2007). Chlamydia: a major challenge for public health. *Euro Surveill* 12(10):E1-2.

Weidner W, Diemer T, Huwe P, Rainer H, Ludwig M. (2002). The role of Chlamydia trachomatis in prostatitis. *Int J Antimicrob Agents* 19(6):466-470.

World Health Organization. (2001). Global prevalence and incidence of selected curable sexually transmitted infections. Overview and estimates. WHO. Geneva

15

Pathogenesis of *Chlamydia pneumonia* Persistent Illnesses in Autoimmune Diseases

Hamidreza Honarmand
Micrbiologist, Cellular and Molecular Research Center,
Guilan University of Medical Sciences
Iran

1. Introduction

Infectious agents have been implicated in the pathogenesis of many autoimmune diseases. In most of these diseases, including those in which specific organisms are known to play a role, the details of pathogenesis remain incompletely defined. Recent studies have aimed to isolate bacterial and viral pathogens from patients with autoimmune diseases, efforts have been made to further define the host immune response to infection, and there have been attempts to develop improved methods of diagnosis and treatment of infectious diseases affecting the Immune system. More recently, *C.pneumonia* has been linked to many autoimmune diseases [20].

Chlamydia pneumoniae is an important respiratory pathogen associated with 5% to 10% of community-acquired cases of pneumonia, pharyngitis, bronchitis, and sinusitis. Infection is most common among children 5 to 14 years of age, and the majority of adults have serologic evidence of past infection. Antibodies have also been found frequently in people in many countries worldwide. The bacterium is an obligatory intracellular pathogen that has the tendency to cause persistent infection, and may drive a chronic inflammatory reaction in coronary vasculature or other tissues. The characteristic feature of all chlamydial species is their tendency to establish a long-lasting parasitic relationship with the host and chronicity is a hallmark of *Chlamydia* infection. Adults are particularly prone to have prolonged illness, with relapses and secondary infections. *Chlamydiae* are known to infect macrophages and monocytes as well as epithelial cells. *C. pneumoniae* also infects endothelial and smooth muscle cells of blood vessels. Tissue injury in all chlamydial diseases appears to be immune mediated [27].

Only one serovar or immunotype has been found, Molecular studies have found only small and probably inconsequential differences among isolates. Despite its recent isolation, it should be said that *C. pneumoniae* is not a new organism. It was not found earlier because it is difficult to isolate and to keep in continuous culture. Retrospective serological studies provides evidence that *C. pneumoniae* was active for years before its isolation. Much of the knowledge of the epidemiology of *C. pneumoniae* infection has been derived from serologic studies utilizing the *C. pneumoniae*-specific microimmunofluorescence (MIF) test. More recent improvements in isolation techniques and the application of the PCR have also greatly improved the capability to detect the organism in clinical specimens and facilitated more detailed microbiologic studies [40].

This review is a brief discussion on recent studies about the association of *C. pneumoniae* infection with illnesses affecting the immune system, with an emphasis on the autoimmune diseases.

2. Autoimmune disorders and infection

2.1 Autoimmune diseases

An autoimmune disorder is a condition that occurs when the immune system mistakenly attacks and destroys healthy body tissue. The immune system is an amazing collection of biological processes designed to defend the body against invasion by infectious pathogens and tumor cells. This system includes innate, adaptive and memory responses that are constantly activated, adapted and improved to meet the challenge of evading pathogens more efficiently. Normally the immune system's army of white blood cells helps protect the body from harmful substances, called antigens. Examples of antigens include bacteria, viruses, toxins, cancer cells, and blood or tissues from another person or species. In addition, the immune system must be tolerant and distinguish between self and nonself, so that substances that are identified as nonself stimulate an immune response, while no harm is inflicted upon self. However, as in any complex system, malfunctions occur, leading to diseases of immune dysregulation. In patients with an autoimmune disorder, the immune system can't tell the difference between healthy body tissue and antigens. The result is an immune response that destroys normal body tissues. This response is a hypersensitivity reaction similar to the response in allergies. In allergies, the immune system reacts to an external substance that it normally would ignore. With autoimmune disorders, the immune system reacts to normal body tissues. Furthermore autoimmunity is a consequence of the breakdown of self-tolerance; the result is an attack of the immune system on various organs and tissues as if they were foreign invaders [61].

There are more than 80 different types of autoimmune disorders. Autoimmune diseases have many causes. Genes, notably genes encoding cell-surface proteins that display peptides for immune recognition, the major histocompatibility complex (MHC), the environment, and the microbial diversity within the human body determine the susceptibility to autoimmune diseases. One mechanism by which infection is linked to the initiation of autoimmunity is termed molecular mimicry. Molecular mimicry describes the phenomenon of protein products from dissimilar genes sharing similar structures that elicit an immune response to both self and microbial proteins. Auto immune diseases (ADs) are the third leading cause of morbidity and mortality, after heart disease and cancer, in the industrialized world. What causes the immune system to no longer tell the difference between healthy body tissues and antigens is not clearly known. Researchers are looking into the role of different factors in the development of autoimmune disorders. It seems that some microorganisms and drugs may trigger some of the changes, especially in people who have genes that make them more likely to get autoimmune disorders. One theory is that, a combination of genetic, immunologic, hormonal and environmental factors, comprising what is known as 'the mosaic of autoimmunity', is required for autoimmune disorders to develop [59]. Among these key elements, the impact of infections on the development of autoimmunity is substantial, and various mechanisms have been suggested to explain this relationship. In recent years, the compound interplay between infections and autoimmunity has been studied extensively [58, 59].

An autoimmune disorder may result in destruction of one or more types of body tissue, abnormal growth of an organ, or changes in organ function. Organs and tissues commonly affected by autoimmune disorders include red blood cells, blood vessels, connective tissues, endocrine glands such as the thyroid or pancreas, muscles, joints, and skin.

Main human autoimmune disorders are Multiple sclerosis, Rheumatoid Arthritis, Scleroderma, and Neurologic autoimmune diseases. With the exception of multiple sclerosis, these diseases are rare. Autoimmune disorders affect people of all genders, races, and ages, but certain people have an increase risk of developing autoimmune disorders. Main risk factors for autoimmune disorders are Gender, Age, Ethnicity, Family history of autoimmune disorders, Exposure to environmental agents and previous infection.

2.2 Autoimmune disorders induced by infection

The high percentage of disease-discordant pairs of monozygotic twins demonstrates the central role of environmental factors in the etiology of autoimmune diseases. Efforts were first focused on the search for triggering factors. The study of animal models has clearly shown that infections may trigger autoimmune diseases, which can also determine its clinical manifestations. Most infectious agents, such as viruses, bacteria and parasites, can induce autoimmunity via different mechanisms. In many cases, it is not a single infection but rather the 'burden of infections' from childhood that is responsible for the induction of autoimmunity. The development of an autoimmune disease after infection tends to occur in genetically susceptible individuals. By contrast, some infections can protect individuals from specific autoimmune diseases [50].

The observation that infection can precipitate an autoimmune disease dates back more than a century. The first human autoimmune disease described, paroxysmal cold hemoglobinuria, was thought of as a late consequence of syphilis, and rheumatic fever is still associated with preceding streptococcal infection.

Bacterial and viral infections are commonplace in a variety of autoimmune and chronic illnesses such as the chronic fatigue syndrome; fibromyalgia syndrome, Gulf war illnesses and rheumatoid conditions. Much attention is focused at present on the role of bacteria and the possible mechanisms of their involvement in the pathogenesis of several diseases. The route of infection and penetration, and the immune responses of the host can not only make any bacterial infection pathogenic but probably can also determine the aggressiveness of the disease and the chance for full recovery [21].

A wide variety of bacterial infections have been associated with autoimmune disorders. For example *M.pneumonia, M.salivarium, and M.fermentas*, has been strongly associated with rheumatoid arthritis. *Proteus mirabilis* has been implicated in the pathogenesis of rheumatoid arthritis and osteoarthritis. Enterobacteriaceae family is associated with some autoimmune conditions such as Kawasaki syndrome and Graves disease. Genitourinary *mycoplasma* infection has been associated with systemic lupus erythematosus. *Campylobacter jejuni, Haemophilus influenza and M. pneumoniae* have been implicated as possible causative of

Guillain-Barre syndrome .Recently it has drawn attention to the putative link of bacterial nasopharyngeal infections with optic neuritis, optochiasmatic arachnoiditis and Multiple Sclerosis. More recently serology and PCR(polymerase chain reaction) have provided ample evidence of *Chlamydia pneumonia ,Borrelia burgdoferi, Mycoplasma* species, human herpesvirus-1 and -6 among others in MS, Amyoyrophic Lateral Sclerosis, Alzheimer's and Parkinson's diseases. A tentative relationship between MS and streptococcal infection has been suggested. And finally acute rheumatic fever, which presents several weeks after infection with *Streptococcus pyogenes* in which, the Molecular resemblance between the bacterial M-protein and human glycoproteins results in a breakdown of self-tolerance in genetically susceptible individuals [24, 58].

Post-infection autoimmunity can be induced by multiple mechanisms, such as molecular mimicry, epitope spreading, bystander activation, viral persistence and polyclonal activation. The induction of a Guillain-Barré syndrome in rabbits after immunization with a peptide derived from *Campylobacter jejuni* is explained by mimicry between *C. jejuni* antigens and peripheral nerve axonal antigens. Triggering of autoimmunity is not always a hit and run event, but rather a cumulative process. The immune system is affected by repeated infections from childhood, and in immune-sensitive individuals, a breakthrough point might occur when the infection burden crosses a crucial level. This breakthrough point might be reached when a specific pathogen load, immune load (i.e. antibody titer) or a unique combination of pathogens is established [23].

Even though there are many tests available, the MIF test is the only currently acceptable serologic test for detection of *C. pneumoniae* antibodies and is widely accepted as the "gold standard" in *C. pneumoniae* Serodiagnonosis [18]. Serologic tests detect antibodies to a specific micro-organism, which indicates that infection with the micro-organism, took place at some point in time. However, absolute proof of the micro-organisms actual involvement in the process atherosclerosis could only come from demonstrating its presence in the vascular wall.

3. *Chlamydia pneumoniae* and autoimmune diseases

3.1 Multiple sclerosis

Multiple sclerosis (MS) is an inflammatory disease leading to disseminated lesions of the central nervous system resulting in both somatomotor and autonomic disturbances. Somatomotor and autonomic disturbances occur with similar frequency. Multiple sclerosis is the most common demyelinating disease of the human central nervous system (CNS), principally affects adults aged 18–50 years. Women are generally affected earlier and more frequently than men. Most patients present with a relapsing disease, progressing over 10- 15 years to a chronic phase with increasing difficulty in movement and co-ordination.

The pathological hallmark of MS is the demyelinating plaque that represents an area of demyelination and gliosis around blood vessels. Acute lesions show perivascular lymphocytic infiltration with infiltration of macrophages and phagocytosis of myelin membranes. Underlying axons are relatively spared, but are nonetheless affected by the inflammatory process; leading to irreversible damage. Current opinion favors the notion that MS is an autoimmune disease directed against self-neural antigens [57].

The disorder is most commonly diagnosed between ages 20 and 40, but can be seen at any age. It is caused by damage to the myelin sheath, the protective covering that surrounds nerve cells. When this nerve covering is damaged, nerve impulses are slowed down or stopped. The nerve damage is caused by inflammation. Inflammation occurs when the body's own immune cells attack the nervous system. Repeated episodes of inflammation can occur along any area of the brain, optic nerve, and spinal cord. People with a family history of MS and those who live in a geographical area where MS is more common have a slightly higher risk of the disease. The disease usually occurs sporadically and studies of identical twins in which one has MS have demonstrated that it occurs in only 30% of second twins [57].

Additional evidence for the role of infection in MS is provided by the presence of increased levels of IgG and the presence of oligoclonal bands with alkaline isoelectric points on electrophoresis gels. Oligoclonal bands occur in. 95% of MS patients, but are also seen in 10% of patients with other infectious diseases of the CNS. This pattern of increased IgG and oligoclonal bands is found almost exclusively in CNS disorders of infectious origin and is thought to represent an intrathecal immune response to an infectious agent with the oligoclonal bands representing antibodies synthesized within the CNS [57]. The bacterium may act to trigger the autoimmune process because antigenic mimicry or from an expansion of self auto reactive T cell clones in response to bacterial or viral superantigens [58].

Chlamydia pneumoniae is the latest pathogen to be associated with MS. A case of CNS infection with *C. pneumoniae* in a patient with rapidly progressive MS has been reported. Antimicrobial therapy directed against this pathogen was accompanied by marked neurological improvement [60]. Subsequent studies found that *C. pneumoniae* is present in the CSF of patients with newly diagnosed relapsing, remitting MS and in patients with progressive MS, but not in other neurological disease controls [61].

Although there is a strong association between *C. pneumoniae* and MS, its role remains unproven. Before a causal relationship with the development or progression of MS can be claimed, the relapsing remitting nature of the disease that later develops into a chronic progressive phase must be explained satisfactorily. Moreover, the immune abnormalities in CSF (increased immunoglobulin synthesis and oligoclonal bands), the sex bias and the geographical distribution of the disease must all be addressed. One of the hallmarks of chlamydial infection is its tissue persistence and the development of chronic infection. *Chlamydiae* are known to infect macrophages and monocytes as well as epithelial cells. *C. pneumoniae* also infects endothelial and smooth muscle cells of blood vessels. Tissue injury in all chlamydial diseases appears to be immune mediated [66].

Recently, it has showed the specificity of intrathecal antibody response to *C. pneumoniae* antigens in relapsing remitting and progressive MS patients [74]. In most of MS patients studied, an elevated antibody titre to *C. pneumoniae* EB antigens was seen and was present in the CSF of them [74]. Increased antibody titres to *C. pneumoniae* were seen in about 20% of other neurological disease controls [24, 38].

Studies carried out by many researchers support a role for *C. pneumoniae* infection of the CNS in the pathogenesis of MS. However, the similarities in clinical disease pattern between known chlamydial diseases and MS do not conclusively establish a causal relationship between *C. pneumoniae* infection of the CNS and the development or progression of MS.

Further evidence to confirm or repudiate the presence of *C. pneumoniae* infection of the CNS in MS patients is needed. Evaluation of brain tissue from MS patients by immunochemical and in-situ PCR staining for *C. pneumoniae* is also necessary. If such studies show *C. pneumoniae* infection of microglial cells or oligodendrocytes in MS plaque or tissues adjacent to plaques, clinical neurologists can then consider treating MS patients with long term antimicrobial agents. The design of an appropriate therapeutic trial may be difficult because of the current absence of experimental animal models for either MS or for *C. pneumoniae* induced inflammation and demyelination of the CNS. Only a well designed therapeutic trial with sufficient statistical power is likely to provide additional answers concerning the relationship between *C. pneumoniae* infection of the CNS and the development or progression of MS [38].

As a large number of individuals are infected with the organism, it is possible that *C. pneumoniae* is the inciting agent of MS in genetically susceptible individuals. Activation of perivascular and parenchymal microglial cells along with the attendant biochemical mediators would lead to destruction of the surrounding myelin. An infectious agent that targeted microglial cells and endothelial cells would be a likely candidate in MS [49].

C. pneumoniae IgM positive cases were more frequent among the patients with rheumatoid arthritis , systemic lupus erythematosus, dermatomyositis/polymyositis , myeloperoxidase-antineutrophil cytoplasmic autoantibody -associated vasculitis , adult onset of Still's disease and giant cell arteritis/Takayasu arteritis than among the controls [24].

3.2 Stroke, an immunopathogenic complication of persistent *C. pneumonia* illness

Etiology of ischemic stroke is multi factorial and infections have emerged as one among them. In the last decade, several reports have shown the association of chronic *C. pneumoniae* infection with atherosclerosis and thrombosis and many studies have incriminated *C. pneumoniae* in the causation of coronary heart disease, stroke and asymptomatic carotid atherosclerosis.

In fact, patients having an infection within a week before the onset of stroke might develop cortical middle cerebral artery infarcts, cardioembolic infarcts and arterial dissections suggesting a differential effect of infection. In older patients, various conventional risk factors (diabetes, hypertension, hypercholesterolemia, etc) play an important role in stroke etiopathogenesis. However, younger patients (aged <45years) usually lack these risk factors, and infections, especially in developing countries, may assume significance [8, 9]. It is therefore relevant to look for the role of infection in contributing to various subgroups of ischemic stroke in young patients [8].

Bandaru *et al* found an association between the presence of *C. pneumoniae* antibodies and ischemic stroke among young Indian patients. They found that positive serum IgG and IgA antibody titer by microimmunofluorescence (MIF) test, against *C. pneumoniae* was significantly more in ischemic stroke patients compared to age and sex matched control subjects [8,9]. This is in agreement with previous studies where *C. pneumoniae* antibody positivity has been noted in young stroke patients [3, 47].

In Cameroon, Njamnshi AK *et al* demonstrated that *C. pneumoniae* infection is significantly associated with ischemic stroke in patients in the < 50 years age group compared to matched controls [47]. Another study also demonstrated that *C. pneumoniae* seropositivity can increase the risk of stroke in young patients aged below 55 years in which, *C. pneumoniae* seropositivity in all ischemic stroke subgroups except stroke of indeterminate etiology is found [8].

C. pneumoniae infection causes atherosclerosis of large arteries by infecting the vascular endothelial cells, activation of the NF-κβ, up regulation of procoagulant activity (tissue factor, plasminogen activator inhibitor), increased platelet count, adhesion molecules and finally thrombosis formation. The positivity of *C. pneumoniae* antibodies in nonatherosclerotic strokes like small artery disease and stroke of other determined etiology caused by pathophylogical changes due to lipohyalinosis or hypercoagulability may be an epiphenomenon.

CRP is a marker of inflammation. Several studies have found that *C. pneumoniae* infection could contribute to elevation of CRP levels and to the instability or progression of atherosclerotic plaques. In the study of Bandaru et al, both *C. pneumoniae* and CRP positivity was found in 29% of patients and it was significantly associated with stroke compared to controls subjects [8]. Hasan found that Chronic *C. pneumoniae* infection demonstrated by positive IgA-type antibody can be considered a significant risk for ischemic stroke [31].

If persistent *C. pneumoniae* infection contributes to vascular events such as stroke, it is interesting from a therapeutic perspective. Although *C .pneumoniae* may contribute to the risk of stroke directly, in most cases, it acts in concordance with the conventional risk factors. In younger individuals with ischemic stroke in whom *C. pneumoniae* found to be a risk factor, eradication of infection by antibiotic treatment may decrease the risk of stroke [3,8,9, 47].

3.3 Alzheimer's disease

Alzheimer's disease (AD) is the most common cause of dementia in the elderly. Symptoms include progressive memory loss, decreased cognition, problems with spacial and perceptual recognition, and impairment of daily living. The hallmark of Alzheimer's disease is the extracellular accumulation and deposition of insoluble amyloid, to be found in the parenchyma in the form of amyloid plaques and in meningeal and cerebral vessels as a congophile angiopathy. Amyloid plaques and neurofibrillary tangles are characteristic, but not specific to Alzheimer's disease. Similar changes can be found in healthy ageing processes and in various other neurodegenerative diseases. It is common to differentiate between an early-onset, familial Alzheimer's disease(FAD) with an established genetic etiology, representing only about 5% of all cases, and the more typical late-onset, sporadic Alzheimer's disease (LOAD)with an age of onset above 65 years and no clear pattern of inheritance [39]. The development of LOAD, the most prevalent form of AD, is believed to be a multifactorial process that may also involve infections with bacterial or viral pathogens. After the first report on the presence of *C. pneumoniae* in brains of patients with AD appeared in 1998, this bacterium has most often been implicated in AD pathogenesis. However, while some studies demonstrate a clear association between *C. pneumoniae* infection and AD, others have failed to confirm these findings [38].

Sporadic, late-onset Alzheimer's disease (LOAD) is actually a non-familial, progressive neurodegenerative disease that is now the most common and severe form of dementia in the elderly. That dementia is a direct result of neuronal damage and loss associated with accumulations of abnormal protein deposits in the brain. Great strides have been made in the past 20 years with regard to understanding the pathological entities that arise in the AD brain, both for familial AD (approximately 5% of all cases) and LOAD (approximately 95% of all cases [39].

Some indirect evidence seems to suggest that infection with *C. pneumoniae* might be associated with the disease. Nucleic acids prepared from those samples were screened by polymerase chain reaction (PCR) assay for DNA sequences from the bacterium and showed that brain areas with typical AD-related neuropathology were positive for the organism in 17/19 AD patients [7, 26, 39]. Electron- and immunoelectron-microscopic studies of tissues from affected AD brain regions identified chlamydial elementary and reticulate bodies, but similar examinations of non-AD brains were negative for the bacterium. Culture studies of a subset of affected AD brain tissues for *C. pneumoniae* were strongly positive, while identically performed analyses of non-AD brain tissues were negative [39]. Reverse transcription (RT)-PCR assays using RNA from affected areas of AD brains confirmed that transcripts from two important *C. pneumoniae* genes were present in those samples but not in controls. Immunohistochemical examination of AD brains, but not those of controls, identified *C. pneumoniae* within pericytes, microglia, and astroglia [7, 26]. Further immunolabelling studies confirmed the organisms' intracellular presence primarily in areas of neuropathology in the AD brain. Thus, *C. pneumoniae* is present, viable, and transcriptionally active in areas of neuropathology in the AD brain, possibly suggesting that infection with the organism is a risk factor for late-onset AD [41]. In other study, Immunohistochemical analyses showed that astrocytes, microglia, and neurons all served as host cells for *C. pneumoniae* in the AD brain, and that infected cells were found in close proximity to both neuritic senile plaques and neurofibrillary tangles in the AD brain [26, 41].

The importance of inflammation in the pathogenesis of neurodegenerative disorders, such as Alzheimer's disease, is increasingly being recognized. Although amyloid-beta is considered to be one of the main initiators of these inflammatory processes, some reports suggest that brain infections may also contribute or even initiate the neuroinflammation [39]. Recent data showed the role of *C. pneumoniae* infection in neuroinflammation and its potential contribution to the pathogenesis of Alzheimer's disease [7].

In an experimental trend, amyloid deposits resembling plaques found in Alzheimer's disease (AD) brains were formed in the brains of non-transgenic BALB/c mice following intranasal infection with *C. pneumoniae*. The mice were infected at 3 months of age with *C. pneumoniae* isolated from an AD brain. Infection was confirmed by light and electron microscopy in olfactory tissues of the mice. *C. pneumoniae* was still evident in these tissues 3 months after the initial infection indicating that a persistent infection had been established [41].

Medications (for example, antibiotics and anti-inflammatory drugs) prescribed to older individuals could affect the phenotypic and persistent nature of the organism, especially in the brains of patients with AD [11]. The proinflammatory response following infection may result in damage to *C. pneumoniae* as a result of evoked bacteriostatic events such as free radical damage in the tissues and/or nutrient starvation of the organisms [39]. In this regard, typical and atypical forms of *C. pneumoniae* were observed in the AD-affected brain. The main phenotypical differences were exhibited in the overall shape and size of the organisms, but immunoreactivity to the organism in the brain was similar to that of *C. pneumoniae* laboratory strains [4].

Inflammation is common in the AD brain in areas of neuropathology. This inflammation has been advanced as a pathogenic mechanism in the disease. Indeed, inflammation has been implicated as an important factor in a number of diseases, and one study indicated that administration of nonsteroidal antiinflammatory drugs could be beneficial in treating AD [11]. Because chlamydial infection engenders a strong inflammatory response, infection by *C. pneumoniae,* in part, may be responsible for the inflammation observed in the AD affected brain [39]. The results of Balin study demonstrated the frequent infection of microglia and astroglia with *C. pneumoniae* in the AD-affected brain [7]. Intriguingly, an animal model, in which low-dose infusion of LPS has been used, revealed remarkable parallels with AD inflammation including APP induction, increased cytokine production with microglial reactivity, and temporal lobe pathology [41].

Microglia are the resident tissue macrophages of the brain, and once activated they, like astroglia, are a source of inflammatory cytokines, including IL-1, TNF, and IL-6. Another study also showed that the infected cells in the AD-affected brains were microglia, astroglia, perivascular pericytes, and macrophages. These findings and an in vitro studies suggest that the glial cells and blood monocytes that traffic into the brain are primarily infected with *C pneumoniae* [39].

The fundamental question that must be answered is whether this organism could be a causative agent or an opportunist that finds its way into damaged tissues. In either case, the organism's presence in AD can affect aspects of symptomatology and progession that have their roots in the inflammation and blood vessel damage currently thought to play significant roles in this disease.

3.4 Vasculitis induced by *Chlamydia pneumoniae*

3.4.1 Giant cell arteritis, polymyalgia rheumatica, temporal arteritis

The possibility of infectious triggers stimulating the development of inflammatory vascular diseases has generated much recent interest. Giant cell arteritis (GCA) is a vasculitis disease affecting medium- to large-sized arteries. The disease is an inflammation of these arteries, mainly of the outermost of their three layers. It is known to be associated with previous upper respiratory tract symptoms. The occurrence of cases is often clustered in certain time periods and geographic locations. It is primarily a disease of the elderly, and is more common in women than in men. Fever of unknown origin is one of the symptoms along with polymyalgia rheumatica (PMR), a related clinical syndrome, that is strongly associated with DR4 positivity [43, 44].

Several recent studies in which activated CD41 T cells were identified in arteries of patients with GCA have strongly suggested that this disease might be antigen driven although the relevant antigens have not been identified as yet. In the search for the disease-inducing antigens in GCA, a number of different parameters have been suggested to be important. For example, the clustering of cases in specific time periods and in particular geographic locations indicates that in addition to genetic predispositions for the disease, environmental or seasonal factors may be significant. Moreover, GCA and polymyalgia rheumatica (PMR) are related clinical syndromes that affect the elderly. This association is supported by the close similarity in the clinical patterns of both, and the striking association of both with DR4 positivity [43, 44, 45].

Importantly, upper respiratory tract symptoms are often recognized as part of the syndrome in both GCA and PMR. In this respect, some reports have suggested that *Chlamydia pneumoniae* might be involved in the pathogenesis of vasculitis. In clinical practice, it is a common observation that the onset of so-called noninfectious vasculitis is often preceded by symptoms of upper respiratory tract infection, although a specific infecting agent is only occasionally recovered in laboratory analysis of such patients. In addition, a number of recent studies have indicated renewed interest in assessing the association between atherosclerosis and vasculitis [44, 45].

Several publications have addressed the interaction among infection, inflammation, and traditional risk factors in atherosclerosis and coronary artery disease [43]. Some clinical and laboratory studies have demonstrated the presence of *C. pneumoniae* in atherosclerotic tissues from diverse anatomic locations, suggesting that this bacterium may be involved in the pathogenesis of that disease [10, 58].

Two studies have presented evidence of a coincidence of cyclic fluctuations of Chlamydia pneumoniae epidemics and cases of GCA [52, 53]. Really conflicting data exist regarding the role of C. pneumoniae in the pathogenesis of GCA. Some authors found a strong correlation between GCA and detection of C. pneumoniae [51]. In another study, 8 of 9 GCA patients were PCR-positive for *C. pneumoniae*, while the only one of nine controls who was positive for *C.pneumonia* had respiratory symptoms [51]. In some of the tissue specimens, *C. pneumoniae* was found outside of cells, "possibly suggesting that the organism was viable and undergoing active vegetative growth in temporal artery tissues in GCA patients" [52, 53].

Positive correlation between the presence of *Chlamydia pneumoniae* in temporal artery biopsy specimens and the diagnosis of temporal arteritis (TA) is found in the study of Regan *et al* using sensitive and specific PCR. Analyses showed that all 90 patients were confirmed to have met the American College of Rheumatology classification criteria for TA [51]. The results of this study and study of Cooper et al [15] do not support a role for *C. pneumoniae* in the pathogenesis of TA.

Kaperonis *et al* investigated the association of inflammation and *Chlamydia pneumoniae* infection with the presence and severity of peripheral arterial disease. This study supports the hypothesis that inflammation (CRP) and chronic *C. pneumoniae* infection (IgA seropositivity), have an important role in lower limb atherosclerosis and correlate with the severity of the disease [37].

3.4.2 Vascular dementia

Vascular dementia is characterized by a loss of cognitive function and social adaptive functions in individuals with cerebrovascular disease. Vascular dementia is the second most common cause of dementia (second only to Alzheimer's disease) and accounts for 10% to 15% of all cases. The clinical presentation of this illness is variable, depending on the site and extent of the lesion or infarct. The pathogenesis of vascular dementia has not been well defined. Chronic inflammation and cytokine dysregulation may play a role similar to that seen in Alzheimer's disease.

Recent data from serological and PCR studies support an association between C. pneumoniae and some cerebrovascular disease. *C.pneumonia* has been associated with stroke, transient cerebral ischemia, and atherosclerosis in the middle cerebral artery in both prospective and case-control studies [13, 64]. Since stroke is an important precursor to vascular dementia, these data raise the possibility that *C.pneumonia* infection may also be a risk factor for vascular dementia.

C.pneumonia serology is an imperfect test of C. pneumoniae exposure and chronic infection. First, the high prevalence of *C.pneumonia* exposure makes it difficult to detect true serological differences between cases and controls. Second, it is unclear what the appropriate serological cut-offs should be for identifying exposure versus chronic infection or recent infections [18]. As a result, different groups have used different criteria making comparisons across studies more difficult. However, the importance of this inconsistency is unclear.

There is an extensive literature supporting an association between *C.pneumonia* and atherosclerosis. Although the majority of these studies initially focused on coronary heart disease [10, 15, 16]. More recent evidence also supports an association with stroke [14]. However, the clinical importance of this association is uncertain. Carusone *et al*, found no significant association between elevated or high C. pneumoniae specific IgG or IgA antibodies and vascular dementia [13]. In this study, the odds ratio estimate for IgA titres was slightly higher than IgG titres, but not statistically different. The meaning of this difference is uncertain. Danesh *et al* suggest that these differences are likely due to chance, selection biases, or selective emphasis on particular reports [16]. The odds ratio estimate for IgA titres is also slightly higher than IgG titres, but not statistically different. Carusone *et al* suggest that the odds ratio estimates for elevated IgA and IgG antibodies do not definitively rule out an association between antibodies and vascular dementia because the relatively small sample[13]. Other studies have suggested that IgA titres are more strongly associated with disease outcomes because they are a better indicator of chronic *C.pneumonia* infection [14].

It is now widely believed that vascular risk factors are also associated with Alzheimer's disease and Alzheimer's and vascular dementia may share many common clinical and pathological characteristics [39]. A number of studies have examined the association between Alzheimer's disease and *C.pneumonia* infection. Balin *et al* found an extremely high association between the presence of *C.pneumonia* in post-mortem brain samples and late-onset Alzheimer's disease [7]. However, more recent studies have not repeated these findings one study has looked for *C.pneumonia* in brain samples of vascular dementia patients. This study, like the later AD studies, did not identify *C.pneumonia* in any of the brain samples [72]. These results suggest that the presence of *C.pneumonia* in the brains is not strongly associated with late-onset Alzheimer's disease or vascular dementia.

Inflammatory responses are also known to be associated with cardiovascular disease and have recently been implicated in dementia. Elevated levels of serum C-reactive protein (CRP), a non-specific marker of inflammation, predict cardiovascular disease and dementia, and have been associated with stroke patients [73]. Although CRP was originally thought to be produced almost exclusively by hepatocytes, CRP is now known to be synthesized in brain cells and upregulated in Alzheimer tissue [73].

3.5 Atherosclerosis and coronary artery disease

An association between coronary artery disease and other Atherosclerotic syndromes and *C. pneumoniae* infection has been suggested by both seroepidemiologic studies and the demonstration of the presence of the organism in athromatous plaque. The initial study indicating a possible association between *C. pneumoniae* and coronary artery disease was performed in Finland and showed that patients with coronary artery disease were significantly more likely to have serologic evidence of past infection with TWAR than were controls [55].

Morphologic and microbiologic evidence of the presence of *C. pneumoniae* in athermanous plaques has been obtained by electron microscopic studies of coronary atheroma, immunocytochemical staining and PCR testing of coronary, carotid, and aortic atheroma [60]. The organism has also been demonstrated in atheromatous tissue removed from patients by directional coronary atherectomy and was found more commonly in restenotic lesions than in primary lesions [12, 68]. Autopsy specimens from young persons (15 to 35 years of age) has offered the opportunity to study coronary arteries from persons without atherosclerosis, an opportunity for control material not available in older adults [12, 68]. The organism was not detected by PCR or immunocytochemical staining in 31 coronary artery specimens that showed no atheroma but was demonstrated in 2 of 11 specimens showing probable early lesions (intimal thickening) and in 6 of 7 specimens with developed atherosclerotic plaques [33]. More recently, *C. pneumonia* seropositivity was associated with enhanced intima-media thickness of arteries. While these studies clearly associate TWAR organisms with atheromatous plaques, the role of TWAR infection in the pathogenesis of atherosclerosis is unknown [10, 36].

Three types of evidence support the association of *C. pneumoniae* with atherosclerosis including seroepidemiological studies, direct detection of bacterial DNA or antigen, or both, in atherosclerotic lesions and isolation of the organism from athermanous tissue. Following the initial report of Saikku *et al* demonstrating an association of *C. pneumoniae* antibody with myocardial infarction and coronary heart disease [55], there have been more than 50 studies demonstrating a sero-epidemiological association between *C. pneumoniae* and cardiovascular disease. The strongest evidence for an association of *C. pneumoniae* with atherosclerosis has been the demonstration of *C. pneumoniae* by PCR, immunocytochemical staining and electron microscopy in atherosclerotic lesions and culture of the organism from atheromata [40, 70]. Within the atherosclerotic lesion, the organism has been detected in foam cells derived from macrophages and smooth muscle cells, a hallmark of early lesion formation, and also in endothelial cells. Although the percentage of atherosclerotic lesions in which the organism has been found covers a wide range and correlation between different detection methods has not been good, more than 45 peer-reviewed publications have confirmed the initial report of Shor *et al* demonstrating the organism in human of 272 atherosclerotic tissues tested and was not found in any of the 52 normal arteries tested [60]. Moreover, *C. pneumoniae* has not been detected in other granulomas, with the exception of sarcoid tissue, and has been found more frequently in atherosclerotic lesions than in other tissues from the same person, suggesting that the organism has a tropism for atheromas. These cumulative observational studies leave no question that *C. pneumoniae* is present in atherosclerotic lesions. Defining the pathogenic mechanisms by which *C. pneumoniae* infection could contribute to atherogenesis must be more investigated.

C. pneumoniae may infect circulatory components, which may attach to the endothelium and smooth muscle cells and kill them by apoptosis. The probable molecular mechanism of atherosclerosis pathogenesis can be explained by up-regulation of expression of heat shock protein 60 (HSP-60) by C. pneumoniae infection, which induces production of cytokines such as TNF-α, IL-1β and IL-6, and MMPs by macrophages. Furthermore, C. pneumoniae could lead to elevation of CRP and contribute to instability or progression of atherosclerotic plaques. The bacterium replicates in endothelial and smooth muscle cells and macrophages, and it can activate CD4+ and CD8+ T lymphocytes. *C.pneumonia* initiates inflammatory activation via the NF-κB pathway, resulting in increased expression of vascular cell adhesion molecule-1, enhanced recruitment of inflammatory leukocytes to the vessel wall, impaired activity of endothelial nitric oxide, increased platelet adhesion to endothelial cells and procoagulant activity in endothelial cells, as well as causing oxidation of LDL-C. Therefore, chronic infection may contribute to the risk of CHD by initiating a high level of immunologic activity, by raising triglyceride levels and decreasing HDL levels, and by increasing the concentrations of acute-phase reactants such as fibrinogen, CRP, and sialic acid [32 , 33].

3.6 Heart diseases, inflammatory diseases

In vivo sites of chlamydial infection demonstrate chronic inflammation characterized by activated monocytes and macrophages. Immunopathogenesis resulting from inflammation is the hallmark for chlamydia-induced disease. Chlamydial infection may elicit the inflammatory response via up-regulated cytokine production in infected or neighboring cells. Ingredients for this elicitation can include direct infection, lipopolysaccharide stimulation (LPS found on the outer surface of *C. pneumoniae*), and/or production of heat shock proteins, such as Hsp60. Proinflammatory cytokines (IL-1, TNF, IL-6) and TH1-associated cytokines such as IFN and IL-12 have been identified at sites of chlamydial infection[49, 50, 68].

Chlamydia infections are epidemiologically linked to human heart disease. A peptide from the murine heart muscle-specific alpha myosin heavy chain that has sequence homology to the 60-kilodalton cysteine-rich outer membrane proteins of *C. pneumoniae, C. psittaci,* and *C. trachomatis* was shown to induce autoimmune inflammatory heart disease in mice [6, 54]. Injection of the homologous Chlamydia peptides into mice also induced perivascular inflammation, fibrotic changes, and blood vessel occlusion in the heart, as well as triggering T and B cell reactivity to the homologous endogenous heart muscle-specific peptide [6, 54]. Chlamydia DNA functioned as an adjuvant in the triggering of peptide-induced inflammatory heart disease. Infection with *C. trachomatis* led to the production of autoantibodies to heart muscle-specific epitopes [6, 54]. Thus, Chlamydia-mediated heart disease is induced by antigenic mimicry of a heart muscle-specific protein [12].

Heart disease is the most prevalent cause of morbidity and mortality in rich countries. Numerous clinical and experimental studies suggest that chronic stages of heart diseases are, at least in part, mediated by autoimmune responses to cardiac antigens [54]. Inflammatory heart disease is caused by a wide variety of pathogens such as viruses, bacteria, and protozoa [54,68]. RNA of the picornavirus Coxsackie B3 (CVB3) is detected in the heart muscle of 40%–50% of patients with dilated cardiomyopathy (DCM), which is defined by enlargement of cardiac chambers, thinning of ventricular walls, and reduced myofibrillar contractility [71]. Several bacterial infections (e.g., with Chlamydia species in particular) are also epidemiologically linked to human heart disease [6, 12, 24].

Because both Coxsackie virus and chlamydial infections are so common in humans, the identification of subsets of patients at risk of progression from acute infections to chronic cardiomyopathy is a large mystery. For example, who would do heart muscle biopsies in a patient with a common cold? Therefore, the challenge will be to identify both genetic and environmental factors that determine the progression to chronic heart disease and the development of DCM. Since autoinflammatory heart disease in humans can be reproduced in mice by immunization with heart muscle myosin, this experimental system has been used to analyze the immune response and host susceptibility.

Infections with bacteria that carry peptides that mimic endogenous heart-specific and heart-pathogenic epitopes lead to activation of autoaggressive lymphocytes. Pathogen-derived DNA contributes to immunactivation. The systemic effects of cytokines allow presentation of short cardiac myosin heavy chain (α-isoform) peptides in association with MHC class II molecules and the up-regulation of adhesion and homing receptors on APC resident within the target organ. The TNF-Rp55 appears to be a crucial receptor that controls target organ susceptibility in autoimmune heart disease via up-regulation of MHC class II on heart interstitial cells. After initiation of the inflammatory process by $CD4^+$ T cells, $CD8^+$ cells and macrophages are recruited into the heart muscle and contribute to disease pathogenesis. In addition, activation of B cells and production of auto antibodies may be involved in the progression of heart disease. This molecular scenario of autoimmunity also suggests that induction of disease depends on a fine balance between activation of self-reactive T cells and target organ susceptibility. The challenge for the development of successful prevention and treatment strategies will be to diagnose those few at risk of developing severe heart disease among the many with chlamydial or Coxsackie virus infections [6,12,54] .

3.7 Juvenile idiopathic arthritis

Infectious agents have been implicated in the pathogenesis of many rheumatologic diseases. In most of these diseases, including those in which specific organisms are known to play a role, the details of pathogenesis remain incompletely defined. Recent studies have aimed to isolate bacterial and viral pathogens from patients with rheumatic diseases, efforts have been made to further define the host immune response to infection, and there have been attempts to develop improved methods of diagnosis and treatment of infectious diseases affecting the musculoskeletal system.

Juvenile idiopathic arthritis (JIA) is a disease that was prominent with increased inflammation response in immune system, appeared mostly with peripheral arthritis. Endogenous and exogenous antigens play a role in the pathogenesis of disease. Two major reasons were thinking to be considerably important. First of them is immunological predisposition and the second one is environmental factors. Infections are considered to be the most important between environmental factors but also stress and trauma are also important in the etiology of the disease. However, the relation between JIA and infections is not clearly defined but the relation between adult chronic arthritis and infections was well-defined [1, 2].

Some investigators have suggested that *C.pneumonia* infection may be associated with atherosclerotic cardiovascular disease, asthma, multiple sclerosis and rheumatoid arthritis that is characterized by chronic inflammation of the synovium. Although *C.pneumonia* has been known to trigger a strong inflammatory response, there is no evidence to indicate a relationship between inflammation of the synovium and *C.pneumonia* [1, 5]. It is also not clear whether this micro-organism can trigger or exacerbate erosive joint damage. Taylor-Robinson *et al* investigated the relationship between JIA and *C.pneumonia* and suggested that larger studies with control groups were needed for more conclusive results [64].

The relationships between chronic synovitis and different bacteria, including mycobacteria, and viruses have been extensively studied by several investigators [1, 35]. Recently, detection methods for genetic material originating from micro-organisms in joint fluids have become readily available. Thus, a hypothesis stating that chronic synovitis is an immunological response to bacterial toxins has become more popular [30, 63].

Villareal focused on the role of *C.pneumonia,* which has a high prevalence amongst the general population, in the pathogenesis of chronic arthritis [65]. It was shown that *C.pneumonia* and C. trachomatis can spread to other anatomical locations by dissemination and cause chronic infections. Hannu evaluated 35 adults with reactive arthritis and demonstrated positive serology for *C.pneumonia* infection in four patients. These investigators also demonstrated that three patients had recently recovered from a lower respiratory tract disease [30]. With these findings, the authors reported that the reactive arthritis of these patients had been triggered by *C.pneumonia,* which could therefore be one of the triggering agents in the etiology of reactive arthritis [30, 64].

Taylor-Robinson *et al* investigated the relationship between JIA and C. pneumoniae in 19 children with JIA and showed that, *C.pneumonia* IgG antibodies were determinable in ten patients, but *C.pneumonia* DNA was found in only one child [64]. The presence of very high antibody titres in synovial fluids from this patient, along with another child with negative results for *C.pneumonia* DNA, suggested that the antibody may have been produced in the synovium [64].

It has been reported that C. pneumoniae can evoke a local inflammatory response when it is carried to the joint fluid. Gerard and Schumacher evaluated 212 patients with arthritis and reported C. pneumoniae DNA was present in synovial tissues of 13 % patients, but it was found in synovial fluids of only 4 % controls [25].

Wilkinson found *C. trachomatis* DNA in rheumatoid arthritis patients and in nearly one-third of unselected patients with undifferentiated oligoarthritis, which further supports the hypothesis that it plays an important role in disease pathogenesis. However, its presence did not correlate with evidence of an antichlamydial immune response. Despite previous anecdotal reports, *C. pneumoniae* does not appear to be a major cause of undifferentiated oligoarthritis or rheumatoid arthritis [69].

3.8 Diabetes

Obesity-associated chronic diseases, such as type 2 diabetes and atherosclerosis, are driven by inflammatory mediators, such as tumour necrosis factor-a (TNF-α) [71], which are also expressed during infection. Epidemiological and pathological evidence has long linked highly prevalent chronic pathogens (i.e., *Chlamydia pneumoniae, Helicobacter pylori, Porphyromonas gingivalis,* hepatitis C virus, human immunodeficiency virus, influenza virus, cytomegalovirus, and herpes simplex virus type 1) to metabolic syndrome, insulin resistance type 2 diabetes, and coronary artery disease. *C.pneumonia* infection occurs with high frequency in virtually all humans during their lifetime, and numerous studies have demonstrated strong links between *C.pneumonia* infection and metabolic syndrome, insulin resistance, and coronary artery disease [46]. However, the cause and relationship has remained inconclusive, and the link was not confirmed in some studies or disappeared after controlling for body weight [17, 22]. Moreover, preventive antibiotic treatment failed to reduce the prevalence of secondary coronary events in large clinical trials, including a 4012-patient trial that tested a 1-year course of weekly azithromycin administration [29, 44- 46].

Murine *C.pneumonia* infection enhanced insulin resistance development in a genetically and nutritionally restricted manner via circulating mediators. The relevance for the current human diabetes epidemic remains to be determined, but this finding is potentially important because of the high prevalence of human *C.pneumonia* infection worldwide.

Fernández *et al* investigated the relationship between *C. pneumoniae* infection and peripheral arterial occlusive disease (PAOD) by analyzing clinical samples from 95 patients with PAD and 100 controls [22]. They did not find significant differences in anti-LPS IgG, anti-LPS IgA and anti-EB IgA between cases and controls but C. *pneumoniae* DNA findings in the vascular wall biopsy showed significant differences between cases and controls. This study showed significantly relationship between C. *pneumoniae* infection with PAD through the detection of anti-EB IgG from serum and bacterial DNA from arterial biopsy [22]. Study of Gutiérrez *et al* also showed that PAOD is significantly associated with *C. pneumoniae* infection through the detection of anti-EB IgG from serum and bacterial DNA from arterial biopsy [29].

3.9 Uveitis

The most common form of uveitis is anterior uveitis, which involves inflammation in the front part of the eye. It is often called iritis because it is usually only effects the iris, the colored part of the eye. The inflammation may be associated with autoimmune diseases, but most cases occur in healthy people. The disorder may affect only one eye. It is most common in young and middle-aged people. Posterior uveitis affects the back part of the uvea, and involves primarily the choroid, a layer of blood vessels and connective tissue in the middle part of the eye. This type of uveitis is called choroiditis. If the retina is also involved it is called chorioretinitis. Anterior uveitis is the most common form, and occurs annually at a frequency of about 8 to 15 cases per 100,000 people. This type of uveitis affects men and women equally. [34, 48].

Numazaki K *et al* found that the prevalence of serum IgA and IgM antibodies to *C. pneumoniae* in patients with endogenous uveitis associated with sarcoidosis was significantly higher than that in patients with other endogenous uveitis [48]. Huhtinen *et al* investigated the prevalence of antibodies to *C. pneumoniae* Hsp60 in patients with acute anterior uveitis

[34]. They did not find significantly difference in frequency and the level of IgG antibodies to *C. pneumoniae* Hsp60 between the patients and control subjects but the levels of IgA antibodies to *C. pneumoniae* Hsp60 were significantly higher in the patients than in the control subjects [48].

4. Conclusion

Immunological studies performed in animal models of autoimmune diseases strongly suggest that infections represent the best candidates for the environmental factors triggering human autoimmune disease. Only limited data are available as yet which show strong indications in this direction. However, the bulk of indirect evidence is serological data and important role of interferon-a in a number of autoimmune diseases, argue in favor of an etiological role for infections. More recently, *C.pneumonia* has been linked to a number of chronic human diseases and many autoimmune diseases with involving chronic inflammation and demyelination. The possible mechanisms of *C.pneumonia* involvement as aetiological agents or in the exacerbation of these diseases have been investigated intensively. Two basic elements are the association between bacterial infection and autoimmune disease and the involvement of the immune system in the disease process. We hope that the numerous studies in progress will provide the possibility of identifying the role of *C.pneumonia* in related autoimmune diseases. This would be important for the understanding of disease pathogenesis. It might prove of crucial clinical interest by opening up major therapeutic perspectives including anti-infectious agents, chemicals and monoclonal antibodies and vaccination.

5. References

[1] Albert LJ (2000). Infection and rheumatoid arthritis: guilt by association? *J Rheumatol* ,Vol.37, pp. 564–566.

[2] Altun, S., Kasapcopur, O., Aslan ,M., *et al* (2004). Is there any relationship between Chlamydophila pneumoniae infection and juvenile idiopathic arthritis? *J Med Microbiol* ,Vol.53, No.8, pp. 787-790

[3] Anzini, A., Cassone, A., Rasura, M., *et al* (2004). *Chlamydia pneumoniae* infection in young stroke patients: a case control study. *Eur J Neurol* , Vol.11, No.5, pp. 321-7.

[4] Arking, EJ.,Appelt, DM., Abrams, JT., Kolbe, S., Hudson, AP., & Balin, BJ (1999). Ultrastructural analysis of *C .pneumoniae* in the Alzheimer's brain. *Pathogen* , Vol.1, pp. 201-211.

[5] Aslan, M., Kasapcopur, O., Yasar, H., *et al* (2011). Do infections trigger juvenile idiopathic arthritis? *Rheumatol Int* , Vol.31, No.2, pp. 215-20.

[6] Bachmaier K., Neu N., de la Maza LM., Pal S., Hessel A., & Penninger, JM (1999). Chlamydia infections and heart disease linked through antigenic mimicry. *Science* , Vol.283, No.5406, pp. 1335-9.

[7] Balin, BJ., Little, CS., Hammond, CJ., Appelt, DM., Whittum-Hudson, JA., Gérard HC., & Hudson AP (2008). *Chlamydophila pneumoniae* and the etiology of late-onset Alzheimer's disease. *J Alzheimers Dis* , Vol.13, No.4, pp. 371-80.

[8] Bandaru, VC., Laxmi, V., Neeraja, M., et al (2008). *Chlamydia pneumoniae* antibodies in various subtypes of ischemic stroke in Indian patients. *J Neurol Sci* , Vol.15, No.272, pp. 115-22

[9] Bandaru, VC., Babu Boddu, D., Laxmi, V., Neeraja M., & Kaul, S (2009). Seroprevalence of *Chlamydia Pneumoniae* Antibodies in Stroke in Young. *Can J Neurological Sci* , Vol.36, No.6, pp. 725-29

[10] Belland, RJ., Ouellette, SP., Gieffers, J., & Byrne, GI (2004). *Chlamydia pneumoniae* and atherosclerosis. *Cell Microbiol* , Vol.6, pp. 117–127.

[11] Breitner, JC (1996). The role of anti-inflammatory drugs in the prevention and treatment of Alzheimer's disease. *Ann Rev Med* , vol.47, pp.401-411.

[12] Campbell, LA., Kuo, C-C., Grayston, JT (1998). *Chlamydia pneumoniae* and cardiovascular disease. *Emerg Infect Dis* , Vol. 4 , pp.571–579

[13] Carusone, SC., Smieja, M., Molloy, W., *et al* (2004) .Lack of association between vascular dementia and *Chlamydia pneumoniae* infection: a case-control study. *BMC Neurol* , Vol. 4 , pp. 15.

[14] Cook, PJ., Honeybourne, D., Lip, GY., Beevers, DG., Wise, R., & Davies, P (1998). *Chlamydia pneumoniae* antibody titers are significantly associated with acute stroke and transient cerebral ischemia: the West Birmingham Stroke Project. *Stroke* , Vol.29 , pp.404–410.

[15] Cooper, RJ ., D'Arcy, S.,Kirby, M., Al-Buhtori, M., Rahman , MJ., Proctor, L., & Bonshek, RE(2008). Infection and temporal arteritis: a PCR-based study to detect pathogens in temporal artery biopsy specimens. *J Med Virol* , Vol. 80, No.3, pp.501-5.

[16] Danesh, J., Whnicup, P., Lewington, S., *et al* (2002). *Chlamydia pneumoniae* IgA titers and coronary heart disease. *Eur Heart J* , Vol.23, No.5, pp. 371-5.

[17] Dart, AM., Martin, JL., & Kay, S (2002). Association between past infection with *Chlamydia pneumoniae* and body mass index, low-density lipoprotein particle size and fasting insulin. *Int J Obes Relat Metab Disord* , Vol.26 , pp.464-8.

[18] Dowell, SF., Boman, J., Carlone, GM., *et al* (2001). Standardizing *Chlamydia pneumoniae* assays: recommendations from the Centers for Disease Control and Prevention (USA) and the Laboratory Center for Diseases (Canada). *Clin infect Dis* , Vol.33, No.4, pp. 492-503.

[19] Engelhart, MJ., Geerlings, MI., Meijer, J., et al (2004). Inflammatory proteins in plasma and the risk of dementia: the Rotterdam Study. *Arch Neurol* , Vol.61, pp.668–672.

[20] Ercolini, AM., & Miller, SD (2009). The role of infections in autoimmune disease. *Clin Exp Immunol* , Vol.155, No.1, pp.1–15.

[21] Fairweather, D., Kaya, Z., Shellam, GR., Lawson, CM., & Rose NR (2001). From infection to autoimmunity. *J Autoimmun* , Vol.16, pp. 175–86.

[22] Fernández-Real, JM., López-Bermejo, A., Vendrell, J., Ferri, MJ., & Recasens, M (2006). Burden of infection and insulin resistance in healthy middle-aged men. *Diabetes Care* , Vol. 29 *pp.*1058-64.

[23] Fujinami, RS., von Herrath, MG.,Christen, U., & Lindsay Whitton J(2006). Molecular Mimicry, Bystander Activation, or Viral Persistence: Infections and Autoimmune Disease. *Clin Microbiol Rev* , Vol.19, No.1, pp.80–94

[24] Fujita, M., Hatachi, S., & Yagita, M (2009). Acute *Chlamydia pneumoniae* infection in the pathogenesis of autoimmune diseases. *Lupus* , Vol.18, No.2, pp. 164-168.

[25] Gerard, HC., Schumacher, HR., El-Gabalawy, H., Goldbach-Mansky, R., & Hudson, AP (2000). *Chlamydia pneumoniae* present in the human synovium are viable and metabolically active. *Microb Pathog* , Vol.29 , pp.17–24.

[26] Gérard, HC., Dreses-Werringloer, U., Wildt, KS., *et al* (2006). *Chlamydophila (Chlamydia) pneumoniae* in the Alzheimer's brain. *FEMS Immunol Med Microbiol* , Vol.48, No.3, pp.355-66.

[27] Grayston JT (1992). Infections caused by *Chlamydia pneumonia* strain TWAR. *Clin Infect Dis* , Vol.15 , pp.757–763.

[28] Grayston, JT., Kronmal, RA., Jackson, LA., *et al* (2005). Azithromycin for the secondary prevention of coronary events. *N Engl J Med,* Vol , 352 *, pp.*637-45.

[29] Gutiérrez, J., Linares, J., Fernández, F., *et al* (2004). Relationship between the peripheral arterial occlusive disease and the infection by *Chlamydophila pneumoniae. Med Clin* (Barc), Vol.123, No.15, pp. 561-6.

[30] Hannu, T, Puolakkainen, M, Leirisalo-Repo, M(1999). *Chlamydia pneumoniae* as a triggering infection in reactive arthritis. *Rheumatology,* Vol.38, pp.411–414.

[31] Hasan ZN (2011). Association of *Chlamydia pneumoniae* serology and ischemic stroke. *South Med J* , Vol.104, No.5, pp. 319-21

[32] Hong, MK. , Mintz, GS., Lee, CW., *et al* (2004). Comparison of coronary plaque rupture between stable angina and acute myocardial infarction: a three-vessel intravascular ultrasound study in 235 patients. *Circulation* , Vol.110, pp.928-933

[33] Hortovanyi, E., Illyes, G., Kadar, A (2003). Early Atherosclerosis and *Chlamydia Pneumoniae* Infection in the Coronary Arteries. *Pathology Oncology Research* , Vol.19, No.1, pp. 42-46

[34] Huhtinen, M., Puolakkainen, M., Laasila, K., Sarvas, M., Karma, A., & Leirisalo -Repo, M (2001). Chlamydial antibodies in patients with previous acute anterior uveitis. *Invest Ophthalmol Vis Sci,* Vol.42, No.8, pp.1816-1819.

[35] Inman, RD., Whittum-Hudson, JA., Schumacher, HR., & Hudson, AP (2000). Chlamydia and associated arthritis. *Curr Opin Rheumatol* ,Vol.12, pp. 254-263.

[36] Kalayoglu, MV, Libby, P, & Byrne, GI (2002). *Chlamydia pneumoniae* as an emerging risk factor in cardiovascular disease. *JAMA* , Vol.288, pp.2724–2731.

[37] Kaperonis, EA., Liapis, CD., Kakisis, JD., *et al* (2006). Inflammation and *Chlamydia pneumoniae* infection correlate with the severity of peripheral arterial disease. Eur *J Vasc Endovasc Surg* , Vol.31, No.5, pp. 509-15.

[38] Koskiniemi, M., Gencay, M., Salonen, O., *et al* (1996). *Chlamydia pneumoniae* associated with central nervous system infections. *Eur J Neurol* , Vol. 36, pp.160–163.

[39] Kratzsch, T., Peters, J., & Frolich, L (2002). Etiology and pathogenesis of Alzheimer dementia. *Wien Med Wochenschr* , Vol.152, No.3-4, pp.72-6.

[40] Kuo, CC , Chen, HH , Wang, P , & Grayston, JT (1986). Identification of an new group of *Chlamydia psittaci* strains called TWAR. *J Clin Microbiol* ,Vol. 24,pp.1034–1037.

[41] Little, CS., Hammond, CJ., MacIntyre, A., Balin, BJ., & Appelt, DM (2004). *Chlamydia pneumoniae* induces Alzheimer-like amyloid plaques in brains of BALB/c mice. *Neurobiol Aging* , Vol.25, No.4, pp.419-29.

[42] Liu, R., Yamamoto, M., Moroi, M., *et al* (2005). *Chlamydia pneumoniae* immunoreactivity in coronary artery plaques of patients with acute coronary syndromes and its relation with serology. *Am Heart J* ,Vol.150 , pp. 681-688.

[43] Ljungstrom, L, Franzen, C, Schlaug, M, Elowson, S, & Viidas, U(1997). Reinfection with *Chlamydia pneumoniae* may induce isolated and systemic vasculitis in small and large vessels. *Scand J Infect Dis* , Vol.104, Suppl pp.37–40.

[44] Mehta, JL., Saldeen, TGP., & Rand, K (1998). Interactive role of infection, inflammation and traditional risk factors in artherosclerosis and coronary artery disease. *J Am Coll Cardiol* , Vol.31,pp.1217–25.

[45] Muhlestein JB (2002). Secondary prevention of coronary artery disease with antimicrobials: current status and future directions. *Am J Cardiovasc Drugs* , Vol.2 , pp.107-18.

[46] Nabipour, I., Vahdat, K., Jafari, SM., Pazoki, R., & Sanjdideh, Z (2006). The association of metabolic syndrome and *Chlamydia pneumoniae, Helicobacter pylori,* cytomegalovirus, and herpes simplex virus type 1: the Persian Gulf Healthy Heart Study. *Cardiovasc Diabetol* ,Vol.5 ,*pp*.25.

[47] Njamnshi, AK., Blackett, KN., Mbagbaw, JN., Gumedze, F., Gupta, S., & Wiysonge, CS (2006). Chronic *Chlamydia pneumoniae* infection and stroke in Cameroon. *Stroke,* Vol.37, No.3, pp. 796-9.

[48] Numazaki, K., Chiba, S., Aoki, K., Suzuki, K., & Ohno, S (1997). Detection of serum antibodies to *Chlamydia pneumoniae* in patients with endogenous uveitis and acute conjunctivitis. *Clin Infect Dis* , Vol.25, pp.928-929.

[49] Peeling, RW., & Brunham, RC(1996). Chlamydiae as pathogens: new species and new issues. *Emerg Infect Dis* , Vol. 2 , pp. 307–319.

[50] Posnett, DN., & Yarilin, D (2005). Amplification of autoimmune disease by infection. *Arthritis Res Ther* , Vol.7, No.2, pp.74–84.

[51] Regan, MJ., Wood, BJ., Hsieh, YH., *et al* (2002). Temporal arteritis and *Chlamydia pneumoniae*: failure to detect the organism by polymerase chain reaction in ninety cases and ninety controls. *Arthritis Rheum,* Vol.46, No.4, pp.1056-60.

[52] Rimenti, GF., Cosentini, BR., Moling, O., Pristera, R., Tarsia, P., Vedovelli, C., & Mian, P (2000).Temporal arteritis associated with *Chlamydia pneumoniae* DNA detected in an artery specimen. *J Rheumatol* ,Vol.27 , pp.2718-2720.

[53] Rimenti, EA., Liapis, CD., Kakisis, JD., *et al* (2006). Inflammation and *Chlamydia pneumoniae* infection correlate with the severity of peripheral arterial disease. Eur *J Vasc Endovasc Surg* , Vol.31, No.5, pp. 509-15.

[54] Rose, NR (1996). Myocarditis: from infection to autoimmunity. *The Immunologist , Vol.* 4 , *pp*.67-75.

[55] Saikku , P., Mattila, K., Nieminen, MS., Makela, PH.,Huttunen, JK., & Valtonen, V(1988). Serological evidence of an association of a novel chlamydia, TWAR, with chronic coronary heart disease and acute myocardial infarction. *Lancet ii,* pp.983–986.

[56] Schneider, R., & Passo, MH (2002). Juvenile rheumatoid arthritis. *Rheum Dis Clin North Am,* Vol. 28 , pp. 503–530.

[57] Scolding, NJ., Zajicek, JP., Wood, N., & Compston, DAS (1994). The pathogenesis of demyelinating disease. *Progr Neurobiol* ; 43: 143–173.

[58] Sherbet, G (2009). Bacterial infections and the pathogenesis of autoimmune conditions. *BJMP* , Vol.2, No.1, pp.6-13.

[59] Shoenfeld Y., *et al* (2008). The mosaic of autoimmunity: hormonal and environ mental factors involved in autoimmune diseases. *Isr Med Assoc J* , Vol.10, pp. 8- 12

[60] Shor, A., Kuo, CC., & Patton, DL (1992). Detection of *Chlamydia pneumoniae* in the coronary artery atheroma plaque. *South Afr Med J* ,Vol.82, pp.158–161

[61] Sinha, AA., Lopez, MT., & McDevitt, HO (1990). Autoimmune diseases: the failure of self tolerance. *Science* , Vol.248 , pp.1380-88.

[62] Sriram, S., Mitchell, W., & Stratton, C (1998). Multiple Sclerosis associated with *Chlamydia Pneumoniae* infection of the CNS. *Neurology* , Vol.50 ,pp. 571-572

[63] Sriram, S., Steratton., CW, Yao., S, *et al* (1999). *Chlamydia Pneumoniae* infection of the Central Nervous System in Multiple Sclerosis. *Ann Neurol* , Vol.46 ,pp. 6-14

[64] Taylor-Robinson, D., Thomas, B., & Rooney, M (1998). Association of *Chlamydia pneumoniae* with chronic juvenile arthritis. *Eur J Clin Microbiol Infect Dis,* Vol.17, pp. 211-212.

[65] Villareal, C., Whittum-Hudson, JA., & Hudson, AP (2002). Persistent *Chlamydiae* and chronic arthritis. *Arthritis Res* , Vol.4 , pp. 5–9.

[66] Virok, D., Kis, Z, Karai, L., et al (2001). *Chlamydia pneumoniae* in artherosclerotic middle cerebral artery. *Stroke* , Vol.32, pp.1973–1976.

[67] Wang C., Gao D., Kaltenboeck B (2009). Acute *Chlamydia pneumoniae* Reinfection Accelerates the Development of Insulin Resistance and Diabetes in Obese C57BL/6 Mice. *Journal of Infectious Diseases* , Vol. 200, No2 , pp. 279-287.

[68] Ward ME (1995). The immunobiology and immunopathology of chlamydial infections. *APMIS,* Vol. 103 , pp.769–796.

[69] Wilkinson, NZ., Kingsley, GH., Sieper, J., Braun, J., & Ward, ME (1998). Lack of correlation between the detection of *Chlamydia trachomatis* DNA in synovial fluid from patients with a range of rheumatic diseases and the presence of an antichlamydial immune response. *Arthritis Rheum* , Vol.41, No.5, pp.845-54

[70] Wimmer, ML, Scandmann-Strupp, R, Saiku, P, & Haberl, RL (1996). Association of chlamydial infection with cardiovascular diseases. *Strok* , Vol. 27, pp. 2207-2210.

[71] Woodruff, JF (1980). Viral myocarditis. A review. *Am J Pathol* , *Vol.*101, pp.425-84.

[72] Wozniak, MA., Cookson, A., Wilcock, GK., & Itzhaki, RF (2003). Absence of *Chlamydia pneumoniae* in brain of vascular dementia patients. *Neurobiol Aging* , Vol.24 , pp.761–765.

[73] xu, H., Barnes, GT., Yang, Q., *et al* (2003). Chronic inflammation in fat plays a crucial role in the development of obesity-related insulin resistance. *J Clin Invest* , Vol.112 ,*pp.*1821-30

[74] Yao, S-Y.,& Sriram S (1999). Reactivity of oligoclonal bands seen in CSF to *C. pneumoniae* antigens in patients with multiple sclerosis. *Neurology* , Vol. 52 (Suppl 2) ,pp. A559.

[75] Yasojima, K., Schwab, C., McGeer, EG., & McGeer, PL (2000). Human neurons generate C-reactive protein and amyloid P: upregulation in Alzheimer's disease. *Brain Res*, Vol.887 , pp.80–89.

16

Chlamydia: Possible Mechanisms of the Long Term Complications

Teoman Zafer Apan
Department of Microbiology and Clinical Microbiology
Kırıkkale University Faculty of Medicine
Turkey

1. Introduction

Chlamydia an insidious intracellular pathogen implicated in various diseases by increasing inflammation and microbial byproducts. Chronic infection may be observed with major types of causative organism initiated disease on ocular, sinopulmonary and reproductive tract.

Chlamydia trachomatis is one of the infectious cause of ocular disease that is endemic in the regions with limited sanitary resources. The infection may start on eye lids and progress to trichiasis, keratoconjunctivitis and corneal opacity, that eventually lead to vision loss. The chronic infection of the same microorganism in female reproductive system may be associated with pelvic inflammatory disease, infertility, ectopic pregnancy and is proposed to induce ovarian cancer by chronic tubal inflammation. The causative microorganism is also demonstrated to be one of the infectious sources of male infertility. *Chlamydia pneumonia,* the other serotype of the microorganism, which is capable of pulmonary infection, has been demonstrated to induce nasal polyps, asthma in pediatric and adult population.

Increasing body of evidence indicates that there is an association between *chlamydial* infection with atherosclerosis and serious related outcomes. Inflammation induced by peroxy-lipid molecules, heat shock protein 60 (HSP 60) and facilitation of the endothelial foam cell formations are the proposed mechanisms.

Interesting findings in several investigations indicate possible association between rheumatoid disease, systemic vasculitis, and certain neurobehavioral diseases such as Alzheimer's disease, multipl sclerosis, seronegative spondylarthritis and Behçet disease and *Chlamydia.*

Chlamydia is an obligatory intra-cytoplasmal gram negative pathogen that requires invading moist epithelial barriers of conjunctiva, sino-bronchial three, and reproductive tract for infection. The organism is capable of chronic infection by modulating host defense, dormancy or by microbial products. Disease could be occur through direct contamination from infected host with touch or dropouts of cough, infected materials or with fly vectors.

1.1 Ocular complications

Trachoma is a keratoconjunctivitis caused by ocular infection of *C. trachomatis*. Serotypes A, B, Ba and C are considered to be responsible for disease in corneal epithelium to initiate the disease. The latent phase of the disease takes about 4-7 days. Reinfection after initial clearance of the organism may occur to clinical signs of the disease. The neonatal form of disease also could occur during labor with vaginal serotypes (D and K). Disease is more common in lower socioeconomic status, and close living with family members and limited access to the clear water resources are indicated as other predisposing factors. Trachoma starts on tarsal conjonctiva of the eyelids, progresses to cause trichitis and entropion. Disease may cause blindness, advancing to the cornea to cause opacity. Trachoma is considered as the primary infectious cause of blindness (Wright, 2007). The global burden of the disease has been calculated to reach about 8 billion US dollars including disability induced loss of work years, payment for caregivers. Active or early disease which is common in the childhood that observed as chronic follicular conjunctivitis, and late cicatricial form results of the recurrent inflammation of the infection which leads to corneal opacity are the clinical features of trachoma. World Health Organization in collaboration with other organizations was initiated to decrease the severe outcomes and disease activity. The program which includes surgery for trichiasis, antibiotic therapy for active disease, face cleaning or personal hygiene and environmental improvements (SAFE) was constituted in 1998 that planned to eliminate these complications at 2020 (Burton, 2007). Convincingly, in a study conducted in the endemic region for trachoma after mass treatment with azithromycin or doxicyclin for *C. trachomatis,* there was no resistance to the antimicrobial treatment (Hong, et al. 2009). Surgical treatment for trichiasis, a late complication of trachoma shows promising results, but requires to be continued with scheduled programs (Burton et al., 2005a). The severity of the ocular pathology in general, influences the duration of the disease that remedy for early intervention in the rural areas such as observed in Ethiopia (Melese et al, 2005). On the other hand, azithromycin treatment after surgery for controlling the relapses has not been changed the outcome (Burton et al, 2005b).

Holland *et al.* demonstrated that the presence of major outer membrane protein to cytotoxic T lymphocytes that specific to the *C. trachomatis* is associated with the current ocular disease with longer duration, but neither indicates estimated load of infection nor leads to presume the course of the disease (Holland et al., 2006). Repeated infections of *Chlamydia* may lead to expression of heat shock proteins (HSP), which closely react with human HSP 60 and are suggested to trigger autoimmune-directed inflammation, which is thought to play role in the pathogenesis of trachoma (Morrison et al., 1989).

In a study based on repeated examination of eyes performed in Australia indicates that *C. pneumoniae* infection was considered as an independent or additional risk factor for age-related macular degeneration possibly by inducing chronic inflammatory reaction (Robman et al., 2005). *C. pneumoniae* has also been demonstrated to induce chorioidal neovascularization by inducing Toll-like receptor 2 in an experimental model indicates a risk factor for age related macular degeneration (Fujimoto et al., 2010).

Ocular adnexial lymhomas constitutes the subgroup of non-hodgkin lymphomas originating from lymphoid tissue of mucosal layer. The association between *C. psittaci* with ocular lymphoma was first determined in a study subjecting Italian patients (Ferreri et al., 2004). *C. psittaci* was also indicated as a possible cause with a varying rate of geographical distribution (Chanudet et al., 2006). However, several studies failed to demonstrate an association between ocular malignancy with *Chlamydiae* (Yakushijin et al., 2007).

1.2 *Chlamydia* and genitourinary tract

Chlamydia trachomatis is able to infect urogenital tract and is one of the most common sexually transmitted diseases in the Western world (Ward, 1995). Other serotypes including L1, L2, L2a and L3 are also capable of infecting monocytes to cause systemic disease called lympogranulomavenereum (Mabey & Peeling, 2002). The genital serovars of *Chlamydiae* are able to migrate to the upper genital tract to induce quiescent infection, which is one of the infectious causes of fallopian tube occlusion, infertility, ectopic pregnancy and salpingitis. The microorganism is deficient in producing energy during life cycle and is required to attach to the host cell through elementary body (EB) to reach to the Golgi apparatus. The EB could be differentiated to the metabolically active non infectious replicative form, namely reticulate body (RB), which is able to inhibit cell apoptosis for long term survival. Mammalian heat shock proteins are evolutionary highly conserved molecular chaperones, which appear to have derived from procaryotic ancestors. Although HSP 60 is primarily considered a mitochondrial protein in mammals, 20 to 40% of cellular HSP 60 occurs in extra-mitochondrial sites. Amino acid sequences of human HSP 60 and *C. trachomatis* HSP 60 (serovar D) are 100% similar. They are identified in four epitopes and 13 other peptides of various lengths with identity between 33% and 75%, and these epitopes were present in all three domain of the molecule (Capello et al., 2009). *Chlamydia trachomatis* also secretes HSP 60 kDalton possibly due to decreasing the external stress to the infection (Morrison, 1991). This molecule itself is capable of inducing strong inflammation in the fallopian tubes and antibody responses and similarly cell mediated immunity to HSP 60 is associated with tubal infertility and ectopic pregnancy. The interaction with human HSP 60, which has 48% homology with *C. trachomatis* HSP 60, may induce loss of pregnancy. Women with asymptomatic tubal infertility have an increased prevalence of antibodies against *C. trachomatis* and anti-HSP 60 (Sziller et al., 2008). Variety types of chlamydial HSP were identified with different properties to induce immunological response (Gérard et al., 2004). The implementation of public health measures to diagnose the recent developed infection in women at reproductive age and treatment is mandatory especially in the case of genital tract infection with the other microorganisms, which may induce the secretion of RB (Caldwell et al., 2003). The relevant data do not support the effectiveness of *Chlamydial* screening in general population younger than 25 years, however, high quality randomized trials are required to determine cost effectiveness or benefits (Low et al., 2009).

It has been suggested by some that exposure to *C. trachomatis* HSP 60 may be a risk factor for development of cancer (Di Felice et al., 2005), while the development of HSP 60 is also proposed to protect against malignancy (Capello et al., 2009). Chronic persistent infection with *C. trachomatis* to the upper genital tract is able to incur significant damage to the reproductive tract and proposed to induce ovarian cancer (Quirk & Kupinski, 2001).

Various mechanisms are suggested for the effect of *C. trachomatis* inducing male infertility. Male reproductive system is separated from innate immunity, which may prevent immunization against one's own sperm. Infections are proposed to disrupt membranes and vascular barriers in testes, epididymis and prostate to initiate autoimmunization through introducing sperm with leucocytes or other inflammatory cells. *C. trachomatis* and *N. gonorrheae* are the most common pathogens for epididymitis and orchitis, which are common in the outpatient setting in men between 14 to 35 years of ages (Trojian et al., 2009). Although many cases of urethritis are idiopathic, *C. trachomatis* has been considered the most common infectious cause with many of these patients being symptomatic during the interview (Wetmore et al., 2009). On the other hand, though there are various studies investigating the relationship, influence of prostatitis induced by *C. trachomatis* on male infertility is uncertain (Cunningham & Beagley, 2008). The surface membrane of sperm has various types of protein including HSP 65 and 70, which react with anti-sperm human IgG antibodies. Three of these proteins were also immunoprecipitated against *C. trachomatis* epitope of HSP 70, suggesting an association between genital tract infection, immunity to HSP 70 and reproductive failure (Naaby-Hansen & Herr, 2010). The influence of leucocytospermia and DNA particles of sexually transmitted diseases (STD) on asymptomatic male infertility was investigated in a study conducted by Bezold *et al.* (Bezold et al., 2007). The incidence of STD was similar between patients with or without leucocytospermia. DNA particles from STD decreased sperm and motile sperm concentration, total sperm count, and neutral α-glucosidase concentration, whereas leucocytospermia was associated with a decrease in total sperm count, % of normal forms, and fructose concentration. In addition to the decrease of spermatogenesis due to the destruction of reproductive system, male infertility seems to be influenced by both the infection itself and increased inflammation. In an in-vitro study, the persistence of *C. trachomatis* was demonstrated in the presence of ciprofloxacin and to a lesser extent of ofloxacin. These results reflect the clinical data that antibacterial susceptibility does not always guarantee the in-vivo success of the therapy (Dreses-Werringloer et al., 2000).

The association between prostate cancer and *C. trachomatis* infection was not determined, however increased seropositivity was found in men with benign prostate hyperplasia, suggesting inflammation-induced or facilitated enlargement (Hracek et al., 2011).

1.3 *Chlamydia* and respiratory system

Respiratory system is an important route of infection for *Chlamydia pneumoniae.* The microorganism is determined to be one of the infectious causes of sinusitis, otitis media, tonsillitis, laryngitis and chronic pharyngitis (Hsahiguchi et al., 1992, Hammaerschlag, 2000). Chronic infection in the upper respiratory tract was demonstrated to cause nasal polyps from the biopsy materials, possibly with increasing inflammation and epithelial cell destruction (Apan et al., 2007).

C. pneumonia is responsible for about 10-15% of community acquired pneumonias. *C. trachomatis* is also able to cause nasopharyngitis and pulmonary infection especially in the newborns. Infection may occur by direct transmission during the vaginal delivery and may be serologically positive in the earlier years of life. However, vertical transmission from the mother may result in the development of the neonatal conjunctivitis and pneumonia (Wu et al., 1999, Darville, 2005). Seropositivity to the *C. pneumonia* was found to be as high as 50% in young adults and 75% for the elderly (Oba & Salzman, 2007).

A substantial body of evidence indicates the role of chronic infections in chronic pulmonary disease. The mechanism of chronic infection in disease process is not clear, but may involve a modification of the airway inflammatory response. Asthma is characterized by T-helper lymphocyte induced eosinophilic response that proceed to airway mucosal damage and increased responsiveness. There was no difference between the subjects who had atypical *C. pneumonia* and those who had nonatypical pneumonia in terms of asthma incidence, indicence being very high in both groups (Sutherland et al., 2004). Both of two serotypes of *Chlamydiacea* family were considered as infectious etiology for asthmatic patients in pediatric populations. Increased prevalence of viable *C. pneumoniae* was detected in samples from bronchoalveolar fluid in pediatric asthmatic patients, which constitutes about the half of the polymerase chain reaction (PCR) positive subjects with the microorganism (Webley et al., 2005). Chlamydia specific DNA strand was detected from bronchoalveolar fluid in about 67 % of pediatric asthmatic patients. On the other hand, this observation is not able to explain 71% positive results obtained from PCR in non-asthmatic patients and increased incidence of asthma that was observed in certain subgroups (Webley et al., 2009).

C. pneumoniae is a causative organism in chronic severe form of asthma (Cook et al., 1998). Raised antibody titer to *C. pneumoniae* IgA was associated with increased neutrophil, monocyte count, and eosinophilic cationic protein in acute exacerbation of asthma (Wark et al., 2002). Elevated IgA antibody levels to *C. pneumoniae* were more commonly encountered in severe and moderate forms of asthma, suggesting chronic infection. However, antibody to *C. pneumoniae* HSP 60 was not considered as a useful marker of such an infection among the asthmatics (Hertzen et al., 2002).

Chronic obstructive pulmonary disease (COPD) is another chronic pulmonary pathology, which is leading cause of morbidity and mortality. There is a strong correlation between disease and smoking habit and about 10-20% of smokers developing COPD. Chronic *C. pneumoniae* infection as determined by persistent elevated IgA levels to the microorganism was associated with COPD and considered as an independent risk factor (Brandén et al., 2005). The relationship between severities of the disease and *C. pneumoniae* IgA antibody was demonstrated in another study, in which peak expiratory flow percentage of the predictive value was inversely correlated with the IgA antibody titers (Falck et al., 2002). On the other hand, the prevalence of IgG and IgM antibodies indicating acute infection was significantly increased in COPD patients when compared to the smoker control subjects, but no significant relation was found with IgA antibodies. Smoking was associated with increased level of *C. pneumoniae* serum antibody levels. It is presumed that smoking may facilitate *C. pneumoniae* infection in lung with chronic epithelial damage or promote deeper penetration into lung tissue to produce a greater antibody response (Karnak et al., 2001). High IgG and IgA antibody titers against *C. pneumonia* are linked with the severity of emphysema high resolution CT and increased IgA titers is also associated with decreased diffusion capacity to carbon monoxide (Kurashima et al., 2005).

Evidence indicates that there is a relation between chronic pulmonary infection with *C. pneumonia* and lung cancers. Antibody titer against to this organism is increased in cancer patients (Littman et al., 2004). The risk of cancer may increase about twofold in patients with elevated Ig A titers, specifically in squamous cell carcinomas and to a lesser extent in small cell and adenomatous cancers (Laurila et al., 1997). Increased seropositivity was found among smoker patients diagnosed with small cell cancer. This point rise concern about infection, which may be facilitated with chronic airway irritation with cigarette or chronic infection combined with increase in epithelial cell turnover that eventually leads to cancer (Samaras et al., 2010).

1.4 *Chlamydia* and atherosclerosis

Atherosclerosis is the main cause of death in the developed countries, inducing coronary heart disease, stroke or advancing organ failure. There are many contributing factor such as cigarette smoking, sedentary life style, increased weight due to hyper caloric, hyper cholesterolemic dietary habit, and low exercise. An association between atherosclerosis and infections has been suggested many times during the past century.

C. pneumonia, one of the infectious etiologies of atherosclerosis, was first demonstrated in the study conducted by Saikku et al. (Saikku et al, 1988). The microorganism first appears in the lower respiratory tract infected alveolar macrophages that transmigrate from the epithelium gain access to the circulation and reach atherosclerotic plaque. *C. pneumonia* may be capable of infecting a variety of cells including macrophages, vascular endothelial and smooth muscles. The lypopolisaccaride (LPS) component of the gram negative bacterial capsule is a potent inflammatory molecule, which changes the biology of the alveolar macrophages to attract low density lipoproteins and change their morphology (Mackman, 2000). The presence of organism on atherosclerotic plaque has been shown by various techniques, including PCR, immunohistochemistry, and electron microscopy (Leinonen & Saikku, 2002, Campbell & Kuo, 2004). The fact that organism is present in the atherosclerotic plaque but is rarely found in the healthy vasculature indicates that microorganism might spread through dissemination from primary infectious site with immune cells, namely T lymphocytes or monocytes (Liu et al., 2005). Also, it possibly requires weak regions between cell connections in endothelial layers for diapedes. Therefore, randomized antimicrobial programs were implemented to eradicate the infectious agent and failed success of long term therapies increased suspicion of atherogenesis theory. However, *C. pneumonia* is one of the possible causative organisms and all microorganisms can not be eradicated with a single antimicrobial agent. Recent cohort studies also indicated that antichlamydial therapy in *Chlamydia* positive patients led to no symptomatic improvement in peripheral vascular disease (Jaff et al., 2009). There is also no association between *C. pneumonia* bacteriophage or its antibody titers and acute coronary events (Patrick et al., 2005).

Beside the contributing factors, atherosclerosis may be initiated not only by direct invasion of microorganism itself but also by increasing and ongoing inflammation with such organisms. Inflammatory stimuli such as lipopolysaccarides of microorganisms may activate toll-like receptors (TLR) from immune response from macrophages and endothelial or smooth muscle cells. Once initiated, TLR are able to initiate inflammatory storm. Inborn deficiency including weaker response to the inflammatory stimuli may protect against cardiovascular diseases (Kiechl et al., 2002). Transient stimuli from certain microorganism had been found to be capable of inducing stimuli to TLR even when causative agent was undetected (Stassen et al., 2008). Leucocyte recruitment and accumulation to the atheroma initiates the second morphological event that accumulates lipid and changes to the foam cells. Smooth muscle cell migration and replication from underlying media to intima and cell death might complicate the atheroma. Volume increase under intima may lead to the rupture of underlying arterial vasa vasorum by restricting adequate oxygen or nutrient intake and hemorrhage may lead to further smooth muscle cell accumulation. The presence of *C. pneumonia* in the plaque may further augment the local inflammatory process. The other possible molecular mechanism induced by *C. pneumonia* is up-regulation and expression of HSP 60, which induces cytokines including tumor necrosis factor-α, interleukine-1β (IL1 β), IL 6, matrix metalloproteinases (MMP) from macrophages. In addition, *C. pneumonia* might increase C reactive protein and contribute to instability or progression of the plaque (Miya et al., 2004). Specific microbial products such as LPS, HSP 60 or other virulence factors may provoke endothelial cell, producing remote infections. Also, the acute inflammation activates coagulation and fibrinolytic system, which changes balance in pro-coagulation site. Rupture of the plaque from its thinned fibrous cap and release of non-occlusive thrombi might produce clinically apparent occlusion in this activated coagulation state (Fazio et al., 2009). Infection with *C. pneumonia* is possibly involved with the pathogenesis of atherosclerosis early in life, such that antichlamydial antibiotic has no influence once inflammation and plaque has been established (Gattone et al., 2001). The organism may accelerate the progression of atherosclerosis by increasing and maintaining inflammation. It has been postulated in mice model that acceleration of atherosclerosis may be mediated through TLR and myeloid differentiation factor with liver X receptor, which is important for cholesterol transportation (Naiki et al., 2008). In another animal model, an anti-oxidant, retinoic acid has been found to be effective against *C. pneumonia*-induced atherosclerosis by reducing foam cell formation in atherosclerotic lesions (Jiang et al., 2008). Recent evidence indicates that *C. pneumonia* may induce apoptosis and endothelial cell necrosis in the latter course of the infection, which is shown by the presence of chlamydial HSP 60 and with high mobility box protein 1, a strong pro-inflammatory molecule (Marino et al., 2008). However, inflammatory reaction seems to be host dependent and polyvalent in etiology. High antibody response is considered to be a more consistent marker for inflammation than seropositivity alone and high antibody response to multiple pathogens is a stronger marker of any single pathogen. Strong association was found between IL-6, CRP and fibrinogen levels with antibody levels (Nazmi et al., 2010). These findings may be partially explained the discrepancy between conflicting results arising on atherosclerosis, in studies which have methodological diversities.

1.5 *Chlamydia* and neurologic disorders

C. pneumonia may contribute to advancing atherosclerotic disease, which eventually leads to ischemic stroke. The presence of *C. pneumonia* was demonstrated in more than 70% of the severely stenotic specimens of carotid artery with immunohistochemical studies (Vink et al., 2001). The antibody titers including IgG and IgA against the organism were found to be higher especially in young stroke patients. Authors indicated that IgA class antibody titers were more important due to the limited half life and determined the persistence of chronic infection (Piechowski-Jóźwiak et al., 2007). There was an association between the risk of ischemic stroke and serum IgA titers, especially in large vessel atherosclerotic and lacunar stroke (Elkind et al., 2006). On the other hand, strong evidence on the relation between IgA titers and chronic infection is lacking because of inter-laboratory differences, limited half life and possible cross reactions with other types or microorganisms. Anti-*C. pneumoniae* antibodies were evaluated in HIV infected patients with coronary atherosclerosis. When atherosclerotic plaques from autopsy specimens were evaluated, there was limited data indicating the presence of *C. pneumoniae* in small cerebral vessels (Voorend et al., 2008). In a study conducted by Maggi et al, (Maggi et al, 2006) no significant difference was found between individuals in terms of IgA and IgG titers and no subject was positive for IgM, which led them to conclude that the damage of the carotid wall in patients infected with HIV-1 was not due to *C. pneumonia*. In contrast, *C. pneumonia* was found to be a risk factor for cardiovascular disease in HIV infected patients with low CD4 level and high HIV load (Tositti et al, 2005). The concurrence of hypercholesterolemia with *C. pneumonia* infection increased the risk of atherosclerosis by about three fold (Gaona-Flores et al, 2008). It has been also suggested that infected carotid plaques contribute to the systemic inflammatory markers in patients with stroke risk. The significant association of lipoprotein and phospholipase-A2 with of *C. pneumoniae* suggests an interaction between them in accelerating inflammation in atherosclerosis (Atik et al, 2010). There is limited data concerning genetic predisposition to the *C. pneumoniae* infection. Strong association was found between HLA B35 allele and serologic markers. Male sex and chronic smoking further increased the possibility of infection (Palikhe et al, 2008).

As an obligatory intracellular pathogen, *C. pneumonia* is able to reside in monocytes and macrophages of tissues and able to be reactivate according to the life cycle and host defense. It was proposed that, long term exposure to inflammatory cytokines and endothelial response may induce certain neurodegenerative disease including Alzheimer's disease, multiple sclerosis (MS), meningoencephalitis and neurobehavioral disorders (Yucesan & Sriram, 2001, Stratton & Sriram, 2003).

Alzheimer's disease (AD) causes dementia with advancing age with the atrophy or death of the certain regions of brain. Two clinical form of disease has been classified as genetically determined: namely, early onset and late onset non-familial and progressive neurodegenerative form, which is the most common and severe form of dementia. The association between AD with *C. pneumoniae* infection was first demonstrated by Balin et al, and 90% positivity was shown in brain specimens using PCR technique. Electron microscopic and immunohisto-chemistry studies also indicated that EB and RB like particles were found in the brains of affected individuals, while no labeling was detected in controls (Balin et al.,1998). These results were further confirmed in a study subjecting brain specimens of AD and controls during autopsy in which increased prevalence of *C. pneumonia* RNA was observed with AD (Gérard HC et al, 2006). Furthermore, strong association was determined between apolipoprotein E ε4 genotype and *C. pneumoniae* (Gérard HC et al., 1999). The olfactory epithelium has been proposed as the primary infectious site and the pathogen seems to reach to the olfactory bulb and olfactory cortex and then neuronal damage may progress (Balin & Appelt, 2001). Long term antibiotic therapy, including doxycycline and rifampin, slowed the course of cognitive impairment (Loeb et al., 2004). Metal protein attenuating compounds have been shown to decrease beta amyloid plaques in animal models and antiprotozoal metal chelator clioquinol was used for treatment (Finefrock et al., 2003, Cahoon, 2009). *C. pneumoniae* is also associated with AIDS-demantia complex, a HIV-induced inflammatory parenchymal disorder of the brain. The presence of microorganism was confirmed at a high rate in using PCR. These findings should be cautiously interpreted as whether the source of infection is reactivation due to immune suppression or superimposed recent infection remains to be clarified (Contini et al., 2003).

Multiple sclerosis (MS), an autoimmune chronic demyelinating disorder of the CNS with unknown etiology appears with episodes of remission and relapse, or is present in progressive forms. Disease has high economic burden and disability potential and affects about 1-2 person in 1000. Perivascular inflammation, gliosis and demyelinating plaque formations are considered as classical the pathologic features (Barnett & Sutton, 2006). Perivascular cell infiltration was presumed to initiate the involvement of glial cells in the earlier and astrocytes in the later phase of the disease. Various types of microorganisms including *Chlamydia* are assumed to induce inflammation through TLR 3 and 4 dependent mechanisms (Joyee & Yang, 2008). Genetic predisposition with a combination of infectious agents has been implicated in MS pathogenesis. The presence of *C. pneumoniae* is still under debate and shows a great variability from 0 to 43% in different studies using PCR techniques (Contini et al., 2010). Several authors indicate that the presence of microorganism may partially influence the occurrence of MS, being linked to the progressive form of the disease (Munger et al, 2003). When compared to the controls, the increased frequency of detection of HSP 60 and 16S rRNA in the CSF samples from MS patients indicates the metabolic activity of the microorganism (Dong-Si et al., 2004). Intrathecal synthesis of anti-chlamydial IgG, indicating the infectious cause, was more frequent in MS patients than in non-infectious neural diseases (Fainardi et al., 2004). The increased presence of *C. pneumonia* was demonstrated in a study investigating autopsy samples of MS patients, which looked for anti-chlamydial monoclonal antibodies using immunohistochemical staining in brain slices. The electron microscopy also detected chlamydial EB in four of ten MS patients but none in the controls (Sriram et al., 2005). A large meta-analysis including 26 studies was not able to conclude that *C. pneumoniae* as a causal relationship with MS (Bagos et al., 2006). Anti microbial therapy in patients with MS requires validated multi-central studies, involving all infectious cycles of the microorganism (Stratton & Wheldon, 2007). The current information indicates that, the causal relationship between *C. pneumoniae* with MS is still controversial. Infection may be activated or supervene in the course of the disease.

There is a paucity of reports regarding the relation of *C. pneumoniae* with meningoencephalitis. These patients are young, have neurological symptoms or radiographic evidence and also have acute symptoms of respiratory infection, and laboratory evidence indicating *C. pneumoniae.* Acute demyelinating encephalitis, cerebellar axatia and Gullian Barre are some of the clinical forms in which faster recovery after antibiotic therapy demonstrates the relation between microorganism and neurological presentations (Contini et al., 2010).

Reports indicating relationship between *C. pneumoniae* and affective and neurobehavioral diseases are also sparse. Autism spectrum disorders (ASD), constitute a group of behavioral diseases such as autism, attention deficit disorder, Asperger's syndrome with unknown etiology. Genetic predisposition, environmental factors, educational and socioeconomic status of the family was determined as possible reasons (Nicholson &

Sztmari, 2003). Infection may be a cofactor in progression of the disease and *C. pneumoniae* is considered as a causative organism along with *Mycoplasma* species or infections from *herpes virus* (Chia & L.Y. Chia, 1999). *Chlamydiacea* family has been postulated to cause of schizophrenia owing to persistence of high IgA levels in subjects. Fellerhoff *et al.* found a significant prevalence of *C. psittaci, C. pneumoniae,* and *C. trachomatis* (50%) compared to the controls (~7%). While antipsycotic drugs were inefficient, treatment including in-vitro activated immune cells and antibiotics showed improvement of the mental illness (Fellerhoff et al., 2005).

1.6 *Chlamydiaceae* and systemic disorders

Reactive arthritis is currently accepted to be associated with *Chlamydial* infections or other enteric or sexually acquired infections.

C. trachomatis and to a lesser extent *C. pneumonia* is determined to be one of the most common infectious etiological agents in reactive arthritis (Carter, 2006, Braun et al, 1994). Specifically, *Chlamydial* source of reactive arthritis was estimated about to be ~5% and 78% of these infections were dormant and asymptomatic during initial infection (Rich et al., 1996). In comparison with osteoarthritis, *Chlamydia* species have been demonstrated to be associated with undifferentiated spondylarthritis (a subgroup of reactive arthritis) using PCR at a higher rate in synovial tissue, than blood serological values. The genetic background influencing predisposition or host defense of *Chlamydia*-induced arthritis remains to be elucidated and HLA-B27 positivity was found to be lower than the other source of reactive arthritis and appeared to be less progressive in HLA-B27 negative patients (Carter et al., 2009). Increased frequency of *C. trachomatis* infection was also detected in patients with ankylosing spondilitis as determined with serologic analysis including immunoblotting (Csango et al., 1987). In addition, psoriatic arthritis (PsA) seems to be a candidate for investigations on the etiologic role of *chlamydial* infections. In their study Silveira *et al* (Silveira et al., 1993) indicated the prevalence of *C. trachomatis* infection in patients with SpA, which demonstrated a significant frequency of positive urogenital *C. trachomatis* culture (22%) as well as elevated levels of IgG antibodies (36%) or IgM antibodies (14%) against *C. trachomatis* in patients with PsA. On the contrary, there was only association of rheumatoid arthritis with *C. trachomatis* in a study investigating the possible infectious etiology in patients with different group of seronegative spondyloarthropathies (Lapadula et al., 1988).

The infectious etiology in diabetes has not been confirmed due to its relatively lower incidence compared with the seropositivity of the possible community acquired microorganisms (Lutsey et al., 2009). Yet, several studies indicate that infection with *C. pneumoniae* might influence the time related outcome of diabetes in a subgroup of patients, thought to be a possible genetic predisposition. *C. pneumoniae* with chronic low grade inflammation induces insulin resistance in healthy middle aged man and correlation increased with body mass index and seropositivity to the multiple microorganisms (Fernández-Real et al., 2006). These results were further confirmed with an animal model demonstrating that *C. pneumoniae* induces long lasting insulin resistance and inflammation in obese mice. Anti TNF-α or antibiotic treatment prevents insulin resistance (Wang et al., 2009). Increased seropositivity to *C. pneumoniae* IgA and IgG in diabetes was associated with the secondary cardiovascular events including myocardial infarction, stroke, or cardiovascular death, having possible relation with chlamydial HSP 60. The relation or role of human HSP 60 in disease progress and complications remains to be determined with large scale prospective studies (Guech-Ongey et al., 2009).

Behçet's disease (BD) is an inflammatory disorder of unknown etiology characterized by recurrent oral aphtous ulcers, genital ulcers, uveitis and skin lesions. Patients with BD demonstrated increased IgA and IgG titers to *C. pneumoniae* when compared with controls (Ayaşlıoğlu et al., 2004). Intestinal lesions of BD expressing interferon-γ, tumor necrosis factor-α, interleukin 12 mRNA and HSP 60 indicates possible involvement of microbial HSP 60 in the pathogenesis of intestinal BD, but the relation with *Chlamydiae* remains to be determined (Imamura et al., 2005).

2. Conclusion

The serotypes of *Chlamydiaceae* tend to cause chronic infection and are involved in various types of disorders. Lacks of standardized methods for diagnosis or laboratory tests that partially reflect the activity of the microorganism is the main problem. Further insight on the life cycle of these ubiquitous bacteria's is mandatory, especially on HSP 60 and interactions with host, to elucidate the therapeutic options better. Genetic predisposition is another issue that needs to be illuminated to determine the individuals who are prone or resistant to disease activity.

3. References

Apan, T.Z., Alpay, D., & Alpay, Y. (2007) The possible association of *Chlamydia pneumoniae* infection with nasal polyps. *European archives of oto-rhino-laryngology,* V.264, No.1, pp.27-31, ISSN: 0937-4477.

Atik, B., Johnstone, C., & Dean D. (2010) Association of carotid plaque Lp-PLA2 with macrophages and Chlamydia pneumoniae infection among patients at risk for stroke. *PLoS ONE* V.5, No.6, e11026, ISSN: 1932-6203.

Ayaşlıoğlu, E., Düzgün, N., Erkek, E, & Inal, A. (2004) Evidence of chronic Chlamydia pneumoniae infection in patients with Behçet's disease. *Scandinavian Journal of Infectious Disase,* V.36, N.6-7, pp.428-30, ISSN: 0036-5548.

Bagos, P.G., Nikolopoulos, G., & Ioannidis, A. (2006) *Chlamydia pneumoniae* infection and the risk of multipl sclerosis: a meta analysis. *Multipl Sclerosis, Vol.*12, N.4, pp.397-411, ISSN: 1352-4585.

Balin, B.J., Gérard, H.C., Arking, E.J., Appelt, D.M., Branigan, P.J., Abrams, J.T., Whittum-Hudson, J.A. & Hudson, A.P. (1998) Identification and localization of *Chlamydia pneumoniae* in the Alzheimer's brain. *Medical Microbiololgy and Immunology* V.187, N.1, pp.23-42, ISSN: 0300-8584.

Balin, B.J. & Appelt D.M. (2001) Role of infection in Alzheimer's disease. *The Journal of the American Osteopathic Association* Vol.101, N.12 suppl Pt1, pp.S1-S6, ISSN: 0098-6151.

Barnett, M.H. & Sutton, I. (2006) The pathology of multiple clerosis: a paradigm shift. *Current Opinion in Neurology* Vol.19, N.3, pp.242-247, ISSN: 1350-7540.

Bezold, G., Politch, J.A., Kiviat, N.B., Kuypers, J.M., Wolff, H., & Anderson, D.J. (2007) Prevalence of sexually transmissible pathogens in semen from asymptomatic male infertility patients with and without leucocytospermia. *Fertility and Sterility* Vol.87, N.5, pp.1087-1097, ISSN: 0015-0282.

Brandén, E., Koyi, H., Gnarpe, J., & Gnarpe, H. (2005) Chronic *Chlamydia pneumoniae* infection is a risk factor for the development of COPD. *Respiratoy Medicine* V.99, N.1, pp.20-26, ISSN: 0954-6111.

Braun, J., Laitko, S., Treharne, J., Eggens, U., Wu, P., Distler, A., & Sieper, J. (1994) Chlamyida pneumoniae--a new causative agent of reactive arthritis and undifferentiated oligoarthritis. *Annals of Rheumatologic Disease* V.53, N.2, pp.100-105, ISSN: 0003-4967.

Burton, M.J. (2007) Trachoma: an overview. *British Medical Bullettin* V.84, pp.99-116, ISSN: 0007-1420.

Burton, M.J., Bowman, R.J.C., Faal, H., Aryee, E.A.N., Ikumapayi, U.N., Alexander, N.D.E., Adegbola, R.A., West, S.K., Mabey, D.C.W., Foster, A., Johnson, G.J., & Bailey, R.L. (2005a) Long term outcome of trichiasis surgery in the Gambia. *The British Journal of Ophtalmology* V.89, N.5, pp.575-579, ISSN: 0007-1161.

Burton, M.J., Kinteh, F., Jallow, O., Sillah, A., Ikumapayi, U.N., Alexander, N.D.E., Adegbola, R.A., Faal, H., Mabey, D.C.W., Foster, A., Johnson; G.J., & Bailey, R.L. (2005b) A randomized controlled trial of azithromycin following surgery for trachomatous trichiasis in the Gambia. *The British Journal of Ophtalmology* Vol.89, N.10, pp.1282-1288, ISSN: 0007-1161.

Cahoon, L. (2009) The curious case of clioquinol. *Nature medicine* V.15, N.5, pp.354-359, ISSN: 1078-8956.

Caldwell, H.D., Wood, H., Crane, D., Bailey, R., Jones, R.B., Mabey, D.;, Maclean, I., Mohammed, Z., Peeling, R., Roshick, C., Schachter, J., Solomon, A.W., Stamm, W.E., Suchland, R.J., Taylor, L., West, S.K., Quinn, T.C., Belland, R.J., & McClarty, G. (2003) Polymorphism in Chlamydia trachomatis tryptophan synthase genes differntiate between genital and ocular isolates. *The Journal of clinical investigation* Vol.111, N. 11, pp.1757–1769, ISSN: 0021-9738.

Campbell, L.A., & Kuo, C.C. (2004) *Chlamydia pneumoniae*-an infectious risk factor for atherosclerosis? *Nature reviews. Microbiology* Vol.2, N.1, pp.23-32, ISSN: 1740-1526.

Capello, F., de Macario, E.C., Di Felice, V., Zummo, G., & Macario, A.J.L. (2009) Chlamydia trachomatis infection and anti-hsp60 immunity: the two sides of the coin. *PLoS pathogens* Vol.5, N.8, e1000552, ISSN: 1553-7366.

Carter, J.D. (2006) Reactive arthritis: defined etiologies, emerging pathophysiology, unresolved treatment. *Infectious Disease Clininics of Noth America* Vol.20, N.4, pp.827-847, ISSN: 0891-5520.

Carter, C.D., Gérard, H.C., Espinoza, L.R., Ricca, L.R., Valeriano, J., Snelgrove, J., Oszust, C., Vasey, F.B., & Hodson, A.P. (2009) Chlamyidae as etiologic agents in chronic undifferentiated spndylartritis. *Arthritis and rheumatism* V.60, N.5, pp.1311-1316, ISSN: 0004-3591.

Chanudet, E., Zhou, Y., Bacon, C.M., Wotherspoon, A.C., Müller-Hermelink, H.K., Adam, P., Dong, H.Y., de Jong, D., Li, Y., Wei, R., Gong, X., Wu, Q., Ranaldi, R., Goteri, G.,

Pileri, S.A., Ye, H., Hamoudi, R.A., Liu, H., Radford, J., & Du, M.Q. (2006) Chlamydia psittaci is variably associated with ocular adnexal MALT lymphoma in different geographical regions. The *Journal of Pathology*. V.209, N.3, pp.344-51, ISSN: 0022-3417.

Chia, J.K.S., & Chia, L.Y. (1999) Chronic *Chlamydia pneumoniae* infection: atreatable cause of chronic fatigue syndrome. *Clinical Infectious Disease* V.29, N.2, pp.452-453, ISSN: 1058-4838.

Contini, C., Fainardi, E., Seraceni, S., Granieri, E., Castellazzi, M., & Cultrera, R. (2003) Molecular identification and antibody testing of *Chlamydophila pneumoniae* in a subgroup of patients with HIV-associated dementia complex, preliminary results. *Journal of neuroimmunology*, V.136, N.1-2, pp.172-177, ISSN: 0165-5728.

Contini, C., Seraceni, S., Cultrera, R., Castellazzi, M., Granieri, M., & Finardi, E. (2010) Chlamydophyla pneumonia: infection and its role in neurological disorders. *Interdisciplinay Perspectives in Infectious Disease* 2010 273573 Epub 2010 Feb 21, ISSN: 1687-708X.

Cook, P.J., Davies, P., Tunnicliffe, W., Ayres, J.G., Honeybourne, D., & Wise, R. (1998) *Chlamydia pneumoniae* and asthma. *Thorax* V.53, N.4, pp.254-259, ISSN: 0040-6376.

Csango, P.A., Upsahl, M.T., Romberg, O., Kornstad, L., & Sarov, I. (1987) Chlamydia trachomatis serology in ankylosing spondylitis. *Clinical Rheumatology,* V.6, N.3, pp.384–90, ISSN: 0770-3198.

Cunningham, K.A. & Beagley, K.W. (2008) Male genital tract Chlamydial infection: implications for pathology and infertility. *Biology of reproduction,* V.79, N.2, pp.180-189, ISSN: 0006-3363.

Darville, T. (2005) *Chlamyida trachomatis* infections in neonates and young children. *Seminars in pediatric infectious diseases*, V.16 N.4, pp.235-44, ISSN: 1045-1870.

Di Felice, V., David, S., Cappello, F., Farina, F., & Zummo, G. (2005) Is chlamydial heat shock protein 60 a risk factor for oncogenesis? *Cellular and molecular life sciences* V.62, N.1, pp.4–9, ISSN: 1420-682X.

Dong-Si, T., Weber, J., Liu, Y.B., Buhmann, C., Bauer, H., Bendl, C., Schnitzler, P., Grond-Ginsbach, C., & Grau, A.J. (2004) Increased prevalence of gene transcription by *Chlamydia pneumoniae* in cerebrospinal fluid of patients with relapsing-remitting multiple sclerosis. *Journal of neurology*, V.251, N.5, pp.542-547, ISSN: 0340-5354.

Dreses-Werringloer, V., Padubrin, I., Jürgens-Saathoff, B., Hudson, A.P., Zeidler, H., & Köhler, L. (2000) Persistence of is induced by ciprofloxacin and ofloxacin in vitro. *Antimicrobial agents and chemotherapy*, V.44, N.12, pp.3288-3297, ISSN: 0066-4804.

Elkind, M.S.V., Tondella, M.L.C., Feikin, D.R., Fields, B.S., Homma, S., & Di Tullio, M.R. (2006) Seropositivity to *Chlamydia pneumoniae* is associated with risk of first ischemic stroke. *Stroke*, V.37, N.3, pp.790-795, ISSN: 0039-2499.

Fainardi, E., Castellazzi, M., Casetta, I., Cultrera, R., Vaghi L, Granieri E, & Contini C. (2004) Intrathecal production of *Chlamydia pneumoniae* –specific high-affinity antibodies is signidficantly associated to a subset of multipl sclerosis patients with progressive forms. *Journal of the neurological sciences*, V.217, N.2, pp.181-188, ISSN: 0022-510X.

Falck, G., Gnarpe, J., Hansson, L.O., Svärdsudd, K., & Gnarpe, H. (2002) Comparison of individuals with and without specific IgA antibodies to *Chlamydia pneumoniae*. *Chest*, V.122, N.5, pp.1587-1593, ISSN: 0012-3692.

Fazio, G., Giovino, M., Gullotti, A., Bacarella, D., Novo, G., & Novo, S. (2009) Atherosclerosis, inflammation and Chlamydia pneumoniae. *World journal of cardiology*, V.1, N.1, pp.31-40, ISSN: 1949-8462.

Fellerhoff, B., Laumbacher, B., & Wank, R. (2005) High risk of schizophrenia and other mental disorders associated with clamydial infections: hypothesis to combine drug treatment and adoptive immunotherapy. *Medical* hypotheses, V.65, N.2, pp.243-252, ISSN: 0306-9877.

Fernández-Real, J.M., Ferri, M.J., López-Bermejo, A., Recasens, M., Vendrell, J., & Ricart, W. (2006) Burden of infection and insulin resistance in healthy middle-aged man. *Diabetes Care*, V.29, N.5, pp.1058-1064, ISSN: 0149-5992.

Ferreri, A.J., Guidoboni, M., Ponzoni, M., De Conciliis, C., Dell'Oro, S., Fleischhauer, K., Caggiari, L., Lettini, A.A., Dal Cin, E., Ieri, R., Freschi, M., Villa, E., Boiocchi, M., & Dolcetti, R. (2004) Evidence for an association between Chlamydia psittaci and ocular adnexal lymphomas. *Journal of the National Cancer Institute*, V.96, N.8, pp.586-94, ISSN: 0027-8874.

Finefrock, A.E., Bush, A.I., & Doraiswamy, P.M. (2003) Current status of metals as therapeutic targets in Alzheimer's disease. *Journal of the American Geriatrics Society*, V.51, N.8, pp.1143-1148, ISSN: 0002-8614.

Fujimoto, T., Somoda, K.H., Hijioka, K., Sato, K., Takeda, A., Hasegawa, E., Oshima, Y., & Ishibashi, T. (2010) Choroidal neovascularization enhanced by *Chlamydia pneumoniae* via Toll-like receptor2 in the retinal pigment epithelium. *Investigative ophthalmology & visual science*, V.51, N.9, pp.4694-702, ISSN: 0146-0404.

Gaona-Flores, V., García-Elorriaga, G., Valerio-Minero, M., González-Veyrand, E., Navarrete-Castro, R., Palacios-Jiménez, N., Del Rey-Pineda, G., González-Bonilla, C., & Monasta, L. (2008) Anti-*Chlamydophila pneumoniae* antibodies as associated factor for carotid atherosclerosis in patients with AIDS. *Current HIV research*, V.6, N.3, pp.267-271, ISSN: 1570-162X.

Gattone, M., Iacoveillo, L., Colombo, M., Castelnuovo, A.D., Soffiantino, F., Gramoni, A., Picco, D., Benedetta, M., & Giannuzzi, P. (2001) *Chlamydia pneumonia* and cytomegalovirus seropositivity, inflammatory markers, and the risk of myocardial infarction at a yound age. *American heart journal*, V.142, N.4, pp.633-640, ISSN: 0002-8703.

Gérard, H.C., Whittum-Hudson, J.A., Schumacher, H.R., & Hudson, A.P. (2004) Differentail expression of three Chlamydia trachomatis hsp-60 encoding genes in active vs. persistent infections. *Microbial pathogenesis*, V.36, N.1, pp.35-39, ISSN: 0882-4010.

Gérard, H.C., Dreses-Werringloer, U., Wildt, K.S., Deka, S., Oszust, C., Balin, B.J., Frey, W.H. 2nd, Bordayo, E.Z., Whittum-Hudson, J.A., & Hudson, A.P. (2006) *Chlamydophila (Chlamydia)* pneumonia in Alzheimer's brain. *FEMS immunology and medical microbiology*, V.48, N.3, pp.355-366, ISSN: 0928-8244.

Gérard, H.C., Wang, G.F., Balin, B.J., Schumacher, H.R., Hudson, A.P. (1999) Frequency of apolipoprotein E (APOE) allele types in patients with *Chlamydia*-associated arthritis and other arthritides. *Microbial pathogenesis*, V.26, N.1, pp.35-43, ISSN: 0882-4010.

Guech-Ongey, M., Brenner, H., Twardella, D., & Rothenbacher, D. (2006) *Chlamydia pneumoniae* heat shock proteins 60 and risk of secondary cardiovascular events in patients with coronary heart disease under special consideration of diabetes: a prospective study. *BMC cardiovascular disorders*, V.6, pp.17, http//www.biomedcentral.com/1471-2261/6/17. ISSN: 1471-2261.

Hammaerschlag, M.R. (2000) The role of *Chlamydia* in upper respiratory tract infections. *Current infectious disease reports*, V.2, N.2, pp.115-120, ISSN: 1523-3847.

Hertzen, L.V., Vasankari, T., Lippo, K., Wahlstöm, E., & Puolakkainen, M. (2002) *Chlamydia pneumoniae* and severity of asthma. *Scandinavian journal of infectious diseases*, V.34, N.1, pp.22-27. ISSN: 0036-5548.

Holland, M.J., Faal, N., Sarr, I., Joof, H., Laye, M., Cameron, E., Pemberton-Pigot, F., Dockrell, H.M., Bailey, R.L., & Mabey, D.C.W. (2006) The frequency of *Chlamydia trachomatis* major outer membrane protein-specific CD8+ T lymphocytes in active trachoma is associated with current ocular infection. *Infection and immunity*, V.74, N.3, pp.1565-1572, ISSN: 0019-9567.

Hong, K.C., Schachter, J., Moncada, J., Zhou, Z., House, J., & Lietman, T.M. (2009) Lack of macrolide resistance in Chlamydia trachomatis after mass azithromycin distributions for trachoma. *Emerging infectious diseases*, V.15, N.7, pp.1088-1090, ISSN: 1080-6040.

Hracek, J., Urban, M., Hamsikova, E., Tachezy, R., Eis, V., Brabec, M., & Heracek, J. (2011) Serum antibodies against genitourinary infectious agents in prostate cancer and benign prostate hyperplasia patients: a case-control study. *BMC Cancer*, V.11: pp.53, ISSN: 1471-2407.

Hsahiguchi, K., Ogawa, H., & Kazuyama, Y. (1992) Seroprevalence of *Chlamydia pneumoniae* infections in otolarygologic diseases. *The Journal of laryngology and otology*, V.106, N.3, pp.208-210, ISSN: 0022-2151.

Imamura, Y., Kurokawa, M.S., Yoshikiwa, H., Nara, K., Takada, E., Masuda, C., Tsukikawa, S., Ozaki, S., Matsuda, T., & Suzuki, N. (2005) Involvement of Th1 cells and heat shock protein in the patogenesis of intestinal Behçet's disease. *Clinical and experimental immunology*, V.139, N.2, pp.371-378, ISSN: 0009-9104.

Jaff, M.R., Dale, R.A., Creager, M.A., Lipicky, R.J., Constant, J., Campbell, L.A., & Hiatt, W.R. (2009) Anti-Chlamydial antibiotic therapy for symptom improvement in peripheral artery disease. *Circulation*, V.119, N3, pp.452-458, ISSN: 0009-7322.

Jiang, S.J., Campbell, L.A., Berry, M.W., Rosenfeld, M.E., & Kou, C.C. (2008) Retinoic acid prevents *Chlamydia pneumoniae* induced foam cell development in a mouse model of atherosclerosis. *Microbes and infection*, V.10, N.12-13, pp.1393-1397, ISSN: 1286-4579.

Joyee, A.G., & Yang, X. (2008) Role of toll-like receptors in immune responses to *chlamydial* infections. *Current pharmaceutical design*, V.14, N.6, pp.593-600, ISSN: 1381-6128.

Karnak, D., Bengisun, S., Beder, S., & Kayacan, O. (2001) *Chlamydia pneumoniae* infection and acute exacerbation of chronic obstructive pulmonary disease (COPD). *Respiratory medicine*, V.95, N.10, pp.811-816, ISSN: 0954-6111.

Kiechl, S., Lorenz, E., Reindl, M., Wiedermann, C.J., Oberhollenzer, F., Bonora, E., Willeit, J., & Schwartz, D.A. (2002) Toll-like 4 polymorphism and atherogenesis. *The New England journal of medicine*, V.347, N.3, pp.185-192, ISSN: 0028-4793.

Kurashima, K., Kanuchi, T., Takayanagi, N., Sato, N., Tokunaga, D., Ubukata, M., Yanagisawa, T., Sugita, Y., & Kanazawa, M. (2005) Serum IgG and IgA antibodies to *Chlamydia pneumoniae* and severity of emphysema. *Respirology*, V.10, N.5, pp.572-578, ISSN: 1323-7799.

Lapadula, G., Covelli, M., & Numo, R. (1988) Antibacterial pattern in seronegative spondyloarthropathies. *Clinical and experimental rheumatology*, V.6, N.4, pp.385-390, ISSN: 0392-856X.

Laurila, A.L., Anttila, T., Läärä, E., Bloigu, A., Virtamo, J., Albanes, D., Leinonen, M., & Saikku, P. (1997) Serological evidence of an association between *Chlamydia pneumoniae* infection and lung cancer. *International journal of cancer*, V.74, N.1, pp.31-34, ISSN: 0020-7136.

Leinonen, M., & Saikku, P. (2002) Evidence for infectious agents in cardiovascular disease and atherosclerosis. *The Lancet infectious diseases*, V.2, N.1, pp.11-17, ISSN: 1473-3099.

Littman, A.J., Thornquist, M.D., White, E., Jackson, L.A., Goodman, G.E., & Vaughan, T.L. (2004) Prior lung disease and risk of lung cancer in a large prospective study. *Cancer causes & control*, V.15, N.8, pp.819-827, ISSN: 0957-5243.

Liu, R., Yamamoto, M., Moroi, M., Kubota, T., Ono, T., Funatsu, A., Komatsu, H., Tsuji, T., Hara, H., Nakamura, M., Hirai, H., & Yamaguchi, T. (2005) Chlamydia pneumonia immunoreactivity in coronary artery plaques of patients with acute coronary syndromes and its relation with serology. *American heart journal*, V.150, N.4, pp.681-688, ISSN: 0002-8703.

Loeb, M.B., Molloy, D.W., Smieja, M., Standish, T., Goldsmith, C.H., Mahony, J., Smith, S., Borrie, M., Decoteau, E., Davidson, W., McDougall, A., Gnarpe, J., O'Donnell, M., & Chernesky, M. (2004) A randomized, controlled trial of doxycycline and rifampin for patients with Alzheimer's disease. *Journal of the American Geriatrics Society*, V.52, N.3, pp.381-387, ISSN: 0002-8614.

Low, N., Bender, N., Nartey, L., Shang, A., & Stephenson, J.M. (2009) Effectiveness of Chlamydia screening: systematic review. *International journal of epidemiology*, V.38, N.2, pp.435-448, ISSN: 0300-5771.

Lutsey, P.L., Pankow, J.S., Beroni, A.G., Szklo, M., & Folsom, A.R. (2009) Serologic evidence of infections and type 2 diabetes: the multiethnic study of antehrosclerosis. *Diabetic medicine*, V.26, N.2, pp.149-152, ISSN: 0742-3071.

Mabey, D., & Peeling, R.W. (2002) Lymphogranuloma venereum. *Sexually transmitted infections*, V.78, N.2, pp.90-92, ISSN: 1368-4973.

Mackman, N. (2000) Lipopolysaccaride induction of gene expression in human monocytic cells. *Immunologic research*, V.21, N.2-3, pp:247-251, ISSN: 0257-277X.

Maggi, P., Monno, R., Chirianni, A., Gargiulo, M., Carito, V., Fumarola, L., Perilli, F., Lillo, A., Bellacosa, C., Panebianco, A., Epifani, G., & Regina G. (2006) Role of *Chlamydia* infection in the pathogenesis of atherosclerotic plaques in HIV-1 positive patients. *In Vivo*, V.20, N.3, pp.409-414, ISSN: 0258-851X.

Marino, J., Stoeckli, I., Walch, M., Latinovic-Golic, S., Sundstroem, H., Groscurth, P., Ziegler, U., & Dumrese, C. (2008) *Chlamydophila pneumoniae* derived from inclusions late in the infectious cycle induce aponecrosis in human aortic endothelial cells. *BMC microbiology*, V.8: pp.32, ISSN: 1471-2180.

Melese, M., West, E.S., Alemayehu, W., Munoz, B., Worku, A., Gaydos, C.A., & West, S.K. (2005) Characteristics of trichiasis patients presenting for surgery in rural Ethiopia. *The British journal of ophthalmology*, V.89, N.9, pp.1084-1088, ISSN: 0007-1161.

Miya, N., Oguchi, S., Watanabe, I., & Kanmatsuse, K. (2004) Relation of secretory phospholipase A(2) and high sensitivity C-reactive protein to *Chlamydia pneumonia* infection in acute coronary syndromes. *Circulation journal*, V.68, N.7, pp.628-633, ISSN: 1346-9843.

Morrison, R.P., Belland, R.J., Lyng, K., & Caldwell, H.D. (1989) *Chlamydial* disease pathogenesis: the 57-kD *chlamydial* hypersensitivity antigen is a stress response protein. *The Journal of experimental medicine*, V.170, N.4, pp.1271-1283, ISSN: 0022-1007.

Morrison, R.P. (1991) Chlamydial hsp60 and immunopathogenesis of chlamydial disease. *Seminars in immunology*, V.3, N.1, pp.25-33, ISSN: 1044-5323.

Munger, K.L., Peeling, W., Hernán, A., Chasan-Taber, L., Olek, M.J., Hankinson, S.E., Hunter, D., & Ascherio, A. (2003) Infection with *Chlamydia pneumoniae* and risk of multipl sclerosis. *Epidemiology*, V.14, N.2 pp.141-147, ISSN: 1044-3983.

Naaby-Hansen, S., Herr, J.C. (2010) Heat shock proteins on the human sperm surface. *Journal of reproductive immunology*, V.84, N,1, pp.32-40, ISSN: 0165-0378.

Naiki, Y., Sorrentino, R., Wong, M.H., Michelsen, K.S., Schimada, K., Chen, S., Yilmaz, A., Slepenkin, A., Schröder, N.W.J., Crother, T.R., Bulut, Y., Doherty, T.M., Bradley, M., Shaposhnik Z., Peterson, E.M., Tontonoz, P., Shah, P.K., & Arditi, M. (2008) TLR/MyD88 and LXRα signaling pathways eciprocally control Chlamydia pneumoniae-induced acceleration of atherosclerosis. *The Journal of immunology*, V.181, N.10, pp.7176-7185, ISSN: 0022-1767.

Nazmi, A., Diez Roux, A.V., Jenny, N.S., Tsai, M.Y., Szklo, M., & Aiello, A.E. (2010) The influence of persistent pathogens on circulating levels of inflammatory markers: a cross-sectional analysis from the multi-ethnic study of atherosclerosis. *BMC Public Health*, V.10, pp.706, ISSN: 1471-2458.

Nicholson, R., & Sztmari, P. (2003) Genetic and neurodevelopmental influences in autistic disorder. *Canadian journal of psychiatry*, V.48, N.8, pp.526-537, ISSN: 0706-7437.

Oba, Y., & Salzman G. (2007) *Chlamydial* pneumonias: overview of infection with the three main *chlamydial* species that cause respiratory disease in humans. *eMedicine*,. http://www.emedicine.com/med/TOPIC341.HTM.

Palikhe, A., Lokki, M.L., Saikku, P., Leinonen, M., Paldanius, M., Seppänen, M., Valtonen, V., Nieminen, M.S., & Sinisalo, J. (2008) Association of *Chlamydia pneumoniae* infection with HLA-B35 in patients with coronary artery disease. *Clinical and vaccine immunology*, V.15, N.1, pp.55-59, ISSN: 1556-6811.

Patrick, D.M., Karunakaran, K., Levy, A.R., Gin, K., Remple, V., Chong, M., Abbey, H., Tarry, L., Shen, C., & Brunham, R.C. (2005) Chlamydia bacteriophage: no role in acute coronary events? *The Canadian journal of infectious diseases & medical microbiology*, V.16, N.5, pp.298-300, ISSN: 1712-9532.

Piechowski-Jóźwiak, B., Mickielewicz, A., Gaciong, Z., Berent, H., & Kwieciński, H. (2007) Elevated levels of anti-*Chlamydia pneumoniae* Ig A and IgG antibodies of young adults with ischemic stroke. *Acta neurologica Scandinavica*, V.116 N.3, pp.144-149, ISSN: 0001-6314.

Quirk, J.T., & Kupinski, J.M. (2001) Chronic infection, inflammation, and epithelial ovarian cancer. *Medical hypotheses*, V.57, N.4, pp.426-428, ISSN: 0306-9877.

Rich, E., Hook, E.W.III, Alarcon, G.S., & Moreland, L.W. (1996) Reactive arthritis in patients attending an urban sexually transmitted diseases clinic. *Arthritis and rheumatism*, V.39, N.7, pp.1172-1177, ISSN: 0004-3591.

Robman, L., Mahdi, O., McCarty, C., Dimitrov, P., Tikellis, G., McNeill, J., Bryne, G., Taylor, H., & Guymer, R. (2005) Exposure to *Chlamydia pneumoniae* infection and progression of age-related macular degeneration. *American journal of epidemiology*, V.161, N.11, pp.1013-1019, ISSN: 0002-9262.

Saikku, P., Leinonen, M., Mattila, K., Ekman, M.R., Nieminen, M.S., Makela, P.H., Huttunen, J.K., & Valtonen, V. (1988) Serological evidence of an association of a novel *Chlamydia* TWAR, with chronic heart disease and acute myocardial infarction. *Lancet*, V.2, N.8618, pp.983-986, ISSN: 0140-6736.

Samaras, V., Rafailidis, P.I., Mourtzoukou, E.G., Peppas, G., & Falagas, M.E. (2010) Chronic bacterial and parasitic infections and cancer: a review. *Journal of infection in developing countries*, V.4, N.5, pp.267-281, ISSN: 2036-6590.

Siveira, L.H., Gutierrez, F., Scopelitis, E., Cuellar, M.L., Citera, G., & Espinoza, L.R. (1993) Chlamydia-induced arthritis. *Rheumatic diseases clinics of North America*, V.19, N.2, pp.351-363, ISSN: 0889-857X.

Sriram, S., Ljunggren-Rose, A., Yao, S-Y., & Whetsell, Jr W.O. (2005) Detection of *chlamydial* bodies and antigens in the central nervous system of patients with multiple sclerosis. *The Journal of infectious diseases*, V.192, N.7, pp.1219-1228, ISSN: 0022-1899.

Stassen, F.R., Vainas, T., & Bruggeman, C.A. (2008) Infection and atherosclerosis. An alternative view of an outdated hypothesis. *Pharmacological reports*, V.60, N.1, pp.85-92, ISSN: 1734-1140.

Stratton, C.W., & Sriram, S. (2003) Association of *Chlamydia pneumoniae* with central nervous system disease. *Microbes and infection*, V.5, N.13, pp.1249-1253, ISSN: 1286-4579.

Stratton, C.W., & Wheldon, D.B. (2007) Antimicrobial treatment of multipl sclerosis. *Infection*, V.35, N.5, pp.383-385, ISSN: 0300-8126.

Sutherland, E.R., Brandıorff, J.M., & Martin, J.M. (2004) Atypical bacterial pneumonia and asthma risk. *The Journal of asthma*, V.41, N.8, pp.863-868, ISSN: 0277-0903.

Sziller, I., Fedorcsak, P., Csapo, Z., Szirmal, K., Linhares, I.M., Papp, Z., & Witkin, S.S. (2008) Cirulating antibodies to a conserved epitope of the Chlamydia trachomatis 60-kDa heat shock protein is associated with decreased spontaneous fertility rate in ectopic pregnant women treated by salpingectomy. *American journal of reproductive immunology*, V.59, N.2, pp. 99-104, ISSN:1046-7408.

Tositti, G., Rassu, M., Fabris, P., Giordani, M., Cazzavillan, S., Reatto, P., Zoppelletto, M., Bonoldi, M., Baldo, V., Manfrin, V., & de Lalla, F. (2005) *Chlamyida pneumoniae* infection in HIV-positive patients: prevalence and relationship with lipid profile. *HIV Medicine, V.*6, N.1, pp.27-32, ISSN: 1464-2662.

Trojian, T.H., Lishnak, T.S., & Heiman, D. (2009) Epididymitis and orchitis: an overwiev. *American family physician*, V.79, N.7, pp.583-587, ISSN: 0002-838X.

Vink, A., Poppen, M., Schoneveld, A.H., Roholl, P.J., de Kleijn, D.P., Borst, C., & Pasterkamp, G. (2001) Distribution of *Chlamydia pneumoniae* in the human arterial system and its relation to the local amount of atherosclerosis within the individual. *Circulation;* V.103, N.12, pp.1613-1617, ISSN: 0009-7322.

Voorend, M., Aan der Ven, A.J.A.M., Kubat, B., Lodder, J., & Bruggeman, C.A. (2008) Limited role for *C. pneumoniae*, CMV, and HSV1 in cerebral large and small vessel atherosclerosis. *The open neurology journal*, V.2, pp.39-44, ISSN: 1874-205X.

Wang, C., Gao, D., & Kaltenboeck, B. (2009) Acute *Chlamydia pneumoniae* reinfection accelerates the development of insulin resistance and diabetes in obese C57BL/6 mice. *The Journal of infectious diseases*, V.200, N.2, pp.279-287, ISSN: 0022-1899.

Ward, M.E. (1995) The immunology and immunopathology of chlamydial infections. *Acta pathologica, microbiologica, et immunologica Scandinavica,* V.103, N.11, pp.769-796, ISSN: 0903-4641.

Wark, P.A.B., Johnston, S.L., Simpson, J.L., Hensley, M.J., & Gibson, P.G. (2002) Chlamydia pneumoniae immunoglobulin A reactivation and airway inflammation in acute asthma. *The European respiratory journal,* V.20, N.4, pp.834-840, ISSN: 0903-1936.

Webley, W.C., Savla, P.S., Andrejewsk, C., Cirino, F., West, C.A., Tilahun, Y., & Stuart, E.S. (2005) The bronchial lavage of pediatric patients with asthma contains infectious chlamydia. *American journal of respiratory and critical care medicine*, V.171, N:10, pp.1083-1088, ISSN: 1073-449X.

Webley, W.C., Tilahun, Y., Lay, K., Patel, K., Stuart, E.S., Andrzejewski, C., & Salva, P.S. (2009) Occurrence of Chlamydia trachomatis and Chlamydia pneumonia in paediatric respiratory infections. *The European respiratory journal*, V.33, N.2, pp.360-367, ISSN: 0903-1936.

Wetmore, C.M., Manhart, L.E., & Golden, M.R. (2009) Idiopathic urethritis in young men in the United States: prevanelnce and comparison to infections with known sexually transmitted pathogens. *The Journal of adolescent health*, V.45, N.5, pp.463-472, ISSN: 1054-139X.

Wright, H.R., Turner, A., & Taylor, H.R. (2007) Trachoma. *Lancet*, V.371, N.9628, pp.1945-1954, ISSN: 0140-6736.

Wu, S., Shen, L., & Liu, G. (1999) Study on vertical transmission of *Chlamydia trachomatis* using PCR and DNA sequencing. *Chinese medical journal,* V.112, N.5, pp.396-399, ISSN: 0366-6999.

Yakushijin, Y., Kodama, T., Takaoka, I., Tanimoto, K., Bessho, H., Sakai, I., Hato, T., Hasegawa, H., & Yasukawa, M. (2007) Absence of chlamydial infection in Japanese patients with ocular adnexal lymphoma of mucosa-associated lymphoid tissue. *International journal of hematology, V.*85, N.3, pp.223-230, ISSN:0925-5710.

Yucesan, C., & Sriram, S. (2001) *Chlamydia pneumoniae* infection of the central nervous system. *Current opinion in neurology,* V.14, N.3, pp.355-359, ISSN: 1350-7540.

Part 3

Classic and Molecular Diagnosis

17

Diagnosis of *Chlamydia trachomatis* Infection

Adele Visser[1] and Anwar Hoosen[2]
[1]*Division Clinical Pathology, Department Microbiology, University of Pretoria, National Health Laboratory Services*
[2]*Department Microbiology, University of Pretoria, National Health Laboratory Services*
South Africa

1. Introduction

With the use of molecular medicine as part of routine laboratory evaluation of patients, the diagnosis of infection with has undergone a metamorphosis in the last 30 years. However, it remains a debated process as molecular testing is to date not accepted as definitive in most clinical settings, and more historic testing methods like cell culture, has not been completely rendered redundant[1]. Infection with *Chlamydia trachomatis* is therefore a complex condition to diagnose, and requires a clear understanding of testing methods and the inherent advantages and disadvantages to each. The modern approach to the diagnosis of *Chlamydia trachomatis* typically involves a combination of assays as part of screening and confirmation[2].

Patients very often manifest very few clinical symptoms and rarely seek medical assistance. For this reason, continued transmission occurs to sexual partners[3] causing *Chlamydia trachomatis* to be the most common sexually transmitted bacterial infection worldwide[3, 4]. Due to these disease and pathogen characteristics, prevalence of this pathogen seems to be increasing in both developing and developed countries[5-8]. Correct diagnosis of infection with *Chlamydia trachomatis* is essential as false negative results may have significant impact on societal health[9]. Chlamydial infections has been associated with a higher risk of acquiring HIV-1 infection[4, 10] as well as cervical cancer[11] and adverse outcomes with pregnancy[12, 13]. For these reasons, early correct diagnosis of infection with Chlamydia trachomatis is essential to prevent long-term sequelae associated with prolonged infection.

2. Specimens, collection and transport

2.1 Clinical specimens

Chlamydia trachomatis is very often asymptomatic in female patients, but may present with cervicitis, endometritis, pelvic inflammatory disease or Bartholin abscesses[14, 15]. Urethritis and proctitis is often a secondary manifestation, found in conjunction with other sites of infection[16]. In heterosexual men, urethral infection accounts for most symptomatic cases[17, 18], with ascending infection causing epididymitis[19]. Among homo- and bisexual men, sites of infection are also predominantly the urethra[20], but further includes the rectum[21]. Infection in infants may cause conjunctivitis as well as pneumonia, particularly in early infancy [22, 23]. Serovars L1-3 is associated with lymphogranulomavenereum (LGV), and is particularly prevalent in areas of Africa, Asia and South America[24]. Clinically, these patients present with a painless genital ulcer, which later progress to lymphadenopathy[24]. They occasionally develop systemic symptoms[25].

2.2 Specimen collection

Chlamydiae are intracellular organisms, and it is therefore essential to obtain host cells with the clinical sample to so ensure yield of organisms[2]. The sensitivity and specificity of any test for *Chlamydia trachomatis,* is highly dependent on sampling and adequacy of the sample obtained[26-28]. This holds true irrespective of testing type, whether it be culture, where viable organisms need to be obtained, or nucleic acid based testing, where non-viable genetic material can be obtained[29]. Although relatively standardized methods for sampling is advocated for direct testing, certain commercially available tests have unique sampling requirements, stipulated in the package insert[2].

In women, the endocervix is most commonly targeted for obtaining samples for culture, by utilizing either a swab or a cytologic brush. In the case of swabs, careful consideration should be taken as certain types of swabs may actually inhibit growth by being directly toxic to either the organisms or the cell culture[30]. Similarly, wooden-shafted swabs also inhibit growth. Optimal sample can be obtained using Dacron, cotton, rayon or calcium alginate-tipped swabs with plastic shafts[31]. Prior to obtaining the sample, the cervical os should be cleared of secretions and discharges, to so reduce bacterial contamination and possible toxicity. This also improves the quality and ease of interpretation of direct fluorescent antibody stains[32, 33]. Sampling should be performed by inserting the swab approximately 1-2 cm into the cervical os, rotating it, and keeping it in situ for 15 to 30 seconds. Using swabs are less likely to induce bleeding[34], which in itself may also inhibit culture, but typically has a lower cell yield than cytological brushes[28]. For this reason, some authors have advocated against the use of a cytological brush, provided sampling with a swab is performed adequately[35]. Furthermore, culture yields have been improved by combining endocervical with urethral sampling[36]. Sampling is similar to male urethral sampling, however, the swab is inserted only 1cm past the urethral opening[2].

In male patients, the anterior urethra is the site of choice for optimal sampling, especially for culture purposes. A dry swab is inserted 3 to 4 cm past the meatal opening of the urethra, rotated and removed. It is important to note that urination should best be avoided for at least 1 hour prior to sampling, as this significantly reduces the yield of cells obtained during sampling[2].

Cases of conjunctivitis should be investigated by first removing the gross purulent discharge. Thereafter, the eye should be swabbed on the palpebral conjunctival surface, to so obtains some epithelial cells[2].

In cases of LGV, sampling can be in the form of swabs from ulcers, saline aspirates from the bubo or biopsies. To ensure adequacy of deep-seated ulcers, these biopsies may be best performed under direct vision through proctoscopy[37].

2.3 Specimen transport

Culture yield is significantly improved if samples are transported to the laboratory for processing within 48 hours, and kept at 2 to 8°C during this time. The practice of freezing samples should be restricted to settings where significant delay is expected, as freezing at -70°C is associated with up to 20% loss in viability, and freezing at -20°C even higher losses[30, 38].

Various formulations of transport media have been used[39-41] as it may improve yield. This is because it typically contains fetal bovine serum to improve viability as well as antimicrobials, to suppress growth by other organisms. The formulation used is similar to transport media used for rickettsiae, but not viral transport media, as this typically contains penicillin[39, 40, 42].

2.4 Sampling for non-culture-based testing

Although typically very similar to culture based testing, non-culture based testing requires sampling and transport as specified by the manufacturers for the particular assay[43, 44]. Urine-based testing has also been advocated for molecular testing. This has the added advantage that simultaneous testing can be performed for other pathogens like *Neisseria gonorrhea* as well as being non-invasive. However, the yield on urine samples are greater if it is a first-catch sample obtained 1 to 2 hours after prior urination, to so increase the amount of columner epithelial cells[45, 46]. If sampling is performed in excess of 3 hours after last void, specificity and sensitivity is reduced in females, but in male patients, controversy still exists[47, 48]. Some authors have reported that preceding cleaning performed in culture samples for females, should not be performed in this setting to so improve yield[46]. Novel testing methods now include sampling the vaginal introitus or vulva with promising results. The major advantage to this is that patients can self-sample[49].

3. Laboratory methods

3.1 Direct detection

3.1.1 Culture-based testing

Historically, culture-based testing was considered the gold standard for diagnosis of *Chlamydia trachomatis*, and specificity was considered to approach 100%[50-52]. This high specificity is at the cost of sensitivity, which in a best-case scenario is estimated at 70 to 85%[52]. Appropriate sampling and transport is absolutely essential to ensure organism viability.

Culture is performed using cell monolayers in dram or shell vials. Cell types permissive to infection include McCoy cells[53-55], HeLa229 cells[56, 57] and BGMK cells[58, 59]. Certain pretreatment steps have been advocated to improve culture yield. These include administration of DEAE-dextran[56, 60], sonication[61] and centrifugation[60]. These cell cultures are maintained using Eagle's minimal essential medium (EMEM) with additional amino acids, vitamins, glucose, foetal calf serum and L-glutamine[2]. Although blind passaging has been shown to improve recovery by 3 to 10%[62], it leads to a significantly delay in obtaining results.

Following culture, the presence of *Chlamydia trachomatis* needs to be confirmed. Firstly, various stains have been used including various Romanovsky stains and iodine staining. These methods lack sensitivity and specificity and require an experienced microscopist[54, 63, 64]. The iodine stain is based on the premise of glycogen binding. However, normal cervical cells also contain glycogen, and therefore may impact on specificity[2]. Fluorescent dye based confirmation shows improved sensitivity and specificity, as it utilizes fluorescently labeled antibodies targeting either the major outer membrane protein (MOMP) or the chlamydial lipopolysaccharide (LPS) following approximately 48 to 72 hours of incubation. Sensitivity seems to be higher with MOMP based assays, as these are more widely distributed on the cells within culture[1]. Alternatively, these methods can also be applied to shell vial based cultures, to so improve turn-around times of results and sensitivity[54, 55].

3.1.2 Antigen detection methods

Wide arrays of validated immunoassays are currently available[65-77]. Direct fluorescent antibody (DFA) testing can be utilized directly on clinical samples. As for culture-based confirmation, two antigenic sites can be utilized as targets, namely the MOMP and LPS. Assays targeting the LPS are specific to Chlamydia spp and are not considered specific to *Chlamydia trachomatis*. These antigens are not as widely distributed as MOMP, and sensitivity of these assays are therefore inferior to those targeting MOMP[2]. The MOMP based assays show specificity for *Chlamydia trachomatis*. These assays are validated for use on endocervical smears and male urethral swabs[78-80] but can be applied to urethral samples[78, 81], conjunctival swabs[82, 83], rectal smears[84] and respiratory samples from infants[85, 86]. DFA testing is a rapid method, with the added advantage providing simultaneous information on the quality of the sample, by way of visualizing presence of columner epithelium in adequate samples. However, the process is laborious and requires an experienced microscopist[2]. Evaluation of DFA methods with external quality programs by the College of American Pathologist (ACP) showed significant variability in results depending on the experience level of the laboratory[80]. It has been clearly established that in the absence of a quality assurance program, more than 10% of samples will be of inadequate quality for processing[27, 35]. For this reason, specimen adequacy can be evaluated by direct examination of the sample - an advantage that only the DFA assays hold.

Immunochemical detection (EIA) can be performed either directly, targeting LPS or indirectly, by detecting anti-Chlamydial antibodies (discussed later). The LPS antigen is more abundant albeit irregularly distributed as compared to MOMP antigen. Prior to performing the EIA assays, samples are lysed, releasing large amounts of LPS thereby improving sensitivity. However, cross-reaction may occur with gram negative organisms to the detriment of specificity[62, 87-89]. To alleviate this issue, some manufacturers produce blocking assays to verify all positive results[90]. With these assays, positive tests are repeated following a pretreatment step where Chlamydial-specific monoclonal antibodies are added to the sample. True positive results will test negative on blocking assays, where false positive results will remain positive[91].

Point-of-Care testing assays are also available. These assays utilize EIA technology targeting LPS, with similar diagnostic problems with poor specificity as with laboratory based testing[65, 92, 93].

Molecular detection of nucleic acids are becoming more common, utilizing various molecular technologies. These can either utilize biological amplification (detection of ribosomal RNA) or laboratory based amplification technology like polymerase chain reaction (PCR)[94]. DNA probes have been designed in commercially available assays targeting the 16S rRNA[95, 96]. These assays are estimated to be 1 log more sensitive as compared to EIA based assays. Specificity is reduced if samples are blood stained, as this may cause autofluorescence[2]. Some manufacturers also produce a confirmatory competitive assay, similar to those described for EIA[44, 97] to improve specificity. Furthermore, certain manufacturers offer combined assays testing for both *Chlamydia trachomatis* and *Neisseria gonorrhea*[98]. Nucleic acid amplification techniques offers the advantage of being highly sensitive and providing a platform for less invasive sampling[52]. Sensitivity may in fact be a diagnostic problem, as DNA amplification techniques have obtained positive results from environmental samples obtained from health care settings[2]. However, provided that sampling is performed with the same care as for culture, this should only be a theoretical diagnostic issue. Commercially available techniques utilized have largely focused on PCR[94, 99, 100], ligase chain reaction[101, 102] and strand displacement assays (SDA)[103], amongst others[104, 105]. Further development into real-time[106, 107] and multiplexed based platforms[108], as well as nesting steps[109] has also improved diagnostic utility.

Inherent to the nature of nucleic acid detection methods, genetic variation may lead to a reduction in sensitivity of assays. A genetic variant was described in Sweden in 2007, which contained a 377bp deletion in the cryptic plasmid[9]. This resulted in false negative results by both the Roche COBAS AMPLICOR and Abbott LCx C trachomatis assays[110, 111], and on a community level, to unrestricted spread to these stains[110, 111]. For this reason, some authorities have called for all diagnostic assays to target at least two genetic sites within the pathogen[112].

3.2 Indirect detection

Historically, serological testing has been used in investigation of women with pelvic inflammatory disease[113], ectopic pregnancies[114], recurrent miscarriages[12] and tubal infertility[115]. Despite this, serological testing to identify Chlamydia specific antibodies is not considered to be useful in the diagnosis of genital tract infection, for a number of reasons. Firstly, these antibodies are long-lived and do not distinguish between previous and current infection. Comparing antibody titers from acute and convalescent sera typically makes this distinction. This sampling window may be required to be as long as 1 month, and this type of diagnostic delay is not acceptable in modern laboratory medicine. Secondly, positivity is not specific for *Chlamydia trachomatis*, but rather Chlamydia spp., rendering interpretation of positive serology even more problematic[2]. Serological testing is considered appropriate in only two clinical settings. Firstly, use of Chlamydia specific IgM in the diagnosis of pneumonitis in infants, and secondly, significant rise in Chlamydial titers (≥ 32) in the diagnosis of LGV[24]. The practical application of this test is more difficult as the initial ulcers are typically painless and patients often do not present at health care facilities in the acute phase[2].

Various testing procedures have been employed in detecting Chlamydial antibodies. Historically, complement fixation (CF) was utilized in many diagnostic laboratories. For this method, a single titer of ≥ 256 is strongly predictive of LGV versus a titer lower than 32 showing good performance as a rule out test[116]. A further consideration with this assay is the requirement of biosafety level (BSL) 3 conditions[117]. Additionally, high quality antigen is not always available as these reagents are usually prepared from guinea pigs, which can be co-infected with *Chlamydia psittaci* [118].

Microscopic immunofluorescence testing (MIF) was long considered the test of choice for the diagnosis of chlamydial pneumonitis in infants, as this was utilized to identify IgM specifically[119, 120]. Historically, it was used in the description of the original 15 serovars described for *Chlamydia trachomatis* [121, 122]. This assay however is laborious and time-consuming and is therefore usually not employed as a routine diagnostic test[2] as this antigen is produced from infected egg yolk in the form of elementary bodies[2].

Enzyme immunoassay methods (EIA) are commercially available, typically targeting the LPS. A positive result in isolation does not distinguish between active or previous infection and may also be due to cross-reaction with antibodies for *Chlamydia pneumonia* or *psittaci*[123, 124]. Generally, EIA based testing is considered to be less sensitive compared to immunofluorescent-based testing[125], however, recently developed assays seem to show adequate sensitivity and specificity for use in a high throughput setting[126]. In a recent study by Baud et al, various serological platforms were evaluated. The CT-IgG-pELISA by Medac (Wedel, Germany) and automated epifluoroscence immunoassay by InoDiag (Signes, France) performed adequately, but still inferior to conventional immunofluorescence assays. The CT pELISA by R-Biopharm (Darmstadt, Germany) had sensitivities and specificities comparable to gold standard assays. These authors therefore considered this assay as an alternative option in a high throughput setting[126].

4. Defining the new "Gold Standard" assay

The FDA expanded its definition of a true positive result in 1992 to include a combination of culture and non-culture based testing[127]. The Centers for Disease Control and Prevention (CDC) classifies diagnosis as definitive, presumptive and suggestive (Table 1)[87].

Definitive Requires either of criteria	1. Culture isolation with confirmation 2. Any two of the following - DFA of exudate - EIA of exudate - NAT testing
Presumptive Requires both criteria	• Presence of clinical symptoms • Detection by non-culture based test
Suggestive Requires 1st criterion with either 2nd or 3rd	• Clinical symptoms • Exclusion of other causes of discharge or exudate • Sexual exposure to person with *C trachomatis* or nongonococcal urethritis, mucopurulent cervicitis or PID

Table 1. Diagnostic criteria for *Chlamydia trachomatis* published by the CDC[87]

The definition of the so-called "Gold Standard" testing assay is important for two reasons. Firstly, all commercially available tests will be measured against this standard to define performance characteristics. In the past, performance was gauged simply on culture results, leading to overestimation of sensitivity[2]. And secondly, this will impact on testing algorithms depending on local epidemiology and prevalence[128]. The issue of prevalence is particularly complex in the case of Chlamydial infection as this not impacts on test performance, but it has also been shown that females in low prevalence settings (defined as ≤5%) seem to have a lower chlamydial load, further reducing testing sensitivity[129-131]. In its most extreme form, asymptomatic patients seem to have the worst sensitivity in testing[132]. Therefore, in these settings, the CDC advocates highly sensitive testing with confirmation of all positive samples[15].

Recently, some authors have not only advocated use of NAT testing as the only gold standard[133], but rather specific assays like the BD ProbeTec ET (Becton Dickinson Diagnostic Systems, Maryland, USA), the COBAS TaqMan ST test v2.0 (Roche Diagnostics, New Jersey, USA) and the Aptima Combo 2 (Gen-Probe, San Diego, USA)[134]. Not only are these assays highly sensitive and specific, these can be easily implemented in a high throughput laboratory[133, 135-138].

5. Comparison of methods

Currently, three molecular assays dominate molecular diagnostics of *Chlamydia trachomatis*. The Gen-Probe Aptima Combo 2 (AC2) targets the 23S rRNA molecule, whereas the Roche Cobas TaqMan CT assay targets both the cryptic plasmid and the *omp*1 gene. The Abbot RealTime CT m2000 PCR targets two parts of the cryptic plasmid[139]. All of these assays can successfully detect the new variant strain, first described in Sweden[140]. Despite very good performance by all these assays, the Gen-Probe assay seems to have superior sensitivity (99.3%) and equally good specificity (99.9%) as the Abbott m2000 assay. The Roche TaqMan assay shows superior specificity (100%), but with sensitivity estimated at 82.4%[139]. These platforms have differing performance characteristics and use different pre-amplification processing steps. Since the quality of results is comparable, the true choice of assay lies by en large in the platform and pre-processing preferences.

6. References

[1] CDC: Sexually transmitted diseases clinical practice guidelines. In. Edited by Prevention CfDCa; 1991.

[2] Black C: Current methods of Laboratory Diagnosis of *Chlamydia trachomatis* Infections. *Clin Microbiol Rev* 1997, 10(1):160-184.

[3] Peipert J: Clinical practice. Genital chlamydial infections. *N Engl J Med* 2003, 349:2424-2430.

[4] Manavi K: A review on infection with *Chlamydia trachomatis*. *Best Pract Res Clin Obstet Gynaecol* 2006, 20:941-951.

[5] Baud D, Jaton K, Bertelli C, Kulling J, Greub G: Low prevalence of *Chlamydia trachomatis* infection in asymptomatic young Swiss men. *BMC Infect Dis* 2008, 8:45.

[6] Fine D, Dicker L, Mosure D, Berman S: Increasing chlamydia positivity in women screened in family planning clinics: do we know why? *Sex Transm Dis* 2008, 35:47-52.

[7] Lind I, Bollerup A, Farhot S, Hoffman S: Laboratory surveillance of urogenital *Chlamydia trachomatis* infections in Denmark 1988-2007. *Scand J Infect Dis* 2009, 41:334-340.

[8] Spiliopoulou A, Lakiotis V, Vittoraki A, Zavou D, Mauri D: *Chlamydia trachomatis*: time for screening? *Clin Microbiol Infect* 2005, 11:687-689.

[9] Rockett R, Goire N, limnios A, Turra M, Higgens G, Lambert S, Bletchly C, Nissen M, Sloots T, Whiley D: Evaluation of the cobas 4800 CT/NG test for detecting *Chlamydia trachomatis* and *Neisseria gonorrhoeae*. *Sex Transm Infect* 2010, 86:470-473.

[10] Sangani P, Rutherford G, Wilkinson D: Population-based interventions for reducing sexually transmitted infections, including HIV infection. *Cochrane Database Syst Rev* 2004, 2:CD001220.

[11] Simonetti A, Melo J, Souza Pd, Bruneska D, Filho JdL: Immunological's host profile for HPV and *Chlamydia trachomatis*, a cervical cancer cofactor. *Microbes Infect* 2009, 11:435-442.

[12] Baud D, Regan L, Greub G: Emerging role of Chlamydia and Chlamydia-like organisms in adverse pregnancy outcomes. *Curr Opin Infect Dis* 2008, 21:70-76.

[13] Mardh P: Influence of infection with *Chlamydia trachomatis* on pregnancy outcome, infant helath and life-long sequelae in infected offspring. *Best Pract Res Clin Obstet Gynaecol* 2002, 16:847-864.

[14] Bleker O, Smalbraak D, Shutte M: Bartholin's abscess: the role of *Chlamydia trachomatis*. *Genitourin Med* 1990, 66:24-25.

[15] CDC: Recommendations for the prevention and management of *Chlamydia trachomatis* infection. *Morbid Mortal Weekly Rep* 1993, 42(RR-12):1-39.

[16] Dunlop E, Goh B, Darougar S, Woodland R: Triple culture tests for the diangosis of Chlamydial infection of the female genital tract. *Sex Transm Dis* 1985, 12:68-71.

[17] Stamm W, Cole B: Asymptomatic *Chalmydia trachomatis* urethritis in men. *Sex Transm Dis* 1986, 13:163-165.

[18] Zelin J, Robinson A, Ridgway G, Allason-Jones E, Williamson P: Chlamydial urethritis in heterosexual men attending a genitourinary medicine clinic: prevalence, symptoms, condom usage and partner change. *Int J STD AIDS* 1995, 6:27-30.

[19] Berger R, Alexander E, Harnish J, Paulsen C, Monda G, Ansell J, Homes K: Etiology and therapy of acute epididymitis: prospective study of 50 cases. *J Urol* 1979, 121:750-754.

[20] Stamm W, Koutsky L, Benedetti J, Jourden J, Brunham R, Holmes K: *Chlamydia trachomatis* urethral infections in men. Prevalence, risk factors, and clinical manifestations. *Ann Intern Med* 1984, 100:47-51.

[21] Rompalo A, Roberts P, Johnson K: Empirical therapy for the management of acute proctitis in homosexual men. *JAMA* 1988, 260:348-353.

[22] Claesson B, Trollfors B, Brolin I, Granstrom M, Henrichsen J, Jodal U, Juto P, Kallings I, Kanclerski K, Lagergard T: Etiology of community-acuired pneumonia in children based on antibody response to bacterial and viral antigens. *Pediatr Infect Dis* 1989, 8:856-862.

[23] Hammerschlag M, Cummings C, Roblin P, Williams T, Delke I: Efficacy of neonatal ocular prophylaxis for the prevention of chlamydial and gonococcal conjunctivitis. *N Engl J Med* 1989, 320(769-772).

[24] Perine P, Osoba A: Lymphogranuloma venereum. In: *Sexually transmitted diseases*. Edited by Holmes K, Mardh P, Sparling P, Wiesner P. New York: McGraw Hill Book Co; 1990: 195-204.

[25] Pearlman M, McNeely S: A review of the microbiology, immunology, and clinical implications of *Chlamydia trachomatis* infections. *Obstet Gynaecol* 1992, 47:448-461.

[26] Howard C, Friedman D, Leete J, Christensen M: Correlation of the precert of positive *Chlamydia trachomatis* direct fluorescent antibody detection tests with the adeuacy of specimen collection. *Diagn Microbiol Infect Dis* 1991, 14:233-237.
[27] Kellogg J, Seiple J, Klinedinst J, Levisky J: Impact of endocervical specimen uality of apparent prevalence of *Chlamydia trachomatis* infections diagnosed using an enzyme-linked immunosorbent assay method. *Arch Pathol Lab Med* 1991, 115:1223-1227.
[28] Moncada J, Schachter J, Shipp M, Bolan G, Wilber J: Cytobrush in collection of cervical specimens for detection of *Chlamydia trachomatis*. *J Clin Microbiol* 1989, 27:1863-1866.
[29] Kellogg J, Seiple J, Klinedinst J, Stroll E: Impact of endocervical specimen quality on apparent prevalance of *Chlamydia trachomatis* infections diagnosed using polymerase chain reaction, abstr. In: *Abstracts of the 95th General Meeting of the American Society for Microbiology 1995 American Society for Microbiology: 1995; Washington DC*. 86.
[30] Mahony J, Chernesky M: Effect of swab type and storage temperature on the isolation of *Chlamydia trachomatis* from clinical specimens. *J Clin Microbiol* 1985, 22(865-867).
[31] Mardh P, Zeeberg B: Toxic effect of sampling swabs and transportation test tubes on the formation of intracytopasmic inclusions of *Chlamydia trachomatis* in McCoy cell cultures. *Br J Vener Dis* 1981, 57:268-272.
[32] Embil J, Thiebaux H, MAnuel F, Pereira L, MacDonald S: Sequencial cervical specimens and the isolation of *Chlamydia trachomatis*: factors affecting detection. *Sex Transm Dis* 1983, 10:62-66.
[33] Hobson D, Karayiannis P, Byng R, Rees E, Tait I, Davies J: Quantitative aspects of chlamydial infection of the cervix. *Br J Vener Dis* 1980, 56:156-162.
[34] Akane A, Matsubara K, Nakumura H, Takahashi S, Kimura K: Identification of the heme compound copurified with deoxyribonucleic acid (DNA) from bloodstains, a major inhibitor of polymerase chain reaction amplication. *J Forensic Sci* 1994, 39:362-372.
[35] Kellogg J, Siple J, Klinedinst J, Levinsky J: Comparison of cytobrushes with swabs for recovery of endocervical cells and for Chlamydiazyme detection of *Chlamydia trachomatis*. *J Clin Microbiol* 1992, 30:2988-2990.
[36] Jones R, Katz B, Vanderpohl B, Caine V, Batteiger B, Newhall W: Effects of blind passage and multiple sampling on recovery of *Chlamydia trachomatis* from urogenital specimens. *J Clin Microbiol* 1986, 24:1029-1033.
[37] Fedorko D, Smith T: Chlamydial infections. In: *Laboratory methods for the diagnosis of sexually transmitted diseases.* Edited by Wentworth B, Judson F, Gilchrist M, 2nd edn. Washington DC: American Public Health Association; 1991: 95-125.
[38] Reeve P, Owen J, Oriel J: Laboratory procedures for the isolation of *Chlamydia trachomatis* from the human genital tract. *J Clin Pathol* 1975, 28:910-914.
[39] Gordon F, Harper I, Quan A, Treharne J, Dwyer R, Garland J: Detection of Chlamydia (Bedsonia) in certain infections of man. 1. Laboratory procedures: comparison of yolk sac and cell culture for detection and isolation. *J Infect Dis* 1969, 120:451-462.
[40] Nash P, Krenz M: Culture media. In: *Manual of clinical microbiology.* Edited by Balows A, Hausler W, Herrmann K, Isenberg H, Shadomy H, 5th edn. Washington DC: American Society for Microbiology; 1991: 1226-1288.

[41] Bovarnick M, Miller J, Snyder J: The influence of certain salts, amino acids, sugars and proteins on the stability of rickettsiae. *J Bacteriol* 1950, 59:509-522.

[42] Salmon V, Kenyon B, OVerall J, Anderson R: USe of a universal transport media in a commercial polymerase chain reaction assay for *Chlamydia trachomatis*, abstr. In: *Abstracts 6f the 10th Annual Clearwater Virology Symposium 1994: 1994*. 33.

[43] Hosein I, Kaunitz A, Craft S: Detection of cervical *Chlamydia trachomatis* and *Neisseria gonorrhoeae* with deoxyribonucleic acid probe assays in obstetric patients. *Am J Obstet Gynecol* 1992, 167:588-591.

[44] Limberger J, Biega R, Evancoe A, McCarthy L, Slivienski L, Kirkwood M: Evaluation of culture and the Gen-Probe PACE 2 assay for detection of *Neisseria gonorrhoea* and *Chlamydia trachomatis* in endocervical specimens transported to a state health laboratory. *J Clin Microbiol* 1992, 30:1162-1166.

[45] Chernesky M, Castriano S, Sellors J, Stewart I, Cunningham I, Landis S: Detection of *Chlamydia trachomatis* antigens in urine as an alternative to swabs and cultures. *J Infect Dis* 1990, 161(124-126).

[46] Chernesky M, Jang D, Chong S, Lee H, Sellors S, Mahony J: Order of urine collection affects the diagnosis of *Chlamydia trachomatis* infection in men by ligase chain reaction, GenProbe Pace II, Chlamydiazyme, and leukocyte esterase testing. In: *Abracts of the 11th Meeting of the International Society for STD Research 1995: 1995*. 180.

[47] Sellors J, Chernesky M, Pickard L, Jang D, Walter S, Krepel J, Mahony J: Effect of time elapsed since previous voiding on the detection of *Chlamydia trachomatis* antigens in urine. *Eur J Clin Microbiol Infect Dis* 1993, 12:285-289.

[48] Sugunendran H, Birley H, Mallinson H, Abbott M, Tong C: Comparison of urine, first and second endourethral swab for PCR based detection of genital *Chlamydia trachomatis* infection in male patients. *Sex Transm Dis* 2001, 77(6):423-426.

[49] Wiesenfeld H, Heine R, DiBiasi F, Repp C, Rideout A, Macio I, Sweet R: Self collection of vaginal introitus specimens: a novel approach to *Chlamydia trachomatis* testing in women, abstr 040. In: *Abstracts of the 11th Meeting of the International Society for STD Research 1995: 1995*. 42.

[50] Chernesky M, Jang D, Lee H, BUrczak J, Hu H, Sellors J, Tomazic-Allen S, Mahony J: Diagnosis of *Chlamydia trachomatis* infections in men and women by testing first-void urine by ligase chain reaction. *J Clin Microbiol* 1994, 32:2682-2685.

[51] Chernesky M, Jang D, Luinstra K, Chong S, Pickard L, Sellors J, Mahony J: Ability of ligase chain reaction and polymerase chain reaction to diagnose female lower genitourinary *Chlamydia trachomatis* infection by testing cervical swabs and first void urine. In: *Chlamydial infections Proceedings of the Eighth International Symposium on Human Chlamydial Infections: 1994; Bologna, Italy*. 326-329.

[52] Lee H, CHernesky M, Schachter J, Burczak J, Andrews W, Muldoon S, Leckie G, Stamm W: Diagnosis of *Chlamydia trachomatis* genitourinary infection in women by ligase chain reaction assay of urine. *Lancet* 1995, 345:213-216.

[53] Smith T, Brown S, Weed L: Diagnosis of *Chlamydia trachomatis* infections by cell cultures and serology. *Lab Med* 1982, 13:92-100.

[54] Stamm W, Tam M, Koester M, Cles L: Detection of *Chlamydia trachomatis* inclusions in McCoy cell cultures with fluorescein-conjugated monoclonal antibodies. *J Clin Microbiol* 1983, 17:666-668.

[55] Yoder B, Stamm W, Doester C, Alexander E: Microtest procedure for isolation of *Chlamydia trachomatis*. *J Clin Microbiol* 1981, 13:1036-1039.

[56] Kuo C, Wang S, Wentworth B, Grayston J: Primary isolation of TRIC organisms in HeLa 229 cells treated with DEAE-dextran. *J Infect Dis* 1972, 125:665-668.

[57] Rota T, Nichols L: Infection of cell culture by trachoma agent. Enhancement by DEAE-dextran. *J Infect Dis* 1971, 124:419-421.

[58] Johnston S, Siegel C: Comparison of Buffalo Green Monkey Kidney cells and McCoy cells for the isolation of *Chlamydia trachomatis* in shell vial centrifugation culture. *Diagn Microbiol Infect Dis* 1992, 15:355-357.

[59] Krech T, Bleckmann M, Paatz R: Comparison of Buffalo Green Monkey cells and McCoy cells for isolation of *Chlamydia trachomatis* in a microtitre system. *J Clin Microbiol* 1989, 27:2364-2365.

[60] Rota T, Nichols R: *Chlamydia trachomatis* in cell culture. 1. Comparison of efficiencies of infection in several chemically defined media, at various pH and temperature values, and after exposure to diethylaminoethyl-dextran. *Appl Microbiol* 1973, 26:560-565.

[61] Warford A, Carter T, Levy R, Rekrut K: Comparison of sonicated and nonsonicated specimens for the isolation of *Chlamydia trachomatis*. *Am J Clin Pathol* 1985, 83:625-629.

[62] Barnes R: Laboratory diagnosis of human chlamydial infections. *Clin Microbiol Rev* 1989, 2:119-136.

[63] Schoenwald E, Schmidt B, Steinmetz G, Hosmann J, Pohla-Gubo G, Luger A, Gasser G: Diagnosis of *Chlamydia trachomatis* infection - culture versus serology. *Eur J Epidemiol* 1988, 4:75-82.

[64] Stephens R, Kuo C, Tam M: Sensitivity of immunofluorescence with monoclonal antigodies for detection of *Chlamydia trachomatis* inclusions in cell culture. *J Clin Microbiol* 1982, 16:4-7.

[65] Skulnick M, Chua R, Simor A, Low D, Khosid H, Fraser S, Lyons E, Legere E, Kitching D: Use of the polymerase chain reaction for the detection of *Chlamydia trachomatis* from endocervical and urine specimens in an asymptomatic low-prevalence population of women. *Diagn Microbiol Infect Dis* 1994, 20:195-201.

[66] Basarab A, Browning D, Lanham S, O'Connell S: Pilot study to assess the presence of *Chlamydia trachomatis* in urine from 18-30-year-old males using EIA/IF and PCR. *Fam Plann Reprod Health Care* 2002, 28(1):36-37.

[67] Altaie S, Meier F, Centor R, Wakabongo M, Toksoz D, Harvey D, Basinger E, Johnson B, Brookman R, Dalton H: Evaluation of two ELISA's for detecting *Chlamydia trachomatis* from endocervical swabs. *Diagn Microbiol Infect Dis* 1992, 15:579-586.

[68] Biro F, Reising S, Doughman J, Kollar L, Rosenthal S: A comparison of diagnostic methods in adolescent girls with and without symptoms of Chlamydia urogenital infection. *Pediatrics* 1994, 93:476-480.

[69] Chan E, Brandt K, Horsman G: A 1-year evaluation of Syva Microtrak Chlamydia enzyme immunoassay with selective confirmation by direct immunofluorescent-antibody assay in a high-volume laboratory. *J Clin Microbiol* 1994, 32:2208-2211.

[70] Clark L, Sierra M, Daidone B, Lopez N, Covino J, McCormack W: Comparison of the Syva Microtrak enzyme immunoassay and Gen-Probe PACE 2 with cell culture for

diagnosis of cervical *Chlamydia trachomatis* infection in a high-prevalence female population. *J Clin Microbiol* 1993, 31:968-971.

[71] Domeika M, Bassiri M, Mardh P: Diagnosis of genital *Chlamydia trachomatis* infection in asymptomatic males by testing urine by PCR. *J Clin Microbiol* 1994, 32:2350-2352.

[72] Gaydos C, Reichart C, Long J, Welsh L, Neumann T, Hook E, Quinn T: Evaluation of Syva enzyme immunoassay for detection of *Chlamydia trachomatis* in genital specimens. *J Clin Microbiol* 1990, 28:1541-1544.

[73] Matthews R, Pandit P, Bonigal S, Wise R, Radcliffe K: Evaluation of an enzyme-linked immunoassay and confirmatory test for the detection of *Chlamydia trachomatis* in male urine samples. *Genitourin Med* 1993, 69:47-50.

[74] Moncada J, Schachter J, Bolan G, Nathan J, Shafer M, Clark A, Schwebke J, Stamm W, Mroczkowski T, Martin D: Evaluation of Syva's enzyme immunoassay for the detection of *Chlamydia trachomatis* in urogenital specimens. *Diagn Microbiol Infect Dis* 1992, 15:663-668.

[75] Moncada J, Schachter J, Shafer M, Williams E, Gouriay L, Lavin B, Bolan G: Detection of *Chlamydia trachomatis* in first catch urine samples from symptomatic and asymptomatic males. *Sex Transm Dis* 1994, 21:8-12.

[76] Talbot H, Romanowski B: Factors affecting urine EIA sensitivity in the detection of *Chlamydia trachomatis* in men. *Genitourin Med* 1994, 70:101-104.

[77] Thomas B, MacLeod E, Hay P, Horner P, Taylor-Robinson D: Limited value of two widely used enzyme immunoassays for detection of *Chlamydia trachomatis* in women. *J Clin Pathol* 1994, 13:651-655.

[78] Tam M, STamm W, Handsfield H, Stephens R, Kuo C, Holmes K, Ditzenberger K, Kreiger M, Nowinski R: Culture-independent diagnosis of *Chlamydia trachomatis* using monoclonal antibodies. *N Engl J Med* 1984, 310:1146-1150.

[79] Thomas B, Gilchrist C, Taylor-Robinson D: Detection of *Chlamydia trachomatis* by direct immunofluorescence improved by centrifugation of specimens. *Eur J Clin Microbiol Infect Dis* 1991, 10:659-662.

[80] Woods G, Bryan J: Detection of *Chlamydia trachomatis* by direct fluorescent antibody staining, Results of the College of American Pathologists proficiency testing program, 1986-1992. *Arch Pathol Lab Med* 1994, 118:483-488.

[81] Stamm W, HAriison H, ALexander E, Cles L, Spence M, Quinn T: Diagnosis of *Chlamydia trachomatis* infection by direct immunofluorescence staining of genital secretions- multicenter trial. *Ann Intern Med* 1984, 101:638-641.

[82] Bell T, Kuo C, Stamm W, Ram M, Stephens R, Holmes K, Grayston J: Direct fluorescent monoclonal antibody stains for rapid detection of infant *Chlamydia trachomatis* infections. *Pediatrics* 1984, 74:224-228.

[83] Rapoza P, Quinn T, Kiessling L, Green W, Taylor H: Assessment of neonatal conjunctivitis witha direct fluorescent monoclonal antibody stain for Chlamydia. *JAMA* 1986, 255:3369-3373.

[84] Rompalo A, Suchland R, Rice C, Stamm W: Rapid diagnosis of *Chlamydia trachomatis* rectal infection by direct fluorescence staining. *J Infect Dis* 1987, 155:1075-1076.

[85] Friis B, Kuo C, Wang S, Mordhorst C, Grayston J: Rapid diagnosis of *Chlamydia trachomatis* pneumonia in infants. *Acta Pathol Microbiol Immunol Scand Sect* 1984, 92:139-143.

[86] Paisley J, Lauer B, Melinkovich P, Bitterman B, Feiten D, Berman S: Rapid diagnosis of *Chlamydia trachomatis* pneumonia in infants by direct immunofluorescence microscopy of nasopharyngeal secretions. *J Pediatr* 1986, 109:653-655.

[87] CDC: False-positive results with the use of chlamydial tests in the evaluation of suspected sexual abuse. *Morbid Mortal Weekly Rep* 1991, 39:932-935.

[88] Kellogg J, Seiple J, Hick M: Cross-reaction of clinial isolates of bacteria and yeasts with the chlamydiazyme test for chlamydial antigen, before and after use of a blocking agent. *Am J Clin Pathol* 1992, 97:309-312.

[89] Stamm W: Diagnosis of *Chlamydia trachomatis* genitourinary infections. *Ann Intern Med* 1988, 108:710-717.

[90] Malenie R, Joshi P, Mathur M: *Chlamydia trachomatis* antigen detection in pregnancy and its verification by antibody blocking assay. *Indian J Med Microbiol* 2006, 24(2):97-100.

[91] Newhall W, DeLisle S, Fine D, Johnson R, Hadgu A, Matsuda B, Osmond D, Campbell J, Stamm W: Head-to-head evaluation of five different nonculture chlamydia tests relative to a quality assured culture standard. *Sex Transm Dis* 1994, 21:S165-166.

[92] Blanding J, Hirsch L, Stranton N, Wright T, Aarnaes S, Maza Ldl, Peterson E: Comparison of the Clearview Chlamydia, the PACE 2 assay, and culture for detection of *Chlamydia trachomatis* from cervical specimens in a low-prevalence population. *J Clin Microbiol* 1993, 31:1622-1625.

[93] Kluytmans J, Goessens W, Mouton J, Rijsoort-Vos Jv, Niesters H, Quint W, Habbema L, Wagenvoort J: Evaluation of Clearview and Magic Lite test, polymerase chain reaction, and cell culture for the detection of *Chlamydia trachomatis* in urethral specimens from males. *J Clin Microbiol* 1993, 32:568-570.

[94] Khan E, Hossain M, Paul S, Mahmud M, Rahman M, Alam M, Hasan M, Mahmud N, Nahar K: Molecular diagnosis of genital *Chlamydia trachomatis* infection by polymerase chain reaction. *Mymensingh Med J* 2011, 20(3):362-365.

[95] Altwegg M, Burger D, Lauper U, Schar G: Comparison of Gen-Probe PACE 2, Amplicor Roche, and a conventional PCR for the detection of *Chlamydia trachomatis* in genital specimens. *Med Microbiol Lett* 1994, 3:181-187.

[96] Kluytmans J, Niesters H, Mouton J, Quint W, Ijpelaar J, Rijsoort Jv, Habbema L, Stoltz E, Michel M, Wagenvoort J: Performance of a nonisotopic DNA probe for detection of *Chlamydia trachomatis* in urogenital specimens. *J Clin Microbiol* 1991, 29:2685-2689.

[97] Stary A, Teodorowicz L, Horting-Muller I, Nerad S, Storch M: Evaluation of the Gen-Prove PACE2 and the Microtrak enzyme immunoassay for diagnosis of *Chlamydia trachomatis* in urogenital samples. *Sex Transm Dis* 1994, 21:26-30.

[98] Melton M, Hale Y, Pawlowicz M, Halstead D, Wright S: Evaluation of the Gen-Probe PACE 2C system for *Chlamydia trachomatis* and *Neisseria gonorrhoea* in a high prevalence population, abstr. In: *Abtracts of the 95th General Meeting of the American Society for Microbiology 1995: 1995; Washington DC.* 138.

[99] Mullis K, Faloona F: Specific synthesis of DNA in votro via a polymerase-catalyzed chain reaction. *Methods Enzymol* 1987, 55:335-350.

[100] Saiki R, Scharf S, Faloona F, Mullis K, Horn G, Erlich H: Enymatic amplification of B-globin genomic sequences and restriction site analysis for diagnosis of sickle cell anaemia. *Science* 1985, 230:1350-1354.

[101] Dille J, Butzen C, Birkenmeyer L: Amplification of *Chlamydia trachomatis* DNA by ligase chain reaction. *J Clin Microbiol* 1993, 31:729-731.

[102] Harinda V, Underhill G, Tobin J: Screening for genital chlamydia infection: DNA amplification techniques should be the test of choice. *Int J STD AIDS* 2003, 14(11):723-726.

[103] Haugland S, Thune T, Fosse B, Wentzel-Larsen T, Hjelmevoll S, Myrmel H: Comparing urine samples and cervical swabs for Chlamydia testing in a female population by means of Strand Displacement Assay (SDA). *BMC Womens Health* 2010, 25(10):9.

[104] Masek B, Arora N, Quinn N, Aumakhan B, Holden J, Hardick A, Agreda P, Barnes M, Gaydos C: Performance of three nucleic acid amplification tests for detection of *Chlamydia trachomatis* and *Neisseria gonorrhoeae* by use of self-collected vaginal swabs obtained via an Internet-based screening program. *J Clin Microbiol* 2009, 47(6):1663-1667.

[105] Matthews-Greer J, McRae K, LaHaye E, Jamison R: Validation of the Roche COBAS Amplicor system for *Chlamydia trachomatis*. *Clin Lab Sci* 2001, 14(2):82-84.

[106] Sevestre H, Mention J, Lefebvre J, Eb F, Hamdad F: Assessment of *Chlamydia trachomatis* infection by Cobas Amplicor PCR and in-house LightCycler assays using PreservCyt and 2-SP media in voluntary legal abortions. *J Med Microbiol* 2009, 58(Pt 1):59-64.

[107] Jaton K, Bille J, Greub G: A novel real-time PCR to detect *Chlamydia trachomatis* in first-void urine or genital swabs. *J Med Microbiol* 2006, 55:1667-1674.

[108] Bhalla P, Baveja U, Chawla R, Saini S, Khaki P, Bhalla K, Mahajan S, Reddy B: Simultaneous detection of *Neisseria gonorrhoeae* and *Chlamydia trachomatis* by PCR in genitourinary specimens from men and women attending an STD clinic. *J Commun Dis* 2007, 39(1):1-6.

[109] Jalal H, Stephen H, Al-Suwaine A, Connex C, Carne C: The superiority of polymerase chain reaction over an amplified enzyme immunoassay for the detection of genital chlamydial infections. *Sex Transm Dis* 2006, 82(1):37-40.

[110] Herrmann B: A new genetic variant of *Chlamydia trachomatis*. *Sex Transm Infect* 2007, 83:253-254.

[111] Unemo M, Olcen P, Agne-Stadling I: Experiences with the new genetic variant of *Chlamydia trachomatis* in Orebra county, Sweden - proportion, characteristics and effective diagnostic solution in an emergent situation. *Euro Surveill* 2007, 12:E5-6.

[112] Whiley D: False-negative results in nucleic acid amplification tests-do we need to routinely use two genetic targets in all assays to overcome problems caused by sequence variation? *Crit Rev Microbiol* 2008, 34:71-76.

[113] Ness R, Soper D, Richter H, Randall H, Peipert J, Nelson D, Schubeck D, McNeley S, Trout W, Bass D *et al*: Chlamydia antibodies, chlamydia heat shock protein, and adverse sequelae after pelvic inflammatory disease: the PID Evaluation and Clinical Health (PEACH) Study. *Sex Transm Dis* 2008, 35:129-135.

[114] Machado A, Guimaraes E, Sakurai E, Fioravante F, Amaral W, Alves M: High titers of *Chlamydia trachomatis* antibodies in Brazilian women with tubal occlusion or previous ectopic pregnancy. *Infect Dis Obstet Gynecol* 2007, 24816.

[115] Arya R, Mannion P, Woodcock K, Haddad N: Incidence of genital *Chlamydia trachomatis* infection in the male partners attending an infertility clinic. *J Obstet Gynaecol* 2005, 25:364-367.

[116] Meyer K, Eddie B: The influence of tetracycline compounds on the development of antibodies in psittacosis. *Am Rev Tuberc* 1956, 74:566-571.

[117] Biosafety in microbiological and biomedical laboratories. In. Edited by Services UDoHaH. Washington DC: US Government Printing Offices; 1988: 88-8395.
[118] Schachter J: Manual of clinical microbiology, 2nd edition edn. Washington DC: American Society for Microbiology; 1980.
[119] Wang S, Grayston J: Immunologic relationship between genital TRIC, lymphogranuloma venereum, and related organisms in a new microtiter indirect immunofluorescence test. *Am J Ophthalmol* 1970, 70:367-374.
[120] Wang S, rayston J, Alexander E, Holmes K: Simplified immunofluorescence test with trachoma-lymphogranuloma venereum (*Chlamydia trachomatis*) antigens for use as a screening test for antibody. *J Clin Microbiol* 1975, 1:250-255.
[121] Lampe M, Suchland R, Stamm W: Nucleotide sequence of the variable domains within the major outer membrane protein gene from serovariants of *Chlamydia trachomatis*. *Infect Immun* 1993, 61:213-219.
[122] Suchland R, Stamm W: Simplified microtiter well cell culture method for rapid immunotyping of *Chlamydia trachomatis*. *J Clin Microbiol* 1991, 29:1333-1338.
[123] Grayston J: Infections cuased by *Chlamydia pneumonia* strain TWAR. *Clin Infect Dis* 1992, 15:757-763.
[124] Moss T, Darougar S, Woodlan R, Nathan M, Dine R, Cathrine V: Antibodies to Chlamydia species in patients attending a genitourinary clinic and the impact of antibodies to *C pneumoniae* and *C psittaci* on the sensitivity and the specificity of *C trachomatis* serology tests. *Sex Transm Dis* 1993, 20:61-65.
[125] Mohony J, Chernesky M, Bromberg K, Schachter J: Accuracy of immunoglobulin M immunoassay for diagnosis of chlamydial infections in infants and adults. *J Clin Microbiol* 1986, 24:731-735.
[126] Baud D, Regan L, Greub G: Comparison of five commercial serological tests for the detection of anti-Chlamydia trachomatis antibodies. *Eur J Clin Microbiol Infect Dis* 2010, 29:669-675.
[127] Schachter J, Stamm W, Chernesky M, Hook E, Jones R, Judson F, Kellogg J, LeBar B, Mardh P, McCormack W: Nonculture tests for genital tract chalmydial infection. What does the package insert mean, and will it mean the same thing tomorrow? *Sex Transm Dis* 1992, 19:243-244.
[128] Sackett D, Haynes R, Tugwell P: Clinical epidemiology. Boston: Little, Brown & Co; 1985.
[129] Hay P, Thomas B, Horner P, MacLeod E, Renton A, Taylor-Robinson D: *Chlamydia trachomatis* in women: the more you look, the more you find. *Genitourin Med* 1994, 70:97-100.
[130] Lin J, Jones W, Yan L, Wirthwin K, Flaherty E, Haivanis R, Rice P: Underdiagnosis of *Chlamydia trachomatis* infection. DIagnostic limitations in patients with low level infection. *Sex Transm Dis* 1992, 19:259-265.
[131] Magder L, Klontz K, Bush L, Barnes R: Effect of patient characteristics on performance of an enzyme immunoassay for detecting cervical *Chlamydia trachomatis* infection. *J Clin Microbiol* 1990, 28:781-784.
[132] Shrier L, Dean D, Klein E, Harter K, Rice P: Limitations of screening tests for the detection of *Chlamydia trachomatis* in asymptomatic adolescent and young adult women. *Am J Obstet Gynecol* 2004, 190(3):654-662.

[133] Gaydos C, Theodore M, Dalesio N, Wood B, Quinn T: Comparison of three nucleic acid amplification tests for detection of *Chlamydia trachomatis* in urine specimens. *J Clin Microbiol* 2004, 41:3041-3045.

[134] Lehmusvuori A, Juntunen E, Tapio A, Rantakokko-Jalava K, Soukka T, Lovgren T: Rapid homogenous PCR assay for the detection of *Chlamydia trachomatis* in urine samples. *J Microbiol Methods* 2010, 83:302-306.

[135] Gaydos C, Quinn T, Willis D, Weissfeld A, Hook E, Martin D, Ferrero D, Schachter J: Performance of the APTIMA Combo 2 assay for detecion of *Chlamydia trachomatis* and *Neisseria gonorrhoeae* in female urine and endocervical swab specimens. *J Clin Microbiol* 2003, 41:304-309.

[136] Hadad R, Fredlund H, Unemo M: Evaluation of the new COBAS TaqMan CT test v2.0 and impact on the proportion of new variant *Chlamydia trachomatis* by the introduction of diagnostic detecting new variant C trachomatis in Orebro county, Sweden. *Sex Transm Infect* 2009, 85:190-193.

[137] Walsh A, Rourke F, Laoi B, Crowley B: Evaluation of the Abbott RealTime CT assay with the BD ProbeTec ET assay for the detection of *Chlamydia trachomatis* in a clinical microbiology laboratory. *Diagn Microbiol Infect Dis* 2009, 64:13-19.

[138] Whiley D, Sloots T: Comparison of three in-house multiplex PCR assays for the detection of *Neisseria gonorrhoeae* and *Chlamydia trachomatis* using real-time and conventional detection methodologies. *Pathology* 2005, 37:364-370.

[139] Moller J, Pedersen L, Persson K: Comparison of the Abbott RealTime CT New Formulation Assay with Two Other Commercial Assays for Detection of Wild-Type and New Variant Strains of *Chlamydia trachomatis*. *J Clin Microbiol* 2010, 48(2):440-443.

[140] Ripa T, Nilsson P: A variant of *Chlamydia trachomatis* with deletion in cryptic plasmid: implications for use of PCR diagnostic tests. *Euro Surveill* 2006, 11:E061109.061102.

Part 4

Prevention of Chlamydia Infections

18

Chlamydia Prevention by Influencing Risk Perceptions

Fraukje E.F. Mevissen[1], Ree M. Meertens[2] and Robert A.C. Ruiter[1]
[1]*Department of Work and Social Psychology, Maastricht University,*
[2]*Department of Health Promotion, Nutrition and Toxicology Research Institute Maastricht (NUTRIM) and Care and Public Health Research Institute (Caphri), Maastricht University,*
The Netherlands

1. Introduction

Worldwide, sexually transmitted infections (STI) are amongst the most serious health problems. More than 340 million new cases of curable STI infections occur every year and in 2007 an estimated 33,2 million people worldwide were infected with HIV (Joint United Nations Program on HIV/AIDS [UNAIDS] & World Health Organisation [WHO], 2007; WHO, 2001). In western countries, *Chlamydia* is one of the most common STI, with heterosexually active (young) adults among the high-risk groups (WHO, 2001). The best way to reduce the likelihood for STI transmissions like *Chlamydia* when being sexually active is by avoiding unsafe sexual contacts, *i.e.*, to use condoms correctly and consistently, or to do an STI test and get treatment before quitting condom use in a monogamous relationship. An alternative risk reduction strategy is to avoid any sexual contacts before staying in a lifelong monogamous relationship.

Condom use and STI screening are often not practiced. One of the reasons for not using condoms or getting tested for STI's like *Chlamydia* is that young adults misjudge the likelihood to get infected with an STI (Crosby et al., 2000; Ethier et al., 2003; Misovich et al., 1997; Schröder et al., 2001). Like with many risky activities, they generally think that 'it won't happen to me' (Harré et al., 2005; Weinstein, 1984). But as long as people do not realize their personal susceptibility to STI, why would condoms be used (Brewer et al., 2007; De Hoog et al., 2005; Gerrard et al., 1996; Weinstein et al., 2007)? Acknowledging ones susceptibility to a health risk is an important first step towards risk reduction (Catania et al., 1990; Conner & Norman, 2005; Milne et al., 2000; Noar, 2007; Van der Pligt, 1998). In order to make young adults feel more susceptible to *Chlamydia* threat and to stimulate preventive actions, it is thus important to communicate the risks of unsafe sex and to enhance awareness of their personal vulnerability to get infected.

The focus of this chapter is on how *Chlamydia*-related susceptibility perceptions can be influenced by using risk communication techniques. We will start with a general outline of risk communication methods (paragraph 1.2) after which two commonly used methods will be discussed in more detail, namely the use of probability-based risk information

(information about the likelihood that it happens or *how often* a risk has negative consequences, paragraph 1.3) and the use of scenario-based risk information (a description of the sequence of events leading to a serious outcome or a description of *how* a risk could happen, paragraph 1.4). Then, the effectiveness of both methods will be compared and the chapter will conclude with some recommendations for *Chlamydia* prevention activities and future research suggestions (paragraph 1.5).

Although the focus of this chapter is on motivating *chlamydia*-preventive behavior by influencing risk perceptions, it is important to note that health-related decisions like safe sex behaviour are not determined by risk perception alone (see, among others, Noar, 2007; Sheeran et al., 1999). Other factors that may influence preventive behaviour are, for example, the perceived benefits and/or the disadvantages of (un)safe sex, social norms, and people's self-confidence and perceived barriers regarding condom use and *chlamydia* screening. However, when people are unaware of their susceptibility for certain health threats like *Chlamydia*, when they do not know or acknowledge that they run a risk, it will be unlikely that they will take preventive actions. Therefore, the understanding of how to influence risk perceptions is an important step in order to motivate preventive behavior.

2. Risk communication methods

The communication of health risks is an essential component of many health prevention activities. Its purpose is to support people in making sensible and healthy risk judgments and decisions. Examples of risk messages can be found in various health-related fields, such as informing people about large-scale industrial accidents, widespread infectious diseases like the severe acute respiratory syndrome (SARS), or communicating the risks of drunk driving, smoking, or someone's risk for getting infected with an STI like *Chlamydia*.

Studies on risk communication are diverse and they have been conducted from many different scientific perspectives, which has resulted in a wide but also scattered knowledge base. There is consensus about the general factors that are important in order for (risk) information to be effective, such as the trustworthiness, understandability, credibility, and relevance of the information (Breakwell, 2000; Glanz & Yang, 1996). But the scientific literature hardly provides clear guideliness on which risk information should be included exactly in the health message. Various methods to communicate (health) risks are provided. We can, for example, communicate risks by providing information about the probability that the risk may happen (Visschers et al., 2009) and frame information in such a way that it positively states the efficacy of the preventive recommendations (Salovey et al., 1998). Stressing the severity of the potential consequences of the risk is an alternative, for example by using so called fear appeals (Ruiter et al., 2001). Another way to communicate health risks is to provide messages that describe the connected chain of events that may cause the risk, like a personal testimonial of somebody describing how he/she was confronted with the risk, to make the hazard more vivid (Koehler, 1991). When informing people about unknown risks, the risk could be compared to hazards with similar dimensional profiles (Freudenburg & Rursch, 1994; Visschers et al., 2007). Apart from these presentation formats, there are factors that may influence the effects of risk information such as the qualitative characteristics of the risk (e.g., dread, likelihood, novelty; Skinner et al., 1999; Slovic, 1987), individual differences (e.g., experience, relevance; Rothman & Schwarz, 1998), the described context in which the risk takes place (e.g., culture, society, surroundings; Weber & Hilton,

1990), or additional information on, for example, how to deal with possible barriers regarding the recommended health actions (Ruiter et al., 2001).

In the remaining part of this chapter, the use of risk probability information and of risk scenario information - two commonly used risk communication approaches - and their impact on influencing *Chlamydia*-related risk perceptions will be discussed in more detail.

3. Risk probability information

Risk probability information is information concerning the likelihood that a certain risky behavior (e.g., unsafe sex) ends up negatively (e.g., getting infected with *Chlamydia*). Probability information is regularly used in risk communication to inform people about the likelihood of risks and aims to improve healthy decision making by presenting the objective facts. Think, for example, of information regarding the chance to develop vascular diseases because of eating unhealthy, or the possibility of getting lung cancer by smoking cigarets.

Probabilities can be described in different ways, using various presentation formats like numerical (frequencies, percentages), verbal ('it is quite likely'), or even visual (*i.e.*, graphs). A lot of research has been done on the effects of different presentation formats of probability information on risk perception and on how to facilitate comprehension and interpretation of this information among lay people (Edwards et al., 2001; Edwards et al., 2002; Rothman & Kiviniemi, 1999; Visschers et al., 2009; Weinstein, 1999). In this chapter, we focus on three of the most frequently used probability formats in health communication, *i.e.*, the use of single incidence probability information, cumulative probability information and personalized probability information to communicate the risk of *Chlamydia* infections.

3.1 Single incidence vs. cumulative probability information

When communicating risk probabilities, health educators generally use one-shot risk information: information about the likelihood of a negative ending with single risk encounters. However, with many health-related behaviours or risky activities, we are often not exposed only once but frequently. And with repeated exposure to the risk, the probability to be confronted with a negative ending increases. In other words, many risks accumulate in time. This surely accounts for the likelihood to get infected with *Chlamydia*: with increasing number of sex partners and increasing number of sexual encounters, the risk to get infected increases as well.

It is shown that people often do not realize that risks accumulate over time but seem to consider each exposure moment as an independent event (Knäuper et al., 2005). Additionally, people make mistakes when asked to estimate the long-term risk based on single-incident risk information (Doyle, 1997; Fuller et al., 2004; Knäuper et al., 2005). Therefore, several authors suggested that the cumulative aspect of risks should be emphasized and explained rather than communicating single incident probabilities (Fuller et al., 2004, p. 618; Holtgrave et al., 1995, p. 136).

We explored this suggestion in the context of sexual risks by presenting single incident rates with or without cumulative risk information on getting infected with *Chlamydia* and investigated if people would feel more susceptible for *Chlamydia* after emphasizing the cumulative aspects of the infection probability (Mevissen et al., 2010a). The probability information was tested using verbal cumulative information ("The more often you have unsafe sex, the higher your probability to get infected with *Chlamydia*", study 1) and numerical cumulative risk information ("the probability of contracting *Chlamydia* after 10 unsafe sexual encounters with an infected person increases to $p = 1 - (1 - 0.7)^{10} = 99\%$, or 99 out of 100 people", study 2). The single incidence information communicated the probability to get infected with *Chlamydia* after a single unprotected sexual encounter with an infected person (70%). The cumulative risk information focused on the increased risk for infection after multiple unsafe sexual encounters with multiple partners.

The effects of this information were tested among a group of sexually experienced young adults, with immediate post-treatment measurement of risk perceptions for *Chlamydia*. It was expected that presenting cumulative probability information, regardless of being verbal or numerical, would result in higher perceived susceptibility to get infected with *Chlamydia* than presenting single incidence information only or than presenting no probability information at all. However, contrary to recommendations and assumptions (Fuller et al., 2004; Holtgrave et al., 1995), the *Chlamydia*-related susceptibility perceptions were not rated higher after presenting cumulative probability information, whether the information was presented in a verbal format or a numerical format. Moreover, the studies showed that stressing the cumulative risk of unsafe sex on *Chlamydia* infections resulted in *lower* perceived susceptibilities compared to a control group that did not receive probability information. The single incident probability information on *Chlamydia* did not influence risk perceptions whatsoever.

The fact that cumulative risk information about *Chlamydia* actually resulted in lower risk perceptions may be related to defensive reactions and denial of one's susceptibility for high probability risks. The high infection probability rates of *Chlamydia* could have been fear arousing, especially because no efficacy information was added (Ruiter et al., 2001). The study showed that even though the probability of getting infected was rated higher than participants thought in advance, and the messages generally were accepted, participants perceived themselves personally less susceptible for *Chlamydia* after receiving cumulative probability information. Even after presenting the high infection probability rates to a group clearly susceptible to *Chlamydia* (study 2 focussed on young women with a serieus risky sexual past), perceived susceptibility was not rated higher but actually lower.

3.2 General vs. personal probability information

In the above described studies, risk probabilities were presented using general risk information aimed at the general public. These studies showed that communicating general risk information does not always have the intended effect on risk perceptions related to oneself. When provided with general risk information, one's personal risk may actually be easily denied by thinking that the information is applicable only for others, but not for oneself, which is confirmed in empirical research (Klar & Ayal, 2004; Price, 2002). Moreover, people seem to favour specific individual risk feedback to general risk information (Bos et al., 2004; Mevissen et al., under review-a). This sounds plausible, as personal risk information describes the risk probabilities based on the individual situation. Personal risk messages that are tailored to the individual thus increase the relevance and accuracy of risk information. This may in turn enhance its persuasiveness. Thus, it may be better to communicate personalized risk probabilities, *i.e.*, how likely is it that *you* are infected or getting infected with an STI like *Chlamydia*?

Several studies showed the effectiveness of personalized risk information in forming adequate risk perceptions (Edwards et al., 2000; Emmons et al., 2004; Kreuter et al., 2000). For example, Emmons and colleagues (2004) developed a computer-based tailored risk communication tool that showed effectiveness in correcting misperceptions regarding personal risk for colorectal cancer among a diverse patient population of a health centre. Kreuter and Strecher (1995) showed that individualized risk feedback effectively increased perceived stroke risk among people who had underestimated their risk.

We also investigated whether it is more effective to increase risk perceptions towards STI using personalized risk information (*i.e.*, risk probability information tailored to the personal circumstances of the individual) as opposed to general, non-tailored risk probability information (Mevissen et al., 2011). In this study, we did not specificly focus on the risk to get infected with *Chlamydia*, but on the risk of STI infection in general. In addition, the risk information was embedded in the context of a larger-scale health intervention program that was developed, implemented and evaluated according to the Intervention Mapping protocol (Bartholomew et al., 2011). Participants not only received information on their STI infection probabilities but they also received a tailored safe sex advice as well as information tailored to their motivation and skills to use condoms or go for STI screening. Using computer tailoring techniques, and based on their indicated sexual experiences, a personal STI risk probability profile was generated and communicated to young adults in starting heterosexual relationships.

In a randomized controlled trial, the interventions' efficacy was compared to a group receiving non-tailored, general information addressing the same determinants and a control group receiving no information. Risk perception for STI infection and intention to use condoms or perform an STI test were measured directly after visiting the intervention. Additionally, a three month follow-up questionnaire measured the behavioural impact (actual condom use or STI screening). The hypothesis was that the tailored intervention with personalized risk feedback would result in higher risk perceptions for STI and higher intention for condom use or to perform an STI test compared to general (non-tailored) information or no information (control group). Also, it was expected that participants in the tailored intervention would have higher rates of condom use and STI-testing.

The results confirmed the hypothesis; perceived susceptibility for STI was rated higher among participants in the tailored intervention group as opposed to participants in the non-tailored group or those in the control group. Moreover, those receiving tailored information had higher intentions to talk about STI testing with their partner (measured directly after the study) as well as higher condom use rates at three month follow-up. It seems that a tailored intervention including personalized probability information is an effective strategy to adequately increase perceived risk probabilities for STI and to enhance protective behaviour. In addition, by providing the information web-based and using computer-tailoring techniques, it also is a cost-effective, easy accessible and anonymous way to deliver the information widespread.

It is important to add, however, that participants not only learned about the probability to get infected with an STI, but also received some guidelines on how to avoid it. Thus, the current setting does not allow us to draw any firm conclusions regarding the explicit impact of personal probability information over general probability information in influencing risk perceptions and behaviour. The potential influence of the additive information provided in both the tailored as well as the non-tailored group may not be ignored. Still, our data suggest that personalized risk communication is a promising method of risk communication.

3.3 Risk scenario information

In everyday reality, statistically-based probability information regarding the prevalence and likelihood of risks is usually unavailable at the moment people have to judge a risky situation. In that case, people use their knowledge and ideas about the event in order to determine its' riskiness. Several authors have suggested that people rely on cognitive strategies in order to decide to take the risk or not, such as simplified representations and heuristics (Gilovich et al., 2006; Katapodi et al., 2005). People might, for instance, recall information from memory about how often similar situations in the past did result in a negative outcome. Thus, susceptibility perceptions are shaped from past-outcomes, information available in one's mind ("availability heuristic"; Tversky & Kahneman, 1982). The cognitive availability of explanations that lead to an event increases the judged likelihood that the event will occur. Another possible judgment strategy is to mentally construct and evaluate potential future scenarios: how could a risky situation possibly result in a negative outcome? The ease with which hypothetical scenario's can be imagined or mentally simulated, influences the judged likelihood that it will happen in reality (Heath et al., 1991; Kahnemann & Tversky, 1982). If an event can be easily constructed in memory, the possibility that it will occur will be perceived as more likely. The cognitive simulation of hypothetical event sequences ("simulation heuristic"; Kahnemann & Tversky, 1982) means that people rely on *how* a particular risk could result in a negative outcome, instead of *how often* a risk has negative consequences.

Providing people with information describing the context in which a risky event might take place and/or can end negatively (scenario information), may aid the construction of a risk image, which, according to the simulation heuristic, could thus influence susceptibility perceptions. Compared to studies on the effects of probability information on risk perceptions, research on scenario-based risk information is scarce (see for a review: Koehler, 1991, p. 506-507). One of the earliest studies on the effects of scenario information - though not related to risky activities - was conducted by Gregory and colleagues (1982). Participants were asked to read and imagine a scenario about subscribing to a cable television service. After the task, they indicated more interest in signing in for such a service compared to people receiving plain information about the cable service. Moreover, subjects who imagined subscribing did actually do so more often than did subjects in the control group. Sherman, Cialdini, Schwartzman, and Reynolds (1985) as well as Broemer (2004) conducted studies demonstrating that it is indeed the *ease* of imagination that influences likelihood estimates. Participants reading and imagining easy-to-imagine disease symptoms rated the probability to contract the disease higher compared to those provided with difficult-to-imagine disease symptoms.

Providing scenario information in order to influence risk perceptions for STI like *Chlamydia* seems a promising alternative method to communicate risks and to motivate preventive behavior. Turner de Palma and colleagues (1996) found that scenario-based risk information increased the imagination of getting infected with HIV though it did not increase HIV-related risk perceptions. They concluded that this could be the result of denial of ones personal susceptibility to a well-known severe disease as simultaneously risk perceptions towards a fake infection with unknown severity did increase. De Wit and colleagues (2008) found higher risk perceptions towards Hepatitis B among homosexual men receiving scenario information compared to people receiving probability information. We conducted several studies using different scenario-formats to see if we could influence perceived susceptibility to *Chlamydia*. The use of one single scenario message will be described first (3.3.1) after which the influence of writing ones own scenario story (3.3.2) and the influence of presenting multiple scenarios (3.3.3) will be presented.

3.3.1 The impact of scenario information on *Chlamydia* risk perceptions

In our first study, we provided a group of young adults with a scenario message concerning a story of a person infected with *Chlamydia* after having unsafe sex with his/her steady partner, a situation generally regarded to be safe by young people and thus condom use is not practiced (Misovich, et al., 1997). The message was selected after a pilot study in which we tested several messages with respect to credibility, personal suitability, and the degree to which people could identify with the situation presented. The message presented the story of a student having unprotected sex with a steady sex partner and discovering that he/she had contracted *Chlamydia*. The student then realizes the risk that is taken because also in former steady relationships condom use had ceased after a while. The main character in the scenario was a young man for male participants, and a young woman for female participants, to make the scenario applicable for both sexes. This lab-based study was conducted among undergraduate students. Self-report questionnaires measuring perceived suceptibility to *Chlamydia* were provided after reading the scenario. It was expected that participants would have higher rates of risk perception after reading the scenario message compared to a control group only receiving general information on *Chlamydia* and not receiving the scenario message.

The results showed that providing young adults with risk scenario information indeed led to higher perceived susceptibility for *Chlamydia* (Mevissen et al., 2009). However, the influence of scenario information on *Chlamydia*-related susceptibility perceptions depended on the relationship status of the recipient: only among participants *without* a steady relationship at time of measurement, perceived susceptibility was rated higher after reading scenario information compared to not reading scenario information. No effect of scenario information was found for participants *with* a relationship.

This relationship-dependent effect may have been caused by some form of denial. The scenario in our study described the story of somebody getting infected with *Chlamydia* by having unsafe sex with a steady partner. The content of the message was thus highly relevant for participants actually having a relationship. Although message relevance generally increases information processing (Petty & Cacioppo, 1986), a strong identification with the message content can also be threatening and may lead to defensive reactions such as message derogation (e.g., denying its' relevance or preventing the information from reaching consciousness) and denial of one's personal susceptibility (Block & Williams, 2002;

Dietz-Uhler, 1999; Liberman & Chaiken, 1992). Due to its' high relevance, the scenario information used in our study may indeed have resulted in denial among people with a relationship. Apart from the message being too threatening because of the content being too relevant an alternative explanation for the limited effects of scenario information could be that not all participants could identify enough with the situation described in the scenario. However, in order to positively influence susceptibility perceptions, it is important to imagine the situation in the scenario very well and be able to identify easily with the character in the story (Anderson, 1983b; Broemer, 2004). It could have been difficult to imagine getting infected with *Chlamydia* within a relationship context for people actually having a relationship (Misovich et al., 1997).

3.3.2 Self-constructed risk scenarios and the role of imaginability

To explore in more detail the above suggested explanation regarding the role of the imaginability and relevance of risk scenarios on feelings of susceptibility, we conducted another study (Mevissen et al., under review-b). A measure rating the imaginability of the described event was included and the mediating effect of imaginability on perceived susceptibility to *Chlamydia* was determined. Additionally, we used a risk scenario with a different story content (*i.e.*, getting infected with *Chlamydia* by having sex with a casual partner instead of by having sex with a steady partner) to see if this scenario could influence risk perceptions not only among participants without a relationship but also among people with a serious relationship. Participants receiving the casual partner story were compared with a group of people who were asked to write their own risk scenario about how they (or somebody like them) could get infected with *Chlamydia*. It seemed plausible that writing your own risk story would more actively trigger the imagination, would be easier to accept and would be less fearful (Aronson, 1999). By making people describe their own risky situation, we could possibly overcome the limited effects of prefabricated risk scenarios on susceptibility perceptions. Risk perception and imaginability measures were scored immediately after the reading or writing assignment. It was expected that reading as well as writing a scenario would increase risk perceptions by making it easier to imagine getting infected with *Chlamydia*. Moreover, it was expected that writing your own risk scenario would make it even easier to imagine the event (e.g., *Chlamydia* infection) and would thus have a stronger influence on risk perceptions.

The results of the study showed that the self-constructed risk scenarios were indeed easier to imagine and this imaginability led to stronger feelings of susceptibility for *Chlamydia* compared to a prefabricated risk scenario message or no risk scenario message, independent of the relationship status of the participant. Additionally, contrary to the prefabricated risk scenario, the self-constructed risk scenario did not cause higher feelings of threat compared to the control group.

To our surprise, however, this time the prefabricated risk scenario did not have any effects on perceived susceptibility whatsoever. As expected, the imaginability of the prefabricated risk scenario was rated lower than the imaginability of the self-constructed scenarios. Moreover, the prefabricated risk scenario indeed led to higher feelings of threat compared to not receiving scenario information. Still, we had expected that the prefabricated scenario would have some influence on risk perceptions. These findings suggest that it is difficult to construct prefabricated risk scenarios in a way that they are easy to imagine for everyone and such that they do not arouse too much fear. The limited effects of risk scenarios in influencing risk perceptions may be partly outweighed if participants create their own risk scenario; scenarios that participants wrote themselves were easier to imagine, less threatening, and increased risk perceptions to *Chlamydia*.

3.3.3 One vs. multiple risk scenario messages

Self-constructed risk scenarios seem to be an effective tool to influence perceived susceptibility to *Chlamydia*. However, it may have difficulties with practical implementation - self-constructed risk scenarios can only be used in face-to-face counseling or a class workshop. We thus explored the efficacy of providing multiple (two) prefabricated risk scenarios in influencing risk perceptions to *Chlamydia* (Mevissen et al., 2010b). The scenario information was presented as two different personal testimonials; one scenario about a *Chlamydia* infection in the context of a serious relationship, the other about a *Chlamydia* infection in the context of a one-night-stand situation. More scenarios signify more examples of possible risky events which could in turn enhance imaginability and perceived susceptibility (Hendrickx et al., 1992; Hendrickx et al., 1989). In addition, when providing multiple risk scenarios, it is more likely that at least one of the messages will be appealing and imaginable for the receiver which may in turn decrease the likelihood for denial of the message content. In an experimental design, undergraduate students were exposed to one or two risk scenario messages or received no scenario message (control group). Risk perception and imaginability measures were rated directly after presenting the scenario messages. The expectation was that reading the scenario information would make people feel more susceptible to *Chlamydia*. Presenting multiple (two) risk scenarios was thought to make it even easier to imagine getting infected with *Chlamydia*, thus resulting in even higher susceptibility perceptions.

The results of the study showed that providing people with only one single risk scenario did not make people feel more susceptible to *Chlamydia*, regardless of the characteristic of the participants (relationship status), or the described event in the scenario message (casual sex or relationship context). However, as hypothesized, providing people with both risk scenarios simultaneously did lead to higher susceptibility perceptions towards *Chlamydia*, independent of relationship status of the participant. This positive effect of two scenarios on perceived susceptibility towards *Chlamydia* was mediated by imaginability. Although again providing just one scenario message did not influence risk perceptions, by providing multiple risk scenarios we could influence susceptibility perceptions to *Chlamydia*. We can say that although the efficacy of scenario-based messages is sensible to several factors, proving multiple scenarios or making people construct their own risk scenario seem effective tools to influence risk perception to *Chlamydia*.

4. Conclusions

In this Chapter, we described the efficacy of different risk communication methods in influencing risk perceptions in order to motivate preventive behavior. More specific, we discussed how probability-based risk information and scenario-based risk information could increase perceived susceptibility for *Chlamydia*. If we consider our studies regarding the influence of probability-based risk information and scenario-based risk information on *chlamydia*-related risk perceptions we can conclude that the effectiviness of both methods depends on the format used. Judgments regarding *Chlamydia* are influenced by different communication formats. We can conclude that:

1. Care should be taken when providing general probability-based risk information in communicating the risk of *Chlamydia* infection. The influence of general probability information (single incident as well as cumulative) on risk perceptions to *Chlamydia* seemed to be less obvious than expected and assumed. It may even lead to unwanted lower instead of the desired higher risk perceptions. We recommend being careful with including (cumulative) probability information in health risk messages and to pilot-test the risk messages properly to prevent unexpected side effects.
2. Personalized probability feedback, on the contrary, seems a promising risk communication strategy to adequately influence risk judgments. A tailored intervention including personalized probability information may effectively increase feelings of susceptibility and positively influence health behaviour change. As face-to-face counselling sessions are an expensive and time-consuming way to deliver tailored information, web-based interventions seem to be a perfect solution for a widespread, cost-effective, and anonymous distribution of personal probability-based risk information. Combined with behavioral recommendations and information tailored to motivation and skills, personalized risk information seems an effective approach to stimulate healthy behavior. More research on whether tailored information regarding motivation and self-efficacy adds to the impact of personalized risk information would increase our understanding on the factors influencing the efficacy of tailored health risk messages.
3. Scenario information is a potentially effective tool to increase feelings of susceptibility towards *Chlamydia*, but its efficacy depends on the characteristics of the person making the risk assessment and the imaginability of the risk scenarios presented.
4. To reduce the likelihood for defensive reactions or a lack of imaginability, it is advisable to make people construct their own risk scenarios or to provide multiple risk scenarios.

Caution when using risk communication methods should be taken. Communicating risks using probability information or scenario information may also induce defensive reactions. The efficacy of cumulative and single incident probability information regarding *Chlamydia* seems to decrease perceived susceptibility. It is thus necessary to thoroughly pretest risk communication messages in experimental studies even when certain presentation frames or strategies seem obviously more effective or better than others. They may cause unexpected and unwanted side effects. More research on which factors trigger defensive reactions and on how to adequately measure them, as well as on how to communicate risk information while avoiding denial, is desirable and necessary.

5. References

Anderson, C. A. (1983b). Imagination and expectation: the effect of imagining behavioral scripts on personal intentions. *Journal of Personality and Social Psychology, 45*, 293-305.

Aronson, E. (1999). The power of self-persuasion. *American Psychologist, 54*(11), 875-884.

Bartholomew, L. K., Parcel, G. S., Kok, G., Gottlieb, N. H., & Fernández, M. E. (2011). *Planning health promotion programs. An interventionmapping approach*. San Francisco: Jossey-Bass.

Block, L. G., & Williams, P. (2002). Undoing the effects of seizing and freezing: decreasing defensive processing of personally relevant messages. *Journal of Applied Social Psychology, 32*(4), 803-833.

Bos, A. E. R., Visser, G. C., Tempert, B. F., & Schaalma, H. P. (2004). Evaluation of the Dutch AIDS information helpline: an investigation of information needs and satisfaction of callers. *Patient Education and Counseling, 54*, 201-206.

Breakwell, G. M. (2000). Risk communication: Factors affecting impact. *British Medical Bulletin, 56*(1), 110-120.

Brewer, N. T., Chapman, G. B., Gibbons, F. X., Gerrard, M., & McCaul, K. D. (2007). Meta-analysis of the relationship between risk perception and health behavior: The example of vaccination. *Health Psychology, 26*(2), 136-145.

Broemer, P. (2004). Ease of imagination moderates reactions to differently framed health messages. *European Journal of Social Psychology, 34*, 103-119.

Catania, J. A., Kegeles, S. M., & Coates, J. T. (1990). Towards an understanding of risk behavior: An AIDS Risk Reduction Model (ARRM). *Health Education Quarterly, 17*(1), 53-72.

Conner, M., & Norman, P. (2005). Predicting health behavior: A social cognition approach. In M. Conner & P. Norman (Eds.), *Predicting Health Behavior* (pp. 1-27). Berkshire: Open University Press.

Crosby, R. A., Newman, D., Kamb, M. L., Zenilman, J., Douglas, J. M., & Iatesta, M. (2000). Misconceptions about STD-protective behavior. *American Journal of Preventive Medicine, 19*(3), 167-173.

De Hoog, N., Stroebe, W., & De Wit, J. B. F. (2005). The impact of fear appeals on processing and acceptance of action recommendations. *Personality and Social Psychology Bulletin, 31*(1), 24-33.

De Wit, J. B. F., Das, E., & Vet, R. (2008). What works best: Objective statistics or a personal testimonial? An assessment of the persuasive effects of different types of message evidence on risk perception. *Health Psychology, 27*(1), 110-115.

Dietz-Uhler, B. (1999). Defensive reactions to group-relevant information. *Group Processes & Intergroup Relations, 2*(1), 17-29.

Doyle, J. K. (1997). Judging cumulative risk. *Journal of Applied Social Psychology, 27*(6), 500-524.

Edwards, A., Elwyn, G., Covey, j., Matthews, E., & Pill, R. (2001). Presenting risk information - A review of the effects of "framing" and other manipulations on patient outcomes. *Journal of Health Communication, 6*, 61-82.

Edwards, A., Elwyn, G., & Mulley, A. (2002). Explaining risks: Turning numerical data into meaningful pictures. *Brittish Medical Journal, 324*, 827-830.

Edwards, A., Hood, K., Matthews, E., Russell, D., Russell, I., Barker, J., et al. (2000). The effectiviness of one-to-one risk-communication interventions in health care: a systematic review. *Medical Decision Making, 20*, 290-297.

Emmons, K. M., Wong, M., Puleo, E., Weinstein, N., Fletcher, R., & Colditz, G. (2004). Tailored computer-based cancer risk communication: correcting colorectal cancer risk perception. *Journal of Health Communication, 9*, 127-141.

Ethier, K. A., Kershaw, T., Niccolai, L., Lewis, J. B., & Ickovics, J. R. (2003). Adolescent women underestimate their susceptibility to sexually transmitted infections. *Sexual Transmitted Infections, 79*(408-411).

Freudenburg, W. R., & Rursch, J. A. (1994). The risks of "putting the numbers in context": a cautionary tale. *Risk Analysis, 14*(6), 949-958.

Fuller, R., Dudley, N., & Blacktop, J. (2004). Older people's understanding of cumulative risks when provided with annual stroke risk information. *Postgraduate Medical Journal, 80*, 677-678.

Gerrard, M., Gibbons, F. X., & Bushman, B. J. (1996). Relation between perceived vulnerability to HIV and precautionary sexual behavior. *Psychological Bulletin, 119*(3), 390-409.

Gilovich, T., Griffin, D., & Kahnemann, D. (Eds.). (2006). *Heuristics and biases. The psychology of intuitive judgment* (4 ed.). New York: Cambridge University Press.

Glanz, K., & Yang, H. (1996). Communicating about risk of infectious diseases. *Journal of the American Medical Association, 275*(3), 253-256.

Gregory, W. L., Cialdini, R. B., & Carpenter, K. M. (1982). Self-relevant scenarios as mediators of likelihood estimates and compliance: does imagining make it so? *Journal of Personality and Social Psychology, 43*(1), 89-99.

Harré, N., Foster, S., & O'Neill, m. (2005). Self-enhancement, crash-risk optimism and the impact of safety advertisements on young drivers. *Brittish Journal of Psychology, 96*, 215-230.

Heath, L., Acklin, M., & Wiley, K. (1991). Cognitive heuristics and AIDS risk assessment among physicians. *Journal of Applied Social Psychology, 21*(22), 1859-1867.

Hendrickx, L., Vlek, C., & Caljé, H. (1992). Effects of frequency and scenario information on the evaluation of large-scale risks. *Organizational Behavior and Human Decision Processes, 52*, 256-275.

Hendrickx, L., Vlek, C., & Oppewal, H. (1989). Relative importance of scenario information and frequency information in the judgment of risk. *Acta Psychologica, 72*, 41-63.

Holtgrave, D. R., Tinsley, B. J., & Kay, L. S. (1995). Encouraging risk reduction. A decision-making approach to message design. In E. Maibach & R. L. Parrott (Eds.), *Designing health messages. Approaches from communication theory and public health pratices* (pp. 24-40). Thousand Oaks: Sage Publications.

Kahnemann, D., & Tversky, A. (1982). The simulation heuristic. In D. Kahnemann, P. Slovic & A. Tversky (Eds.), *Judgment under uncertainty: Heuristics and biases* (pp. 201-208). New York: Cambridge University Press.

Katapodi, M. C., Facioneb, N. C., Humphreysc, J. C., & Dodda, M. J. (2005). Perceived breast cancer risk: heuristic reasoning and search for a dominance structure *Social Science & Medicine, 60*(2), 421-432.

Klar, Y., & Ayal, S. (2004). Event frequency and comparative optimism: Another look at the indirect elicitation method of self-others risks. *Journal of Experimental Social Psychology, 40*, 805-814.

Knäuper, B., Kornik, R., Atkinson, K., Guberman, C., & Aydin, C. (2005). Motivation influences the underestimation of cumulative risk. *Personality and Social Psychology Bulletin, 31*(11), 1511-1523.

Koehler, D. J. (1991). Explanation, imagination, and confidence in judgment. *Psychological Bulletin, 110*(3), 499-519.

Kreuter, M. W., Farrell, D., Olevitch, L., & Brennan, L. (2000). *Tailoring health messages: Customizing communication with computer technology*. Mahwah, NJ: Erlbaum.

Kreuter, M. W., & Strecher, V. J. (1995). Changing inaccurate perceptions of health risk: Results from a randomized trial. *Health Psychology, 14*(1), 56-63.

Liberman, A., & Chaiken, S. (1992). Defensive processing of personally relevant health messages. *Personality and Social Psychology Bulletin, 18*(6), 669-679.

Mevissen, F. E. F., Eiling, E., Bos, A. E. R., Tempert, B., Mientjes, M., & Schaalma, H. P. (under review-a). Evaluation of the dutch AIDS STI information helpline: differential outcomes of telephone versus online counseling.

Mevissen, F. E. F., Meertens, R. M., Ruiter, R. A. C., Feenstra, H., & Schaalma, H. (2009). HIV/STI Risk communication: The effects of scenario-based risk information and frequency-based risk information on perceived susceptibility to Chlamydia and HIV. *Journal of Health Psychology, 14*(1), 78-87.

Mevissen, F. E. F., Meertens, R. M., Ruiter, R. A. C., & Schaalma, H. P. (2010a). Testing implicit assumptions and explicit recommendations. The effects of probability information on risk perception. *Journal of Health Communication, 15*, 578-589.

Mevissen, F. E. F., Meertens, R. M., Ruiter, R. A. C., & Schaalma, H. P. (under review-b). Bedtime Stories. The effects of self-constructed risk scenarios on imaginability and perceived susceptibility to sexually transmitted infections.

Mevissen, F. E. F., Ruiter, R. A. C., Meertens, R. M., & Schaalma, H. P. (2010b). The Effects of Scenario-Based Risk Information on Perceptions of Susceptibility to Chlamydia and HIV. *Psychology & Health, 25*, 1161-1174.

Mevissen, F. E. F., Ruiter, R. A. C., Meertens, R. M., Zimbile, F., & Schaalma, H. P. (2011). Justify your love: Testing an online STI-risk communication intervention designed to promote condom use and STI-testing. *Psychology & Health, 26*, 205-221.

Milne, S., Sheeran, P., & Orbell, S. (2000). Prediction and intervention in health-related behavior: A meta-analytic review of protection motivation theory. *Journal of Applied Social Psychology, 30*, 106-143.

Misovich, S. J., Fisher, J. D., & Fisher, W. A. (1997). Close relationships and elevated hiv risk behavior: Evidence and possible underlying psychological processes. *Review of General Psychology, 1*(1), 72-107.

Noar, S. M. (2007). An interventionist's guide to AIDS behavioral theories. *AIDS Care, 19*(3), 392-402.

Petty, R. E., & Cacioppo, J. T. (1986). The elaboration likelihood model of persuasion. In L. Berkowitz (Ed.), *Advances in experimental social psychology* (Vol. 19, pp. 123-205). Orlando, FL: Academic Press.

Price, P. C., Pentecost, H.C., Voth, R.D. (2002). *Perceived event frequency and the optimistic bias: Evidence for a Two-process model of personal risk judgments. Journal of Experimental Social Psychology, 38*, 242-252.

Rothman, A. J., & Kiviniemi, M. T. (1999). Treating people with information: An analysis and review of approaches to communicating health risk information. *Journal of the National Cancer Institute Monographs, 25*, 44-51.

Rothman, A. J., & Schwarz, N. (1998). Constructing Perceptions of vulnerability: Personal relevance and the use of experiental information in health judgments. *Personality and Social Psychology Bulletin, 24*(10), 1053-1064.

Ruiter, R. A. C., Abraham, C., & Kok, G. (2001). Scary warnings and rational precautions: A review of the psychology of fear appeals. *Psychology and Health, 16*, 613-630.

Salovey, P., Rothman, A. J., & Rodin, J. (1998). Health behavior. In D. T. Gilbert, S. T. Fiske & G. Lindzey (Eds.), *The handbook of social psychology* (4th ed., pp. 633-683). Boston: McGraw-Hill.

Schröder, K. E. E., Hobfoll, S. E., & Jackson, A. P. (2001). Proximal and distal predictors of Aids risk behaviors among inner-city african american and european american women. *Journal of Health Psychology, 6*(2), 169-190.

Sheeran, P., Abraham, C., & Orbell, S. (1999). Psychosocial correlates of heterosexual condom use: a meta-analysis. *Psychological Bulletin, 125*(1), 90-132.

Sherman, S. J., Cialdini, R. B., Schwartzman, D. F., & Reynolds, K. D. (1985). Imagining can heighten or lower the perceived likelihood of contracting a disease: the mediating effect of ease of imagery. *Personality and Social Psychology Bulletin, 11*(1), 118-127.

Skinner, C. S., Campbell, M. K., Rimer, B. K., Curry, S., & Prochaska, J. O. (1999). How effective is tailored print communication? *Annals of Behavioral Medicine, 21*(4), 290-298.

Slovic, P. (1987). *Perception of risk. Science, 236*, 280-285.

Turner DePalma, M., McCall, M., & English, G. (1996). Increasing perceptions of disease vulnerability through imagery. *Journal of American College Health, 44*(5), 226-234.

Tversky, A., & Kahneman, D. (1982). Availability: a heuristic for judging frequency and probability. In D. Kahneman, P. Slovic & A. Tversky (Eds.), *Judgment under uncertainty: heuristics and biases*. Cambridge: Cambridge University Press.

UNAIDS, & WHO. (2007). AIDS epidemic update. December 2007. Retrieved November 2008

Van der Pligt, J. (1998). Perceived risk and vulnerability as predictors of precautionary behaviour. *British Journal of Health Psychology, 3*, 1-14.

Visschers, V., Meertens, R. M., Passchier, W., & de Vries, N. K. (2007). How do the general public evaluate risk information? The impact of associations with other risks. *Risk Analysis, 27*(3), 715-727.

Visschers, V., Meertens, R. M., Passchier, W., & DeVries, N. K. (2009). Probability information in risk communication: A review of the research literature. *Risk Analysis, 29*, 267-287.

Weber, E. U., & Hilton, D. J. (1990). Contextual effects in the interpretations of probability words: Perceived base rate and severity of events. *Journal of Experimental Psychology: Human Perception and Performance., 16*(4), 781-789.

Weinstein, N. D. (1984). Why it won't happen to me: perceptions of risk factors and susceptibility. *Health Psychology, 3*(5), 431-457.

Weinstein, N. D. (1999). What does it mean to understand a risk? Evaluating Risk comprehension. *Journal of the National Cancer Institute Monographs, 25*, 15-20.

Weinstein, N. D., Kwitel, A., McCaul, K. D., Magnan, R. E., Gerrard, M., & Gibbons, F. X. (2007). Risk perceptions: assessment and relationship to influenza vaccination. *Health Psychology, 26*(2), 146-151.

WHO. (2001). *Global prevalence and incidence of selected curable sexually transmitted infections. Overview and estimates*. Geneva: World Health Organisation.